MW00843830

GROUP SEQUENTIAL METHODS with APPLICATIONS to CLINICAL TRIALS

GROUP SEQUENTIAL METHODS with APPLICATIONS to CLINICAL TRIALS

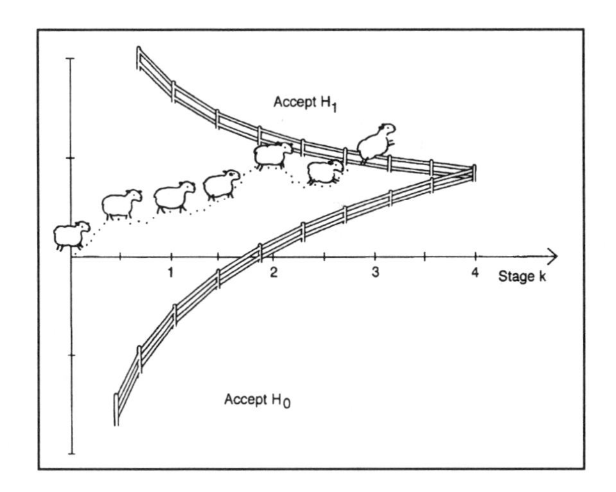

Christopher Jennison

Professor of Statistics
Department of Mathematical Sciences
University of Bath, UK.

and

Bruce W. Turnbull

Professor of Statistics
School of Operations Research & Industrial Engineering
Department of Statistical Science
Cornell University, USA.

CHAPMAN & HALL/CRC

Boca Raton London New York Washington, D.C.

Library of Congress Cataloging-in-Publication Data

Turnbull, Bruce W.
Group sequential methods with applications to clinical trials / Bruce W. Turnbull, Christopher Jennison.
p. cm.
Includes bibliographical references and index.
ISBN 0-8493-0316-8 (alk. paper)
1. Clinical trials—Statistical methods. I. Title. II. Jennison, Christopher, 1956–.
[DNLM: 1. Decision Theory. 2. Statistics—methods. 3. Clinical Trials—methods.
4. Models, Statistical. QA 279.7T942g 1999]
R853.C55 T87 1999
615′.19′0727 21—dc21 99-043218
CIP

Direct all inquiries to CRC Press LLC, 2000 N.W. Corporate Blvd., Boca Raton, Florida 33431.

International Standard Book Number 0-8493-0316-8
Library of Congress Card Number 99-043218
Printed in the United States of America 5 6 7 8 9 0
Printed on acid-free paper

To

Debbie and Marty

Contents

List of figures

List of tables

Preface

In one of our favorite books *Notes from a Small Island**, the American writer Bill Bryson reports that the term *statistics* was coined in 1834 by Sir John Sinclair, a "local worthy" of Thurso in the northern tip of Scotland, although Bryson did hasten to add that "things have calmed down there pretty considerably since". A check of an etymological dictionary might suggest a more classical than Gaelic origin of the word. Be that as it may, like the word *statistics*, the writing of this book has had a lengthy and much-travelled history. For one of us (BWT), it started in 1971, when as a fledgling assistant professor at Stanford University Medical School, he was responsible for the data management of an important clinical trial. The sequential nature of the study became rapidly apparent, when the Principal Investigator, a leading surgeon, would stop by the office every few days to report on a patient who had just relapsed or died that day and to ask the question "whether he could report the results yet?" While much of this book was written in Ithaca in upstate New York or on Claverton Down, Bath, U.K., various parts have origins from far and wide — from Bradford on Avon in Wiltshire to Tucson, Arizona, from North Ryde in New South Wales to Oak Ridge, Tennessee.

We wish to thank Alan Peacock for the pastoral cover illustration; Stuart Barber for assistance with the calculations for Table 9.3; Catalin Starica for assistance with the example in Section 10.5; and Rebecca Betensky, John Bryant, Jonathan Denne and Patricia Grambsch for helpful comments on an early draft of the manuscript. We are also grateful to support from grants from the U.S. National Cancer Institute (R01 CA-66218) and from the U.K. Science and Engineering Research Council/ Engineering and Physical Sciences Research Council.

We are indebted to many people who have strongly influenced us, in particular at Cornell, to Bob Bechhofer who introduced us to the fascination of statistics as an academic subject and to Jack Kiefer for our first introduction to sequential analysis which he taught in a graduate seminar. BWT is also indebted to Rupert Miller and to Toby Mitchell who taught him, by example, how to bring together theory and practice of statistics in real-world biomedical applications. Sadly, Bob Bechhofer, Jack Kiefer, Rupert Miller and Toby Mitchell have all passed on — taken before their time. BWT must also credit Dr Larry Clark of the University of Arizona Cancer Center for supplying a long and taxing stream of important, difficult and highly motivating statistical questions that he encountered in the day to day conduct of the clinical trials and epidemiological studies in which

* Bill Bryson, *Notes from a Small Island*, Avon Books, New York, 1995, p.292

he was engaged. Finally and above all, we are indebted to the patience of our families, Debbie, Marty, Kenneth and Douglas, who were amazed when we announced that the book was finally complete! Things have calmed down here pretty considerably since.

Bath and Ithaca
July 1999

Christopher Jennison
Bruce Turnbull

Glossary

ASN	average sample number
cdf	cumulative distribution function
DSMB	data and safety monitoring board
GST	group sequential test
ITN	inferior treatment number
LD	Lan and DeMets
LR	likelihood ratio
LSD	least significant difference
LSE	least squares estimate
MLE	maximum likelihood estimate
NK	Newman-Keuls
OBF	O'Brien and Fleming
OS	one-sided (in connection with error spending test)
RBO	relative betting odds
RCI	repeated confidence interval
SCP	stochastically curtailed procedure
SPRT	sequential probability ratio test
UMVUE	uniformly minimum variance unbiased estimator
$\mathcal{I}$	information level
J	number of treatment arms in a multi-armed trial
K	number of groups (analyses, looks, stages) in a group sequential procedure
R	ratio of maximum information level for a group sequential test to that required by a fixed sample test with the same α and β
$\boldsymbol{X}^T$	transpose of vector or matrix $\boldsymbol{X}$
$t_{\nu,\alpha}$	upper α tail point of a Student's t-distribution with ν degrees of freedom
z_α	upper α tail point of a standard normal distribution, i.e. $z_\alpha = \Phi^{-1}(1-\alpha)$
α	Type I error probability
β	Type II error probability
$\boldsymbol{\beta}$ (boldface)	vector of regression coefficients
Φ	standard normal cumulative distribution function
ϕ	standard normal density function

Vectors and matrices are indicated by boldface type.

CHAPTER 1

Introduction

1.1 About This Book

This book describes statistical methodology for the group sequential design of studies in which interim analyses will be performed. The principal context in which we illustrate the methods will be that of clinical trials. However, application can be found in almost any area where an experiment or survey can be carried out in phases or where its duration is long enough to permit periodic interim analyses. In the medical field this includes animal studies and also epidemiological studies; in industrial applications, there are established sequential and group sequential designs for acceptance sampling in quality control and for life testing in reliability. Clearly, interim analyses may be called for in any long-term follow-up study, be it a field test of product reliability, a parolee recidivism evaluation of correctional programs, or a surveillance program for monitoring the occurrence of chronic disease in an occupational cohort. The examples described in Section 1.4 will illustrate the breadth of possible applications.

Since many of our examples will be stated in terms of clinical trials, we need to explain a little of the terminology for those unfamiliar with this field. A new therapy may go through various stages of testing in human subjects after showing promise in laboratory and animal studies before it is accepted by the medical community. Phase I trials are exploratory and are concerned with aspects of clinical pharmacology and toxicity. An objective is to find a suitable dose level that avoids unacceptable adverse side effects. Usually the sample consists of between 20 and 80 healthy volunteers, often pharmaceutical company employees or medical students. Phase II pilot studies are of moderate size, involving 100 to 300 diseased patients, and are concerned with evaluating both efficacy and safety aspects. A Phase III trial is the definitive evaluation for the proposed new therapy in which effectiveness is verified and the presence of any long-term adverse side effects is monitored. Patients suffering from the disease in question are randomly assigned either to the new treatment or to the current standard, or possibly placebo, treatment. Phase III trials often involve more than 1000 patient volunteers and last three to five years, or maybe longer depending on recruitment rates and the necessary follow-up time. Occasionally, more than two treatments will be compared in the same study. It is in the comparative Phase III study that the statistical design and analysis come under the most attention and scrutiny (although of course careful statistical planning and evaluation are called for in any research endeavor). Phase IV refers to the additional testing and monitoring of experience with the new treatment after it has been accepted and approved for general use, sometimes referred to as post-marketing surveillance.

This categorization is not a strict one, and a trial's purposes can overlap the boundary definitions, especially in phases II and III. Sometimes these stages are subdivided into finer categories (see Burdette & Gehan, 1970). This nomenclature was introduced for *therapeutic* trials but is now also used in disease *prevention* trials. There, the subjects in Phase II and III might be patients at high risk; for example, in a trial for the prevention of skin cancer by dietary supplementation, subjects might have a prior history of skin lesions or high sun exposure.

We think of clinical trials as being conducted to find improved or superior therapies. However, many trials are *equivalence* studies, designed to show that a new treatment's efficacy or safety is "the same as" or "at least no worse than" that of a standard treatment. Such trials are common in pharmaceutical applications where it may be desired to compare two formulations of the same drug. For a text on bioequivalence studies in pharmaceutical trials, we refer the reader to Chow & Liu (1992). Dunnett & Gent (1977) give an example of a randomized trial in the area of patient management, originally reported by Spitzer et al. (1974), with the objective of determining whether certain aspects of the health care provided by nurse-practitioners could be considered equivalent to conventional care methods requiring a greater commitment of the physician's time. It should be noted that if the goal is to demonstrate equivalence, then the trial should be designed as such. A clear distinction must be made between failure to find evidence of a treatment difference, perhaps due to the low power of a small study, and the active demonstration of "equivalence" by confirming that the treatment difference lies within some acceptable region; see Freiman et al. (1978), Simon (1986) and Durrleman & Simon (1990). We look specifically at designs for equivalence studies in Chapter 6.

In medical trials the term "endpoint" is often used to denote a response variable. These variables can be of various types. A binary response of success or failure is common, especially in Phase II trials. A quantitative response variable is one measured on a continuous scale and is often modeled by a normal distribution. Examples might include the plasma level of a particular biochemical, or the initial second forced expiratory volume (FEV_1) lung function measure in a trial of respiratory disorder. A survival endpoint refers to the time it takes for some event of interest to occur, such as death, failure or relapse. It is an elapsed time, usually measured from the date of each patient's entry to the study. Of course, for some patients the event of interest has not occurred by the time the analysis is performed, possibly because they have withdrawn from the trial or died from causes unrelated to the trial. In this case, we say the patient's survival time is *right censored* and note the partial information that the time to event exceeds the observed follow-up time. Some endpoints are more complex; for example, they could consist of multivariate, repeated measure or growth curve data. We illustrate a variety of response types with examples in Section 1.4.

This book is not intended to be a comprehensive treatment of the conduct of medical trials. There are several admirable books on this subject, including Burdette & Gehan (1970); Pocock (1983); Friedman, Furberg & DeMets (1998); Piantadosi (1997) and Chow & Liu (1998). In addition, there are several collections of papers by well-known authors on various aspects of clinical trials;

these include volumes edited by Tygstrup, Lachin & Juhl (1982); Miké & Stanley (1982); Shapiro & Louis (1983) and Buyse, Staquet & Sylvester (1984). We shall not be covering topics such as organization, protocols, eligibility requirements, randomization techniques, ethics, blinding, placebos and data management. These and many other related issues are well covered in the above references. Similarly, there are many textbooks concerning design and analysis of epidemiological studies: just a few are Breslow & Day (1980 and 1987); Kleinbaum, Kupper & Morgenstern (1982); Checkoway, Pearce & Crawford-Brown (1989) and Rothman & Greenland (1998). For a textbook on the design and analysis of long-term animal experiments, the reader is referred to Gart et al. (1986). In addition, there are several excellent books on general medical statistics, including Armitage & Berry (1987), Fleiss (1986) and Altman (1991).

We shall assume the reader has some familiarity with the classical design of multi-factor experiments, an important topic in the repertoire of every consulting statistician not only in agricultural and industrial applications, for which the subject was first developed, but also in biomedical experiments. Classic books on design include Cochran & Cox (1957) and a more modern treatment is provided by Box, Hunter & Hunter (1978). Although the practicalities of long-term Phase III trials usually preclude complicated designs and organizers typically aim to make the protocol as straightforward as possible, it is certainly possible to use some simple factorial designs. Beck et al. (1991) describe the use of a 2^2 design to investigate the effects of diet and blood pressure control on glomerular filtration function in a renal disease trial. Blot et al. (1993) report a one-half replicate of a 2^4 factorial design used to test effects of combinations of four nutrient groups in prevention of cancer incidence and cancer mortality among populations in Linxian County, China.

1.2 Why Sequential Methods

In any experiment or survey in which data accumulate steadily over a period of time, it is natural to monitor results as they occur with a view to taking action such as early termination or some modification of the study design. The period of experiment involved might be measured in terms of hours in the context of industrial acceptance sampling. In contrast, a clinical trial concerning disease prevention or an epidemiological cohort study of occupational exposure may run on a time scale of tens of years.

The many reasons for conducting interim analyses of accumulating data can be loosely categorized in three classes: *ethical*, *administrative* and *economic*. In trials involving human subjects, there is an ethical need to monitor results to ensure that individuals are not exposed to unsafe, inferior or ineffective treatment regimens. Even in negative trials where there appears to be no difference in the performance of two therapies, there is an ethical imperative to terminate a trial as soon as possible so that resources can be allocated to study the next most promising treatment waiting to be tested. Ethical considerations prescribe that accumulating data be evaluated frequently, not only with regard to internal comparisons of safety and efficacy, but also in the light of new information from outside the trial. In animal trials, ethics are also an important consideration, and interim monitoring is indicated there, too.

Included in the administrative reasons for interim analyses is the need to ensure that the experiment is being executed as planned, that the subjects or experimental units are from the correct population and satisfy eligibility criteria and that the test procedures or treatments are as prescribed in the protocol. An early examination of interim results will sometimes reveal the presence of problems which can be remedied before too much expense is incurred. As an example, in an accelerated life test of electronic components in helicopter parts, a rash of early failures indicated that the stress conditions had been incorrectly calibrated. In another application area, a randomized clinical trial to investigate the effect of a nutritional supplement of selenium on the prevention of skin cancer, a discovery that plasma selenium levels were not rising as expected in some patients in the supplement group indicated a possible non-compliance problem. Failure of some subjects to receive the prescribed amount of selenium supplement would have led to a loss of power to detect a significant benefit, if present, and action was therefore taken to initiate a run-in period whereby potential non-compliers could be identified and eliminated from the study prior to randomization. Another administrative reason for early examination of study results is to check on assumptions made in designing the trial. In an experiment where the primary response variable is quantitative, the sample size is often set assuming this variable to be normally distributed with a certain variance. For binary response data, sample size calculations rely on an assumed value for the background incidence rate; for time-to-event data when individuals enter the trial at staggered intervals, an estimate of the subject accrual rate is important in determining the appropriate accrual period. An early interim analysis can reveal inaccurate assumptions in time for adjustments to be made to the design. We shall describe in Chapter 14 how such adjustments can be made in an objective fashion, based on statistical considerations.

Sequential statistical methods were originally developed in order to obtain economic benefits. For a trial with a positive result, early stopping means that a new product can be exploited sooner. If a negative result is indicated, early stopping ensures that resources are not wasted, referred to as "abandoning a lost cause" by Gould (1983). Sequential methods typically lead to savings in sample size, time and cost when compared with standard fixed sample procedures. The early sequential analysis literature stressed this aspect, as we shall do in this book. Interim analyses also enable informed management decisions to be made concerning the continuing allocation of limited research and development funds. Thus, a manager of a large diverse research program might require interim progress reports for this purpose.

In pharmaceutical industry clinical trials, there have been moves toward the formal requirement of interim analyses and also regulations governing reporting of their results. In the U.S. the *Federal Register* (1985) published regulations for new drug applications (NDAs) which included (Section 314.146.b.7) the requirement that the analysis of a Phase III trial "assess . . . the effects of any interim analyses performed". This statement was further elaborated in a Guideline (Food and Drug Administration, 1988, p. 64):

> The process of examining and analyzing data accumulating in a clinical trial, either formally or informally, can introduce bias. Therefore all interim analyses, formal or informal, by any study participant, sponsor staff member, or data monitoring group should be described in full even if treatment groups were not identified. The need for statistical adjustment because of such analyses should be addressed. Minutes of meetings of the data monitoring group may be useful (and may be requested by the review division).

The Guideline also proposed that the plan for interim analyses appear on the protocol cover sheet for the NDA. Responses to the Guideline by representatives of the pharmaceutical industry were published (Enas et al., 1989; PMA Biostatistics and Medical Ad Hoc Committee on Interim Analysis, 1993). The Food and Drug Administration (1985) also required periodic monitoring and reporting of adverse drug experiences in Phase IV trials.

The FDA guidelines were updated by publication of "E9 Statistical Principles for Clinical Trials" in the *Federal Register* of 16 September, 1998 (Vol. 63, No. 179, pp. 49583–49598). This document was prepared under the auspices of the International Conference on Harmonization of Technical Requirements for Registration of Pharmaceuticals for Human Use. It gives a comprehensive list of recommendations for all aspects of statistical principles and methodology applied to clinical trials in the pharmaceutical industry. Of direct relevance for this book, Section III.4 of the document advocates use of group sequential designs and Section IV gives detailed recommendations for trial conduct, including trial monitoring, interim analysis, early stopping, sample size adjustment and the role of an independent data and safety monitoring board (DSMB). Although intended for pharmaceutical industry trials, many of the recommendations apply equally well to government-sponsored clinical trials.

Whereas continuous monitoring is desirable, it is often impractical. In fact, most of the possible benefits of sequential monitoring can be obtained by examining the data at periodic intervals, about 5 to 10 times during the course of the experiment. Such schemes are called "multi-stage" or "group sequential" and many studies can be naturally phased in this way. DSMBs of large multi-center clinical trials will only meet to examine the collected data at periodic intervals. In a rodent carcinogenicity study, the sample size in each stage might be the maximum number of animals that can be accommodated in the laboratory's cages and started on treatment at one time. In industrial acceptance sampling procedures, such as those prescribed in MIL-STD-105E (1989), successive equally sized batches of items are inspected and a lot is accepted or rejected as soon as there is sufficient evidence to make a decision. This book is about these *group sequential* procedures.

1.3 A Short History of Sequential and Group Sequential Methods

Introductory texts on statistics mention little or nothing about sequential design and analysis, even though interim analyses of experimental data are common in many branches of scientific research. Similarly, with a few exceptions (see Section 1.6) the widely used statistical computer software packages currently offer little assistance. As stated by Armitage (1993, p. 392):

> The classical theory of experimental design deals predominantly with experiments of predetermined size, presumably because the pioneers of the subject, particularly R. A. Fisher, worked in agricultural research, where the outcome of a field trial is not available until long after the experiment has been designed and started. It is interesting to speculate how differently statistical theory might have evolved if Fisher had been employed in medical or industrial research.

The sequential approach has been a natural way to proceed throughout the history of experimentation. Perhaps the earliest proponent was Noah, who on successive days released a dove from the Ark in order to test for the presence of dry land during the subsidence of the Flood. The 17th and 18th century work of Huyghens, James Bernoulli, DeMoivre, Laplace and others who studied gambling systems might also be considered precursors; see, for example, Barnard (1946, p. 7). The formal application of sequential procedures started in the late 1920s in the area of statistical quality control in manufacturing production. Shewhart (1931) introduced control charts for process control. Dodge & Romig (1929) defined a two-stage acceptance sampling plan for components which could be tested and classified as effective or defective. Their plan has six parameters: the sample sizes for each stage (n_1 and n_2), acceptance numbers (c_1 and c_2), and rejection numbers (d_1 and d_2), where $d_1 > c_1 + 1$ and $d_2 = c_2 + 1$. In implementing the plan, one first takes an initial sample of n_1 items, and if this contains c_1 defectives or fewer, the lot is accepted; but if d_1 defectives or more are found, the lot is rejected. Otherwise, the decision is deferred until a second sample of size n_2 is inspected, and the lot is then accepted if the total cumulative number of defectives is less than or equal to c_2 and rejected if this number is greater than or equal to d_2. This idea is easily generalized to that of a multi-stage or multiple sampling plan in which up to K stages are permitted (Bartky, 1943). The multi-stage plans subsequently developed by the Columbia University Research Group (Freeman et al., 1948) went on to form the basis of the U.S. military standard for acceptance sampling, MIL-STD-105E (1989). A similar problem arises in the early stages of drug screening and in Phase II clinical trials, where the aim is to identify drugs with at least a certain level of therapeutic efficacy.

The modern theory of sequential analysis has stemmed from the work of Abram Wald (1947) in the U.S., and of George Barnard (1946) in Great Britain, who were participating in industrial advisory groups for war production and development from about 1943. In particular, the major influence on the subject has been the work of Wald (1947) related to his sequential probability ratio test (SPRT). Suppose observations are from a distribution whose probability density or mass function is known apart from a parameter θ. In its basic form for testing a simple null hypothesis H_0: $\theta = \theta_0$ against a simple alternative H_1: $\theta = \theta_1$, successive observations are taken as long as the likelihood ratio remains in a certain interval (a, b); otherwise the experiment is stopped and the appropriate hypothesis selected. The constants a and b can be chosen so that the probabilities of a Type I error (selecting H_1 when H_0 is true) and of a Type II error (selecting H_0 when H_1 is true) are approximately equal to pre-specified values α and β, respectively. This procedure typically leads to lower sample sizes than fixed sample tests. In fact, Wald & Wolfowitz (1948) proved the SPRT has the theoretical optimal property that, among all tests with error probabilities not exceeding α and β, it attains the smallest possible expected sample size or "average sample number" (ASN) when either H_0 or H_1 is true. However, the SPRT is an "open" procedure, i.e., the sample size is not bounded, and a consequence of this is that the distribution of sample size can be quite skewed with a large variance. Also the ASN can be large when θ is not equal to θ_0 or θ_1. These disadvantages led to consideration of non-parallel, curved boundaries for which the critical boundary values a and b are no longer constant but depend on the cumulative sample size, n, and which are "closed" in the sense that $a_{n^*} = b_{n^*}$ for some n^*, ensuring an upper limit on the sample size. One simple modification discussed by Wald is to truncate the SPRT at a certain sample size; Aroian (1968) and Aroian & Robison (1969) showed how to compute the operating characteristic (the probability of accepting H_0 as a function of θ) and ASN curves for such plans using numerical integration.

Another class of sequential tests is based on triangular continuation regions which approximately minimize the maximum ASN; see Kiefer & Weiss (1957), Anderson (1960), Lai (1973) and Lorden (1976). Good discussions of generalizations of the SPRT and corresponding theoretical optimality properties can be found in Siegmund (1985), Wetherill & Glazebrook (1986) and Lai (1991). The mathematical statistics journals now contain a vast literature on the subject of sequential analysis; a detailed chronology up to 1990 can be found in Ghosh (1991).

The SPRT and related procedures are concerned primarily with the problem of selecting one of two competing hypotheses. The problem of selecting from among more than two hypotheses is more difficult and has attracted less attention. A classic book in the area is that by Bechhofer, Kiefer & Sobel (1968). An important application is in the field of communication theory, where problems include target detection in multiple-resolution radar (Marcus & Swerling, 1962) and infrared systems (Emlsee et al., 1997), signal acquisition (Veeravalli & Baum, 1996) and pattern recognition (Fu, 1968). For the multi-hypothesis problem, Baum & Veeravalli (1994) have developed a procedure that generalizes the SPRT which they term the MSPRT.

Another important area is that of the sequential *design* of experiments in which the experimenter is allowed to choose the type of observation to take at each stage. It is desirable to choose that type of observation which yields the most information for the ultimate decision of which hypothesis to accept, but the best type of observation to choose usually depends on the unknown true hypothesis. Accruing observations can help guide the selection of observations in an optimal manner; see Chernoff (1972, Sections 13 to 15) and Blot & Meeter (1973). The so-called two-armed or multi-armed bandit problems (see Berry & Fristedt, 1985; Gittins, 1989) are special cases of this problem. Zelen (1969) introduced the "play-the-winner" rule for allocating treatments to subjects entering a medical study on the basis of previously observed responses, and various modifications to this rule have since been proposed. A highly controversial application of the play-the-winner design was the ECMO study; see the article by Ware (1989) and accompanying discussion, where the issues are explored in detail. We shall discuss some aspects of data-dependent treatment allocation in Chapter 17, especially as it might be applied in medical trials.

As noted above, early multi-stage or "group sequential" designs were proposed for industrial acceptance sampling with a binary response, effective or defective. Two-stage and three-stage procedures for normal responses were developed by Armitage & Schneiderman (1958), Schneiderman (1961), Dunnett (1961) and Roseberry & Gehan (1964). A review of specifically two-stage procedures is provided by Hewett & Spurrier (1983). It is noteworthy that, in this early work, repeated numerical integration is used to calculate operating characteristic and ASN curves of multi-stage procedures for normal data. This device now provides the key tool in the construction of many group sequential tests and forms the basis of methods designed to handle unpredictable group sizes and for the calculation of significance levels and confidence intervals following a group sequential test. Because of the discreteness of the sample space, calculations for binary responses are more straightforward and there is a large literature on group sequential designs for drug screening experiments and Phase II clinical trials: see, for example, Schultz et al. (1973), Elashoff & Beal (1976), Herson (1979), Lee et al. (1979), Fleming (1982), Jennison & Turnbull (1983) and Duffy & Santner (1987). Group sequential methods are by no means restricted to binary or normal responses, however, and in later chapters we shall describe methods for monitoring t-statistics, the odds ratio of survival data, multivariate test statistics and more.

Armitage (1954, 1958b, 1975) and Bross (1952, 1958) pioneered the use of sequential methods in the medical field, particularly for comparative clinical trials. Initially these plans were fully sequential and did not receive widespread acceptance, perhaps because continuous assessment of study results was often impractical. In his discussion printed following the paper by Cutler et al. (1966), Shaw proposed the use of group sequential methods for a clinical trial, using the term "block sequential analysis". The shift to formal group sequential methods for clinical trials did not occur until the 1970s. Elfring & Schultz (1973) specifically used the term "group sequential design" to describe their procedure for comparing two treatments with binary response; McPherson (1974) suggested that the repeated significance tests of Armitage, McPherson & Rowe (1969) might be used to analyze clinical trial data at a small number of interim analyses; Canner (1977) used Monte Carlo simulation to find critical values of a test statistic in a survival study with periodic analyses. However, the major impetus for group sequential methods came from Pocock (1977), who gave clear guidelines for the implementation of group sequential experimental designs attaining Type I error and power requirements. Pocock also demonstrated the versatility of the approach, showing that the nominal significance levels of repeated significance tests for normal responses can be used reliably for a variety of other responses and situations.

In an article that appeared shortly after Pocock's paper, O'Brien & Fleming (1979) proposed a different class of group sequential tests based on an adaptation of a truncated SPRT. These tests have conservative stopping boundaries at very early analyses and give a decision rule similar to the fixed sample test if the last stage is reached, features which have turned out to be very appealing to practitioners. Later papers by Slud & Wei (1982) and Lan & DeMets (1983) were very important, as they showed that group sequential methods can be employed when group sizes are unequal and even unpredictable, a common situation in clinical trials but not a problem usually encountered in industrial sampling applications. The papers by Pocock (1977), O'Brien & Fleming (1979) and Lan & DeMets (1983) have been particularly influential and together form the starting point for recent methodological research and the basis of current practice in clinical trial design. Of course, these authors built on foundations laid by others, particularly the work of Armitage (1975).

It became clear in the 1980s, with the growing number of large-scale clinical trials and increasing use and influence of policy advisory boards or DSMBs to police the progress and conduct of a trial, that formal statistical procedures for interim monitoring of efficacy and safety data were required. Protocols of nearly all major long-term clinical trials now contain statements of formal group sequential procedures for statistical monitoring of accruing results. The practical demands have led to rapid progress in statistical methodology since 1980. The development and acceptance of group sequential methods also benefited from concurrent advances in biostatistical methods, especially in survival analysis (see Kalbfleisch & Prentice, 1980; Miller, 1981; Cox & Oakes, 1984), and from easy availability of high-powered computers, facilitating both the data management and data analyses necessary for interim analyses.

The recent rapid developments can be illustrated in the simplest setting of a comparison between two treatments. A group sequential test monitors a statistic summarizing the difference in primary responses between the two treatment groups at a series of times during the trial. If the absolute value of this statistic exceeds some specified critical value, the trial is stopped and the null hypothesis of no difference between the groups is rejected, usually regarded as a "positive" result. The critical values form a boundary for the sequence of test statistics, the null hypothesis being rejected if this boundary is crossed. If the statistic stays within the testing boundary until the trial's planned termination, then the null hypothesis is accepted (a "negative" result). Armitage, McPherson & Rowe (1969) pointed out that if the usual fixed sample critical values are used at each analysis, the false positive, or Type I, error probability is greatly increased over the nominal level of, say, $\alpha = 0.05$. Early developments by Pocock (1977), O'Brien & Fleming (1979), Fleming, Harrington & O'Brien (1984) and Wang & Tsiatis (1987) concerned methods of adjusting the critical values to maintain the overall false positive rate at an acceptable level; further calculations determine the sample size needed for the group sequential test to attain a desired power.

Subsequent researchers modified the two-sided testing boundary by inserting an "inner wedge" to permit early stopping to accept the null hypothesis; see, for example, Gould & Pecore (1982), Whitehead & Stratton (1983, Section 5) and Emerson & Fleming (1989, Section 4). It should be noted that the idea of an "inner wedge" originated in the fully sequential methods for binary data proposed by Bross (1952) and Armitage (1957).

As different testing boundaries were being investigated, theoretical research and simulation studies extended group sequential methodology to endpoints other than a simple normal response. Notably, increasingly more general results were obtained justifying normal approximations to the joint distribution of test statistics arising in the analysis of survival data. The work of Slud & Wei (1982), Lan & DeMets (1983) and Kim & DeMets (1987a) permitted methods to be extended to the often more realistic setting in which group sizes, or more generally increments in information, are unequal and unpredictable, the typical situation in clinical trials with survival endpoints and staggered entry.

The group sequential tests referred to above are for the "two-sided" problem in which the null hypothesis of no difference between treatments A and B is tested against the alternative of a difference in either direction. Sometimes it is more appropriate to test the hypothesis of treatment equality against the one-sided alternative that one particular treatment, A say, is superior, and this leads to consideration of "one-sided" group sequential tests. Early stopping may arise with a decision in favor of treatment A or to accept the null hypothesis, which now represents the case that treatment A is equal or inferior to treatment B. Some problems have the further asymmetry that early stopping is only appropriate under one conclusion. Suppose, for example, treatment A is a new therapy for a non-life-threatening condition and treatment B a standard therapy. Gould (1983) remarks that in such a trial, if interim findings indicate that A is better than B, the study should continue to completion in order to provide adequate information on safety, tolerability and secondary aspects of the efficacy of treatment A; see also Berry & Ho (1988). A similar asymmetry occurs in a Phase II trial when a safety endpoint is being monitored.

Although group sequential tests are formulated in terms of tests between particular hypotheses, it is possible to draw more general inferences on termination of a trial. These include calculation of interval estimates (e.g., Siegmund, 1978, 1985; Tsiatis, Rosner & Mehta 1984; Kim & DeMets, 1987b), of P-values (e.g., Fairbanks & Madsen, 1982; Madsen & Fairbanks, 1983) and of point estimates (e.g., Whitehead, 1986a). Since different outcomes to a sequential test have varying numbers of observations, the monotone likelihood ratio property does not apply and there is some freedom in defining the sample space orderings which underlie the construction of confidence intervals and P-values. This has led to a substantial literature defining and assessing different proposals.

A recurrent problem in sequential analysis is the dominant role of the stopping rule. All the methods mentioned in the preceding paragraphs rely for their justification on adherence to a statistical stopping rule. However, it cannot be guaranteed that a monitoring committee will abide by such a rule in practice. We have seen that there are many reasons to monitor a trial and there are just as many to decide to stop or continue a trial. In medical applications, these might include side effects, financial cost, quality of patients' lives or the availability of new promising treatments unknown at the start of the trial. The decision to stop the experiment is *not* primarily statistical; rather it is highly complex, involving many subjective factors. Meier (1975, p. 26) claims the problem is political rather than medical, legal or statistical. Because of its complex and subjective nature, the decision to terminate or continue a trial can be a cause of considerable controversy. One example was the UGDP study (Kolata, 1979); more recent examples include the Physicians' Health Study, the NSABP trial on tamoxifen for breast cancer prevention and the CDC study in Thailand on the use of short-course zidovudine (AZT) to prevent mother to child transmission of HIV.

Standard sequential statistical analysis is not well equipped to handle a non-rigid stopping rule and some recent research has involved more flexible approaches. Methods proposed within the frequentist paradigm include stochastic curtailment and repeated confidence intervals. The former approach monitors the probability that a specific fixed sample test will achieve a significant result; see Lan, Simon & Halperin (1982), Choi, Smith & Becker (1985) and Spiegelhalter, Freedman & Blackburn (1986). Repeated confidence intervals (Jennison & Turnbull, 1984, 1989) allow interval estimates to be constructed for the parameter of interest, such as treatment difference, at any stage independently of any stopping rule. The Bayesian approach (see, for example, Spiegelhalter, Freedman & Parmar, 1994) also affords the possibility of flexible monitoring of trial results, and we shall contrast and compare the Bayesian and frequentist approaches in Chapter 18. There has been related research into the decision theoretic basis for group sequential designs by, for example, Bather (1985) and Eales & Jennison (1992, 1995).

This section is by no means intended to be a complete survey and chronology of statistical methodology for sequential design and analysis. For this, the reader is referred to the book by Wetherill & Glazebrook (1986) and the volume edited by Ghosh & Sen (1991), in particular the first chapter (Ghosh, 1991). However, much of the development of *group sequential* methods will be reviewed in detail in the chapters that follow.

1.4 Some Examples

To follow the development of the methods in this volume, it is useful to have some typical examples in mind.

1.4.1 Acute Binary Response: Comparison of Proportions

Here, two treatments are compared with respect to a binary outcome measure taking one of two possible values, "success" or "failure". Let p_A and p_B denote the probabilities of success on the two treatments. The parameter of interest can be the difference $p_A - p_B$, the ratio p_A/p_B or the log odds ratio

$$\log\left\{\frac{p_A(1-p_B)}{p_B(1-p_A)}\right\}.$$

Here, as in later chapters, we use $\log(x)$ to denote the natural logarithm of x.

Kim & DeMets (1992) cite the example of the Thrombolytic Intervention in Myocardial Infarction Trial (The TIMI Study Group, 1985) which compared the effectiveness of two agents in breaking down blood clots in coronary vessels. Here, the dichotomous outcome is determined by whether or not the agent succeeds in re-opening these vessels.

The randomized trial described by Martinez et al. (1996) is an equivalence trial comparing two methods of treating acute diarrhea in young children in rural Mexico. One treatment is an easily available, home based rice-powder beverage, the other the standard oral rehydration solution (ORS) recommended by the World Health Organization. The response, successful rehydration or not, is known within a few hours. Because of the practical advantages of the rice-powder beverage, the trial organizers hoped to demonstrate that it has a success probability equal to, or at least not too much lower than, the standard ORS.

1.4.2 Comparison of Proportions with Strata

Consider the monitoring of incidence data in a prospective stratified intervention study. A pilot study under the direction of Dr L. Clark conducted in Qidong county in the People's Republic of China investigated the effect of a dietary supplement of selenium on the prevention of liver cancer. The full design called for a study population of 40 townships of approximately 30,000 people each. On the basis of demographic and other characteristics, the 40 townships were to be grouped in 20 matched pairs. One township in each pair was to be chosen at random to receive a supplement of selenium in the salt supply. The response variable is the number of deaths from liver cancer during the study period. Here the summary parameter of interest might again be the log odds ratio, assumed approximately constant across the strata (township pairs), i.e.,

$$\theta = \log\left\{\frac{p_{Aj}(1-p_{Bj})}{p_{Bj}(1-p_{Aj})}\right\}, \quad j = 1, \ldots, 20,$$

where p_{Aj} and p_{Bj} are the probabilities of dying of liver cancer for individuals on treatments A and B, respectively, in the jth township pair. The study was planned to last for 10 years but with interim reports to be made annually.

Similar data arose in the study U.S. Air Force Project Ranch Hand II, which assessed the effects of the herbicide Agent Orange. Here, each case, a pilot exposed to Agent Orange, was matched to several controls consisting of unexposed pilots of otherwise similar characteristics. It was mandated that reports be made by the Air Force to the U.S. Congress annually for 20 years.

1.4.3 Normally Distributed Responses

The normal distribution can often be used to approximate the distribution of a continuous outcome, sometimes after a logarithmic or power transformation. In order to gain the full benefits of sequential analysis, the response should be available shortly after treatment is administered, at least relative to the study duration. Examples of such a response might be tumor shrinkage, blood pressure, lung function, or concentration of some chemical in the blood or urine.

In a two-sample problem, the parameter of interest is the difference in the mean responses of the two treatments. Facey (1992) describes a placebo-controlled efficacy trial investigating a new treatment for hypercholesterolemia where the primary response, reduction in total serum cholesterol level over a 4-week period, is assumed to be normally distributed.

A one-sample problem in which the parameter of interest is simply the mean response can occur in a Phase I or II trial when there is no control or comparison group. Comparisons within pair-matched patients or between two measurements on the same patient in a crossover study (see, for example, Jones & Kenward, 1989) lead to essentially the same analysis as the simple one-sample problem. Armitage (1975, p. 119) gives an example where responses represent differences in recovery times for pairs of patients treated with two competing hypotensive agents. Recovery times were measured in minutes and thus responses can be considered to be immediate relative to the length of the trial.

1.4.4 Survival Data

A "survival" endpoint such as time to death or time to disease progression is very common in Phase III clinical trials for chronic diseases such as cancer or AIDS. Patients can enter the trial at different calendar dates and the outcome measure is the elapsed time from the patient's entry, the date of randomization say, to the occurrence of the event of interest. Response times are often of the same order of magnitude as the duration of the study, leading to right censoring when a patient has not experienced the event by the time of an interim or final analysis. Other patients' response times may be censored because of early withdrawal from the study for reasons unrelated to treatment.

Response time data also arise in industrial life testing and reliability studies. Cox & Oakes (1984, p. 7) give an example of an experiment where 60 springs were tested under cycles of repeated loading and failure time was measured in units of 10^3 cycles. The springs were subjected to different stress levels and at the lower stress levels, where failure times are longer, testing was abandoned before many units had failed, again giving rise to censored observations. The reliability and life-testing plans in MIL-STD-781C (1977) involve sequential monitoring of such failure time data.

1.4.5 Recurrent Event Data

In some studies the event of interest can occur repeatedly over time in the same patient. Studies of asthma attacks and of epileptic seizures are obvious examples. The outcome data for each patient consist of a series of failure times which can be viewed as the realization of a stochastic point process. In the Nutritional Prevention of Cancer Trial (see Clark et al., 1996; Jiang, Turnbull & Clark, 1999), over 1000 high-risk patients were randomly allocated to selenium supplementation or placebo and followed for up to ten years. Each patient was monitored at a dermatology clinic where the time from entry to each new occurrence of a squamous or basal cell carcinoma was recorded. In another application, Prentice, Williams & Peterson (1981) discuss a study of the frequencies of infections in patients following bone marrow transplantation.

In engineering, such repeated event data also arise in experiments and field studies concerning the reliability of repairable systems (e.g., see Ascher & Feingold, 1984).

1.4.6 Longitudinal Data

Sometimes the outcome for an individual subject consists of a series of repeated measurements. In a trial of treatments for prevention of osteoporosis in post-menopausal women, we may wish to compare a control group with various intervention groups taking estrogen, calcium or other supplements, measuring patient status by the Spinal Deformity Index (SDI). If the patients enter the study at staggered times during the accrual period and then undergo spine examinations at irregular intervals, the data for each patient will consist of a series of SDI values, taken at varying intervals and with unequal numbers for each patient.

Wu & Lan (1992) describe a sequential design for the Lung Health Study (Anthonisen, 1989), a three-armed study of the effect of an intensive anti-smoking program, with or without bronchodilators, on chronic obstructive pulmonary disease. Almost 6000 smokers with early airway obstruction were recruited over two years by 10 clinical centers. The primary outcome variable is the series of initial second forced expiration volumes measured at baseline and at each of five annual follow-up visits.

Armitage, Stratton & Worthington (1985) give an example of sequential testing in a clinical trial of toothpastes, in which the series of annual increments in the counts of decayed, missing or filled teeth forms the response variable.

1.4.7 Multivariate Data

In almost any trial, many outcome variables are examined. As an example, in the Nutritional Prevention of Cancer Trial mentioned in Section 1.4.5, the DSMB was provided with information on some 200 endpoints at each interim analysis. Usually a single most important variable, mortality for example, is designated of primary interest. However, there will sometimes be several endpoints of equal interest *a priori*. Variables of a similar type can be combined to give a univariate score or summary statistic, as O'Brien (1984) suggests for a randomized trial of treatments for diabetes in which nerve function was measured by 34 electromyographic variables.

In other instances, variables may be combined to reduce the outcome measure to a small number of components, each of a different type, and for which further reduction to a univariate statistic is inappropriate. Suppose, for example, we reduce a set of variables to a bivariate outcome whose two components measure overall "efficacy" and "safety". We may wish to treat these variables differently in a sequential design, stopping early if the new treatment appears greatly superior or inferior to the standard in terms of efficacy, but only stopping early on grounds of safety to reject the new treatment if it is substantially less safe than the standard; see Jennison & Turnbull (1993c). Group sequential methods for multiple endpoints are treated in Chapter 15.

1.5 Chapter Organization: A Roadmap

There are two main threads of development through this book. On the one hand we consider different formulations of testing problems and the many facets of group sequential testing such as initial experimental design, coping with unpredictable sample sizes and analysis on termination. The other thread concerns application of all types of group sequential procedure to a wide range of response distributions. Fortunately, there is a central example, that of normally distributed responses with known variance, which links both strands and there is no need to address every combination of group sequential procedure and data type. Initially, we need to introduce the key elements both of group sequential tests and of the joint distribution of a sequence of statistics. We do this in Chapters 2 and 3 in the context of two-sided tests; thereafter, chapters fall more clearly into one of the two categories noted above.

In Chapter 2, we describe basic group sequential procedures for comparing results from two parallel treatment arms. Specifically, outcomes are assumed to be immediately available and normally distributed with known variance. It is desired to test the null hypothesis, H_0, of equality of the two mean responses against a two-sided alternative. Observations are to be taken in up to K equally sized groups, but the experiment can stop early to reject H_0 if the observed difference is sufficiently large. Even though this is a very simple situation, unrealistic for many applications, it serves to illustrate the ideas of Type I and Type II error probabilities and choice of sample size and stopping criteria that are fundamental to group sequential procedures. We consider the same form of testing problem in Chapter 3 but adapt the tests of Chapter 2 to a variety of new data types.

We begin Chapter 3 by describing a unified formulation of group sequential problems based on sequences of standardized test statistics and information levels. This formulation will be used throughout the remainder of the book: it has the benefit of encompassing many common situations with normally distributed data, including two-treatment parallel designs, balanced or unbalanced, the one-treatment-arm designs common in Phase I and II trials, paired sample designs, crossover designs, general linear models used to adjust for covariates or factor variables, and longitudinal studies involving repeated measures or growth curve data. The same formulation also applies approximately to parametric models amenable to standard maximum likelihood analysis and to some special data types, in particular survival data. We continue Chapter 3 by explaining the "significance level approach", a key device in adapting group sequential tests defined in the idealized setting of Chapter 2 to other situations; this approach is used to deal with unequal group sizes, linear model data, the log-rank test for survival data and, very importantly, group sequential t-tests for normal data of unknown variance. All of these applications to different response distributions are presented in the context of a two-sided test. However, the same basic principles allow us to extend the use of other types of group sequential test from the simple case of normal data with known variance to the full range of response variables.

Chapters 4 to 6 concern other forms of hypothesis test. In Chapter 4 we present one-sided group sequential tests appropriate when a null hypothesis is to be tested against departures in one specific direction because those in the other direction are either implausible or not of interest. In Chapter 5 we introduce two-sided tests with an inner wedge allowing early stopping to accept the null hypothesis. Early acceptance of H_0 is not permitted in the two-sided tests of Chapters 2 and 3, but even though the ethical motivation may not be not so strong, there are sound financial reasons to curtail a study heading toward a negative conclusion; such curtailment can also benefit future patients by releasing experimental resources for the earlier exploration of further promising treatments. The goal of some clinical trials, particularly in pharmaceutical applications, is to establish "equivalence" between two treatments rather than to prove the superiority of one over the other. This goal leads to a reversal of the roles of null and alternative hypotheses and to another class of group sequential procedures. We describe group sequential equivalence tests in Chapter 6, illustrating these with examples of tests for "average equivalence" and "individual equivalence". The tests in Chapters 4 to 6 are introduced in a form appropriate for equally sized groups of normal observations with known variance, but in each case, we show how to use the techniques of Chapter 3 to adapt to unequal group sizes and unknown variance.

Chapters 7 to 10 continue with generic methods, usually described for the standard case of normal observations but readily applicable to other responses. An adaptive approach is needed to construct testing boundaries when group sizes, or more generally increments in information between analyses, are unequal and unpredictable; such unpredictability is not uncommon and is certainly to be expected in survival studies, where observed information depends on subject accrual, dropout and baseline event rates. In Chapter 7 we describe "error spending" methods for dealing with these problems in both one-sided and two-sided tests. These error spending methods require numerical computation for their implementation, a topic discussed briefly in Chapter 7 and at greater length in Chapter 19. In Chapter 8, we discuss the full statistical analysis to be performed upon conclusion of a group sequential study, including the construction of P-values and confidence intervals which retain their standard frequentist properties despite the unusual sample space.

Chapter 9 concerns sequences of "repeated confidence intervals" and "repeated P-values" which enable results to be reported and assessed at any interim stage, irrespective of whether or not the study design calls for termination. These sequences possess the important feature that their validity does not depend on the stopping rule used. As well as providing data summaries with well-defined properties when a formal stopping rule is not adhered to, repeated confidence intervals and P-values are suitable for presentation at professional meetings during the course of a trial as they automatically protect against "over-interpretation" of interim results. Chapter 10 explores the idea of stochastic curtailment, an informal approach to interim monitoring based on predictions of the outcome of a single, fixed-sample analysis to be conducted at the end of the study when a specified time or sample size is reached. At any interim stage, it is natural to consider the probability that a particular decision will eventually be made when the trial reaches its planned conclusion, given trends in the data seen so far. If a certain decision is inevitable, it is reasonable to stop or "curtail" the trial. Stopping a trial because a particular decision, while not inevitable, is highly likely is referred to as "stochastic curtailment".

The next three chapters take up the complementary thread of applying group sequential procedures defined for an idealized form of normal data to other response types. In Chapter 11, we derive the general theory for normal linear models which underlies the "unified formulation" of Chapter 3. This theory extends to correlated data and the mixed effects models which often arise in longitudinal and repeated measures studies. We also present theory for the case of unknown variance, and this provides the exact joint distribution of sequences of t-statistics, justifying more general use of the group sequential t-tests presented earlier. Section 11.6 addresses general parametric models satisfying the conditions for standard maximum likelihood theory, and these include generalized linear models as an important special case. The theory shows that standardized statistics have, asymptotically, the same multivariate normal joint distribution as statistics from a normal linear model, supporting the extension of the unified formulation of Chapter 3.

Chapter 12 concerns binary data. We describe methods of exact calculation for group sequential tests with small or moderate sample sizes for which the normal approximations of Chapter 11 may be inaccurate. This chapter also discusses more complex applications involving binary data, such as inference for logistic regression models and stratified 2×2 tables. The latter, commonly found in epidemiological cohort studies and matched pair case-control studies, lead to group sequential versions of the Mantel-Haenszel and McNemar tests. The primary response in many clinical trials is a survival time or time to occurrence of an event such as failure, relapse or remission of symptoms. In Chapter 13 the group sequential log-rank test, already introduced in Section 3.7, is generalized to allow the effects of covariates through use of Cox's (1972) proportional hazards regression model; this is illustrated with an extensive example. Also in this chapter, methods are described for inference concerning Kaplan-Meier (1958) estimates of survival probabilities and quantiles. As an example, a repeated confidence interval of a two-year survival probability or median survival time might provide a useful data summary for consideration by a DSMB at an interim analysis.

In setting the sample size for a study, the power calculation may require knowledge of an unknown parameter, such as a response variance or event rate. In Chapter 14, we discuss studies with an initial "internal pilot" phase, the results of which are used to estimate parameters affecting sample size and, hence, to modify the planned overall sample size. In Chapter 15, we consider the topic of multiple endpoints, i.e., multivariate responses, and the examination of a number of patient outcome measures at interim analyses. Because of the considerable overhead expense in setting up a large clinical trial, there are economies of scale and savings in time if several competing treatments can be compared in the same trial. Accordingly, it is increasingly more common for trials to be conducted with three or more treatment arms. Methodology for such multi-armed trials is the subject of Chapter 16.

In a parallel design comparing two treatments, it is not unusual for unequal randomization or dropout of some subjects to produce unbalanced numbers of observations on the two treatment arms. In Chapter 17, we consider designs with intentional imbalance between treatments achieved by modifying treatment allocation at each stage in response to previously observed outcomes. Such designs are said to use stage-wise data-dependent or stage-wise adaptive sampling rules and their usual purpose is to reduce the number of subjects assigned to the inferior treatment, although of course the identity of this treatment is initially unknown.

This book is primarily concerned with frequentist inference for group sequential tests. A very different framework for the design and analysis of group sequential trials arises if inference is made in the Bayesian paradigm. The Bayesian approach is discussed in Chapter 18.

Finally, in Chapter 19, we present details of the numerical computations required to design and evaluate group sequential tests. These computational methods were used to obtain the many tables and figures appearing throughout the book.

1.6 Bibliography and Notes

Since the classic book of Armitage (1975), there have been very few books on the specific topic of sequential statistical procedures for clinical trials. An exception is the book by Whitehead (1997) which concentrates mostly on developing the theory and application of the triangular tests we shall describe in Sections 4.5 and 5.3. A number of case studies can be found in the book edited by Peace (1992) and in the proceedings of two workshops, one on practical issues in data monitoring sponsored by the U.S. National Institutes of Health in 1992, the other on early stopping rules held at Cambridge University in 1993. These proceedings were published as special issues of the journal *Statistics in Medicine* (Issues 5 and 6 of Volume 12 in March 1993 and Issues 13 and 14 of Volume 13 in July 1994). The review paper by Fleming (1992) and accompanying discussion contain descriptions of several case studies of sequentially monitored trials in cancer and AIDS. In particular, Fleming describes an experience which illustrates the perils and undesirable consequences of an unstructured approach to interim monitoring, and another in which premature release of interim results had a harmful effect. Another lesson to be learned from the experiences reported in Fleming (1992) is that group sequential methods are important in indicating when a trial should *not* be stopped.

Although the tests in Chapters 2 to 6 can be applied with a minimum of calculation, this is not the case for error spending tests and inferences on termination of a group sequential test. The description given in Chapter 19 of numerical integration methods can serve as a basis for writing special purpose software, and we have made some of our own FORTRAN programs available at the website `http://www.bath.ac.uk/~mascj/` to assist the reader.

There are two commercial computer software packages currently available for use in the sequential design and analysis of clinical trials. The package PEST 3 (Brunier & Whitehead, 1993) is based on the tests described by Whitehead in his 1997 book; a new version, PEST 4, is scheduled to be released in the year 2000. The other package, EaSt, is developed by Cytel Software Corporation (1992) and a new version, EaSt for Windows (Cytel Software Corporation, 1999), is due to be released soon. We discuss the capabilities of these packages in Section 19.7.

A module S+SeqTrial based on the Splus statistical software (MathSoft, 1998) is in development at the time of writing. FORTRAN routines for use in implementing error spending tests have been made available at `http://www.medsch.wisc.edu/landemets/` by the authors, David Reboussin, David DeMets, KyungMann Kim and K. K. Gordon Lan.

CHAPTER 2

Two-Sided Tests: Introduction

2.1 Two-Sided Tests for Comparing Two Treatments with Normal Response of Known Variance

The name *two-sided test* is given to a test of a hypothesis against a two-sided alternative. In this chapter we restrict attention to testing for a difference in the mean response of two treatments when observations are normally distributed with common, known variance. Denoting the difference in means by θ, the null hypothesis H_0: $\theta = 0$ states that responses follow the same distribution under both treatments. The alternative hypothesis, H_A: $\theta \neq 0$, contains two cases, $\theta < 0$ and $\theta > 0$, which correspond to one treatment being superior to the other and vice versa.

In this comparison, the standardized test statistic, Z, is distributed symmetrically about 0 under H_0, and a fixed sample test rejects H_0 if $|Z| > c$ for some constant c. The sign of Z determines which treatment is to be preferred when H_0 is rejected. A test's *Type I error probability* is defined to be the probability of wrongly rejecting the null hypothesis,

$$Pr_{\theta=0}\{|Z| > c\}.$$

The *power* of a test is the probability of rejecting the null hypothesis when it does not hold, $Pr_\theta\{|Z| > c\}$, for values of $\theta \neq 0$. The power depends on θ, increasing as θ moves away from 0, but it is convenient to state a power requirement at a specific value or values of θ, for example,

$$Pr_{\theta=\delta}\{|Z| > c\} = Pr_{\theta=-\delta}\{|Z| > c\} = 1 - \beta, \tag{2.1}$$

where δ represents a treatment difference that the investigators would hope to detect with high probability. The small probability β is referred to as the *Type II error probability* at $\theta = \pm\,\delta$. In practical terms, it is not desirable to reject H_0 in favor of $\theta < 0$ when actually $\theta > 0$ as this would imply a recommendation of the inferior of the two treatments. With this in mind, the above power requirement can be replaced by

$$Pr_{\theta=\delta}\{Z > c\} = Pr_{\theta=-\delta}\{Z < -c\} = 1 - \beta. \tag{2.2}$$

Fortunately, for values of c and δ that we shall consider, the probabilities $Pr_{\theta=\delta}\{Z < -c\}$ and $Pr_{\theta=-\delta}\{Z > c\}$ are extremely small and the two requirements (2.1) and (2.2) are equal for all practical purposes.

We present the standard non-sequential test for this problem in Section 2.2, and in the remainder of the chapter we describe and compare group sequential tests that achieve specified Type I and Type II errors. There is no loss of generality in introducing two-sided tests for the particular problem of a two-treatment comparison. We shall explain in Chapter 3 how the same forms of group sequential tests can be used in other problems including paired comparisons, crossover trials and a two-treatment comparison with allowance for the effects of covariates.

The assumption of normal observations with known variance can also be relaxed. We discuss application of the same tests to general parametric models in Section 3.5, and consider tests for binary data and survival data in subsequent sections. Binary responses and survival data are also discussed in greater detail in Chapters 12 and 13, respectively. The assumption of a known variance for normal observations is often unrealistic but we start by deriving tests under this assumption for simplicity and because the resulting tests can, in fact, be adapted to more realistic problems. We discuss two-sided group sequential t-tests for normal data with unknown variance in Section 3.8 and consider the problem of re-computing sample size during the course of a study to meet a stated power requirement in Section 14.3.2.

2.2 A Fixed Sample Test

Let X_{Ai} and X_{Bi}, $i = 1, 2, \ldots$, denote the responses of subjects allocated to two treatments, A and B. Suppose responses of subjects receiving treatment A are normally distributed with variance σ^2 and mean μ_A, which we write $X_{Ai} \sim N(\mu_A, \sigma^2)$, $i = 1, 2, \ldots$. Likewise, suppose $X_{Bi} \sim N(\mu_B, \sigma^2)$, $i = 1, 2, \ldots$, and all observations are independent. Consider the problem of testing the null hypothesis of no treatment difference H_0: $\mu_A = \mu_B$ against the two-sided alternative $\mu_A \neq \mu_B$ with Type I error probability α and power $1 - \beta$ at $\mu_A - \mu_B = \pm\delta$.

If n subjects are allocated to each treatment, the standardized statistic

$$\begin{aligned} Z &= \frac{1}{\sqrt{(2n\sigma^2)}} \left(\sum_{i=1}^{n} X_{Ai} - \sum_{i=1}^{n} X_{Bi} \right) \\ &\sim N((\mu_A - \mu_B)\sqrt{\{n/(2\sigma^2)\}}, 1). \end{aligned}$$

Thus $Z \sim N(0, 1)$ under H_0 and the symmetric two-sided test with Type I error probability α rejects H_0 if $|Z| > \Phi^{-1}(1 - \alpha/2)$, where Φ denotes the standard normal cumulative distribution function (cdf). To satisfy the power requirement, we also need

$$Pr\{|Z| > \Phi^{-1}(1 - \alpha/2)\} = 1 - \beta$$

when $Z \sim N(\pm\delta\sqrt{\{n/(2\sigma^2)\}}, 1)$. As explained in Section 2.1, we can ignore the very small probabilities that $Z < -\Phi^{-1}(1 - \alpha/2)$ when $\mu_A - \mu_B = \delta$ or $Z > \Phi^{-1}(1 - \alpha/2)$ when $\mu_A - \mu_B = -\delta$; thus we need

$$E(Z) = \Phi^{-1}(1 - \alpha/2) + \Phi^{-1}(1 - \beta)$$

at the positive alternative, $\mu_A - \mu_B = \delta$, and equating this expected value to $\delta\sqrt{\{n/(2\sigma^2)\}}$ we find the necessary sample size to be

$$n_f(\alpha, \beta, \delta, \sigma^2) = \{\Phi^{-1}(1 - \alpha/2) + \Phi^{-1}(1 - \beta)\}^2 2\sigma^2/\delta^2 \qquad (2.3)$$

subjects per treatment arm. In practice, n_f must, of course, be rounded to an integer sample size.

As an example, suppose $\sigma^2 = 4$, so $X_{Ai} \sim N(\mu_A, 4)$ and $X_{Bi} \sim N(\mu_B, 4)$, $i = 1, 2, \ldots$, and it is required to test H_0: $\mu_A = \mu_B$ with Type I error $\alpha = 0.05$ and power $1 - \beta = 0.9$ at $\mu_A - \mu_B = \pm 1$. From (2.3), the fixed sample test for this problem needs $\{\Phi^{-1}(0.975) + \Phi^{-1}(0.9)\}^2 \times 2 \times 4 = 84.1$ subjects on each treatment, which we round up to 85. The null hypothesis is rejected if

$$\left| \sum_{i=1}^{85} X_{Ai} - \sum_{i=1}^{85} X_{Bi} \right| \geq 1.96 \sqrt{(85 \times 2 \times 4)} = 51.1$$

and accepted otherwise. We shall return to this example to illustrate and compare different types of group sequential test.

2.3 Group Sequential Tests

The key feature of a group sequential test, as opposed to a fully sequential test, is that the accumulating data are analyzed at intervals rather than after every new observation. Continuous data monitoring can be a serious practical burden, and the introduction of group sequential tests has led to much wider use of sequential methods. Their impact has been particularly evident in clinical trials, where it is standard practice for a monitoring committee to meet at regular intervals to assess various aspects of a study's progress and it is relatively easy to add formal interim analyses of the primary patient response. Not only are group sequential tests convenient to conduct, they also provide ample opportunity for early stopping and can achieve most of the benefits of fully sequential tests in terms of lower expected sample sizes and shorter average study lengths.

Although earlier suggestions for group sequential medical studies had been made by Elfring & Schultz (1973), McPherson (1974) and Canner (1977), the major impetus to group sequential testing came with the papers of Pocock (1977) and O'Brien & Fleming (1979). These two papers describe group sequential two-sided tests which are easy to implement and can be readily adapted to a variety of response distributions. In the basic two-treatment comparison, a maximum number of groups, K, and a group size, m, are chosen, subjects are allocated to treatments according to a constrained randomization scheme which ensures m subjects receive each treatment in every group and the accumulating data are analyzed after each group of $2m$ responses. For each $k = 1, \ldots, K$, a standardized statistic Z_k is computed from the first k groups of observations, and the test terminates with rejection of H_0 if $|Z_k|$ exceeds a critical value c_k. If the test continues to the Kth analysis and $|Z_K| < c_K$, it stops at that point and H_0 is accepted. The sequence of critical values, $\{c_1, \ldots, c_K\}$, is chosen to achieve a specified Type I error, and different types of group sequential test give rise to different sequences. The group size, m, is determined separately by a power condition.

We introduce the Pocock and O'Brien & Fleming tests in Sections 2.4 and 2.5, and we compare properties of these two types of test in Section 2.6. We present two other types of test in Section 2.7, the Wang & Tsiatis (1987) family of tests, which include Pocock and O'Brien & Fleming tests as special cases as well as other tests with boundaries of intermediate shapes, and the "Haybittle-Peto" test, which uses a very simple criterion for early stopping. We present tabulated properties of a range of tests to assist in choosing the most suitable type of test and number of groups of observations for a particular application.

Although the assumption of equal numbers of observations in each group can be relaxed a little, the tests described in this chapter do require approximate equality of group sizes. More flexible methods for handling unequal and unpredictable group sizes will be described in Chapter 7. A possibility which we do not consider at this stage is early stopping to *accept* the null hypothesis; tests with this property will be discussed in Chapter 5.

All the tests introduced in this chapter can be viewed as *repeated significance tests* since, at each analysis, the null hypothesis is rejected if a non-sequential test of H_0 is significant at or below a certain level. In the case of the Pocock test, the same significance level is applied at each analysis, whereas for other tests, the constants c_k decrease and the nominal significance levels increase over the course of the study. This representation provides a convenient mechanism for generalizing the tests. In Chapter 3 we shall extend the basic methods to other two-sided testing problems, to slightly unequal group sizes and to data from other response distributions, by applying tests of the null hypothesis at the same sequences of significance levels. Our method of specifying the group size required to attain a given power also generalizes easily. A group sequential test's maximum sample size is calculated by multiplying the group size needed in a fixed sample test by a factor, which we provide, appropriate to the type of test, the number of groups and the specified error probabilities. The same factors apply to other two-sided testing problems and are approximately correct when group sizes are slightly unequal or when non-normal response distributions give rise to approximately normal test statistics.

2.4 Pocock's Test

2.4.1 Definition of Pocock's Test

Pocock (1977) adapted the idea of a "repeated significance test" at a constant nominal significance level to analyze accumulating data at a relatively small number of times over the course of a study. Patient entry is divided into K equally sized groups containing m subjects on each treatment, and the data are analyzed after each new group of observations has been observed.

For simplicity, we shall first consider the case where treatment allocation within each group is random subject to the constraint that m subjects receive each treatment. More sophisticated randomization methods, such as stratification with respect to prognostic factors, can be used instead, in which case the analysis falls under the general treatment for linear models described later on in Section 3.4. For the testing problem of Section 2.2, observations $X_{Ai} \sim N(\mu_A, \sigma^2)$ and $X_{Bi} \sim N(\mu_B, \sigma^2)$, $i = 1, 2, \ldots$, are available from treatment groups A and B, respectively. Pocock's test uses the standardized statistic after each group of observations,

$$Z_k = \frac{1}{\surd(2mk\sigma^2)} \left(\sum_{i=1}^{mk} X_{Ai} - \sum_{i=1}^{mk} X_{Bi} \right), \quad k = 1 \ldots, K. \tag{2.4}$$

If, at the kth analysis, $k = 1, \ldots, K$, the absolute value of Z_k is sufficiently large, the study stops with rejection of H_0. If H_0 has not been rejected by the final analysis, K, it is accepted. It is not appropriate simply to apply a level-α two-sided test at each analysis since the multiple looks at the data would lead to a Type I error well in excess of α; for example, Armitage, McPherson & Rowe (1969, Table 2) report that the probability under H_0 that $|Z_k|$ exceeds $\Phi^{-1}(0.975) = 1.96$ for *at least* one k, $k = 1, \ldots, 5$, is 0.142, nearly three times the 0.05 significance level applied at each individual analysis.

Pocock's test retains the general form of a repeatedly applied significance test, rejecting H_0 at stage k if $|Z_k| \geq C_P(K, \alpha)$, $k = 1, \ldots, K$, but the critical value $C_P(K, \alpha)$ is chosen to give overall Type I error α, i.e.,

$$Pr_{\mu_A - \mu_B = 0}\{\text{Reject } H_0 \text{ at analysis } k = 1, k = 2, \ldots, \text{or } k = K\} = \alpha.$$

Formally, the test is

$$\begin{array}{lll} \text{After group } k = 1, \ldots, K-1 & & \\ \quad \text{if } |Z_k| \geq C_P(K, \alpha) & \text{stop, reject } H_0 & \\ \quad \text{otherwise} & \text{continue to group } k+1, & \\ \text{after group } K & & \\ \quad \text{if } |Z_K| \geq C_P(K, \alpha) & \text{stop, reject } H_0 & \\ \quad \text{otherwise} & \text{stop, accept } H_0. & \end{array} \tag{2.5}$$

This is an example of the general group sequential test in which H_0 is rejected after group k if $|Z_k| \geq c_k$, and in this case the critical values c_k, $k = 1, \ldots, K$, are constant and equal to $C_P(K, \alpha)$. The constants $C_P(K, \alpha)$ displayed in Table 2.1 for $\alpha = 0.01, 0.05$ and 0.1 were computed numerically using the joint distribution of the sequence of statistics $Z_1, \ldots, Z_K$. Details of this computation, which need not concern us at this point, are described in Chapter 19. Values for $K = 1$, the non-sequential case, are included in Table 2.1 for comparison.

Note that at each analysis, the test rejects H_0 if the two-sided significance level of a non-sequential test of H_0 using the data available at that time is below $\alpha' = 2[1 - \Phi\{C_P(K, \alpha)\}]$. Hence, this is a repeated significance test with constant "nominal significance level" α'. As an example, if $K = 5$ and $\alpha = 0.05$, the nominal significance level applied at each analysis is $\alpha' = 2\{1 - \Phi(2.413)\} = 0.0158$. A nominal significance level below the overall Type I error probability is essential in order to avoid the "multiple-looks" problem mentioned earlier.

Table 2.1 *Pocock tests: constants $C_P(K, \alpha)$ for two-sided tests with K groups of observations and Type I error probability α*

	$C_P(K, \alpha)$		
K	$\alpha = 0.01$	$\alpha = 0.05$	$\alpha = 0.10$
1	2.576	1.960	1.645
2	2.772	2.178	1.875
3	2.873	2.289	1.992
4	2.939	2.361	2.067
5	2.986	2.413	2.122
6	3.023	2.453	2.164
7	3.053	2.485	2.197
8	3.078	2.512	2.225
9	3.099	2.535	2.249
10	3.117	2.555	2.270
11	3.133	2.572	2.288
12	3.147	2.588	2.304
15	3.182	2.626	2.344
20	3.225	2.672	2.392

2.4.2 *Satisfying the Power Requirement*

The test defined by (2.5) has Type I error probability α for any group size, m. It is the power requirement

$$Pr_{\mu_A - \mu_B = \pm\delta}\{\text{Reject } H_0\} = 1 - \beta$$

that determines the appropriate group size. The maximum sample size that the group sequential test may need depends on K, α and β and is proportional to σ^2/δ^2. Since the sample size of a fixed sample test with the same Type I error α and power $1-\beta$ at $\mu_A - \mu_B = \pm\delta$ is also proportional to σ^2/δ^2, it is sufficient to specify the ratio $R_P(K, \alpha, \beta)$ of the group sequential test's maximum sample size to the fixed sample size, and this ratio will then apply for all δ and σ^2. We shall also see that the same ratios can be used in other two-sided testing problems and with other data types. The values of $R_P(K, \alpha, \beta)$ in Table 2.2 were found by the same type of numerical calculation used to determine the $C_P(K, \alpha)$. Again, details of their derivation can be found in Chapter 19. For brevity, we have tabulated $C_P(K, \alpha)$ and $R_P(K, \alpha, \beta)$ only for selected values of K; accurate estimates of constants for $K = 13$, 14 and $16, \ldots, 19$ can be obtained by linear interpolation both here and for other tests to be presented later.

The sample size per treatment arm, $n_f(\alpha, \beta, \delta, \sigma^2)$, required by a fixed sample test with Type I error α and power $1-\beta$ at $\mu_A - \mu_B = \pm\delta$ is given by (2.3). A Pocock group sequential test with K groups needs a maximum of $R_P(K, \alpha, \beta)\, n_f(\alpha, \beta, \delta, \sigma^2)$ observations per treatment arm and groups of $m = R_P(K, \alpha, \beta)\, n_f(\alpha, \beta, \delta, \sigma^2)/K$ observations on each treatment. Rounding

Table 2.2 *Pocock tests: constants $R_P(K, \alpha, \beta)$ to determine group sizes for two-sided tests with K groups of observations, Type I error probability α and power $1-\beta$*

	$R_P(K,\alpha,\beta)$					
	$1-\beta=0.8$			$1-\beta=0.9$		
K	$\alpha=0.01$	$\alpha=0.05$	$\alpha=0.10$	$\alpha=0.01$	$\alpha=0.05$	$\alpha=0.10$
1	1.000	1.000	1.000	1.000	1.000	1.000
2	1.092	1.110	1.121	1.084	1.100	1.110
3	1.137	1.166	1.184	1.125	1.151	1.166
4	1.166	1.202	1.224	1.152	1.183	1.202
5	1.187	1.229	1.254	1.170	1.207	1.228
6	1.203	1.249	1.277	1.185	1.225	1.249
7	1.216	1.265	1.296	1.197	1.239	1.266
8	1.226	1.279	1.311	1.206	1.252	1.280
9	1.236	1.291	1.325	1.215	1.262	1.292
10	1.243	1.301	1.337	1.222	1.271	1.302
11	1.250	1.310	1.348	1.228	1.279	1.312
12	1.257	1.318	1.357	1.234	1.287	1.320
15	1.272	1.338	1.381	1.248	1.305	1.341
20	1.291	1.363	1.411	1.264	1.327	1.367

m to an integer value will have a slight effect on the test's actual power, and it is usual to round m upward to obtain a conservative test, i.e., with power a little larger than $1-\beta$.

2.4.3 An Example

To illustrate Pocock's test, we return to the example of Section 2.2 where it was required to test H_0: $\mu_A = \mu_B$ with Type I error $\alpha = 0.05$ and power $1-\beta = 0.9$ at $\mu_A - \mu_B = \pm 1$ when observations have variance $\sigma^2 = 4$. From (2.3), the fixed sample size is $n_f(0.05, 0.1, 1, 4) = 84.1$ observations per treatment arm. From Table 2.2, $R_P(5, 0.05, 0.1) = 1.207$. Hence, a Pocock test with five groups of observations has maximum sample size per treatment arm

$$R_P(5, 0.05, 0.1)\, n_f(0.05, 0.1, 1, 4) = 1.207 \times 84.1 = 101.5$$

and the necessary group size is $m = 101.5/5 = 20.3$ per treatment, which we round up to 21. The test stops with rejection of the null hypothesis at analysis k, $k = 1, \ldots, 5$, if

$$\left| \sum_{i=1}^{21k} X_{Ai} - \sum_{i=1}^{21k} X_{Bi} \right| \geq 2.413 \sqrt{(21k \times 2 \times 4)} = 31.28 \sqrt{k}.$$

If the null hypothesis has not been rejected by analysis 5, it is accepted at that point.

Figure 2.1 *A Pocock test for five groups of observations*

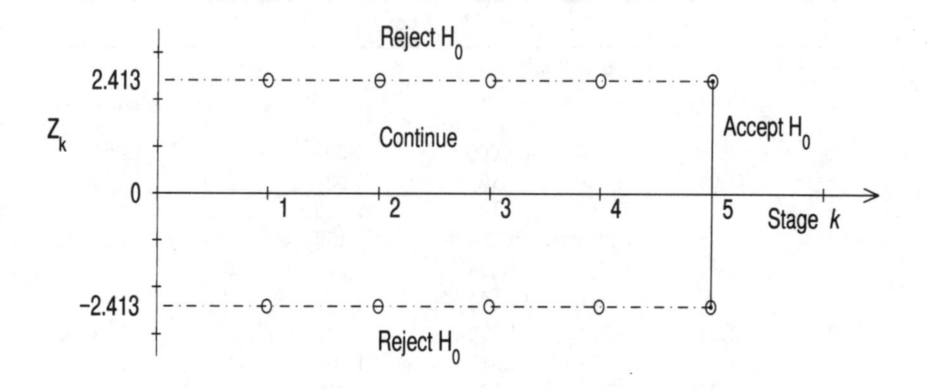

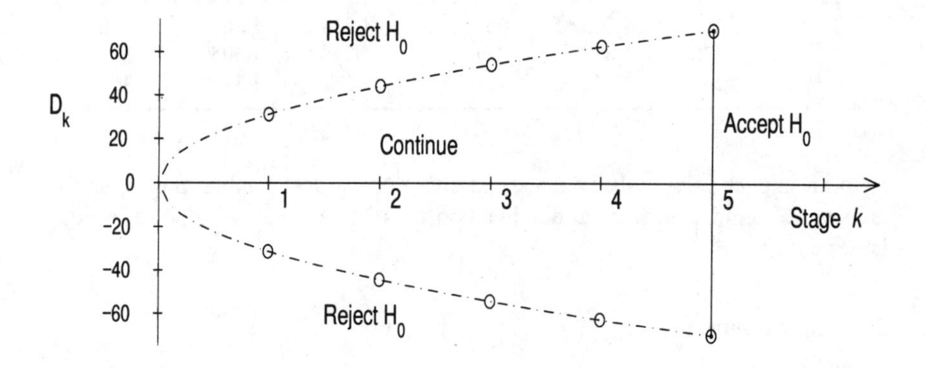

The boundary of the Pocock test for this example is illustrated in Figure 2.1. The first diagram shows the critical values applied to the standardized statistics Z_k, which are constant over the five analyses for the Pocock test. In the second diagram, the same test is expressed in terms of the unstandardized differences of sample sums on treatments A and B, $D_k = \sum_{i=1}^{21k} X_{Ai} - \sum_{i=1}^{21k} X_{Bi}$, $k = 1, \ldots, 5$, and in this representation the Pocock boundary points lie on a square-root-shaped curve, $C_P(K, \alpha)\sqrt{\{42\, k\sigma^2\}}$.

Note that the maximum total number of subjects over both treatment arms that may be required using Pocock's test is 210. This is somewhat greater than the 170 needed for a fixed sample test, but the benefit is a smaller expected number of subjects for the group sequential test when $|\mu_A - \mu_B|$ is sufficiently large. Numerical comparisons of expected sample size will be seen in Section 2.6.

Table 2.3 *O'Brien & Fleming tests: constants $C_B(K,\alpha)$ for two-sided tests with K groups of observations and Type I error probability α*

	$C_B(K,\alpha)$		
K	$\alpha = 0.01$	$\alpha = 0.05$	$\alpha = 0.10$
1	2.576	1.960	1.645
2	2.580	1.977	1.678
3	2.595	2.004	1.710
4	2.609	2.024	1.733
5	2.621	2.040	1.751
6	2.631	2.053	1.765
7	2.640	2.063	1.776
8	2.648	2.072	1.786
9	2.654	2.080	1.794
10	2.660	2.087	1.801
11	2.665	2.092	1.807
12	2.670	2.098	1.813
15	2.681	2.110	1.826
20	2.695	2.126	1.842

2.5 O'Brien & Fleming's Test

2.5.1 Definition of O'Brien & Fleming's Test

As an alternative to the repeated significance test with constant nominal significance levels, O'Brien & Fleming (1979) proposed a test in which the nominal significance levels needed to reject H_0 at each analysis increase as the study progresses. Thus, in their test it is more difficult to reject H_0 at the earliest analyses but easier later on. As in Pocock's test, subjects are allocated to treatments in groups, and the accumulating data are analyzed after complete groups of data become available. The O'Brien & Fleming test is also defined in terms of the standardized statistics Z_k of (2.4), and H_0 is rejected after group k if $|Z_k| \geq c_k$ for a sequence of critical values $c_1, \ldots, c_K$. Formally, the test is

$$\begin{array}{lll} \text{After group } k = 1, \ldots, K-1 & & \\ \quad \text{if } |Z_k| \geq C_B(K,\alpha)\sqrt{(K/k)} & \text{stop, reject } H_0 & \\ \quad \text{otherwise} & \text{continue to group } k+1, & \\ \text{after group } K & & \quad (2.6) \\ \quad \text{if } |Z_K| \geq C_B(K,\alpha) & \text{stop, reject } H_0 & \\ \quad \text{otherwise} & \text{stop, accept } H_0. & \end{array}$$

Thus, $c_k = C_B(K,\alpha)\sqrt{(K/k)}$, $k = 1, \ldots, K$. Values of $C_B(K,\alpha)$ which ensure an overall Type I error probability α are provided in Table 2.3. In terms of nominal significance levels, H_0 is rejected at analysis k, $k = 1, \ldots, K$, if the

Table 2.4 *O'Brien & Fleming tests: constants $R_B(K, \alpha, \beta)$ to determine group sizes of two-sided tests with K groups of observations, Type I error probability α and power $1-\beta$*

	$R_B(K, \alpha, \beta)$					
	$1-\beta=0.8$			$1-\beta=0.9$		
K	α=0.01	α=0.05	α=0.10	α=0.01	α=0.05	α=0.10
1	1.000	1.000	1.000	1.000	1.000	1.000
2	1.001	1.008	1.016	1.001	1.007	1.014
3	1.007	1.017	1.027	1.006	1.016	1.025
4	1.011	1.024	1.035	1.010	1.022	1.032
5	1.015	1.028	1.040	1.014	1.026	1.037
6	1.017	1.032	1.044	1.016	1.030	1.041
7	1.019	1.035	1.047	1.018	1.032	1.044
8	1.021	1.037	1.049	1.020	1.034	1.046
9	1.022	1.038	1.051	1.021	1.036	1.048
10	1.024	1.040	1.053	1.022	1.037	1.049
11	1.025	1.041	1.054	1.023	1.039	1.051
12	1.026	1.042	1.055	1.024	1.040	1.052
15	1.028	1.045	1.058	1.026	1.042	1.054
20	1.030	1.047	1.061	1.029	1.045	1.057

two-sided significance level of H_0 is below $\alpha'_k = 2[1 - \Phi\{C_B(K,\alpha)\surd(K/k)\}]$. Since $C_B(K,\alpha)\surd(K/k)$ decreases with increasing k, α'_k increases. For $K = 5$ and $\alpha = 0.05$ the nominal significance levels applied at analyses 1 to 5 are $\alpha'_1 = 0.000005$, $\alpha'_2 = 0.0013$, $\alpha'_3 = 0.0084$, $\alpha'_4 = 0.0225$ and $\alpha'_5 = 0.0413$.

Since $c_K = C_B(K,\alpha)$, comparing $C_B(K,\alpha)$ with $C_B(1,\alpha)$ shows how much larger the critical value for $|Z_K|$ is than the critical value that would be applied in a fixed sample analysis of the final data set. It is evident that this increase is quite small for O'Brien & Fleming tests.

2.5.2 *Satisfying the Power Requirement*

Table 2.4 contains constants $R_B(K, \alpha, \beta)$ for use in sample size calculations and these play the same role as the $R_P(K, \alpha, \beta)$ do for the Pocock test. The maximum sample size on each treatment arm is $R_B(K, \alpha, \beta)\, n_f(\alpha, \beta, \delta, \sigma^2)$ where $n_f(\alpha, \beta, \delta, \sigma^2)$, given by (2.3), is the number of observations per treatment needed by a fixed sample size test with the same Type I error and power. Thus, the necessary group size is $m = R_B(K, \alpha, \beta)\, n_f(\alpha, \beta, \delta, \sigma^2)/K$ per treatment arm, suitably rounded.

In general, O'Brien & Fleming's test requires a smaller group size than Pocock's test to satisfy the same power requirement. To understand why this should be the case, note that from (2.4), the effect of $(\mu_A - \mu_B)$ on $E(Z_k)$ increases with k and so power is gained primarily from the later analyses. O'Brien & Fleming boundaries are wide early on but narrow at the last few analyses, where they are able to gain more power than Pocock boundaries with the same group sizes. Thus, for a fixed power requirement, the O'Brien & Fleming test needs a smaller group size.

2.5.3 *An Example*

We return again to our previous example of testing H_0: $\mu_A = \mu_B$ with Type I error $\alpha = 0.05$ and power $1 - \beta = 0.9$ at $\mu_A - \mu_B = \pm 1$ when observations have variance $\sigma^2 = 4$. From (2.3), the fixed sample size required is $n_f(0.05, 0.1, 1, 4) = 84.1$ observations per treatment arm and, from Table 2.4, $R_B(5, 0.05, 0.1) = 1.026$. Hence, an O'Brien & Fleming test with five groups of observations has maximum sample size per treatment arm

$$R_B(5, 0.05, 0.1)\, n_f(0.05, 0.1, 1, 4) = 1.026 \times 84.1 = 86.3$$

and the necessary group size is $m = 86.3/5 = 17.3$ per treatment, which rounds up to 18. The test stops to reject the null hypothesis at analysis k, $k = 1, \ldots, 5$, if

$$\left| \sum_{i=1}^{18k} X_{Ai} - \sum_{i=1}^{18k} X_{Bi} \right| \geq 2.040\, \sqrt{(5/k)}\, \sqrt{(18k \times 2 \times 4)} = 54.74$$

and accepts H_0 if it has not been rejected by analysis 5.

The maximum total number of subjects over both treatment arms that may be required by O'Brien & Fleming's test is 180, a small increase over the 170 needed for a fixed sample test. Just as for Pocock's test, the expected number of subjects is reduced substantially when $|\mu_A - \mu_B|$ is sufficiently large.

The boundary of the O'Brien & Fleming test for this example is illustrated in Figure 2.2. In the first diagram, where the test is described in terms of critical values for the standardized statistics, Z_k, the boundary values decrease markedly at successive analyses. The second diagram shows the same test expressed in terms of the unstandardized differences of sample sums, $D_k = \sum_{i=1}^{mk} X_{Ai} - \sum_{i=1}^{mk} X_{Bi}$, $k = 1, \ldots, 5$, and on this scale the O'Brien & Fleming test has horizontal boundaries.

2.6 Properties of Pocock and O'Brien & Fleming Tests

2.6.1 *Comparing Group Sequential Tests*

A number of properties can be considered when comparing group sequential tests. Qualitative differences between the two types of test are apparent in Figures 2.1 and 2.2: the Pocock test has narrower boundaries initially, affording a greater opportunity for very early stopping, whereas the O'Brien & Fleming test has the narrower boundaries at later analyses and a smaller maximum sample size. For quantitative comparisons, a number of criteria are available. Error probabilities are a crucial property of any test, and it is important to compare properly "matched" tests. However, once the Type I and Type II error probabilities are specified, a test's power is largely determined over the range of possible parameter values, and there is little to be gained by investigating any remaining differences between

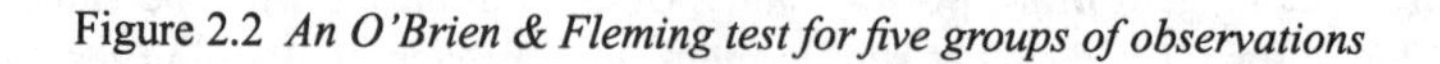

Figure 2.2 *An O'Brien & Fleming test for five groups of observations*

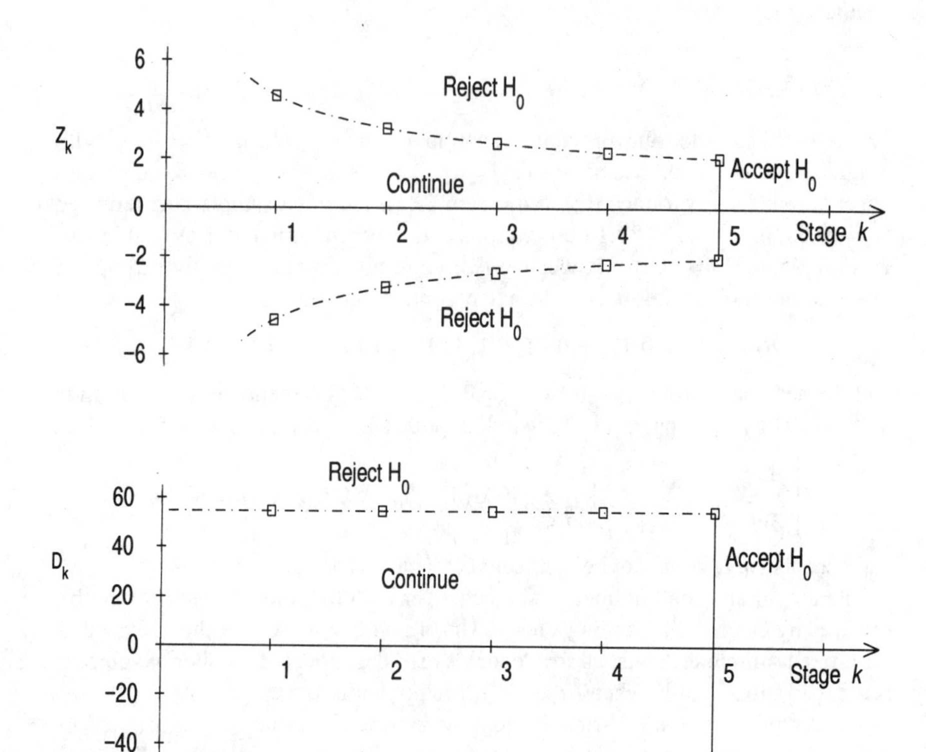

tests. A principal reason for using a sequential test is to reduce sample size. In the example we have been considering, the sample size distribution depends on the value of $\mu_A - \mu_B$, and one should consider the sample size over a range of values of $\mu_A - \mu_B$ when drawing comparisons. While it is convenient to summarize the sample size distribution under a particular value of $\mu_A - \mu_B$ by its expectation, other features of the distribution should not be ignored. In particular, the maximum possible sample size is a useful indication of what may happen in the worst case, and this sample size will occur quite often since it must arise whenever the null hypothesis is accepted.

We start by comparing the Pocock and O'Brien & Fleming tests in the previously studied example with five groups of observations. In Section 2.6.4, we explain how these comparisons generalize to other examples with five groups of observations. In Section 2.6.5 we present properties of tests with different numbers of groups which can be referred to when choosing a suitable number of groups of observations for a specific study.

Table 2.5 *Fixed sample, Pocock and O'Brien & Fleming tests: power functions, expected sample sizes and standard deviations of the sample size. Tests have five groups of observations and are designed to have Type I error* $\alpha = 0.05$ *and power* $1 - \beta = 0.9$ *at* $|\mu_A - \mu_B| = 1$. *Observations on each treatment are normal with variance* $\sigma^2 = 4$.

	Fixed sample test	*Pocock test*	*O'Brien & Fleming test*
		$Pr\{\text{Reject } H_0\}$	
$\|\mu_A - \mu_B\| = 0.0$	0.050	0.050	0.050
0.5	0.371	0.351	0.378
1.0	0.903	0.910	0.912
1.5	0.998	0.999	0.999
		$E\{\text{Number of observations}\}$	
$\|\mu_A - \mu_B\| = 0.0$	170.0	204.8	178.7
0.5	170.0	182.3	167.9
1.0	170.0	116.9	129.8
1.5	170.0	70.1	94.4
		St. dev.{Number of observations}	
$\|\mu_A - \mu_B\| = 0.0$	0.0	26.1	8.6
0.5	0.0	50.8	24.7
1.0	0.0	57.9	35.5
1.5	0.0	34.1	25.7

2.6.2 An Example with Five Groups

Table 2.5 shows properties of the fixed sample test and the Pocock and O'Brien & Fleming tests with five groups of observations for the example described in Sections 2.2, 2.4.3 and 2.5.3. All values shown here and in subsequent examples were obtained by numerical computation and are accurate to the number of decimal places shown. Differences between the tests in power at $|\mu_A - \mu_B| = 1$ are due to the rounding of group sizes to integer values, and this rounding is also partly responsible for differences in power at other values of $|\mu_A - \mu_B|$. These differences in power are of minor interest, and we shall concentrate on comparisons of the sample size distributions of different tests.

The fixed sample size of 170 subjects provides a benchmark against which sequential tests can be compared. Both group sequential tests have higher expected sample sizes at $\mu_A - \mu_B = 0$ than this baseline value, but this is to be expected since the group sequential tests must continue to their maximum sample sizes, 210 for Pocock's test and 180 for O'Brien & Fleming's test, in order to accept H_0. However, the ethical imperative for stopping a clinical trial early is greatest when the treatment difference is large, since an early decision avoids the randomization

Table 2.6 *Sample size distributions for Pocock and O'Brien & Fleming tests for five groups of observations. Tests are designed to have Type I error* $\alpha = 0.05$ *and power* $1 - \beta = 0.9$ *at* $|\mu_A - \mu_B| = 1$. *Observations on each treatment are normal with variance* $\sigma^2 = 4$.

Pocock test

		Probability of sample size =				
		42	84	126	168	210
$\lvert\mu_A - \mu_B\rvert =$	0.0	0.016	0.012	0.009	0.007	0.956
	0.5	0.055	0.071	0.075	0.076	0.723
	1.0	0.214	0.268	0.210	0.138	0.171
	1.5	0.507	0.352	0.110	0.025	0.006

O'Brien & Fleming test

		Probability of sample size =				
		36	72	108	144	180
$\lvert\mu_A - \mu_B\rvert =$	0.0	0.000	0.001	0.008	0.017	0.974
	0.5	0.000	0.015	0.078	0.134	0.773
	1.0	0.001	0.134	0.354	0.282	0.229
	1.5	0.010	0.472	0.415	0.089	0.013

of further subjects to an inferior treatment. The group sequential tests offer reductions in expected sample size over the fixed sample test when $|\mu_A - \mu_B|$ is sufficiently far from zero, and the Pocock test has the advantage of lower expected sample sizes under extreme values of $|\mu_A - \mu_B|$.

The table also shows standard deviations of the sample size, and we see that values for the Pocock test are uniformly higher than those for the O'Brien & Fleming test. This difference between the two tests is easily explained, as the Pocock test offers greater opportunity to stop early with a low sample size, and when it continues to the final analysis, it has a higher maximum sample size.

2.6.3 *Significance of the Maximum Sample Size*

Continuing with the preceding example, Table 2.6 shows the complete distribution of the sample size upon termination of the Pocock and O'Brien & Fleming tests. Both tests give rise to considerable random variation in sample size and a substantial probability of continuing to observe all five groups even if $\mu_A - \mu_B \neq 0$.

In some applications, the greater variance in the Pocock test's sample size may be unappealing and its higher maximum sample size may be regarded as a serious disadvantage. Suppose our example concerns the treatment of a rare disease and subjects are expected to enter the study at a rate of 40 per year. The maximum study duration is then 4.25 years for the fixed sample test, 4.5 years for the O'Brien

& Fleming test and 5.25 years for the Pocock test. Despite the savings in *average* sample size, a cautious investigator might be deterred from using the Pocock test by the possibility of waiting 5.25 years to reach a conclusion when a fixed sample study can guarantee a conclusion one year earlier.

We have approached the testing problem by specifying Type I and Type II error probabilities, supposing it will be feasible to work with the group sizes determined by the calculations of Sections 2.4.2 and 2.5.2. This approach will not be realistic in some studies where time constraints or limitations on resources impose a maximum duration and a maximum sample size for any test. If sequential tests are to be used in such situations, they must sacrifice some of the available power in order to reduce expected sample size. If in our example the maximum sample size were fixed at 170 subjects altogether, i.e., 85 on each treatment arm, the fixed sample test with Type I error probability 0.05 would achieve power 0.903 at $\mu_A - \mu_B = \pm 1$. Group sequential tests with five groups of observations would have to take group sizes of $m = 17$ per treatment arm: the five-group O'Brien & Fleming test with $m = 17$ and Type I error probability 0.05 would achieve power 0.896 at $\mu_A - \mu_B = \pm 1$, and the five-group Pocock test with $m = 17$ and Type I error probability 0.05 would have a power of only 0.84 at $\mu_A - \mu_B = \pm 1$. Since, in many clinical trials, it is difficult to achieve a sample size large enough to guarantee minimal power requirements, this point should not be taken lightly.

2.6.4 *Generalizing from a Single Example*

There are important relationships between tests of a given type with the same number of groups and the same Type I error rate. In the two-treatment comparison with observations $X_{Ai} \sim N(\mu_A, \sigma^2)$ and $X_{Bi} \sim N(\mu_B, \sigma^2)$, $i = 1, 2, \ldots$, consider Pocock tests of H_0: $\mu_A = \mu_B$ with K groups of observations and Type I error probability α. Suppose also that the group size m is chosen to give power $1-\beta$ at $\mu_A - \mu_B = \pm\,\delta_1$. The procedure described in Section 2.4.2 for satisfying a power requirement at $\mu_A - \mu_B = \pm\,\delta$ defines the group size to be proportional to σ^2/δ^2. We now compare two tests defined for different values of δ and σ^2. Test 1 is for observations X_{Ai} and X_{Bi} with variance σ_1^2 and achieves power $1-\beta$ at $\mu_A - \mu_B = \pm\,\delta_1$ with groups of m_1 observations per treatment arm. Test 2 is for observations X'_{Ai} and X'_{Bi} with variance σ_2^2 and attains power $1-\beta$ at $\mu_A - \mu_B = \pm\,\delta_2$ with groups of m_2 observations per treatment arm. We denote the sequence of standardized statistics for Test 1 by $\{Z_1^1, \ldots, Z_K^1\}$, where

$$Z_k^1 = \frac{1}{\sqrt{(2m_1k\sigma_1^2)}}\left(\sum_{i=1}^{m_1k} X_{Ai} - \sum_{i=1}^{m_1k} X_{Bi}\right), \quad k = 1\ldots, K,$$

and denote those for Test 2 by $\{Z_1^2, \ldots, Z_K^2\}$, where

$$Z_k^2 = \frac{1}{\sqrt{(2m_2k\sigma_2^2)}}\left(\sum_{i=1}^{m_2k} X'_{Ai} - \sum_{i=1}^{m_2k} X'_{Bi}\right), \quad k = 1\ldots, K.$$

It follows from results we shall present in Section 3.1 that for any value of ξ, the joint distribution of the sequence $\{Z_1^1, \ldots, Z_K^1\}$ when $\mu_A - \mu_B = \xi\delta_1$

and observations have variance σ_1^2 is the same as that of $\{Z_1^2, \ldots, Z_K^2\}$ when $\mu_A - \mu_B = \xi\delta_2$ and the variance is σ_2^2. Since Z_k^1 and Z_k^2 are compared to the same critical value, $c_k = C_P(K, \alpha)$, we see that for each $k = 1, \ldots, K$ the probability that Test 1 rejects H_0 at stage k when $\mu_A - \mu_B = \xi\delta_1$ and $\sigma^2 = \sigma_1^2$ is equal to the probability that Test 2 rejects H_0 at stage k when $\mu_A - \mu_B = \xi\delta_2$ and $\sigma^2 = \sigma_2^2$. Application of this result in the case $\xi = 0$ confirms that both tests have the same Type I error. Consideration of the case $\xi = 1$ shows that Test 1 has the same power at $\mu_A - \mu_B = \pm\delta_1$ when $\sigma^2 = \sigma_1^2$ as Test 2 has at $\mu_A - \mu_B = \pm\delta_2$ when $\sigma^2 = \sigma_2^2$, and this justifies our method for determining group sizes to meet a power requirement for general δ and σ^2. The power functions of the two tests also match up at other points, the power of Test 1 at $\mu_A - \mu_B = \xi\delta_1$ when $\sigma^2 = \sigma_1^2$ equaling that of Test 2 at $\mu_A - \mu_B = \xi\delta_2$ when $\sigma^2 = \sigma_2^2$.

In practice, the need for integer group sizes may mean that m_2 cannot be exactly equal to $m_1\sigma_2^2\delta_1^2/(\sigma_1^2\delta_2^2)$ and the sequences $\{Z_1^1, \ldots, Z_K^1\}$ and $\{Z_1^2, \ldots, Z_K^2\}$ have slightly different distributions. In order to obtain more general comparisons of different types of test, it is helpful to suppress such problems and evaluate tests assuming that groups of m observations are permissible for all values of m. Results for one pair of values for δ and σ^2 can then be generalized to other pairs, and only slight departures from this idealized case will arise from rounding to integer group sizes.

Another consequence of the above relation between $\{Z_1^1, \ldots, Z_K^1\}$ and $\{Z_1^2, \ldots, Z_K^2\}$ is that the distribution of the number of groups before termination is the same for both Test 1 and Test 2 under the given conditions, $\mu_A - \mu_B = \xi\delta_1$ and $\sigma^2 = \sigma_1^2$ for Test 1 and $\mu_A - \mu_B = \xi\delta_2$ and $\sigma^2 = \sigma_2^2$ for Test 2. Hence, the expected sample sizes of the two tests differ by a factor $m_2/m_1 = \sigma_2^2\delta_1^2/(\sigma_1^2\delta_2^2)$ in such situations. This relationship allows us to quote expected sample sizes at values of $\mu_A - \mu_B$ equal to stated multiples of the value δ at which the power requirement is set. Expected sample sizes can then be deduced for tests of the same type and with the same number of groups at other values of δ and σ^2 although, again, rounding to integer group sizes will produce small perturbations.

There is nothing specific to Pocock's test in the above arguments. Properties of other two-sided tests can be presented for general δ and σ^2 in the same way, and we shall follow a similar approach in describing properties of one-sided tests in later chapters.

2.6.5 Choosing the Number of Groups

As well as choosing the type of test to use, an experimenter must decide on the number of groups in which observations are to be taken. A larger number of groups usually implies smaller expected sample sizes at the values of $\mu_A - \mu_B$ of most interest, but this advantage has to be balanced against the effort required to carry out more frequent interim analyses. Tables 2.7 and 2.8 show how maximum and expected sample sizes vary with the number of groups in Pocock and O'Brien & Fleming tests. Results are for tests with $\alpha = 0.05$ and power $1 - \beta = 0.8$ and 0.9 at $\mu_A - \mu_B = \pm\delta$. Entries in the table are 100 × the ratios of maximum and expected sample sizes to $n_f(\alpha, \beta, \delta, \sigma^2)$, the number of observations required

Table 2.7 *Pocock tests: maximum and expected sample sizes of tests with K groups of observations, Type I error probability $\alpha = 0.05$ and power $1-\beta$ at $\mu_A - \mu_B = \pm\delta$. Values are expressed as percentages of the fixed sample size, $n_f(\alpha, \beta, \delta, \sigma^2)$.*

		$\alpha = 0.05$			
	Sample size as percentage of fixed sample size				
K	*Maximum sample size*	*Expected sample size at $\mu_A - \mu_B =$* 0	$\pm 0.5\delta$	$\pm\delta$	$\pm 1.5\delta$
$1-\beta = 0.8$					
1	100.0	100.0	100.0	100.0	100.0
2	111.0	109.4	103.9	85.3	65.0
3	116.6	114.3	106.7	81.9	56.0
4	120.2	117.5	108.8	80.5	52.2
5	122.9	119.8	110.4	79.9	50.1
10	130.1	126.3	115.3	79.5	46.2
15	133.8	129.7	118.1	80.0	45.1
20	136.3	131.9	120.0	80.5	44.7
$1-\beta = 0.9$					
1	100.0	100.0	100.0	100.0	100.0
2	110.0	108.4	100.9	77.6	59.2
3	115.1	112.8	102.6	72.1	48.2
4	118.3	115.6	104.1	69.7	43.7
5	120.7	117.7	105.2	68.5	41.2
10	127.1	123.4	109.0	66.6	36.7
15	130.5	126.4	111.2	66.4	35.4
20	132.7	128.4	112.8	66.5	34.8

for a fixed sample size test with the same Type I error and power. It should be remembered that, since n_f depends on β, the entries for $\beta = 0.8$ and 0.9 have been divided by different values of n_f. The tabulated values do not take account of the small effect of rounding group sizes to integer values, but apart from this, they apply to all pairs of δ and σ^2.

It is clear from these tables that the introduction of one or two interim analyses is quite effective in reducing expected sample sizes at $\mu_A - \mu_B = \pm\,\delta$ and $\pm\,1.5\delta$, and even if interim analyses require little effort, designs with only four or five analyses will often be sufficient. Whereas expected sample sizes of O'Brien & Fleming tests at the larger values of $|\mu_A - \mu_B|$ continue to decrease as K increases, those for Pocock tests start to increase again. (The tabulated ratios vary smoothly with K, and expected sample sizes for values of $K < 20$ not given in the table are well approximated by interpolation.) Also, for Pocock tests, the maximum sample

Table 2.8 *O'Brien & Fleming tests: maximum and expected sample sizes of tests with K groups of observations, Type I error probability $\alpha = 0.05$ and power $1-\beta$ at $\mu_A - \mu_B = \pm\delta$. Values are expressed as percentages of the fixed sample size, $n_f(\alpha, \beta, \delta, \sigma^2)$.*

	$\alpha = 0.05$				
	Sample size as percentage of fixed sample size				
K	*Maximum sample size*	*Expected sample size at $\mu_A - \mu_B =$* 0	$\pm 0.5\delta$	$\pm\delta$	$\pm 1.5\delta$
$1-\beta = 0.8$					
1	100.0	100.0	100.0	100.0	100.0
2	100.8	100.5	99.0	90.2	71.9
3	101.7	101.2	98.3	85.6	68.0
4	102.4	101.7	98.0	83.1	64.1
5	102.8	102.1	97.9	81.8	61.9
10	104.0	103.1	97.9	79.1	58.1
15	104.5	103.5	97.9	78.3	56.9
20	104.7	103.7	97.9	77.9	56.3
$1-\beta = 0.9$					
1	100.0	100.0	100.0	100.0	100.0
2	100.7	100.5	98.2	85.1	63.3
3	101.6	101.1	96.9	79.9	61.0
4	102.2	101.6	96.4	76.7	57.3
5	102.6	101.9	96.1	75.0	54.8
10	103.7	102.8	95.6	71.8	50.8
15	104.2	103.2	95.5	70.8	49.5
20	104.5	103.4	95.5	70.3	48.9

size and expected sample sizes when $\mu_A - \mu_B$ is near zero increase significantly with the number of groups. Thus, while it may be reasonable to choose as many as 10 groups for an O'Brien & Fleming test, there is little reason to take more than about 5 groups in a Pocock test. The same patterns are observed in results for $\alpha = 0.01$ and 0.1 with similar implications for choice of the number of groups.

2.6.6 Discussion

Both types of group sequential test considered so far have their advantages. Pocock tests have lower expected sample sizes than O'Brien & Fleming tests when $|\mu_A - \mu_B|$ is large and the ethical imperative for early stopping is greatest. Against this, Pocock tests have rather high maximum sample sizes and their expected sample sizes are higher than the fixed sample test when $|\mu_A - \mu_B|$ is small. O'Brien & Fleming tests sacrifice little of the available power for a given maximum sample size, and since the nominal significance level applied at the final analysis is close to the Type I error probability, the confusing situation in which the null hypothesis is accepted when a fixed sample analysis of the final set of data would have rejected H_0 is unlikely to arise.

The O'Brien & Fleming tests apply extremely low nominal significance levels at the first few analyses. There are practical reasons to prefer group sequential tests with wide early boundaries that make it unlikely that a study will terminate at a very early stage. Problems in data quality most often arise at the start of a study as data recording procedures are introduced and participants gain experience in administering new treatments. It is difficult to check distributional assumptions on a small set of data. Most importantly perhaps, investigators are aware that the broader scientific community is likely to be skeptical of conclusions based on only a few observations. On the other hand, these issues will be of lesser concern if the sample sizes, even at the earlier stages, are quite substantial. In such circumstances, for ethical reasons a DSMB may be reluctant to continue a trial upon observing a high Z-value at an early stage, even though an O'Brien & Fleming boundary has not been crossed. The tests that will be described in the following section can be considered as compromises — enjoying many of the benefits of both the Pocock and the O'Brien & Fleming tests.

2.7 Other Tests

2.7.1 Wang & Tsiatis Tests

Wang & Tsiatis (1987) proposed a family of two-sided tests indexed by a parameter Δ which offers boundaries of different shapes, including Pocock and O'Brien & Fleming tests as special cases. The test with parameter Δ rejects H_0 after group k if $|Z_k| \geq c_k = C_{WT}(K, \alpha, \Delta)(k/K)^{\Delta-1/2}$, $k = 1, \ldots, K$. Formally, the test is

$$
\begin{array}{ll}
\text{After group } k = 1, \ldots, K-1 & \\
\quad \text{if } |Z_k| \geq C_{WT}(K, \alpha, \Delta)(k/K)^{\Delta-1/2} & \text{stop, reject } H_0 \\
\quad \text{otherwise} & \text{continue to group } k+1, \\
\text{after group } K & \\
\quad \text{if } |Z_K| \geq C_{WT}(K, \alpha, \Delta) & \text{stop, reject } H_0 \\
\quad \text{otherwise} & \text{stop, accept } H_0.
\end{array}
\tag{2.7}
$$

For consistency with our descriptions of other tests, we have adopted a different parameterization from that used by Wang & Tsiatis. However, the role of Δ is unchanged, so the test with parameter Δ defined by (2.7) is still the Wang & Tsiatis test with parameter Δ.

Taking $\Delta = 0.5$ gives Pocock's test and $\Delta = 0$ gives O'Brien & Fleming's test; values of Δ between 0 and 0.5 give tests with boundaries of intermediate shapes. The constants $C_{WT}(K, \alpha, \Delta)$ are chosen to ensure a specific Type I error α. Since $C_{WT}(K, \alpha, 0.5) = C_P(K, \alpha)$ and $C_{WT}(K, \alpha, 0) = C_B(K, \alpha)$, values for

Table 2.9 *Wang & Tsiatis tests: constants $C_{WT}(K, \alpha, \Delta)$ for two-sided tests with K groups of observations and Type I error probability* $\alpha = 0.05$

	$C_{WT}(K, \alpha, \Delta)$		
	$\alpha = 0.05$		
K	$\Delta = 0.1$	$\Delta = 0.25$	$\Delta = 0.4$
1	1.960	1.960	1.960
2	1.994	2.038	2.111
3	2.026	2.083	2.186
4	2.050	2.113	2.233
5	2.068	2.136	2.267
6	2.083	2.154	2.292
7	2.094	2.168	2.313
8	2.104	2.180	2.329
9	2.113	2.190	2.343
10	2.120	2.199	2.355
11	2.126	2.206	2.366
12	2.132	2.213	2.375
15	2.146	2.229	2.397
20	2.162	2.248	2.423

these cases can be obtained from Tables 2.1 and 2.3. Constants for $\alpha = 0.05$ and $\Delta = 0.1$, 0.25 and 0.4 are given in Table 2.9; constants for $\alpha = 0.01$ and $K \leq 5$, in Wang & Tsiatis' parameterization, can be found in Wang & Tsiatis (1987).

The constants $R_{WT}(K, \alpha, \beta, \Delta)$ listed in Table 2.10 determine the group size needed to satisfy a power requirement in the same way as the constants $R_P(K, \alpha, \beta)$ and $R_B(K, \alpha, \beta)$ for Pocock and O'Brien & Fleming tests. A test with Type I error α and power $1 - \beta$ at $\mu_A - \mu_B = \pm\delta$ requires a maximum sample size per treatment arm of $R_{WT}(K, \alpha, \beta, \Delta)\, n_f(\alpha, \beta, \delta, \sigma^2)$, where $n_f(\alpha, \beta, \delta, \sigma^2)$, given by (2.3), is the sample size per treatment required by a fixed sample size test with the same Type I error α and power $1 - \beta$ at $\mu_A - \mu_B = \pm\delta$. The necessary group size is therefore $m = R_{WT}(K, \alpha, \beta, \Delta)\, n_f(\alpha, \beta, \delta, \sigma^2)/K$ per treatment arm, suitably rounded.

As an illustration, consider the five-group test with $\Delta = 0.25$ applied to the example of Section 2.2, testing H_0: $\mu_A = \mu_B$ with Type I error $\alpha = 0.05$ and power $1-\beta = 0.9$ at $\mu_A - \mu_B = \pm 1$ when observations have variance $\sigma^2 = 4$. The fixed sample test requires $n_f(0.05, 0.1, 1, 4) = 84.1$ observations per treatment arm; hence the Wang & Tsiatis test with $\Delta = 0.25$ has a maximum sample size per treatment of

$$R_{WT}(5, 0.05, 0.1, 0.25)\, n_f(0.05, 0.1, 1, 4) = 1.066 \times 84.1 = 89.7.$$

Dividing by 5 and rounding to an integer gives a group size of 18 per treatment arm, the same as that required by an O'Brien & Fleming test but smaller than

Table 2.10 *Wang & Tsiatis tests: constants $R_{WT}(K, \alpha, \beta, \Delta)$ to determine group sizes for two-sided tests with K groups of observations, Type I error probability $\alpha = 0.05$ and power $1 - \beta$*

	$R_{WT}(K, \alpha, \beta, \Delta)$					
	$\alpha = 0.05$					
	$1-\beta = 0.8$			$1-\beta = 0.9$		
K	Δ=0.1	Δ=0.25	Δ=0.4	Δ=0.1	Δ=0.25	Δ=0.4
1	1.000	1.000	1.000	1.000	1.000	1.000
2	1.016	1.038	1.075	1.014	1.034	1.068
3	1.027	1.054	1.108	1.025	1.050	1.099
4	1.035	1.065	1.128	1.032	1.059	1.117
5	1.040	1.072	1.142	1.037	1.066	1.129
6	1.044	1.077	1.152	1.041	1.071	1.138
7	1.047	1.081	1.159	1.044	1.075	1.145
8	1.050	1.084	1.165	1.046	1.078	1.151
9	1.052	1.087	1.170	1.048	1.081	1.155
10	1.054	1.089	1.175	1.050	1.083	1.159
11	1.055	1.091	1.178	1.051	1.085	1.163
12	1.056	1.093	1.181	1.053	1.086	1.166
15	1.059	1.097	1.189	1.055	1.090	1.172
20	1.062	1.101	1.197	1.058	1.094	1.180

the value 21 of a Pocock test; without the effects of rounding, the Wang & Tsiatis group size would lie between those of the O'Brien & Fleming and Pocock tests. The boundary also has an intermediate shape. Critical values for the Pocock test are constant at 2.413; for the O'Brien & Fleming test, $c_k = C_B(5, 0.05)(5/k)^{0.5} = 2.040\,(5/k)^{0.5}$, $k = 1, \ldots, 5$, giving the sequence of critical values 4.562, 3.226, 2.634, 2.281, 2.040; for the Wang & Tsiatis test with $\Delta = 0.25$, $c_k = C_{WT}(5, 0.05, 0.25)(k/5)^{-0.25} = 2.136\,(k/5)^{-0.25}$, $k = 1, \ldots, 5$, and the sequence of critical values is 3.194, 2.686, 2.427, 2.259, 2.136. Note that the Wang & Tsiatis test reduces the first two very high critical values, $c_1 = 4.562$ and $c_2 = 3.226$, of the O'Brien & Fleming test, with only a small increase in the final critical value, c_5.

Table 2.11 shows maximum and expected sample sizes of Wang & Tsiatis tests with $\Delta = 0.1$, 0.25 and 0.4, Type I error $\alpha = 0.05$ and power $1 - \beta = 0.8$ when $\mu_A - \mu_B = \pm\delta$. Table 2.12 gives the same quantities for $1 - \beta = 0.9$. As before, sample sizes are expressed as percentages of the corresponding fixed sample sizes $n_f(\alpha, \beta, \delta, \sigma^2)$. Comparison of these tables with Tables 2.7 and 2.8 shows that Wang & Tsiatis tests with $\Delta = 0.1$ have lower expected sample sizes at $|\mu_A - \mu_B| = \delta$ and 1.5δ than O'Brien & Fleming tests, with only a small increase in maximum sample size. Tests with $\Delta = 0.4$ offer similar low expected sample sizes at $|\mu_A - \mu_B| = \delta$ and 1.5δ to Pocock tests but with significantly lower maximum sample size and expected sample sizes at $|\mu_A - \mu_B| = 0$ and 0.5δ.

Table 2.11 *Wang & Tsiatis tests: maximum and expected sample sizes of tests with K analyses, Type I error probability* $\alpha = 0.05$ *and power* $1-\beta = 0.8$ *at* $\mu_A - \mu_B = \pm\delta$. *Values are expressed as percentages of the fixed sample size,* $n_f(\alpha, \beta, \delta, \sigma^2)$.

	$\alpha = 0.05,\ 1-\beta = 0.8$				
	Sample size as percentage of fixed sample size				
K	*Maximum sample size*	*Expected sample size at* $\mu_A-\mu_B=$ 0	$\pm 0.5\delta$	$\pm\delta$	$\pm 1.5\delta$
$\Delta = 0.1$					
1	100.0	100.0	100.0	100.0	100.0
2	101.6	101.1	99.0	88.2	69.0
3	102.7	102.0	98.5	84.1	64.7
4	103.5	102.7	98.4	81.8	61.5
5	104.0	103.1	98.3	80.4	59.4
10	105.4	104.2	98.4	77.9	55.5
15	105.9	104.7	98.5	77.1	54.2
20	106.2	105.0	98.5	76.7	53.7
$\Delta = 0.25$					
1	100.0	100.0	100.0	100.0	100.0
2	103.8	103.0	99.7	86.0	66.1
3	105.4	104.4	99.6	82.0	60.0
4	106.5	105.2	99.7	79.9	57.1
5	107.2	105.8	99.8	78.7	55.2
10	108.9	107.3	100.2	76.2	51.3
15	109.7	108.0	100.4	75.4	50.0
20	110.1	108.3	100.5	75.0	49.4
$\Delta = 0.4$					
1	100.0	100.0	100.0	100.0	100.0
2	107.5	106.2	101.6	85.1	64.8
3	110.8	109.1	102.8	81.2	56.9
4	112.8	110.8	103.6	79.3	53.4
5	114.2	112.0	104.2	78.3	51.4
10	117.5	114.9	105.8	76.3	47.5
15	118.9	116.2	106.5	75.7	46.2
20	119.7	116.9	107.0	75.4	45.5

Table 2.12 *Wang & Tsiatis tests: maximum and expected sample sizes of tests with K analyses, Type I error probability* $\alpha = 0.05$ *and power* $1 - \beta = 0.9$ *at* $\mu_A - \mu_B = \pm\delta$. *Values are expressed as percentages of the fixed sample size,* $n_f(\alpha, \beta, \delta, \sigma^2)$.

$\alpha = 0.05,\ 1 - \beta = 0.9$

	Sample size as percentage of fixed sample size				
K	Maximum sample size	Expected sample size at $\mu_A - \mu_B =$ 0	$\pm 0.5\delta$	$\pm\delta$	$\pm 1.5\delta$
$\Delta = 0.1$					
1	100.0	100.0	100.0	100.0	100.0
2	101.4	101.0	97.9	82.5	61.0
3	102.5	101.8	96.9	77.7	57.0
4	103.2	102.4	96.4	74.9	54.2
5	103.7	102.8	96.1	73.2	52.0
10	105.0	103.9	95.8	70.0	47.9
15	105.5	104.3	95.7	69.0	46.6
20	105.8	104.6	95.7	68.5	46.0
$\Delta = 0.25$					
1	100.0	100.0	100.0	100.0	100.0
2	103.4	102.6	98.0	79.5	59.0
3	105.0	103.9	97.4	74.5	51.9
4	105.9	104.7	97.1	71.9	49.1
5	106.6	105.3	97.0	70.4	47.3
10	108.3	106.7	96.9	67.2	43.3
15	109.0	107.3	97.0	66.2	41.9
20	109.4	107.6	97.0	65.7	41.3
$\Delta = 0.4$					
1	100.0	100.0	100.0	100.0	100.0
2	106.8	105.5	99.3	77.8	58.7
3	109.9	108.1	99.6	72.4	48.9
4	111.7	109.7	100.0	69.9	45.1
5	112.9	110.8	100.2	68.4	42.9
10	115.9	113.4	101.2	65.5	38.8
15	117.2	114.6	101.7	64.5	37.4
20	118.0	115.2	102.0	64.1	36.6

In general, as Δ increases, expected sample sizes at higher values of $|\mu_A - \mu_B|$ decrease but at the cost of larger maximum sample size and expected sample sizes at values of $|\mu_A - \mu_B|$ closer to zero. Thus, the Wang and Tsiatis family introduces a useful extra degree of freedom in choosing a group sequential test to balance the conflicting aims of low maximum sample size and low expected sample size over a range of values of $\mu_A - \mu_B$.

2.7.2 Haybittle-Peto tests

Haybittle (1971) and Peto et al. (1976) suggested a simple form of sequential monitoring in which H_0 is rejected at an analysis $k < K$ only if $|Z_k| \geq 3$. If the number of interim analyses is small, early stopping is unlikely under H_0, and it is approximately correct to carry out a fixed sample analysis at the final stage with no allowance for the interim analyses. One can, however, adjust the final critical value for $|Z_K|$ to give an overall Type I error exactly equal to α, and this is the approach we shall adopt. Formally, the Haybittle-Peto test with a maximum of K groups of observations is

$$
\begin{array}{lll}
\text{After group } k = 1, \ldots, K-1 & & \\
\quad \text{if } |Z_k| \geq 3 & \text{stop, reject } H_0 & \\
\quad \text{otherwise} & \text{continue to group } k+1, & \\
\text{after group } K & & \qquad (2.8) \\
\quad \text{if } |Z_K| \geq C_{HP}(K, \alpha) & \text{stop, reject } H_0 & \\
\quad \text{otherwise} & \text{stop, accept } H_0. &
\end{array}
$$

Thus, the test applies critical values $c_1 = \ldots = c_{K-1} = 3$ and $c_K = C_{HP}(K, \alpha)$.

We shall restrict attention to the case $\alpha = 0.05$ where the choice of $c_k = 3$ for $k = 1, \ldots, K-1$ is most appropriate. (Calculations show that for $K \geq 7$, in which case $c_1 = \ldots = c_6 = 3$, the probability under H_0 of rejecting H_0 at or before the sixth analysis is 0.0107, so it is not possible to achieve an overall Type I error as low as 0.01.) Table 2.13 gives values of $C_{HP}(K, \alpha)$ for $\alpha = 0.05$ and constants $R_{HP}(K, \alpha, \beta)$ which determine the group size needed to achieve power $1-\beta$ at $|\mu_A - \mu_B| = \delta$ in the usual way. Table 2.14 shows maximum and expected sample sizes of Haybittle-Peto tests expressed as percentages of the corresponding fixed sample sizes, $n_f(\alpha, \beta, \delta, \sigma^2)$. Expected sample sizes at $|\mu_A - \mu_B| = \delta$ and 1.5δ are at most a little higher than those of O'Brien & Fleming tests and Wang & Tsiatis tests with $\Delta = 0.1$. Although the Haybittle-Peto test uses high critical values, $c_k = 3$, up to the penultimate analysis, these are less extreme than the first few O'Brien & Fleming critical values (for example, the five-group O'Brien & Fleming test has $c_1 = 4.562$ and $c_2 = 3.226$); thus the low expected sample sizes at larger values of $|\mu_A - \mu_B|$ are not surprising.

Figure 2.3 illustrates the differences in boundary shape of three tests in the Wang & Tsiatis family and the Haybittle-Peto test. The figure shows critical values for standardized statistics Z_k in tests with 10 groups of observations and Type I error rate $\alpha = 0.05$. At one extreme, the Haybittle-Peto test and the Wang & Tsiatis test with $\Delta = 0$, which is also the O'Brien & Fleming test, have very wide

Table 2.13 *Haybittle-Peto tests: constants* $C_{HP}(K, \alpha)$ *and* $R_{HP}(K, \alpha, \beta)$ *for two-sided tests with K groups of observations and Type I error probability* $\alpha = 0.05$

		$\alpha = 0.05$	
K	$C_{HP}(K, \alpha)$	$R_{HP}(K, \alpha, \beta)$	
		$1-\beta=0.8$	$1-\beta=0.9$
1	1.960	1.000	1.000
2	1.967	1.003	1.003
3	1.975	1.007	1.007
4	1.983	1.011	1.010
5	1.990	1.015	1.014
6	1.997	1.019	1.017
7	2.003	1.023	1.021
8	2.010	1.027	1.024
9	2.016	1.030	1.027
10	2.021	1.033	1.030
11	2.027	1.037	1.033
12	2.032	1.040	1.035
15	2.046	1.048	1.043
20	2.068	1.061	1.055

early boundaries and a final critical value close to that of 1.96 applied in a fixed sample analysis. The Wang & Tsiatis test with $\Delta = 0.5$, which is also the Pocock test, has constant critical values $c_k = 2.555$, $k = 1, \ldots, 10$, while the test with $\Delta = 0.25$ is intermediate to these extremes, its critical values decreasing steadily to $c_{10} = 2.199$ at the final analysis.

Although Haybittle-Peto tests do not attain the maximum possible reductions in expected sample size, this is not always the key issue. In some studies, investigators wish to continue sampling in order to learn more about aspects of a new treatment other than its primary efficacy. A new treatment will not necessarily be approved as soon as it has been shown to be effective in a single study: further data may be required to demonstrate the treatment's safety relative to a standard treatment or placebo, or it may be necessary to reproduce evidence of efficacy under other experimental conditions. It is also important to consider the contribution a study will make to meta-analyses in which data from a number of studies are analyzed together. This is particularly relevant to treatments for diseases, such as many types of cancer, for which effective therapies are available and extremely large sample sizes are needed to detect the modest improvements that a new treatment is likely to offer. In such cases, the investigators' objective is really to gather as much information as possible on all aspects of a treatment, and there is little incentive for early stopping apart from the ethical need to cease randomizing patients to a clearly inferior treatment.

There has been some discussion of "administrative analyses" in clinical trials;

Table 2.14 *Haybittle-Peto tests: maximum and expected sample sizes of tests with K groups of observations, Type I error probability* $\alpha = 0.05$ *and power* $1-\beta$ *at* $\mu_A - \mu_B = \pm\delta$. *Values are expressed as percentages of the fixed sample size,* $n_f(\alpha, \beta, \delta, \sigma^2)$.

	$\alpha = 0.05$				
	Sample size as percentage of fixed sample size				
K	*Maximum sample size*	*Expected sample size at* $\mu_A - \mu_B =$ 0	$\pm 0.5\delta$	$\pm\delta$	$\pm 1.5\delta$
$1-\beta = 0.8$					
1	100.0	100.0	100.0	100.0	100.0
2	100.3	100.2	99.2	92.5	75.7
3	100.7	100.5	98.9	89.2	68.1
4	101.1	100.8	98.8	87.2	64.0
5	101.5	101.1	98.8	85.9	61.5
10	103.3	102.5	99.3	83.0	55.6
15	104.8	103.7	100.0	81.8	53.3
20	106.1	104.8	100.7	81.3	51.9
$1-\beta = 0.9$					
1	100.0	100.0	100.0	100.0	100.0
2	100.3	100.2	98.7	88.2	66.6
3	100.7	100.4	98.1	83.4	58.0
4	101.0	100.7	97.8	80.6	53.5
5	101.4	100.9	97.6	78.8	50.8
10	103.0	102.2	97.6	74.5	44.7
15	104.3	103.2	97.9	72.7	42.3
20	105.5	104.1	98.3	71.8	41.0

see, for example, Enas et al. (1989) and Fleming & DeMets (1993). These are analyses at which the monitoring committee reviews various aspects of the trial such as patient recruitment, compliance to the specified treatment regimens, data recording procedures and data quality. Although there may be no intention to terminate the study on such an occasion, a regulatory body can require that a formal stopping rule for these analyses be stated in the protocol. The Haybittle-Peto criterion of early stopping at analysis k only if $|Z_k| \geq 3$ has the advantage of fulfilling this requirement with little effect on subsequent analyses. A similar approach may be taken in monitoring a secondary endpoint when the main objective is to gather data on a primary response. For example, a Haybittle-Peto rule could be applied to the safety variable in a study where treatment efficacy is the primary endpoint but where there is an ethical need to cease allocating subjects to a treatment which has proved to cause excessive toxicity.

Figure 2.3 *Boundaries of four two-sided tests for ten groups of observations: Pocock* (○), *O'Brien & Fleming* (□), *Haybittle-Peto* (∗), *and Wang & Tsiatis with* $\Delta = 0.25$ (×)

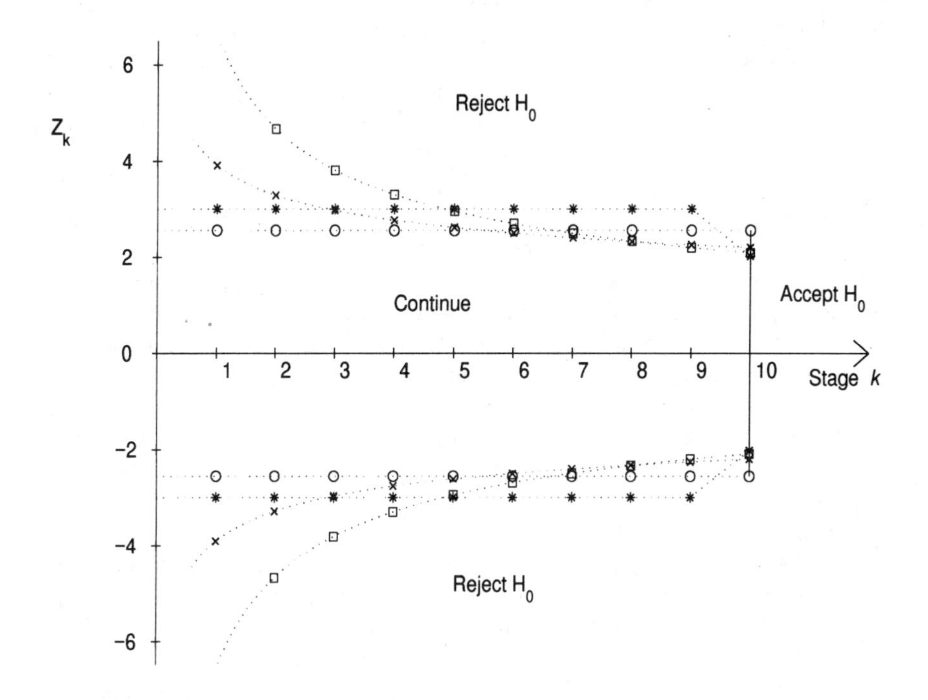

2.8 Conclusions

In this chapter we have presented easily implemented tests and provided constants which define the tests and determine the group sizes required to satisfy a power condition. We have done this for the most common cases of Type I error $\alpha = 0.05$ and power $1 - \beta = 0.8$ and 0.9 for all the tests considered. Constants for other cases can be computed using the methods described in Chapter 19. The tables of maximum and expected sample sizes aid in choosing the test best suited to a particular application and in selecting an appropriate number of groups of observations. Other forms of group sequential tests have been proposed; see, for example, Fleming, Harrington & O'Brien (1984).

In Section 2.6.6, we discussed the practical benefits of tests having wide early boundaries, such as the O'Brien & Fleming tests. However it was also stated there that a DSMB may be unwilling for ethical reasons to continue a trial upon observing a high Z-value at an early stage even though the stopping boundary has not been crossed. For example, at the first analysis of a four-stage O'Brien & Fleming test with Type I error $\alpha = 0.05$, the critical value is 4.048 corresponding to a nominal two-sided significance of less than 0.0001. As long as the sample size is large enough that validity of model assumptions and the phenomenon of "bad news traveling faster than good news" are not of concern, the DSMB may feel compelled to stop the trial in the face of a Z_1-value as great as $Z_1 = 4$, say. If this is the case, such a group sequential design is not the appropriate one to use. It is recommended that at its initial meeting before inspection of any data, the DSMB discuss the choice of criteria for stopping the trial. In particular, its members should discuss circumstances under which they would be uncomfortable in agreeing to continue the trial. Of course, not all eventualities can be foreseen — see also the comments in Section 9.1. However, it is invaluable to have such a a discussion among the members of the DSMB, with written records kept. Although current opinion in the U.S. favors the O'Brien & Fleming test, the tests of Wang & Tsiatis with parameter Δ in the region of 0.25, have much to be commended. They have wide boundaries at early stages but they are no so extreme. They have much of the benefit of the Pocock test of having low expected sample sizes at alternatives that are important. They also enjoy much of the benefits of the O'Brien & Fleming test, which has a low maximum sample size and critical values close to those to the fixed test if the final analysis is reached.

The Wang & Tsiatis tests form a rich class, including the Pocock and O'Brien & Fleming tests as special cases. The experimenter is free to select a suitable member of the family, balancing reductions in expected sample size when θ is away from zero against a higher maximum sample size, which will usually be needed if $\theta = 0$. Optimality results of Pocock (1982) and Eales & Jennison (1995) show there is not much opportunity for further reductions in expected sample size at values of θ away from zero. However, we shall see in Chapter 5 that allowing early termination to *accept* H_0 can reduce expected sample size when θ is close to zero.

Although we have introduced tests in this chapter in the particular context of a two-sample comparison, these tests are readily generalized to other two-sided testing problems and other data types; we shall describe such generalizations in Chapter 3. The one limitation of the tests considered so far is their need for at least approximately equal group sizes. We shall show in Section 3.3 that small differences between groups, suitably handled, have negligible effects on error probabilities, but if larger differences are unavoidable, the specialized methods for unequal and unpredictable group sizes presented in Chapter 7 should be used.

CHAPTER 3

Two-Sided Tests: General Applications

3.1 A Unified Formulation

In Chapter 2 we presented two-sided tests for a two-treatment comparison when normally distributed observations of common known variance are collected in equally sized groups. The tests were defined in terms of significance levels for testing the null hypothesis after each new group of observations, and power was guaranteed by setting the maximum sample size as a multiple of that required by a fixed sample test. We shall see that group sequential tests described in this manner can be applied to other testing problems with little or no modification. The reason for this lies in the common form of the joint distribution of the sequence of standardized test statistics, $\{Z_1, \ldots, Z_K\}$.

Suppose a group sequential study with up to K analyses yields the sequence of test statistics $\{Z_1, \ldots, Z_K\}$. We say that these statistics have the *canonical joint distribution* with information levels $\{\mathcal{I}_1, \ldots, \mathcal{I}_K\}$ for the parameter θ if:

$$\begin{array}{ll} \text{(i)} & (Z_1, \ldots, Z_K) \text{ is multivariate normal,} \\ \text{(ii)} & E(Z_k) = \theta\sqrt{\mathcal{I}_k}, \quad k = 1, \ldots, K, \quad \text{and} \\ \text{(iii)} & Cov(Z_{k_1}, Z_{k_2}) = \sqrt{(\mathcal{I}_{k_1}/\mathcal{I}_{k_2})}, \quad 1 \le k_1 \le k_2 \le K. \end{array} \tag{3.1}$$

Note this implies that $\{Z_1, \ldots, Z_K\}$ is a Markov sequence, and this will be important in simplifying calculations for group sequential tests. In this section we show that several common testing problems give rise to sequences of test statistics with this joint distribution.

It should be noted that (3.1) specifies the *conditional* distribution of $\{Z_1, \ldots, Z_K\}$ given $\{\mathcal{I}_1, \ldots, \mathcal{I}_K\}$. When, for some reason, there is an element of randomness in the sample sizes observed at analyses 1 to K, we consider properties of tests conditional on the sequence of $\mathcal{I}_k$ values actually observed. Thus, as a group sequential test progresses, it is important to ensure that the value of $\mathcal{I}_k$ is not influenced by the values of statistics $Z_1, \ldots, Z_{k-1}$ seen previously, as this could destroy the property (3.1) on which error rate calculations are based; this is a subtle point which need not trouble us now, but we shall consider it in greater depth in Section 7.4 and Chapter 17.

The following examples illustrate a general result that sequences of standardized test statistics obtained from maximum likelihood estimates of a parameter in a normal linear model follow the canonical joint distribution (3.1). We shall discuss this result in Section 3.4 and prove it later in Section 11.3. The general result also extends to the case of correlated observations, hence the same joint distribution arises in the group sequential analysis of longitudinal data in which repeated measurements on the same subject are correlated. We shall see in Section 11.6 that (3.1) arises, approximately, in the maximum likelihood analysis of data following many parametric models, including generalized linear models. Further, (3.1) applies asymptotically in other special situations, including the analysis of right-censored survival data using a group sequential log-rank test or by repeatedly fitting Cox's proportional hazards regression model, and the analysis of accumulating data in multiple 2×2 tables using a repeated Mantel-Haenszel test.

3.1.1 *Parallel Two-Treatment Comparison*

We generalize the example of Chapter 2 and allow different variances and unequal numbers of subjects on the two treatment arms. Thus, we have responses $X_{Ai} \sim N(\mu_A, \sigma_A^2)$, $i = 1, 2, \ldots$, for subjects allocated to treatment A and $X_{Bi} \sim N(\mu_B, \sigma_B^2)$, $i = 1, 2, \ldots$, for those on treatment B. For $k = 1, \ldots, K$, let n_{Ak} and n_{Bk} denote the cumulative number of observations on treatments A and B, respectively, at the time of the kth analysis. The natural estimate of $\mu_A - \mu_B$ is

$$\begin{aligned}\bar{X}_A^{(k)} - \bar{X}_B^{(k)} &= \frac{1}{n_{Ak}} \sum_{i=1}^{n_{Ak}} X_{Ai} - \frac{1}{n_{Bk}} \sum_{i=1}^{n_{Bk}} X_{Bi} \\ &\sim N(\mu_A - \mu_B, \frac{\sigma_A^2}{n_{Ak}} + \frac{\sigma_B^2}{n_{Bk}}).\end{aligned}$$

Note that, here, the stated distribution of $\bar{X}_A^{(k)} - \bar{X}_B^{(k)}$ is simply the marginal distribution for given n_{Ak} and n_{Bk}, not, for example, the conditional distribution of $\bar{X}_A^{(k)} - \bar{X}_B^{(k)}$ given that the test continues up to analysis k, which arises in calculations of a group sequential test's error probabilities. We shall follow the same practice elsewhere, so, unless explicitly stated otherwise, the "distribution" of an estimate or test statistic should be taken to mean its marginal distribution.

We define the information for $\mu_A - \mu_B$ to be

$$\mathcal{I}_k = (\sigma_A^2/n_{Ak} + \sigma_B^2/n_{Bk})^{-1},$$

the reciprocal of our estimate's variance, and use this to create the standardized statistic at analysis k for testing H_0: $\mu_A = \mu_B$,

$$Z_k = (\bar{X}_A^{(k)} - \bar{X}_B^{(k)})\sqrt{\mathcal{I}_k}, \quad k = 1, \ldots, K.$$

The vector $(Z_1, \ldots, Z_K)$ is multivariate normal since each Z_k is a linear combination of the independent normal variates X_{Ai} and X_{Bi}, $i = 1, 2, \ldots$, and marginally,

$$Z_k \sim N(\theta\sqrt{\mathcal{I}_k}, 1), \quad k = 1, \ldots, K,$$

where $\theta = \mu_A - \mu_B$. It remains to establish the covariance of the Z_ks. For $k_1 \le k_2$,

$$\begin{aligned}Cov(Z_{k_1}, Z_{k_2}) &= Cov(\{\bar{X}_A^{(k_1)} - \bar{X}_B^{(k_1)}\}\sqrt{\mathcal{I}_{k_1}}, \{\bar{X}_A^{(k_2)} - \bar{X}_B^{(k_2)}\}\sqrt{\mathcal{I}_{k_2}}) \\ &= (\frac{1}{n_{Ak_1}} \frac{1}{n_{Ak_2}} n_{Ak_1}\sigma_A^2 + \frac{1}{n_{Bk_1}} \frac{1}{n_{Bk_2}} n_{Bk_1}\sigma_B^2)\sqrt{\mathcal{I}_{k_1}}\sqrt{\mathcal{I}_{k_2}} \\ &= (\mathcal{I}_{k_2})^{-1}\sqrt{\mathcal{I}_{k_1}}\sqrt{\mathcal{I}_{k_2}} = \sqrt{(\mathcal{I}_{k_1}/\mathcal{I}_{k_2})},\end{aligned}$$

as required. Thus, $\{Z_1, \ldots, Z_K\}$ have the canonical joint distribution with information levels $\{\mathcal{I}_1, \ldots, \mathcal{I}_K\}$ for $\theta = \mu_A - \mu_B$.

3.1.2 *Testing the Mean of a Single Population*

Suppose observations $X_i \sim N(\mu, \sigma^2)$, $i = 1, 2, \ldots$, are independent, σ^2 is known, and we wish to test the hypothesis H_0: $\mu = \mu_0$. If n_k observations are available at analysis k, we estimate μ by

$$\bar{X}^{(k)} = \frac{1}{n_k} \sum_{i=1}^{n_k} X_i \sim N(\mu, \frac{\sigma^2}{n_k})$$

and define $\mathcal{I}_k = \{Var(\bar{X}^{(k)})\}^{-1} = n_k/\sigma^2$, the information for μ at analysis k. The standardized test statistics are then

$$Z_k = (\bar{X}^{(k)} - \mu_0)\sqrt{\mathcal{I}_k}, \quad k = 1, \ldots, K.$$

Since each Z_k is a linear combination of the independent normal variates X_i, the vector $(Z_1, \ldots, Z_K)$ is multivariate normal. Marginally,

$$Z_k \sim N(\theta\sqrt{\mathcal{I}_k}, 1), \quad k = 1, \ldots, K,$$

where $\theta = \mu - \mu_0$. Finally, for $k_1 \leq k_2$,

$$\begin{aligned} Cov(Z_{k_1}, Z_{k_2}) &= Cov(\{\bar{X}^{(k_1)} - \mu_0\}\sqrt{\mathcal{I}_{k_1}}, \{\bar{X}^{(k_2)} - \mu_0\}\sqrt{\mathcal{I}_{k_2}}) \\ &= \frac{1}{n_{k_1}} \frac{1}{n_{k_2}} n_{k_1} \sigma^2 \sqrt{\mathcal{I}_{k_1}} \sqrt{\mathcal{I}_{k_2}} = \sqrt{(\mathcal{I}_{k_1}/\mathcal{I}_{k_2})} \end{aligned}$$

and we see that $\{Z_1, \ldots, Z_K\}$ have the canonical joint distribution with information levels $\{\mathcal{I}_1, \ldots, \mathcal{I}_K\}$ for $\theta = \mu - \mu_0$.

3.1.3 *Paired Two-Treatment Comparison*

In a two-treatment comparison, it can be advantageous to control the variance in response attributable to known prognostic factors by using a "matched pairs" design. Subjects are paired so that both subjects in the same pair have similar values of the prognostic factors; one subject in each pair is randomly selected to receive treatment A and the other receives treatment B. Let X_{Ai} and X_{Bi} denote the responses of the subjects in pair i receiving treatments A and B, respectively. We suppose the differences within pairs are normally distributed,

$$X_{Ai} - X_{Bi} \sim N(\mu_A - \mu_B, \tilde{\sigma}^2), \quad i = 1, 2, \ldots , \tag{3.2}$$

and the variance, $\tilde{\sigma}^2$, is known. If the variance of an individual observation is σ^2 and the correlation between the responses of subjects in the same pair is ρ, then $\tilde{\sigma}^2 = 2(1-\rho)\sigma^2$. Thus, if matching of subjects within pairs achieves a moderately large positive correlation, $\tilde{\sigma}^2$ can be significantly less than the variance, $2\sigma^2$, of the difference in response between two randomly selected subjects allocated to treatments A and B. We consider the problem of testing the null hypothesis H_0: $\mu_A = \mu_B$ in a group sequential test where observations are taken in up to K

groups. If n_k pairs of observations are available at the kth analysis, we estimate $\theta = \mu_A - \mu_B$ by

$$\frac{1}{n_k}\sum_{i=1}^{n_k}(X_{Ai} - X_{Bi}) \sim N(\mu_A - \mu_B, \frac{\tilde{\sigma}^2}{n_k}),$$

the information for θ is $\mathcal{I}_k = n_k/\tilde{\sigma}^2$, the reciprocal of this estimate's variance, and the standardized test statistic is

$$Z_k = \frac{1}{\sqrt{(n_k\tilde{\sigma}^2)}}\sum_{i=1}^{n_k}(X_{Ai} - X_{Bi}), \quad k = 1, \ldots, K. \tag{3.3}$$

The differences $X_{Ai} - X_{Bi}$ play the same role as the observations X_i in the single-population situation of Section 3.1.2, and essentially the same argument shows that $\{Z_1, \ldots, Z_K\}$ have the canonical joint distribution with information levels $\{\mathcal{I}_1, \ldots, \mathcal{I}_K\}$ for $\theta = \mu_A - \mu_B$.

3.1.4 Two-Period Crossover Trial

If between-patient variation is high but it is possible to observe a single subject's response to more than two treatments, the necessary sample size may be reduced by using a crossover design in which inferences are based on within-patient comparisons. Here, we describe group sequential analysis of a two-treatment comparison in a two-period crossover trial. General results for group sequential analysis of linear models, which we shall present in Section 3.4, can be applied to give a similar sequential treatment of more complex crossover designs.

In a two-treatment, two-period crossover trial each subject is allocated treatments A and B in a randomly chosen order. After a subject's response to each treatment has been observed, one calculates the difference (Response on treatment A)–(Response on treatment B). Let X_i, $i = 1, 2, \ldots$, denote the values of this difference for subjects receiving treatment A first and Y_i, $i = 1, 2, \ldots$, the values for subjects who receive treatment B first. The usual normal model is then $X_i \sim N(\theta + \phi, \sigma^2)$ and $Y_i \sim N(\theta - \phi, \sigma^2)$, $i = 1, 2, \ldots$, where θ represents the treatment difference and ϕ a period effect. We consider a group sequential test of $H_0\colon \theta = 0$ when the variance σ^2 is assumed known.

For each $k = 1, \ldots, K$, suppose observed values $X_1, \ldots, X_{n_{Xk}}$ and $Y_1, \ldots, Y_{n_{Yk}}$ are available at the kth analysis. We can estimate θ by

$$\frac{1}{2}(\bar{X}^{(k)} + \bar{Y}^{(k)}) = \frac{1}{2}\left(\frac{1}{n_{Xk}}\sum_{i=1}^{n_{Xk}} X_i + \frac{1}{n_{Yk}}\sum_{i=1}^{n_{Yk}} Y_i\right)$$

$$\sim N(\theta, \frac{\sigma^2}{4n_{Xk}} + \frac{\sigma^2}{4n_{Yk}}),$$

the information for θ is the reciprocal of the above variance,

$$\mathcal{I}_k = 4\left(\frac{\sigma^2}{n_{Xk}} + \frac{\sigma^2}{n_{Yk}}\right)^{-1}, \tag{3.4}$$

and the standardized statistic for testing H_0: $\theta = 0$ is

$$Z_k = \frac{1}{2}(\bar{X}^{(k)} + \bar{Y}^{(k)})\sqrt{\mathcal{I}_k}. \tag{3.5}$$

It is straightforward to check that $(Z_1, \ldots, Z_K)$ is multivariate normal,

$$Z_k \sim N(\theta\sqrt{\mathcal{I}_k}, 1), \quad k = 1, \ldots, K,$$

and

$$Cov(Z_{k_1}, Z_{k_2}) = \sqrt{(\mathcal{I}_{k_1}/\mathcal{I}_{k_2})}, \quad 1 \le k_1 \le k_2 \le K.$$

So we see, once again, that $\{Z_1, \ldots, Z_K\}$ have the canonical joint distribution with information levels $\{\mathcal{I}_1, \ldots, \mathcal{I}_K\}$ for θ.

3.2 Applying the Tests with Equal Group Sizes

3.2.1 General Form of the Tests

Suppose it is required to test a null hypothesis H_0: $\theta = 0$ with two-sided Type I error probability α and power $1 - \beta$ at $\theta = \pm\delta$. We consider group sequential tests in which up to K analyses are permitted and standardized statistics Z_k, $k = 1, \ldots, K$, are available at these analyses. For a general testing problem, we assume $\{Z_1, \ldots, Z_K\}$ have the canonical joint distribution (3.1) with information levels $\{\mathcal{I}_1, \ldots, \mathcal{I}_K\}$ for θ. We start by considering the case of equal group sizes which produce equally spaced information levels.

When a fixed sample test is based on a standardized statistic with distribution $Z \sim N(\theta\sqrt{\mathcal{I}}, 1)$, Type I error α is obtained by rejecting H_0 if $|Z| > \Phi^{-1}(1-\alpha/2)$. Here Φ denotes the standard normal cdf. Setting $\mathcal{I}$ equal to

$$\mathcal{I}_{f,2} = \{\Phi^{-1}(1 - \alpha/2) + \Phi^{-1}(1 - \beta)\}^2/\delta^2 \tag{3.6}$$

ensures that $E(Z) = \pm\{\Phi^{-1}(1-\alpha/2)+\Phi^{-1}(1-\beta)\}$ for $\theta = \pm\delta$ and, hence, power $1 - \beta$ is attained at $\theta = \pm\delta$. The subscript 2 in $\mathcal{I}_{f,2}$ is used to distinguish the two-sided case from the one-sided case, which we shall consider in Chapter 4. A group sequential test requires a larger maximum sample size and we set a maximum information level, $\mathcal{I}_{max} = R\mathcal{I}_{f,2}$, where R is greater than one and depends on K, α, β and the type of group sequential boundary being used. With equally spaced information levels, we then have

$$\begin{aligned} \mathcal{I}_k &= (k/K)\mathcal{I}_{max} = (k/K)R\mathcal{I}_{f,2} \\ &= \frac{kR}{K}\frac{\{\Phi^{-1}(1 - \alpha/2) + \Phi^{-1}(1 - \beta)\}^2}{\delta^2}, \quad k = 1, \ldots, K. \end{aligned}$$

Under H_0: $\theta = 0$, the standardized statistics $\{Z_1, \ldots, Z_K\}$ have the null joint distribution:

$$\begin{aligned} &\text{(i)} \quad (Z_1, \ldots, Z_K) \text{ is multivariate normal,} \\ &\text{(ii)} \quad E(Z_k) = 0, \quad k = 1, \ldots, K, \quad \text{and} \\ &\text{(iii)} \quad Cov(Z_{k_1}, Z_{k_2}) = \sqrt{(k_1/k_2)}, \quad 1 \le k_1 \le k_2 \le K. \end{aligned} \tag{3.7}$$

The following alternate distribution arises when $\theta = \pm\delta$:

$$\begin{array}{ll} \text{(i)} & (Z_1, \ldots, Z_K) \text{ is multivariate normal,} \\ \text{(ii)} & E(Z_k) = \pm\{\Phi^{-1}(1-\alpha/2) + \Phi^{-1}(1-\beta)\}\sqrt{(kR/K)}, \\ & k = 1, \ldots, K, \quad \text{and} \\ \text{(iii)} & Cov(Z_{k_1}, Z_{k_2}) = \sqrt{(k_1/k_2)}, \quad 1 \le k_1 \le k_2 \le K. \end{array} \tag{3.8}$$

Each of the tests introduced in Chapter 2 has the form:

$$\begin{array}{ll} \text{After group } k = 1, \ldots, K-1 & \\ \quad \text{if } |Z_k| \ge c_k & \text{stop, reject } H_0 \\ \quad \text{otherwise} & \text{continue to group } k+1, \\ \text{after group } K & \\ \quad \text{if } |Z_K| \ge c_K & \text{stop, reject } H_0 \\ \quad \text{otherwise} & \text{stop, accept } H_0. \end{array} \tag{3.9}$$

Since the null hypothesis is rejected at stage k if $|Z_k|$, a standard normal variate under H_0, exceeds the critical value c_k, such tests can be interpreted as "repeated significance tests", applying the two-sided significance level $2\{1 - \Phi^{-1}(c_k)\}$ to the data at analysis k.

A test's Type I error probability is

$$Pr\{|Z_k| \ge c_k \text{ for some } k = 1, \ldots, K\},$$

evaluated when $\{Z_1, \ldots, Z_K\}$ follow the null distribution (3.7). Each type of test, Pocock, O'Brien & Fleming, etc., uses a different sequence of critical values, $\{c_1, \ldots, c_K\}$, but all are chosen to ensure the Type I error probability is equal to the specified value, α, when (3.7) holds.

The power of the test at $\theta = \pm\delta$ is

$$Pr\left\{\bigcup_{k=1}^{K} (|Z_j| < c_j \text{ for } j = 1, \ldots, k-1 \text{ and } |Z_k| \ge c_k)\right\} \tag{3.10}$$

evaluated when $\{Z_1, \ldots, Z_K\}$ follow the distribution (3.8). For practical testing boundaries, the probability in (3.10) arises almost wholly from outcomes which terminate at an analysis k with $Z_k \ge c_k$ when $\theta = \delta$ and with $Z_k \le c_k$ when $\theta = -\delta$. For given K, α, β and critical values $\{c_1, \ldots, c_K\}$, a value of R can be found for which (3.10) is equal to $1 - \beta$ when $\{Z_1, \ldots, Z_K\}$ follow (3.8). The factors $R_P(K, \alpha, \beta)$, $R_B(K, \alpha, \beta)$, $R_{WT}(K, \alpha, \beta, \Delta)$ and $R_{HP}(K, \alpha, \beta)$, presented in Tables 2.2, 2.4, 2.10 and 2.13, are those appropriate to Pocock, O'Brien & Fleming, Wang & Tsiatis and Haybittle-Peto tests, respectively. Although these factors were introduced as multipliers of the sample size of each treatment group in a parallel comparison, the general theory implies that the same multiples of $\mathcal{I}_{f,2}$ provide the correct maximum information levels for group sequential tests to achieve power $1 - \beta$ in general testing problems.

Five-Step Summary

The general method can be summarized in the following five steps:

(1) Identify the statistical model for the data to be observed and the parameter θ which is to have value zero under the null hypothesis. Specify δ, α and β. The test of H_0: $\theta = 0$ will have Type I error probability α and power $1 - \beta$ at $\theta = \pm\delta$.

(2) Choose the type of test, Pocock, O'Brien & Fleming, etc., and the maximum number of analyses, K.

(3) Define the standardized test statistics Z_k, and find an expression for the information levels $\mathcal{I}_k$ in terms of the numbers and types of observations available at each analysis, $k = 1, \ldots, K$.

(4) Find the factor R for the chosen test and number of analyses, K. Calculate the information levels required at each analysis, $\mathcal{I}_k = (k/K) R \mathcal{I}_{f,2}$, $k = 1, \ldots, K$, where $\mathcal{I}_{f,2}$ is given by (3.6). Design the experiment so that these levels will be attained.

(5) Run the experiment applying the stopping rule (3.9).

3.2.2 Examples

Paired Comparison

As a first example, consider the paired comparison of two treatments described in Section 3.1.3. Pairs of observations X_{Ai} and X_{Bi} yield differences with mean $\mu_A - \mu_B$. We define $\theta = \mu_A - \mu_B$ since we wish to test the null hypothesis of no treatment difference. Suppose $|\mu_A - \mu_B| = 1$ represents a clinically important treatment difference and we decide to test H_0: $\theta = 0$ with Type I error probability $\alpha = 0.05$ and power $1 - \beta = 0.9$ at $\theta = \pm 1$ using an O'Brien & Fleming test with five groups of observations.

The standardized test statistics are given by (3.3) and information levels are $\mathcal{I}_k = n_k/\tilde{\sigma}^2$ at analyses $k = 1, \ldots, 5$, where n_k is the number of pairs of observations in the first k groups and $\tilde{\sigma}^2 = Var(X_{Ai} - X_{Bi})$. Suppose it is known that $\tilde{\sigma}^2 = 6$. Equation (3.6) gives $\mathcal{I}_{f,2} = (1.960 + 1.282)^2/1^2 = 10.51$ and, taking $R = R_B(5, 0.05, 0.1) = 1.026$ from Table 2.4, we find the desired information levels to be

$$\mathcal{I}_k = n_k/6 = (k/5)1.026 \times 10.51, \quad k = 1, \ldots, 5.$$

This requires $n_k = 12.94\,k$, i.e, 12.9 pairs of observations per group, which we round up to 13.

The critical values for an O'Brien & Fleming test are $c_k = C_B(5, 0.05)(5/k)^{1/2}$, and we find $C_B(5, 0.05) = 2.040$ from Table 2.3. Thus, at analyses $k = 1, \ldots, 5$, the test stops to reject H_0: $\theta = 0$ if

$$\left| \frac{1}{\sqrt{(13k \times 6)}} \sum_{i=1}^{13k} (X_{Ai} - X_{Bi}) \right| \geq 2.040 \sqrt{\frac{5}{k}},$$

i.e., if $\left| \sum_{i=1}^{13k} (X_{Ai} - X_{Bi}) \right| \geq 40.29$, and H_0 is accepted if it has not been rejected by analysis 5.

Crossover Trial

For our second example, we take a two-treatment, two-period crossover trial, as described in Section 3.1.4. With the notation of that section, suppose it is required to test H_0: $\theta = 0$ with Type I error probability $\alpha = 0.05$ and power $1 - \beta = 0.8$ at $\theta = \pm 0.6$. We shall use a Wang & Tsiatis test, as defined in Section 2.7.1, with $\Delta = 0.25$ and four groups of observations. The standardized test statistics $\{Z_1, \ldots, Z_K\}$ are given by (3.5). Assuming we know $\sigma^2 = 9$ and equal numbers will be allocated to each sequence of treatments so $n_{Xk} = n_{Yk} = n_k$, say, for $k = 1, \ldots, 4$, the information levels given in (3.4) become $\mathcal{I}_k = 2n_k/9$. Equation (3.6) gives $\mathcal{I}_{f,2} = (1.960 + 0.842)^2/0.6^2 = 21.81$, and we find $R = R_{WT}(4, 0.05, 0.2, 0.25) = 1.065$ from Table 2.10. Hence, we require

$$\mathcal{I}_k = 2n_k/9 = (k/4)1.065 \times 21.81, \quad k = 1, \ldots, 4,$$

i.e., $n_k = 26.1\,k$, $k = 1, \ldots, 4$. Rounding up to integer values, we see that each group should consist of 27 subjects on each treatment sequence.

The critical values for the Wang & Tsiatis test with $\Delta = 0.25$ are $c_k = C_{WT}(4, 0.05, 0.25)(k/4)^{0.25-1/2}$, $k = 1, \ldots, 4$, where, from Table 2.9, $C_{WT}(4, 0.05, 0.25) = 2.113$. Applying the rule (3.9), the test stops to reject H_0 at analysis k if

$$\left| \frac{1}{2}\left(\bar{X}^{(k)} + \bar{Y}^{(k)}\right)\sqrt{\frac{2n_k}{9}} \right| \geq 2.113\,(k/4)^{-0.25} = 2.988\,k^{-0.25}.$$

Substituting $n_k = 27k$ and simplifying, this condition becomes

$$\left| \sum_{i=1}^{27k} X_i + \sum_{i=1}^{27k} Y_i \right| \geq \sqrt{2} \times 3 \times \sqrt{27k} \times 2.988\,k^{-0.25} = 65.87\,k^{0.25}.$$

If H_0 has not been rejected by analysis 4, it is accepted at this point.

In both these examples, information is proportional to sample size and standard sample size formulae provide an alternative route to calculating the group sizes. Consider the second example, a crossover trial yielding observations $X_i \sim N(\theta + \phi, \sigma^2)$ and $Y_i \sim N(\theta - \phi, \sigma^2)$. The number of subjects following each treatment sequence needed for a fixed sample test of H_0: $\theta = 0$ with Type I error α and power $1 - \beta$ at $\theta = \pm\delta$ is

$$n_f = \{\Phi^{-1}(1 - \alpha/2) + \Phi^{-1}(1 - \beta)\}^2 \sigma^2/(2\delta^2) = 98.11.$$

It follows that the maximum number of observations of each type required for the group sequential test is $R\,n_f$ where $R = R_{WT}(4, 0.05, 0.2, 0.25) = 1.065$; hence the number of observations of each type per group is $R\,n_f/K = 1.065 \times 98.11/4 = 26.1$, which rounds to 27.

The crossover trial example also serves to demonstrate another feature of sequential testing. In deriving a group sequential test, we have assumed a statistical model before observing any data. This particular model does not include a treatment-by-period interaction term, which could be present due to a "carry-over" effect of the first treatment into the second period. It may be desirable to check for the presence of such an interaction, using the separate responses of each subject on treatments A and B, before interpreting evidence of a treatment difference θ. Such a test has low power if the between-subject variation is high, as is usually the case when a crossover design is adopted; thus group sequential analysis is most appropriate when an interaction is known to be unlikely *a priori*. Even so, it may be wise to use a test with wide early boundaries, so that extreme evidence of a treatment main effect is required to terminate the study before there is at least a modest chance of detecting a treatment by period interaction.

3.3 Applying the Tests with Unequal Increments in Information

In practice, it is often not possible to guarantee the equal group sizes needed to produce the equally spaced information levels assumed in Section 3.2. We now present an approximate but simple way of dealing with this problem. A more sophisticated treatment which can handle highly unpredictable information levels will be presented in Chapter 7.

Our objective remains as before, to test a null hypothesis H_0: $\theta = 0$ with two-sided Type I error probability α and power $1 - \beta$ at $\theta = \pm\delta$ in a group sequential test with up to K analyses. We assume the standardized statistics at these analyses, $\{Z_1, \ldots, Z_K\}$, have the canonical joint distribution (3.1) with information levels $\{\mathcal{I}_1, \ldots, \mathcal{I}_K\}$ for θ but now these information levels may be unequally spaced.

At the design stage, some assumptions must be made about the sequence of information levels that will be observed, and it is often sensible to suppose these will be equally spaced. One can then follow the five steps of the procedure laid out at the end of Section 3.2.1, defining statistics Z_k, information levels $\mathcal{I}_k$, and target values for the $\mathcal{I}_k$. Even though one expects observed information levels to depart from their intended values, analyses should still be planned so that target levels will be met as closely as possible. In particular, the final information level, $\mathcal{I}_K$, should be close to its target, $R\,\mathcal{I}_{f,2}$, since the value of $\mathcal{I}_K$ has a major influence on a test's power.

As analyses are conducted during the experiment, the observed information levels are found using the numbers of observations actually recorded at each stage. Standardized statistics Z_k are calculated from the data available at each analysis and the test is conducted using the rule (3.9) just as before. Note that, since each Z_k, $k = 1, \ldots, K$, has a marginal $N(0, 1)$ distribution under H_0, the criterion for terminating with rejection of H_0 at analysis k is still that a single hypothesis test based on Z_k should reject H_0 at a two-sided significance level less than or equal to $2\{1 - \Phi(c_k)\}$. This "significance level" interpretation can be helpful in implementing a group sequential test, and we shall see later that it provides a useful starting point for generalizing a group sequential test for normal data to other response distributions.

For each k, we assume the value of $\mathcal{I}_k$ may be influenced by external factors, such as the accrual rate of suitable subjects, but not by the previously observed test statistics $Z_1, \ldots, Z_{k-1}$. In this case, the sequence $\{Z_1, \ldots, Z_K\}$ has the standard distribution (3.1) conditional on the observed information levels $\{\mathcal{I}_1, \ldots, \mathcal{I}_K\}$, and we can compute a test's properties conditional on $\{\mathcal{I}_1, \ldots, \mathcal{I}_K\}$.

Differences between the observed information levels and their target values lead to deviations from the planned Type I error probability and power. As an example, consider the parallel two-treatment comparison of Chapter 2 where responses $X_{Ai} \sim N(\mu_A, \sigma^2)$ and $X_{Bi} \sim N(\mu_B, \sigma^2)$, $i = 1, 2, \ldots$, are observed. Suppose it is known that $\sigma^2 = 4$, and we wish to test H_0: $\mu_A = \mu_B$ against $\mu_A \neq \mu_B$ with Type I error probability $\alpha = 0.05$ and power $1 - \beta = 0.9$ at $\mu_A - \mu_B = \pm 1$ using a group sequential test with five groups of observations. We saw in Chapter 2 that, if groups contain m observations on each treatment, the Pocock test requires $m = 21$, and the O'Brien & Fleming test and Wang & Tsiatis test with $\Delta = 0.25$ both require $m = 18$. Suppose one such test is planned, and when the data are analyzed, cumulative sample sizes on the two treatments are equal at each analysis, taking the values n_k, $k = 1, \ldots, K$, but these differ from the planned sample sizes $m \times k$. At the kth analysis we simply calculate the standardized test statistic from the data that are available,

$$Z_k = \left(\frac{1}{n_k} \sum_{i=1}^{n_k} X_{Ai} - \frac{1}{n_k} \sum_{i=1}^{n_k} X_{Bi} \right) \sqrt{\frac{n_k}{2\sigma^2}}, \quad k = 1, \ldots, K,$$

and stop to reject H_0 if $|Z_k| > c_k$ using the original sequence of critical values $\{c_1, \ldots, c_K\}$.

Table 3.1 shows the Type I error probability and power actually achieved by these tests for a variety of sequences of cumulative sample sizes on each treatment, $\{n_1, \ldots, n_5\}$. Results were obtained by numerical computation. The first example for each test follows the original design, Type I error is exactly 0.05 and power at $\mu_A - \mu_B = \pm 1$ is a little greater than 0.9 because of upward rounding of the group sizes to integer values. Examples 2 and 3 for each test have equal group sizes and, since $\{Z_1, \ldots, Z_5\}$ still have the standard null joint distribution (3.7), Type I error is equal to 0.05; power is affected by the group sizes, increasing as n_K increases. In Examples 4 and 5, the final sample size is exactly as planned and power is close to its value in Example 1 for each test. The unequal group sizes have a greater effect on the Type I error: if the cumulative sample sizes are bunched together, as in each Example 4, test statistics at the five analyses are more highly correlated and the Type I error rate decreases, whereas the patterns of cumulative sample sizes in each Example 5 reduce correlations and increase Type I error. The effects on Type I error are smallest for the O'Brien & Fleming test in which values c_k are high for small k and there is little probability of rejecting H_0 at the early analyses. Finally, Examples 6 and 7 for each test show haphazard variations in group size; in each case the Type I error probability is very close to 0.05 and, since the final sample size is close to its design value, power is close to 0.9.

It is evident from (3.1) that the observed information levels $\{\mathcal{I}_1, \ldots, \mathcal{I}_K\}$ determine the joint distribution of $\{Z_1, \ldots, Z_K\}$ and, hence, a test's attained Type I error probability and power. Thus, the results of Table 3.1 also apply to other applications of the same tests when the same sequences $\{\mathcal{I}_1, \ldots, \mathcal{I}_5\}$ arise.

Table 3.2 shows further results from a systematic study of the effects of variations in observed information on attained error probabilities. Experiments were designed for Pocock or O'Brien & Fleming tests with Type I error probability

Table 3.1 *Type I error probability and power achieved by group sequential tests when group sizes are not equal to their design values. Tests are two-treatment comparisons with* $\sigma^2 = 4$ *and total numbers of observations in the first k groups on each treatment arm* $n_{Ak} = n_{Bk} = n_k$, $k = 1, \ldots, K$. *The first example for each test has group sizes equal to their design values.*

Pocock test

	$\{n_k;\ k = 1, \ldots, K\}$	*Type I error*	*Power at* $\mu_A - \mu_B = \pm 1$
1	21, 42, 63, 84, 105	0.050	0.910
2	18, 36, 54, 72, 90	0.050	0.860
3	23, 46, 69, 92, 115	0.050	0.934
4	30, 50, 55, 86, 105	0.046	0.909
5	12, 31, 57, 81, 105	0.054	0.909
6	13, 42, 56, 78, 99	0.051	0.892
7	26, 40, 63, 96, 110	0.049	0.923

O'Brien & Fleming test

	$\{n_k;\ k = 1, \ldots, K\}$	*Type I error*	*Power at* $\mu_A - \mu_B = \pm 1$
1	18, 36, 54, 72, 90	0.050	0.912
2	16, 32, 48, 64, 80	0.050	0.877
3	20, 40, 60, 80, 100	0.050	0.937
4	26, 39, 50, 76, 90	0.049	0.911
5	10, 27, 55, 66, 90	0.051	0.912
6	11, 38, 59, 65, 83	0.049	0.888
7	27, 40, 57, 73, 96	0.051	0.928

Wang & Tsiatis test, $\Delta = 0.25$

	$\{n_k;\ k = 1, \ldots, K\}$	*Type I error*	*Power at* $\mu_A - \mu_B = \pm 1$
1	18, 36, 54, 72, 90	0.050	0.901
2	16, 32, 48, 64, 80	0.050	0.864
3	20, 40, 60, 80, 100	0.050	0.929
4	26, 39, 50, 76, 90	0.049	0.901
5	10, 27, 55, 66, 90	0.052	0.901
6	11, 38, 59, 65, 83	0.048	0.875
7	27, 40, 57, 73, 96	0.050	0.919

Table 3.2 *Properties of two-sided tests designed for information levels* $\mathcal{I}_k = (k/K)\mathcal{I}_{max}$, $k = 1, \ldots, K$, *but applied with* $\mathcal{I}_k = \pi(k/K)^r\mathcal{I}_{max}$, $k = 1, \ldots, K$. *Attained Type I error probabilities and power are shown for Pocock and O'Brien & Fleming tests with K analyses, designed to achieve Type I error rate* $\alpha = 0.05$ *and power* $1 - \beta = 0.9$ *at* $\theta = \pm\delta$.

	r	π	*Pocock tests* Type I error	*Pocock tests* Power	*O'Brien & Fleming* Type I error	*O'Brien & Fleming* Power
$K = 2$						
	0.80	0.9	0.048	0.868	0.049	0.867
		1.0	0.048	0.901	0.049	0.900
		1.1	0.048	0.926	0.049	0.925
	1.00	0.9	0.050	0.867	0.050	0.867
		1.0	0.050	0.900	0.050	0.900
		1.1	0.050	0.926	0.050	0.925
	1.25	0.9	0.052	0.865	0.050	0.868
		1.0	0.052	0.899	0.050	0.900
		1.1	0.052	0.925	0.050	0.925
$K = 5$						
	0.80	0.9	0.047	0.867	0.048	0.866
		1.0	0.047	0.901	0.048	0.899
		1.1	0.047	0.927	0.048	0.925
	1.00	0.9	0.050	0.866	0.050	0.867
		1.0	0.050	0.900	0.050	0.900
		1.1	0.050	0.927	0.050	0.925
	1.25	0.9	0.053	0.864	0.052	0.868
		1.0	0.053	0.899	0.052	0.900
		1.1	0.053	0.926	0.052	0.925
$K = 10$						
	0.80	0.9	0.046	0.866	0.048	0.866
		1.0	0.046	0.901	0.048	0.899
		1.1	0.046	0.928	0.048	0.924
	1.00	0.9	0.050	0.865	0.050	0.867
		1.0	0.050	0.900	0.050	0.900
		1.1	0.050	0.927	0.050	0.925
	1.25	0.9	0.055	0.863	0.053	0.869
		1.0	0.055	0.899	0.053	0.901
		1.1	0.055	0.926	0.053	0.926

0.05, power 0.9 at $\theta = \pm\delta$, and 2, 5 or 10 groups of observations. The target information levels are $\mathcal{I}_k = (k/K)\mathcal{I}_{max}$, $k = 1, \ldots, K$, where $\mathcal{I}_{max}$ is the multiple of $\mathcal{I}_{f,2}$ needed to meet the power requirement. Information levels actually observed are $\mathcal{I}_k = \pi(k/K)^r \mathcal{I}_{max}$, $k = 1, \ldots, K$. Since $\mathcal{I}_K = \pi\,\mathcal{I}_{max}$, π controls the final information level, and we see that this factor plays the major role in determining power. The attained power lies within 0.001 of its nominal level in all cases where $\pi = 1$ and increases as π, and hence $\mathcal{I}_{max}$, increases: in all cases with $\pi = 0.9$, power is close to the value 0.868 attained by a fixed sample test with 0.9 times the required information, $\mathcal{I}_{f,2}$, and when $\pi = 1.1$, power is close to the value 0.925 achieved by a fixed sample test with information $1.1 \times \mathcal{I}_{f,2}$.

The exponent r governs the spacing of the $\mathcal{I}_k$: information levels are equally spaced if $r = 1$, bunched together toward $\mathcal{I}_{max}$ if $r < 1$, and more widely separated at the higher values of k if $r > 1$. As an example, values $\mathcal{I}_k = 10k$, $k = 1, \ldots, 5$, when $r = 1$ become $\mathcal{I}_k = \{14, 24, 33, 42, 50\}$ if $r = 0.8$, and $\mathcal{I}_k = \{7, 16, 26, 38, 50\}$ if $r = 1.25$. The Type I error probability is reduced below its nominal value for $r < 1$ and increased for $r > 1$; but these effects are slight, the attained Type I error rate lying between 0.046 and 0.055 in all cases.

We conclude from these results that this approximate treatment of unequal group sizes will be satisfactory in many applications. The O'Brien & Fleming test and Wang & Tsiatis tests with low values of Δ are particularly insensitive to variations in early group sizes, as they allocate very little Type I error probability to the first few analyses. Proschan, Follmann & Waclawiw (1992) have investigated the maximum possible increase in Type I error probability under certain restrictions on the observed group sizes, finding this error rate to be robust to many types of departure from equal group sizes but capable of rising to unacceptably high levels in some extreme cases. Thus, if very unequal group sizes are anticipated, the alternative methods which we shall describe in Chapter 7 should be considered.

The tests we have described are in no way limited to the response types considered thus far. We illustrate some of the wide variety of experimental settings and data types to which they can be applied in the remainder of this chapter. In Section 3.4 we state theoretical results which provide a basis for the group sequential analysis of normal linear models and apply this theory to a crossover trial, a two-treatment comparison with adjustment for covariates and a longitudinal study with correlated repeated measurements. We address general parametric models in Section 3.5, summarizing asymptotic results and explaining how these may be used to implement group sequential tests. We present tests for binary data in Section 3.6, introduce the group sequential log-rank test for comparing two survival distributions in Section 3.7 and describe group sequential t-tests in Section 3.8.

3.4 Normal Linear Models

3.4.1 Theory for Independent Observations

In the general normal linear model, we suppose observations X_i, $i = 1, 2, \ldots$, are independent and normally distributed, with expectations depending linearly on a parameter vector $\boldsymbol{\beta} = (\beta_1, \ldots, \beta_p)^T$. Consider a study in which data are collected group sequentially in a maximum of K groups and the first k groups contain a total of n_k observations, $k = 1, \ldots, K$. Let $\boldsymbol{X}^{(k)} = (X_1, \ldots, X_{n_k})^T$ denote the vector of observations available at the kth analysis. At each interim analysis, $k = 1, \ldots, K$, we have

$$\boldsymbol{X}^{(k)} \sim N(\boldsymbol{D}^{(k)}\boldsymbol{\beta},\ \boldsymbol{I}_{n_k}\sigma^2),$$

where $\boldsymbol{D}^{(k)}$ denotes the design matrix for the first n_k observations and $\boldsymbol{I}_{n_k}$ the $n_k \times n_k$ identity matrix. Assuming $\boldsymbol{\beta}$ to be estimable at each analysis, its least squares estimate based on the first k groups of observations is

$$\widehat{\boldsymbol{\beta}}^{(k)} = (\boldsymbol{D}^{(k)T}\boldsymbol{D}^{(k)})^{-1}\boldsymbol{D}^{(k)T}\boldsymbol{X}^{(k)}$$

and it is well known that this is normally distributed with expectation $\boldsymbol{\beta}$ and

$$\mathbf{Var}(\widehat{\boldsymbol{\beta}}^{(k)}) = (\boldsymbol{D}^{(k)T}\boldsymbol{D}^{(k)})^{-1}\sigma^2.$$

In Section 11.3 we shall establish the joint distribution of the sequence of estimates of $\boldsymbol{\beta}$, proving that $\{\widehat{\boldsymbol{\beta}}^{(1)}, \ldots, \widehat{\boldsymbol{\beta}}^{(K)}\}$ is multivariate normal with

$$E(\widehat{\boldsymbol{\beta}}^{(k)}) = \boldsymbol{\beta}, \quad 1 \le k \le K, \tag{3.11}$$

and

$$\mathbf{Cov}(\widehat{\boldsymbol{\beta}}^{(k_1)}, \widehat{\boldsymbol{\beta}}^{(k_2)}) = \mathbf{Var}(\widehat{\boldsymbol{\beta}}^{(k_2)}), \quad 1 \le k_1 \le k_2 \le K. \tag{3.12}$$

Suppose an experimenter is mainly interested in β_1, the first element of the parameter vector $\boldsymbol{\beta}$, and wishes to test the null hypothesis H_0: $\beta_1 = 0$ against a two-sided alternative, with Type I error α and power $1 - \beta$ at $\beta_1 = \pm\delta$. Such a test might be conducted when β_1 represents a treatment effect and the other elements of $\boldsymbol{\beta}$ are covariates which affect response but are not themselves of primary interest. The group sequential test of H_0: $\beta_1 = 0$ is based on the sequence of estimates, $\{\hat{\beta}_1^{(1)}, \ldots, \hat{\beta}_1^{(K)}\}$. At the kth analysis, the variance of $\hat{\beta}_1^{(k)}$ is the (1, 1) element of the variance matrix

$$\mathbf{Var}(\widehat{\boldsymbol{\beta}}^{(k)}) = (\boldsymbol{D}^{(k)T}\boldsymbol{D}^{(k)})^{-1}\sigma^2$$

and $\mathcal{I}_k$, the "Fisher information" for β_1 after k groups of observations, is the reciprocal of this variance. Thus,

$$\mathcal{I}_k = \{Var(\hat{\beta}_1^{(k)})\}^{-1} = [\{(\boldsymbol{D}^{(k)T}\boldsymbol{D}^{(k)})^{-1}\}_{11}\sigma^2]^{-1}, \quad k = 1, \ldots, K.$$

The standardized statistic for testing H_0 after the kth group of observations is

$$Z_k = \frac{\hat{\beta}_1^{(k)}}{\sqrt{Var(\hat{\beta}_1^{(k)})}} = \hat{\beta}_1^{(k)}\sqrt{\mathcal{I}_k}, \quad k = 1, \ldots, K.$$

It follows from the multivariate normality of the vector $\{\widehat{\boldsymbol{\beta}}^{(1)}, \ldots, \widehat{\boldsymbol{\beta}}^{(K)}\}$ that $(\hat{\beta}_1^{(1)}, \ldots, \hat{\beta}_1^{(K)})$ is multivariate normal with

$$E(\hat{\beta}_1^{(k)}) = \beta_1, \quad 1 \le k \le K,$$

and

$$Cov(\hat{\beta}_1^{(k_1)}, \hat{\beta}_1^{(k_2)}) = Var(\hat{\beta}_1^{(k_2)}), \quad 1 \le k_1 \le k_2 \le K.$$

Hence, $(Z_1, \ldots, Z_K)$ is multivariate normal with

$$E(Z_k) = \beta_1 \sqrt{\mathcal{I}_k}, \quad k = 1, \ldots, K,$$

and

$$Cov(Z_{k_1}, Z_{k_2}) = \sqrt{(\mathcal{I}_{k_1}/\mathcal{I}_{k_2})}, \quad 1 \le k_1 \le k_2 \le K,$$

i.e., the sequence of standardized statistics has the canonical joint distribution (3.1) with information levels $\{\mathcal{I}_1, \ldots, \mathcal{I}_K\}$ for $\theta = \beta_1$.

Test statistics with the same joint distribution also arise when testing a hypothesis of the form H_0: $\boldsymbol{c}^T \boldsymbol{\beta} = \gamma$, where $\boldsymbol{c}$ is a $p \times 1$ vector and γ a scalar. Suppose a two-sided test is required with Type I error α and power $1 - \beta$ at $\boldsymbol{c}^T \boldsymbol{\beta} = \gamma \pm \delta$. The standardized test statistic at analysis k is

$$Z_k = \frac{\boldsymbol{c}^T \widehat{\boldsymbol{\beta}}^{(k)} - \gamma}{\sqrt{Var(\boldsymbol{c}^T \widehat{\boldsymbol{\beta}}^{(k)})}} = (\boldsymbol{c}^T \widehat{\boldsymbol{\beta}}^{(k)} - \gamma)\sqrt{\mathcal{I}_k}, \quad k = 1, \ldots, K,$$

where now

$$\mathcal{I}_k = \{Var(\boldsymbol{c}^T \widehat{\boldsymbol{\beta}}^{(k)})\}^{-1} = [\boldsymbol{c}^T (\boldsymbol{D}^{(k)T} \boldsymbol{D}^{(k)})^{-1} \boldsymbol{c} \sigma^2]^{-1}$$

is the Fisher information for $\boldsymbol{c}^T \boldsymbol{\beta}$ at analysis k. Again it follows from the multivariate normality of $\{\widehat{\boldsymbol{\beta}}^{(1)}, \ldots, \widehat{\boldsymbol{\beta}}^{(K)}\}$ that $(Z_1, \ldots, Z_K)$ is multivariate normal and it is straightforward to show that

$$E(Z_k) = (\boldsymbol{c}^T \boldsymbol{\beta} - \gamma)\sqrt{\mathcal{I}_k}, \quad k = 1, \ldots, K,$$

and

$$Cov(Z_{k_1}, Z_{k_2}) = \sqrt{(\mathcal{I}_{k_1}/\mathcal{I}_{k_2})}, \quad 1 \le k_1 \le k_2 \le K.$$

Setting $\theta = \boldsymbol{c}^T \boldsymbol{\beta} - \gamma$, we once again obtain the canonical joint distribution (3.1).

This general theory explains the common features seen in the examples of Sections 3.1.1 to 3.1.4. Since the theory applies in generality, it justifies application of the group sequential tests already described to a great many other statistical models. Having established that the sequence of standardized test statistics follows the canonical joint distribution, we find ourselves in the situation addressed in Section 3.2 if information levels are equally spaced and in Section 3.3 in the case of unequally spaced information levels.

We recommend designing a study under the assumption of equally spaced information levels, following the five steps listed at the end of Section 3.2.1. Further assumptions about the likely form of the design matrix $\boldsymbol{D}^{(k)}$ at each analysis, $k = 1, \ldots, K$, may be needed in order to determine the numbers of observations necessary to achieve specified information levels $\mathcal{I}_k$. Failure of these assumptions will cause the Type I error to differ from its design value, but increments in information must be highly unequal for this to be a serious problem. Since the final information level, $\mathcal{I}_K$, plays a key role in determining the attained power, care should be taken to ensure $\mathcal{I}_K$ is as close as possible to its target, $R\mathcal{I}_{f,2}$. As the study proceeds, statistics $Z_k, k = 1, \ldots, K$, will be calculated from the data available at each analysis and the test conducted using rule (3.9).

3.4.2 Examples

Crossover Trial

The two-treatment, two-period crossover trial of Section 3.1.4 provides an interesting example to represent in general linear model form. With observations $X_i, i = 1, 2, \ldots$, and $Y_i, i = 1, 2, \ldots$, as previously defined and parameter vector $\boldsymbol{\beta} = (\theta, \phi)^T$, the observation vector and design matrix at analysis k are

$$\boldsymbol{X}^{(k)} = \begin{pmatrix} X_1 \\ \vdots \\ X_{n_{X1}} \\ Y_1 \\ \vdots \\ Y_{n_{Y1}} \\ \\ \vdots \\ \\ X_{n_{X,k-1}+1} \\ \vdots \\ X_{n_{Xk}} \\ Y_{n_{Y,k-1}+1} \\ \vdots \\ Y_{n_{Yk}} \end{pmatrix} \quad \text{and} \quad \boldsymbol{D}^{(k)} = \begin{pmatrix} 1 & 1 \\ \vdots & \vdots \\ 1 & 1 \\ 1 & -1 \\ \vdots & \vdots \\ 1 & -1 \\ \\ \vdots & \vdots \\ \\ 1 & 1 \\ \vdots & \vdots \\ 1 & 1 \\ 1 & -1 \\ \vdots & \vdots \\ 1 & -1 \end{pmatrix}.$$

A little algebra shows that

$$\widehat{\boldsymbol{\beta}}^{(k)} = (\boldsymbol{D}^{(k)T}\boldsymbol{D}^{(k)})^{-1}\boldsymbol{D}^{(k)T}\boldsymbol{X}^{(k)} = \begin{pmatrix} (\bar{X}^{(k)} + \bar{Y}^{(k)})/2 \\ (\bar{X}^{(k)} - \bar{Y}^{(k)})/2 \end{pmatrix}$$

where

$$\bar{X}^{(k)} = \frac{1}{n_{Xk}} \sum_{i=1}^{n_{Xk}} X_i \quad \text{and} \quad \bar{Y}^{(k)} = \frac{1}{n_{Yk}} \sum_{i=1}^{n_{Yk}} Y_i, \quad k = 1, \ldots, K.$$

Thus $\hat{\theta}^{(k)} = (\bar{X}^{(k)} + \bar{Y}^{(k)})/2$, $\mathcal{I}_k = 4(\sigma^2/n_{Xk} + \sigma^2/n_{Yk})^{-1}$ and $Z_k = \hat{\theta}^{(k)}\sqrt{\mathcal{I}_k}$, in agreement with the results of Section 3.1.4.

Two-Treatment Comparison Adjusting for Covariates

We now have the necessary theoretical tools to consider group sequential monitoring of a clinical trial with randomized treatment allocation and allowance for baseline variables when making treatment comparisons.

One commonly used method for allocating treatments in clinical trials is the "randomly permuted block design". For a block size of $2m$, the sequence of treatment labels is created by combining strings of length $2m$, each of which is a random permutation of m As and m Bs. Patients are assigned the treatments denoted by these labels in the order of admission to the study. Treatment allocation may also be balanced with respect to a small number of patient characteristics, each with two or three levels. If the total number of such categories is fairly small, a randomly permuted block design can be used within each category defined by a set of such "stratification" variables. When there are several stratification variables, it is preferable to use the strategy known as "minimization", in which each new subject's treatment is chosen to equalize, as far as possible, the numbers on treatments A and B within each level of each stratification variable. More detailed descriptions of these and other treatment allocation schemes can be found in textbooks on the general practice of clinical trials; see, for example, Chapter 5 of Pocock (1983) or Chapter 2 of Whitehead (1997).

When testing for a treatment effect, it is usually desirable to model the effects of stratification variables and possibly other baseline variables not involved in the treatment allocation rule. Suppose responses are assumed to be independent and normally distributed with the ith patient's response:

$$X_i \sim N(\sum_{j=1}^{p} d_{ij}\beta_j, \sigma^2), \quad i = 1, 2, \ldots . \qquad (3.13)$$

Setting $d_{i1} = 0$ if patient i receives treatment A and $d_{i1} = 1$ if he or she receives treatment B defines β_1 as the treatment effect. Other terms in $\sum d_{ij}\beta_j$ may include an overall constant or intercept term, additive effects associated with particular levels of categorical variables and linear terms in suitably transformed baseline variables.

If n_k responses have been observed at the time of the kth analysis, the data vector is

$$\boldsymbol{X}^{(k)} = (X_1, \ldots, X_{n_k})^T \sim N(\boldsymbol{D}^{(k)}\boldsymbol{\beta},\ \boldsymbol{I}_{n_k}\sigma^2),$$

where $\boldsymbol{\beta} = (\beta_1, \ldots, \beta_p)^T$ and $\boldsymbol{D}^{(k)}$ is the $n_k \times p$ matrix with (i, j)th element d_{ij}. The maximum likelihood estimate of $\boldsymbol{\beta}$ at this point is

$$\widehat{\boldsymbol{\beta}}^{(k)} = (\boldsymbol{D}^{(k)T}\boldsymbol{D}^{(k)})^{-1}\boldsymbol{D}^{(k)T}\boldsymbol{X}^{(k)} \sim N(\boldsymbol{\beta}, (\boldsymbol{D}^{(k)T}\boldsymbol{D}^{(k)})^{-1}\sigma^2)$$

and the estimated treatment effect is

$$\hat{\beta}_1^{(k)} \sim N(\beta_1, \mathcal{I}_k^{-1}),$$

where $\mathcal{I}_k = [\{(\boldsymbol{D}^{(k)T}\boldsymbol{D}^{(k)})^{-1}\}_{11}\sigma^2]^{-1}$. The standardized statistic for testing H_0: $\beta_1 = 0$ is simply $Z_k = \hat{\beta}_1^{(k)}\sqrt{\mathcal{I}_k}$.

As a numerical example, suppose it is desired to test H_0: $\beta_1 = 0$ with Type I error $\alpha = 0.05$ using an O'Brien & Fleming test with six analyses. Further suppose that $\beta_1 = \pm 0.5$ is regarded as a clinically significant treatment difference which the test should have power 0.8 to detect, and it is known from previous studies that $\sigma^2 = 1.2$. In practice, it is usual to estimate a variance from the current study, even when an estimate from previous data is available, and then a test for a normal response with unknown variance is needed. We shall deal with the topic of group sequential t-tests in Section 3.8 and return to this example in Section 3.8.2, but for now we proceed under the simplifying assumption of known σ^2 in order to give a self-contained account of this example using the methods already introduced.

From (3.6), the fixed sample test for this comparison requires Fisher information for β_1,

$$\mathcal{I}_{f,2} = \{\Phi^{-1}(0.975) + \Phi^{-1}(0.8)\}^2 / 0.5^2 = 31.40.$$

Taking $R = R_B(6, 0.05, 0.2) = 1.032$ from Table 2.4, we see that the group sequential test must have a maximum information level for β_1 of $1.032 \times 31.40 = 32.40$. Dividing this equally between the six analyses gives the required information levels:

$$\mathcal{I}_k = 32.40\,k/6 = 5.40\,k, \quad k = 1, \ldots, 6. \tag{3.14}$$

Since $\sigma^2 = 1.2$, the study should be designed to ensure

$$\{(\boldsymbol{D}^{(k)T}\boldsymbol{D}^{(k)})^{-1}\}_{11} = \frac{1}{\mathcal{I}_k \sigma^2} = \frac{1}{5.40\,k \times 1.2} = \frac{0.154}{k}, \quad k = 1, \ldots, 6.$$

For a general design matrix $\boldsymbol{D}^{(k)}$, numerical computation is usually required to evaluate elements of $(\boldsymbol{D}^{(k)T}\boldsymbol{D}^{(k)})^{-1}$. However, if treatment allocation is well balanced with respect to covariates, the estimated treatment effect $\hat{\beta}_1^{(k)}$ will be, approximately, the difference between mean patient responses on treatments A and B. Then, if n_k patients, divided equally between treatments A and B, are observed by analysis k,

$$Var(\hat{\beta}_1^{(k)}) \approx 4\sigma^2/n_k, \quad k = 1, \ldots, 6,$$

implying

$$\mathcal{I}_k = \{Var(\hat{\beta}_1^{(k)})\}^{-1} \approx n_k/(4\sigma^2), \quad k = 1, \ldots, 6,$$

and substituting into (3.14), we obtain the requirement

$$n_k = 4\sigma^2 \times 5.40\,k = 25.9\,k, \quad k = 1, \ldots, 6,$$

i.e., about 26 patients per group. Since this sample size has been calculated under the assumption of perfectly balanced treatment allocation with respect to all covariates in the model (3.13), it would be advisable to plan for a slightly higher sample size in order to guard against loss of information on β_1 through imbalance in some variables. The target patient recruitment should also be increased to allow for loss of observations through patient ineligibility, failure to record a response or any of the other problems that can occur in a clinical trial.

Implementation of the O'Brien & Fleming test follows the standard pattern. At each analysis $k = 1, \ldots, 6$, the statistic $Z_k = \hat{\beta}_1^{(k)}\sqrt{\mathcal{I}_k}$ is compared with the critical value $c_k = C_B(6, 0.05)(6/k)^{1/2} = 2.053\,(6/k)^{1/2} = 5.029\,k^{-1/2}$ and the test terminates with rejection of H_0 if $|Z_k| \geq 5.029\,k^{-1/2}$. If H_0 has not been rejected by analysis 6, the test concludes with acceptance of H_0.

In a large, multi-center study, the dates of interim analyses are usually set in advance for administrative reasons, and it is only to be expected that observed information levels will deviate somewhat from their target values. If these deviations are of the same magnitude as those in the examples of Section 3.3, attained error probabilities will be quite close to their nominal values, particularly the Type I error, which is only affected by ratios of information levels. The attained power is more likely to vary, as this depends on overall information levels, which in turn depend on the rate at which eligible patients present themselves and are enrolled in the trial.

3.4.3 Theory for Correlated Observations

We now consider normal linear models for correlated observations. Suppose $\boldsymbol{X}^{(k)}$ and $\boldsymbol{D}^{(k)}$, $k = 1, \ldots, K$, and $\boldsymbol{\beta}$ are as previously defined, but now

$$\boldsymbol{X}^{(k)} \sim N(\boldsymbol{D}^{(k)}\boldsymbol{\beta}, \boldsymbol{\Sigma}^{(k)}\sigma^2),$$

where $\boldsymbol{\Sigma}^{(k)}$ and σ^2 are known. The maximum likelihood estimate of $\boldsymbol{\beta}$ at analysis k is

$$\widehat{\boldsymbol{\beta}}^{(k)} = (\boldsymbol{D}^{(k)T}\boldsymbol{\Sigma}^{(k)-1}\boldsymbol{D}^{(k)})^{-1}\boldsymbol{D}^{(k)T}\boldsymbol{\Sigma}^{(k)-1}\boldsymbol{X}^{(k)},$$

which has a multivariate normal distribution with mean $\boldsymbol{\beta}$ and variance $(\boldsymbol{D}^{(k)T}\boldsymbol{\Sigma}^{(k)-1}\boldsymbol{D}^{(k)})^{-1}\sigma^2$.

The proof in Section 11.3 that the sequence of estimates $\{\widehat{\boldsymbol{\beta}}^{(1)}, \ldots, \widehat{\boldsymbol{\beta}}^{(K)}\}$ is multivariate normal with the expectations and covariances given in (3.11) and (3.12) holds in the correlated as well as the uncorrelated case. It therefore follows, as in Section 3.4.1, that if a group sequential test of H_0: $\boldsymbol{c}^T\boldsymbol{\beta} = \gamma$ is based on the sequence of standardized statistics

$$Z_k = \frac{\boldsymbol{c}^T\widehat{\boldsymbol{\beta}}^{(k)} - \gamma}{\sqrt{Var(\boldsymbol{c}^T\widehat{\boldsymbol{\beta}}^{(k)})}}, \quad k = 1, \ldots, K,$$

the information for $\theta = \boldsymbol{c}^T\boldsymbol{\beta} - \gamma$ at analysis k is

$$\mathcal{I}_k = \{Var(\boldsymbol{c}^T\widehat{\boldsymbol{\beta}}^{(k)})\}^{-1} = \{\boldsymbol{c}^T(\boldsymbol{D}^{(k)T}\boldsymbol{\Sigma}^{(k)-1}\boldsymbol{D}^{(k)})^{-1}\boldsymbol{c}\sigma^2\}^{-1}$$

and $\{Z_1, \ldots, Z_K\}$ have the canonical joint distribution with information levels $\{\mathcal{I}_1, \ldots, \mathcal{I}_K\}$ for θ. Thus, the Z_k conform to the standard pattern and group sequential tests can be applied in the usual way.

3.4.4 Sequential Comparison of Slopes in a Longitudinal Study

As an example with correlated responses, we consider a longitudinal study in which repeated measurements are made on each patient over a period of time. Suppose a patient's mean response is expected to change linearly over time, and interest focuses on the effect of treatment on the rate of change. A simple linear regression model for observations $X_{i1}, \ldots, X_{ip}$ on patient i recorded at times $t_{i1}, \ldots, t_{ip}$ is

$$X_{ij} = a_i + b_i t_{ij} + \epsilon_{ij}, \quad j = 1, \ldots, p,$$

where the ϵ_{ij} are independent, distributed as $N(0, \sigma_e^2)$. If slopes are expected to vary between patients, we may suppose $b_i \sim N(\mu_A, \sigma_b^2)$ for patients on treatment A and $b_i \sim N(\mu_B, \sigma_b^2)$ for those on treatment B. We can then write

$$X_{ij} = a_i + (\mu_{T(i)} + \delta_i)t_{ij} + \epsilon_{ij}, \quad j = 1, \ldots, p,$$

where $T(i) \in \{A, B\}$ denotes the treatment received by patient i and the δ_i are independent, distributed as $N(0, \sigma_b^2)$. If n patients have been treated and p_i measurements recorded on patient i, $i = 1, \ldots, n$, we have a *random effects* model in which the data $\{X_{ij}; i = 1, \ldots, n, j = 1, \ldots, p_i\}$ are multivariate normal with

$$E(X_{ij}) = a_i + \mu_{T(i)} t_{ij}, \quad i = 1, \ldots, n, \; j = 1, \ldots, p_i,$$

$$Var(X_{ij}) = t_{ij}^2 \sigma_b^2 + \sigma_e^2, \quad i = 1, \ldots, n, \; j = 1, \ldots, p_i,$$

and

$$Cov(X_{ij}, X_{i'j'}) = \begin{cases} 0 & \text{if } i \neq i', \\ t_{ij} t_{ij'} \sigma_b^2 & \text{if } i = i' \text{ and } j \neq j'. \end{cases}$$

Rearranging the X_{ij}s in a single-column vector, this model can be expressed as a normal linear model in which repeated observations on the same subject are positively correlated.

When a longitudinal study of this type is analyzed group sequentially, both the total number of subjects and the numbers of measurements on each subject may increase between analyses. If $\boldsymbol{X}^{(k)}$ denotes the observation vector at analysis k, containing responses from n_k different subjects, we can write

$$\boldsymbol{X}^{(k)} \sim N(\boldsymbol{D}^{(k)} \boldsymbol{\beta}^{(k)}, \boldsymbol{\Sigma}^{(k)} \sigma_e^2),$$

where $\boldsymbol{\beta}^{(k)} = (\mu_A, \mu_B, a_1, \ldots, a_{n_k})^T$ is the parameter vector for "fixed effects" at this analysis, $\boldsymbol{D}^{(k)}$ is the appropriate design matrix and the matrix $\boldsymbol{\Sigma}^{(k)}$ involves the ratio σ_b^2/σ_e^2. The maximum likelihood estimate of $\boldsymbol{\beta}$ is then

$$\widehat{\boldsymbol{\beta}}^{(k)} = (\boldsymbol{D}^{(k)T} \boldsymbol{\Sigma}^{(k)-1} \boldsymbol{D}^{(k)})^{-1} \boldsymbol{D}^{(k)T} \boldsymbol{\Sigma}^{(k)-1} \boldsymbol{X}^{(k)},$$

and to investigate $\theta = \mu_A - \mu_B$, we extract $\hat{\theta}^{(k)} = \boldsymbol{d}_k^T \widehat{\boldsymbol{\beta}}^{(k)}$ where the contrast vector $\boldsymbol{d}_k = (1, -1, 0, \ldots, 0)^T$. The Fisher information for θ at this point is $\mathcal{I}_k = \{Var(\boldsymbol{d}_k^T \widehat{\boldsymbol{\beta}}^{(k)})\}^{-1}$, and the standardized statistic for testing H_0: $\theta = 0$ is $Z_k = \hat{\theta}^{(k)} \sqrt{\mathcal{I}_k}$.

Although the parameter vector $\boldsymbol{\beta}^{(k)}$ grows as intercepts a_i are added for additional subjects, successive estimates of μ_A and μ_B, and hence of θ, still follow the standard joint distribution (see the discussion of this point in Section 11.3). Consequently, $\{Z_1, \ldots, Z_K\}$ has the canonical joint distribution with information levels $\{\mathcal{I}_1, \ldots, \mathcal{I}_K\}$ for θ, and group sequential tests can be applied in the usual way.

If a group sequential test is to satisfy given Type I error and power requirements, it must be designed so that the information levels $\mathcal{I}_k$ reach specified values. The formula

$$\mathcal{I}_k = \{Var(\boldsymbol{d}_k^T \widehat{\boldsymbol{\beta}}^{(k)})\}^{-1} = \{\boldsymbol{d}_k^T (\boldsymbol{D}^{(k)^T} \boldsymbol{\Sigma}^{(k)^{-1}} \boldsymbol{D}^{(k)})^{-1} \boldsymbol{d}_k \, \sigma_e^2\}^{-1}$$

allows numerical computation of $\mathcal{I}_k$ for particular data sets but provides little insight into just how $\mathcal{I}_k$ depends on the numbers and times of measurements on each subject available at analysis k.

Suppose that for $i = 1, \ldots, n_k$ we have $p_i(k)$ measurements on patient i taken at times $t_{i1}, \ldots, t_{ip_i(k)}$ available at analysis k. In discussing this problem, Lan, Reboussin & DeMets (1994) note that $\hat{b}_i^{(k)}$, the usual least squares estimate of b_i from the $p_i(k)$ measurements on subject i, has expectation $\mu_{T(i)}$ and variance

$$V_i(k) = \sigma_b^2 + \frac{\sigma_e^2}{\sum_{j=1}^{p_i(k)} (t_{ij} - \bar{t}_{i.}(k))^2},$$

where $\bar{t}_{i.}(k) = (t_{i1} + \ldots + t_{ip_i(k)})/p_i(k)$. They then propose estimating μ_A and μ_B by the weighted averages of estimates $\hat{b}_i^{(k)}$ for subjects receiving treatments A and B, respectively, weights being inversely proportional to the variance of each $\hat{b}_i^{(k)}$. It can be shown that this method does, in fact, produce the maximum likelihood estimates of μ_A and μ_B, and so we can use it to find a more helpful expression for $\mathcal{I}_k$. We have

$$\begin{aligned} Var(\hat{\mu}_A^{(k)}) &= Var\left(\frac{\sum_{i=1}^{n_k} I(T(i) = A)\, \hat{b}_i^{(k)} / V_i(k)}{\sum_{i=1}^{n_k} I(T(i) = A)/V_i(k)}\right) \\ &= \left\{\sum_{i=1}^{n_k} I(T(i) = A)\{V_i(k)\}^{-1}\right\}^{-1}, \end{aligned}$$

where I is the indicator variable, and similarly

$$Var(\hat{\mu}_B^{(k)}) = \left\{\sum_{i=1}^{n_k} I(T(i) = B)\{V_i(k)\}^{-1}\right\}^{-1}.$$

Since $\hat{\mu}_A^{(k)}$ and $\hat{\mu}_B^{(k)}$ are based on separate, uncorrelated sets of variables, we conclude that

$$\mathcal{I}_k = \{Var(\hat{\theta}^{(k)})\}^{-1} = \{Var(\hat{\mu}_A^{(k)}) + Var(\hat{\mu}_B^{(k)})\}^{-1}.$$

We have tacitly assumed in describing this example that σ_b^2 and σ_e^2 are known. In practice, this is unlikely to be the case and these variance components will have to be estimated during the study. An estimate of the ratio σ_b^2/σ_e^2 can be substituted in $\boldsymbol{\Sigma}^{(k)}$ for use in computing $\hat{b}_i^{(k)}$ at each analysis. However, σ_b^2 and σ_e^2 also govern the variance of $\hat{b}_i^{(k)}$ and the value of $\mathcal{I}_k$ for each $k = 1, \ldots, K$. If the ratio σ_b^2/σ_e^2 were known, we would have a normal linear model with variance known up to a single scale factor, a situation we shall address in Section 3.8; applying methods for this case with estimates of σ_b^2/σ_e^2 substituted at each analysis provides an approximate solution to this problem.

3.5 Other Parametric Models

3.5.1 General Theory

In Section 11.6 we consider the group sequential analysis of observations whose distribution depends on a parameter vector $\boldsymbol{\beta}$ for which maximum likelihood estimates are obtained at analyses $k = 1, \ldots, K$. There we state an asymptotic result proved by Jennison & Turnbull (1997a) that, under certain regularity conditions concerning the statistical model and the covariate values for observed data, the sequence of estimates $\{\widehat{\boldsymbol{\beta}}^{(1)}, \ldots, \widehat{\boldsymbol{\beta}}^{(K)}\}$ is approximately multivariate normal with

$$E(\widehat{\boldsymbol{\beta}}^{(k)}) = \boldsymbol{\beta}, \quad k = 1, \ldots, K,$$

and

$$Cov(\widehat{\boldsymbol{\beta}}^{(k_1)}, \widehat{\boldsymbol{\beta}}^{(k_2)}) = Var(\widehat{\boldsymbol{\beta}}^{(k_2)}), \quad 1 \le k_1 \le k_2 \le K,$$

when sample sizes are sufficiently large. Thus, the joint distribution of successive estimates of the parameter vector matches that seen for normal linear models in Section 3.4. Furthermore, the inverse of the Fisher information matrix for $\boldsymbol{\beta}$ at analysis k provides a consistent estimate of $Var(\widehat{\boldsymbol{\beta}}^{(k)})$.

Precise conditions under which this theory applies depend on the particular statistical model in question, but in all cases they reduce to the conditions required to derive standard maximum likelihood theory at each individual analysis. Thus, the scope of the group sequential theory for parametric models is as broad as that of the underlying fixed sample maximum likelihood theory. The sample size necessary for these results to hold accurately is problem specific, and in a group sequential analysis it is advisable to ensure the first group of observations is sufficiently large that the asymptotic approximation holds adequately at the first analysis.

We illustrate the general theory with two simple applications to binary response data in Section 3.6. Many further applications arise in the group sequential analysis of generalized linear models, including the important examples of logistic regression for a binary response (see Section 12.5 for an example), probit regression, multiplicative models for Poisson count data and normal linear models with non-linear link functions.

3.5.2 Implementing Group Sequential Tests

Suppose it is required to test the hypothesis H_0: $\boldsymbol{c}^T\boldsymbol{\beta} = \gamma$ with two-sided Type I error probability α and power $1 - \beta$ at $\boldsymbol{c}^T\boldsymbol{\beta} = \gamma \pm \delta$. We assume that at each analysis $k = 1, \ldots, K$, we have an estimate $\widehat{\boldsymbol{\beta}}^{(k)}$ and an estimated variance matrix $\widehat{Var}(\widehat{\boldsymbol{\beta}}^{(k)})$. Many statistical computer packages routinely produce such estimates after fitting a model to data, and it is straightforward to use output from such packages for group sequential testing. Our estimate of $\theta = \boldsymbol{c}^T\boldsymbol{\beta} - \gamma$ at analysis k is $\hat{\theta}^{(k)} = \boldsymbol{c}^T\widehat{\boldsymbol{\beta}}^{(k)} - \gamma$, and we approximate its distribution as

$$\hat{\theta}^{(k)} \sim N(\theta, \boldsymbol{c}^T\widehat{Var}(\widehat{\boldsymbol{\beta}}^{(k)})\boldsymbol{c}).$$

Thus, the estimated information for θ is $\mathcal{I}_k = \{c^T \widehat{Var}(\widehat{\beta}^{(k)})c\}^{-1}$ and the standardized test statistic $Z_k = \hat{\theta}^{(k)}\sqrt{\mathcal{I}_k}$ is distributed, approximately, as $N(\theta\sqrt{\mathcal{I}_k}, 1)$.

It follows from the joint distribution of $\{\widehat{\beta}^{(1)}, \dots, \widehat{\beta}^{(K)}\}$ that the statistics $\{Z_1, \dots, Z_K\}$ have the canonical joint distribution (3.1) with information levels $\{\mathcal{I}_1, \dots, \mathcal{I}_K\}$ for θ. We can therefore obtain a group sequential test with the required properties by following the five steps listed at the end of Section 3.2.1 in the usual way.

In order to attain its desired power, the experiment must be designed to yield the appropriate sequence of information levels. To achieve this requires some understanding of the relationship between information and sample size for the assumed statistical model. When available, formulae or tables that provide sample sizes needed to attain specified Type I error and power in a fixed sample experiment, can be used to aid the planning a group sequential study. Assuming information is proportional to sample size, one sets the maximum sample size to be the corresponding fixed sample size multiplied by the factor R, i.e., one of the constants $R_P(K, \alpha, \beta)$, $R_B(K, \alpha, \beta)$, etc., as appropriate to the form of group sequential test being used. If analyses are arranged so that $\mathcal{I}_K = R\,\mathcal{I}_{f,2}$, where $\mathcal{I}_{f,2}$ is given by (3.6), and $\mathcal{I}_1, \dots, \mathcal{I}_K$ are equally spaced, the target Type I error and power will be attained accurately. Deviations from the desired pattern of information levels will have roughly the same effect as we saw for normal data in Section 3.3, and if it is particularly difficult to control information levels, the more flexible methods of Chapter 7 may be preferred.

3.5.3 Parameter Estimates, Wald Statistics and Score Statistics

Although we have defined group sequential tests in terms of the standardized statistics $\{Z_1, \dots, Z_K\}$, this is not the only possibility. Consider a study yielding data $X_i \sim N(\theta, 1)$, $i = 1, 2, \dots,$ with n_k observations available at the kth analysis, $k = 1, \dots, K$. Denote the sample sum at analysis k by $S_k = X_1 + \ldots + X_{n_k}$, then $\hat{\theta}^{(k)} = S_k/n_k$, $\mathcal{I}_k = \{Var(\hat{\theta}^{(k)})\}^{-1} = n_k$ and the standardized statistic for testing H_0: $\theta = 0$ is $Z_k = \hat{\theta}^{(k)}\sqrt{\mathcal{I}_k}$. Each of the sequences $\{\hat{\theta}^{(1)}, \dots, \hat{\theta}^{(K)}\}$, $\{Z_1, \dots, Z_K\}$ and $\{S_1, \dots, S_K\}$ is multivariate normal, with

$$
\begin{aligned}
\hat{\theta}^{(k)} &\sim N(\theta, \mathcal{I}_k^{-1}) && \text{and} \quad Cov(\hat{\theta}^{(k_1)}, \hat{\theta}^{(k_2)}) = \mathcal{I}_{k_2}^{-1}, \\
Z_k &\sim N(\theta\sqrt{\mathcal{I}_k}, 1) && \text{and} \quad Cov(Z_{k_1}, Z_{k_2}) = \sqrt{(\mathcal{I}_{k_1}/\mathcal{I}_{k_2})}, \\
S_k &\sim N(\theta\,\mathcal{I}_k, \mathcal{I}_k) && \text{and} \quad Cov(S_{k_1}, S_{k_2}) = \mathcal{I}_{k_1},
\end{aligned}
\tag{3.15}
$$

for $k = 1, \dots, K$ and $1 \le k_1 \le k_2 \le K$.

More generally, suppose $\theta = c^T\beta - \gamma$ where β is the parameter vector in a normal linear model. Given $\hat{\theta}^{(k)} \sim N(\theta, \mathcal{I}_k^{-1})$, we can define $Z_k = \hat{\theta}^{(k)}\sqrt{\mathcal{I}_k}$ and $S_k = \hat{\theta}^{(k)}\mathcal{I}_k$, and the three sequences $\{\hat{\theta}^{(1)}, \dots, \hat{\theta}^{(K)}\}$, $\{Z_1, \dots, Z_K\}$ and $\{S_1, \dots, S_K\}$ also have the above joint distributions.

For other parametric models satisfying the appropriate regularity conditions, the theory of Section 11.6 shows that the sequence of maximum likelihood estimates $\hat{\theta}^{(k)} = c^T\widehat{\beta}^{(k)} - \gamma$, $k = 1, \dots, K$, has, approximately, the joint distribution stated above with $\mathcal{I}_k$ given by the Fisher information for θ at analysis k. The statistics $Z_k = \hat{\theta}^{(k)}\sqrt{\mathcal{I}_k}$ are called the Wald statistics for testing $\theta = 0$. The statistics $S_k = \hat{\theta}^{(k)}\mathcal{I}_k$, $k = 1, \ldots, K$, are asymptotically equivalent to the "efficient score statistics" for testing H_0: $\theta = 0$, which are obtained from the derivative of the log likelihood function evaluated at the maximum likelihood estimate of $\boldsymbol{\beta}$ subject to the constraint $\boldsymbol{c}^T\boldsymbol{\beta} = \gamma$ (by "asymptotically equivalent" we mean that the difference between suitably standardized versions of the statistics converges in probability to zero and, hence, properties of tests based on each statistic agree to the first order). It follows from the joint distribution of $\{\hat{\theta}^{(1)}, \ldots, \hat{\theta}^{(K)}\}$ that both $\{Z_1, \ldots, Z_K\}$ and $\{S_1, \ldots, S_K\}$ have, approximately, the joint distributions stated above.

Many authors have defined group sequential boundaries in terms of the statistics $\{S_1, \ldots, S_K\}$. The O'Brien & Fleming test for equally sized groups was defined by comparing each $|S_k|$, $k = 1, \ldots, K$, against a constant critical value. Wang & Tsiatis defined their tests by comparing $|S_k|$ against boundary values proportional to k^{Δ}, which explains why critical values for Z_k are proportional to $k^{\Delta-1/2}$ in our description of these tests. Figure 3.1 shows Pocock and O'Brien & Fleming tests for four groups of observations designed to achieve Type I error rate $\alpha = 0.05$ with boundaries expressed in terms of both Z_k and S_k, $k = 1, \ldots, 4$. In each case, critical values are plotted against information levels $\mathcal{I}_k$ chosen to guarantee power $1 - \beta = 0.9$ at $\delta = 0.2$. It should be noted that these information levels are higher for the Pocock test since its maximum information level is a larger multiple of the information $\mathcal{I}_{f,2}$ needed for a fixed sample test.

Whitehead (1997) defines tests in terms of the sequences of observed pairs $(S_k, \mathcal{I}_k)$ using the symbols Z for S_k and V for $\mathcal{I}_k$ in his notation. The sequence $\{S_1, \ldots, S_K\}$ has a certain mathematical appeal as its increments S_1, $S_2 - S_1$, $S_3 - S_2$, etc., are independent. This sequence can also be viewed as a Brownian motion with drift θ observed at times $\{\mathcal{I}_1, \ldots, \mathcal{I}_K\}$. Lan & Zucker (1993) note the relationship between the three processes $\{\hat{\theta}^{(k)}\}$, $\{Z_k\}$ and $\{S_k\}$ and their link with Brownian motion, pointing out the consequent freedom to express a group sequential test derived for one sequence of statistics in terms of a different sequence.

The properties of a group sequential test remain the same whether it is expressed through a boundary for $\hat{\theta}^{(k)}$, Z_k or S_k, and numerical computations of error probabilities and expected sample sizes are just as easy to implement using one statistic as another. We have chosen to express tests in terms of the standardized statistics Z_k as these are used commonly in applied work. Also, the method described in Section 3.3 for adapting tests designed for equally spaced information levels to other information sequences is most simply defined in terms of standardized statistics. But, whichever sequence of statistics is used to define a test, it is a simple exercise to use the relations $S_k = Z_k\sqrt{\mathcal{I}_k} = \hat{\theta}^{(k)}\mathcal{I}_k$ to re-express the test in terms of another set of statistics.

Figure 3.1 *Pocock and O'Brien & Fleming tests for four groups of observations expressed in terms of* Z_k *and* S_k

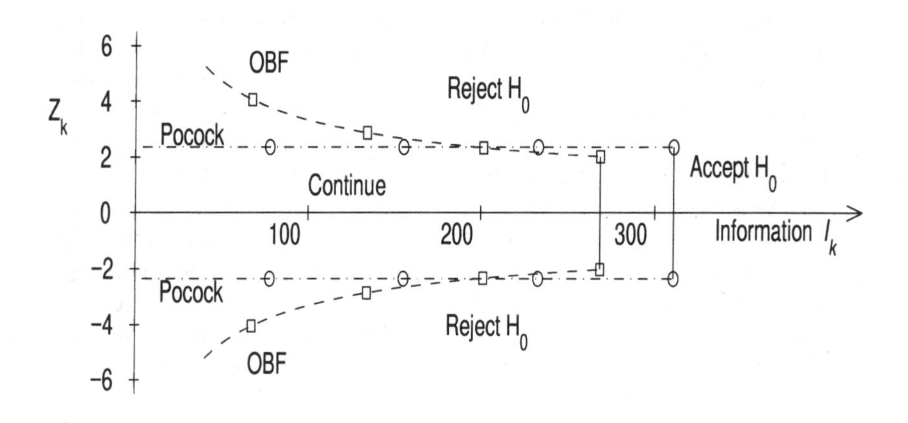

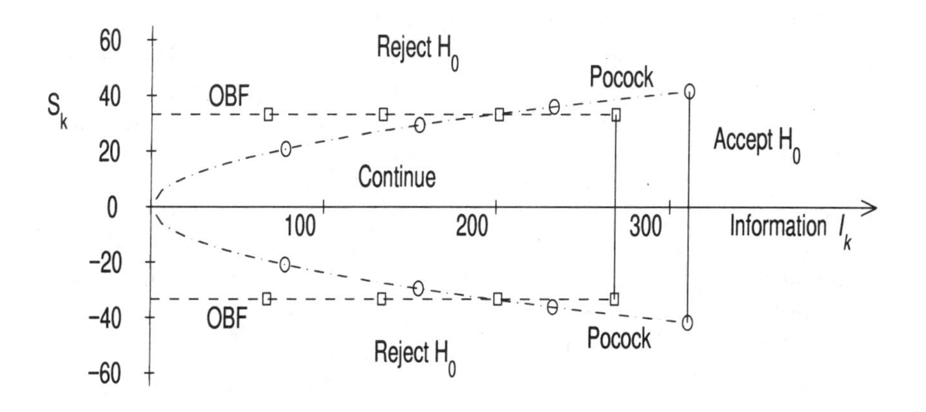

3.5.4 *Further Special Results*

Even when standard maximum likelihood methods are not directly applicable, it is sometimes possible to show that sequences of parameter estimates $\{\hat{\theta}^{(1)}, \ldots, \hat{\theta}^{(K)}\}$, standardized statistics $\{Z_1, \ldots, Z_K\}$ or score statistics $\{S_1, \ldots, S_K\}$ follow the appropriate canonical joint distribution approximately for large sample sizes. In all these cases, it is straightforward to design and implement group sequential tests following the approach we have laid out. This generalization applies not only to the two-sided tests seen so far, but also to the one-sided tests and two-sided tests with early stopping to accept H_0 to be described in Chapters 4 and 5, to the "equivalence tests" of Chapter 6 and to tests defined through "error spending functions" which we shall introduce in Chapter 7.

The major endpoint in many clinical trials is survival time, right censored for those patients alive at the time of each analysis. The proportional hazards regression model proposed by Cox (1972) is widely used for modeling the dependence of survival on treatment and other baseline covariates but, since this model is only semi-parametric, maximum likelihood estimation is not a viable option. Nevertheless, sequences of parameter estimates obtained by maximum partial likelihood estimation (Cox, 1975) do follow the usual pattern of maximum likelihood estimates for parametric models, and so can form the basis of group sequential tests as described in Section 3.5.2. We shall describe the Cox model in detail and illustrate its group sequential application in Chapter 13.

If data arise as multiple 2×2 tables with a common odds ratio and the number of tables increases with the number of observations, standard maximum likelihood theory is not applicable due to the increasing number of nuisance parameters. Here, it is convenient to base tests on the Mantel-Haenszel estimate of the odds ratio, and we shall see in Section 12.3 that the sequence of such estimates is approximately multivariate normal with the standard covariance structure. Hence, tests can be implemented in the usual manner.

The log-rank test is commonly used for comparing two survival distributions without adjustment for covariates. Under a proportional hazards assumption, the sequence of log-rank statistics obtained from accumulating data has, approximately, the canonical joint distribution of a sequence of score statistics, and a group sequential test can be applied in the standard way. We describe the group sequential log-rank test in detail in Section 3.7.

For normal data, it is usually necessary to estimate both the mean and variance and, hence, a group sequential t-test is required. We explain in Section 3.8 how the two-sided tests previously defined for normal data with known variance can be adapted to give group sequential t-tests with approximately the same Type I error probability, and power dependent on the true mean and variance. The general theory which underlies these group sequential t-tests is presented later in Section 11.4.

3.6 Binary Data: Group Sequential Tests for Proportions

3.6.1 The One-Sample Problem

Binary data arise when each observation can take one of two possible values. An example of a binary outcome is whether or not a subject responds to a given treatment; another is whether a patient experiences severely toxic side-effects. Coding responses as zero or one, we obtain a Bernoulli distribution, denoted $B(p)$, in which the value one occurs with probability p and the value zero with probability $1 - p$. We first consider the case of a single Bernoulli distribution where p is to be compared with a standard value by testing the null hypothesis H_0: $p = p_0$.

Let $X_1, X_2, \ldots,$ denote a sequence of $B(p)$ observations. If data are collected group sequentially with total numbers of observations $n_1, \ldots, n_K$ at analyses 1 to

K, the usual estimate of p at analysis k,

$$\hat{p}^{(k)} = \frac{1}{n_k} \sum_{i=1}^{n_k} X_i,$$

has expectation p and variance $p(1-p)/n_k$. The general theory discussed in Section 3.5.1 implies that the sequence of estimates $\{\hat{p}^{(1)}, \ldots, \hat{p}^{(K)}\}$ is approximately multivariate normal with

$$Cov(\hat{p}^{(k_1)}, \hat{p}^{(k_2)}) = Var(\hat{p}^{(k_2)}), \quad 1 \le k_1 \le k_2 \le K.$$

If, also, p is close to p_0,

$$Var(\hat{p}^{(k)}) \simeq p_0(1-p_0)/n_k, \quad k = 1, \ldots, K.$$

Let $\theta = p - p_0$. We define the information for θ at analysis k to be the reciprocal of the null variance of $\hat{p}^{(k)}$, $\mathcal{I}_k = n_k/\{p_0(1-p_0)\}$, and the standardized statistics are $Z_k = (\hat{p}^{(k)} - p_0)\sqrt{\mathcal{I}_k}$, $k = 1, \ldots, K$. Then, for p close to p_0, the sequence $\{Z_1, \ldots, Z_K\}$ has, approximately, the canonical joint distribution (3.1) with information levels $\{\mathcal{I}_1, \ldots, \mathcal{I}_K\}$ for θ. Hence, the group sequential tests of Chapter 2 can be applied directly to create a group sequential two-sided test of H_0.

As an example, suppose it is desired to test H_0: $p = 0.6$ against the two-sided alternative $p \neq 0.6$ with Type I error $\alpha = 0.05$ and power $1 - \beta = 0.9$ at $p = 0.4$ and $p = 0.8$. We shall do this using a Pocock test with four groups of observations. Using (3.6) with $\delta = 0.2$, we find the information for p required by a fixed sample test with these error probabilities to be

$$\mathcal{I}_{f,2} = \{\Phi^{-1}(0.975) + \Phi^{-1}(0.9)\}^2/0.2^2 = 262.7,$$

and hence the group sequential test's final information level should be

$$R_P(4, 0.05, 0.1) \times 262.7 = 1.183 \times 262.7 = 310.8.$$

Since $\mathcal{I}_k = n_k/\{p_0(1-p_0)\} = n_k/(0.6 \times 0.4)$, we solve $n_4/0.24 = 310.8$ to obtain $n_4 = 74.6$, and rounding this to a multiple of four gives the sample size requirement $n_4 = 76$, i.e., four groups of 19 observations. The standardized test statistics are

$$Z_k = (\hat{p}^{(k)} - 0.6)\sqrt{\mathcal{I}_k} = (\hat{p}^{(k)} - 0.6)\sqrt{(19\,k/0.24)}, \quad k = 1, \ldots, 4,$$

and we reject H_0 at analysis k if $|Z_k| \ge C_P(4, 0.05) = 2.361$, i.e., if

$$|\hat{p}^{(k)} - 0.6| \ge 0.265/\sqrt{k}, \quad k = 1, \ldots, 4.$$

If H_0 has not been rejected by the fourth analysis, it is accepted.

We shall return to this example in Section 12.1. One point that merits further discussion is the dependence of $Var(\hat{p}^{(k)})$, and hence $\mathcal{I}_k$, on the value of p. In the above treatment, we used the approximation

$$Var(\hat{p}^{(k)}) = p_0(1-p_0)/n_k = 0.24/n_k$$

in both Type I error and power calculations, whereas the lower variance of $0.16/n_k$ when $p = 0.8$ actually leads to greater power at this alternative than the stated value of 0.9. Another feature of binary data is their discreteness, and this is not well modeled by a normal approximation when sample sizes are small. We shall show in Chapter 12 that exact calculation of properties of group sequential tests for binary responses is quite straightforward and can be used to fine-tune tests obtained under normal approximations.

3.6.2 Comparing Two Proportions

We now suppose observations X_{Ai} and X_{Bi} are Bernoulli responses of subjects receiving two different treatments with $X_{Ai} \sim B(p_A)$ and $X_{Bi} \sim B(p_B)$, $i = 1, 2, \ldots$. We shall consider tests of the null hypothesis of no treatment difference, H_0: $p_A = p_B$, when data are collected group sequentially.

Denote the total numbers of observations on treatments A and B at analyses $k = 1, \ldots, K$ by n_{Ak} and n_{Bk}, respectively. Let $\bar{p} = (p_A + p_B)/2$ and define the estimates of p_A and p_B,

$$\hat{p}_A^{(k)} = \frac{1}{n_{Ak}} \sum_{i=1}^{n_{Ak}} X_{Ai} \quad \text{and} \quad \hat{p}_B^{(k)} = \frac{1}{n_{Bk}} \sum_{i=1}^{n_{Bk}} X_{Bi}, \quad k = 1, \ldots, K.$$

Under H_0, $p_A = p_B = \bar{p}$, and the information for $p_B - p_A$ at analysis k is the reciprocal of $Var(\hat{p}_B^{(k)} - \hat{p}_A^{(k)})$,

$$\mathcal{I}_k = \{\bar{p}(1 - \bar{p})(n_{Ak}^{-1} + n_{Bk}^{-1})\}^{-1}.$$

Estimating the common response probability $\bar{p}$ under H_0 by

$$\tilde{p}_k = \frac{\sum_{i=1}^{n_{Ak}} X_{Ai} + \sum_{i=1}^{n_{Bk}} X_{Bi}}{n_{Ak} + n_{Bk}},$$

we obtain the estimated information level at analysis k:

$$\widehat{\mathcal{I}}_k = \{\tilde{p}_k(1 - \tilde{p}_k)(n_{Ak}^{-1} + n_{Bk}^{-1})\}^{-1}, \quad k = 1, \ldots, K. \tag{3.16}$$

We base our test of H_0 on the standardized statistics

$$Z_k = (\hat{p}_B^{(k)} - \hat{p}_A^{(k)})\sqrt{\widehat{\mathcal{I}}_k}, \quad k = 1, \ldots, K.$$

The general theory of Section 3.5.1 implies that, if $p_B - p_A$ is small, the sequence of statistics $\{Z_1, \ldots, Z_K\}$ follows, approximately, the canonical joint distribution (3.1) with information levels $\{\widehat{\mathcal{I}}_1, \ldots, \widehat{\mathcal{I}}_K\}$ for $\theta = p_B - p_A$. Hence, we can apply any of the group sequential tests of Chapter 2.

As an example, suppose we wish to test H_0: $p_A = p_B$ against a two-sided alternative with Type I error probability $\alpha = 0.05$ and power $1 - \beta = 0.8$ at $|p_B - p_A| = 0.2$ using an O'Brien & Fleming test with eight groups of observations. From (3.6), the information required by a fixed sample test with these error probabilities is

$$\mathcal{I}_{f,2} = \{\Phi^{-1}(0.975) + \Phi^{-1}(0.8)\}^2/0.2^2 = 196.2,$$

and the final information level needed by the group sequential test is, therefore,

$$R_B(8, 0.05, 0.2) \times 196.2 = 1.037 \times 196.2 = 203.5.$$

It is evident from (3.16) that information depends on the value of $\bar{p}$, which is unknown at the design stage. However, since $\mathcal{I}_k$ varies slowly as a function of $\bar{p}$ for values away from zero and 1, a highly accurate estimate of $\bar{p}$ is not usually necessary. We shall continue this example assuming the worst case value, $\bar{p} = 0.5$, so any error will be in the direction of too large a group size and attained power greater than stipulated. Under this assumption, and supposing $n_{Ak} = n_{Bk}$ for each $k = 1, \ldots, 8$, we find $\mathcal{I}_8 = \{0.25 \times 2/(n_8)\}^{-1} = 2n_8$, where n_8 denotes the common value of n_{A8} and n_{B8}. Solving $\mathcal{I}_8 = 203.5$ gives $n_8 = 101.7$, which we round to 104 to obtain a multiple of 8, and we see that eight groups of 13 observations per treatment should be planned.

The standardized test statistic at analysis k is then

$$Z_k = (\hat{p}_B^{(k)} - \hat{p}_A^{(k)})\sqrt{\widehat{\mathcal{I}}_k} = (\hat{p}_B^{(k)} - \hat{p}_A^{(k)})\sqrt{\{6.5\,k/(\tilde{p}_k(1-\tilde{p}_k))\}},$$

and H_0 is rejected at this analysis if $|Z_k| \geq C_B(8, 0.05) = 2.072\sqrt{(8/k)}$, i.e., if

$$|\hat{p}_B^{(k)} - \hat{p}_A^{(k)}| \geq \frac{2.30\sqrt{\{\tilde{p}_k(1-\tilde{p}_k)\}}}{k}, \quad k = 1, \ldots, 8.$$

If H_0 has not been rejected by the eighth analysis, it is accepted.

As for the one-sample problem, we defer discussion of the variance-mean relationship and the possibility of exact calculation of a test's properties until Chapter 12. Another issue, which we shall return to in Section 14.3.1, is the adaptive re-computing of sample sizes in response to increasingly accurate estimates of $\bar{p}$. The important conclusion for the moment is that the general theory for parametric models is easily applied to specific non-normal data types.

3.7 The Group Sequential Log-Rank Test for Survival Data

The most important outcome in many clinical trials is the length of time from treatment to an event such as death, relapse or remission. Suppose the primary outcome is time until death, then survival time is right censored if a subject is alive at the time of an analysis since his or her ultimate survival time is still unknown. In group sequential studies, this effect is seen repeatedly at successive analyses, but with the length of follow-up on each patient increasing as the study progresses. Follow-up also varies between patients according to their time of entry to the study. A separate form of "competing risk" censoring can occur when patients are lost to follow-up, for example, if a subject moves to another part of the country and cannot be traced by the experimenters.

A key element of survival analysis is the hazard rate of a distribution. Let T be a continuous, positive random variable with probability density function $f(t)$, $t \geq 0$. The corresponding survival function is defined as

$$S(t) = Pr\{T > t\} = \int_t^\infty f(u)du, \quad t \geq 0,$$

and the hazard rate is

$$h(t) = \frac{f(t)}{S(t)}, \quad t \geq 0.$$

Note that $h(t)$ can be interpreted as the limit, as δt tends to zero, of

$$\frac{1}{\delta t} Pr\{T \in (t, t+\delta t) \mid T > t\}.$$

A convenient assumption in modeling survival data is that the hazard rates for different observations are affected multiplicatively by explanatory variables. In the proportional hazards model for a two-treatment comparison, we assume the hazard rate is $h(t)$ for subjects receiving treatment A and $\lambda h(t)$ for those receiving treatment B. Interest then focuses on the hazard ratio, λ, while the unknown function $h(t)$ is usually of secondary interest. The "log-rank" test of Mantel (1966) and Peto & Peto (1972) is commonly used to test the null hypothesis of no difference in survival between two treatments which occurs when $\lambda = 1$.

In a group sequential study, let d_k, $k = 1, \ldots, K$, denote the total number of uncensored failures observed when analysis k is conducted. Assuming no ties, we denote the survival times of these subjects by $\tau_{1,k} < \tau_{2,k} < \ldots < \tau_{d_k,k}$, where the $\tau_{i,k}$ represent elapsed times between entry to the study and failure. Let the numbers known at analysis k to have survived up to time $\tau_{i,k}$ after treatment be $r_{iA,k}$ and $r_{iB,k}$ on treatments A and B, respectively. Then, the log-rank score statistic at analysis k is

$$S_k = \sum_{i=1}^{d_k} \left\{ \delta_{iB,k} - \frac{r_{iB,k}}{r_{iA,k} + r_{iB,k}} \right\}, \tag{3.17}$$

where $\delta_{iB,k} = 1$ if the failure at time $\tau_{i,k}$ was on treatment B and $\delta_{iB,k} = 0$ otherwise.

The variance of S_k when $\lambda = 1$ can be approximated by the sum of the conditional variances of the $\delta_{iB,k}$ given the numbers $r_{iA,k}$ and $r_{iB,k}$ at risk on each treatment just before time $\tau_{i,k}$. This variance is also the information for $\theta = \log(\lambda)$ when $\lambda = 1$, so we have

$$\mathcal{I}_k = \widehat{Var}(S_k) = \sum_{i=1}^{d_k} \frac{r_{iA,k}\, r_{iB,k}}{(r_{iA,k} + r_{iB,k})^2}. \tag{3.18}$$

For λ close to unity and, thus, $\theta = \log(\lambda)$ close to zero, we can use the approximation $S_k \sim N(\theta \mathcal{I}_k, \mathcal{I}_k)$, given a sufficiently large $\mathcal{I}_k$. Furthermore, conditional on the observed information sequence $\{\mathcal{I}_1, \ldots, \mathcal{I}_K\}$, the joint distribution of $\{S_1, \ldots, S_K\}$ approximates the standard form for a sequence of score statistics described in Section 3.5.3. Alternatively, defining estimates $\hat{\theta}^{(k)} = S_k/\mathcal{I}_k$ or standardized statistics $Z_k = S_k/\sqrt{\mathcal{I}_k}$, $k = 1, \ldots, K$, yields sequences $\{\hat{\theta}^{(1)}, \ldots, \hat{\theta}^{(K)}\}$ or $\{Z_1, \ldots, Z_K\}$ with the standard joint distributions given in (3.15). Whichever sequence of statistics one chooses to work with, a group sequential test can be developed in the usual way. These joint distributions of sequences of log-rank and associated statistics have been established asymptotically by Harrington, Fleming & Green (1982) and Tsiatis (1982), and their small sample accuracy is demonstrated in simulation studies by Gail, DeMets & Slud (1982); Jennison & Turnbull (1984); DeMets & Gail (1985) and Jennison (1992).

As an illustrative example, consider the design of an O'Brien & Fleming test of H_0: $\lambda = 1$ with five analyses, to achieve two-sided Type I error probability 0.05 and power 0.8 at $\lambda = 1.5$ or 0.667, i.e., at $\theta = \pm 0.405$. Following the general approach laid out in Sections 3.2 and 3.3, we first find the information for θ required by the corresponding fixed sample test:

$$\mathcal{I}_{f,2} = \{\Phi^{-1}(0.975) + \Phi^{-1}(0.8)\}^2/0.405^2 = 47.85.$$

Hence, the target for the final information level is

$$47.85 \times R_B(5, 0.05, 0.2) = 47.85 \times 1.028 = 49.19,$$

where the value 1.028 of $R_B(5, 0.05, 0.2)$ is taken from Table 2.4. The study should therefore be designed to produce observed information levels as close as possible to the values $\mathcal{I}_k = 49.19(k/5)$, $k = 1, \ldots, 5$. In practice, it will be difficult to attain these levels accurately since observed information depends on the realized pattern of deaths and censoring times. However, if the numbers at risk in each treatment group remain nearly equal over time, as is to be expected if λ is close to unity, $r_{iA,k} \approx r_{iB,k}$ for each i, and we can use the approximation $\mathcal{I}_k \approx d_k/4$. Thus, a total of about $4 \times 49.19 \approx 197$ deaths is needed by the end of the study, and the sample size for each treatment arm and study duration should be chosen to achieve this, bearing in mind the likely rates of competing risk and end-of-study censoring.

Implementation of the O'Brien & Fleming test is straightforward. Taking the constant $C_B(5, 0.05) = 2.040$ from Table 2.3, we see that the test should stop to reject H_0 at analysis k if

$$|Z_k| = |S_k/\sqrt{\mathcal{I}_k}| \geq 2.040\sqrt{(5/k)}, \quad k = 1, \ldots, 5,$$

and H_0 is accepted if it has not been rejected by the fifth analysis. As explained in Section 3.3, the Type I error probability will be close to 0.05 as long as the information levels $\mathcal{I}_1, \ldots, \mathcal{I}_5$ are approximately equally spaced, but the attained power depends primarily on the final information level $\mathcal{I}_5$.

When a study's monitoring committee is scheduled to meet at fixed calendar times, it is quite possible that increases in information levels between analyses will be highly uneven. In this case the "error spending" approach (see Chapter 7) offers an attractive alternative to the significance level method we have described here since it yields tests that satisfy the Type I error requirement precisely, conditional on the observed sequence of information levels. We illustrate the application of an error spending test to survival data in Section 7.2.3 and discuss methods for survival endpoints more generally in Chapter 13.

3.8 Group Sequential t-Tests

3.8.1 Implementation

When observations follow a normal linear model, it is usually necessary to estimate the variance, σ^2, as well as the parameter vector $\boldsymbol{\beta}$. In the setting described in Section 3.4, estimates $\widehat{\boldsymbol{\beta}}^{(1)}, \ldots, \widehat{\boldsymbol{\beta}}^{(K)}$ are obtained at analyses 1 to K. Let $\boldsymbol{V}_1, \ldots, \boldsymbol{V}_K$ be such that $Var(\widehat{\boldsymbol{\beta}}^{(k)}) = \boldsymbol{V}_k\sigma^2$ and denote by s_k^2,

$k = 1, \ldots, K$, the usual unbiased estimates of σ^2 which follow $\sigma^2 \chi^2_{n_k - p}/(n_k - p)$ marginal distributions. At each analysis $k = 1, \ldots, K$, the estimate of $\boldsymbol{c}^T \boldsymbol{\beta}$ is

$$\boldsymbol{c}^T \widehat{\boldsymbol{\beta}}^{(k)} \sim N(\boldsymbol{c}^T \boldsymbol{\beta}, \boldsymbol{c}^T \boldsymbol{V}_k \boldsymbol{c} \sigma^2),$$

the Z-statistic for testing H_0: $\boldsymbol{c}^T \boldsymbol{\beta} = \gamma$ when σ^2 is known is

$$Z_k = \frac{\boldsymbol{c}^T \widehat{\boldsymbol{\beta}}^{(k)} - \gamma}{\sqrt{\{\boldsymbol{c}^T \boldsymbol{V}_k \boldsymbol{c} \sigma^2\}}},$$

and the t-statistic for testing H_0 is

$$T_k = \frac{\boldsymbol{c}^T \widehat{\boldsymbol{\beta}}^{(k)} - \gamma}{\sqrt{\{\boldsymbol{c}^T \boldsymbol{V}_k \boldsymbol{c}\, s_k^2\}}}. \tag{3.19}$$

Suppose an experimenter wishes to test the hypothesis H_0: $\boldsymbol{c}^T \boldsymbol{\beta} = \gamma$ in a two-sided group sequential test with Type I error probability α. In adapting one of the known variance tests of Chapter 2 to the unknown variance problem, we follow the approach suggested by Pocock (1977). We take the two-sided significance levels, $2\{1 - \Phi(c_k)\}$, defined for the Z-statistics (here Φ denotes the standard normal cumulative distribution function) but apply these to the t-statistics $T_1, \ldots, T_K$. Since T_k has a marginal $t_{n_k - p}$ distribution, we reject H_0 at analysis k if

$$|T_k| \geq t_{n_k - p, 1 - \Phi(c_k)}, \quad k = 1, \ldots, K,$$

where $t_{\nu,q}$ denotes the upper q tail-point of a t-distribution on ν degrees of freedom, i.e., $Pr\{T > t_{\nu,q}\} = q$ when $T \sim t_\nu$. If H_0 has not been rejected by analysis K, it is accepted.

Here $\{c_1, \ldots, c_K\}$ can be any of the sequences of critical values from Chapter 2. Since these were derived for a sequence of Z-statistics, this form of test satisfies the Type I error requirement only approximately. Nevertheless, investigations have shown that this approximation is remarkably accurate.

Guaranteeing power at a specified value of $\boldsymbol{c}^T \boldsymbol{\beta} - \gamma$ is more difficult since power depends on the unknown value of σ^2, and so one is obliged to design a study choosing group sizes on the basis of an estimated value of σ^2. However, we can find a good approximation to this power for any given value of σ^2 and, hence, check that adequate power will be achieved at a stated alternative $\boldsymbol{c}^T \boldsymbol{\beta} - \gamma = \pm\delta$ if σ^2 lies in some plausible range.

The information for $\boldsymbol{c}^T \boldsymbol{\beta}$ at the final analysis is

$$\{Var(\boldsymbol{c}^T \widehat{\boldsymbol{\beta}}^{(K)})\}^{-1} = (\boldsymbol{c}^T \boldsymbol{V}_K \boldsymbol{c} \sigma^2)^{-1}.$$

By analogy with the case of known variance, we expect the group sequential t-test's power at a given alternative to be approximately that of a fixed sample t-test with $1/R(K, \alpha, \beta)$ times this information for $\boldsymbol{c}^T \boldsymbol{\beta}$, where $R(K, \alpha, \beta)$ is the appropriate sample size factor for the test as tabulated in Chapter 2. Thus, we need to find the power of a fixed sample test with estimator $\widehat{\boldsymbol{\beta}}$ for which

$$Var(\boldsymbol{c}^T \widehat{\boldsymbol{\beta}}) = R(K, \alpha, \beta)\, Var(\boldsymbol{c}^T \widehat{\boldsymbol{\beta}}^{(K)}).$$

If there are $n_K - p$ degrees of freedom to estimate σ^2, the fixed sample test statistic has a t_{n_K-p} distribution under H_0 and when $\boldsymbol{c}^T\boldsymbol{\beta} - \gamma = \delta$ it has a $T(n_K - p; \delta/\sqrt{\{R(K,\alpha,\beta)\, \boldsymbol{c}^T \boldsymbol{V}_K \boldsymbol{c} \sigma^2\}})$ distribution, where $T(\nu; \xi)$ denotes a non-central t-distribution with ν degrees of freedom and non-centrality parameter ξ. The probability of rejecting H_0 with a large, negative t-statistic is negligible when $\boldsymbol{c}^T\boldsymbol{\beta} - \gamma = \delta > 0$. So, this fixed sample test has power

$$Pr\{T(n_K - p; \delta/\sqrt{\{R(K,\alpha,\beta)\, \boldsymbol{c}^T \boldsymbol{V}_K \boldsymbol{c} \sigma^2\}}) \geq t_{n_K-p,1-\alpha/2}\}, \tag{3.20}$$

and this is our approximation to the group sequential t-test's power, when $\boldsymbol{c}^T\boldsymbol{\beta} - \gamma = \delta$ and the variance is σ^2. By symmetry the power at $\boldsymbol{c}^T\boldsymbol{\beta} - \gamma = -\delta$ is the same. If $n_K - p$ is large, we may choose to disregard the error in estimating σ^2, leading to the cruder but simpler estimate of power

$$\Phi\left(\frac{\delta}{\sqrt{\{R(K,\alpha,\beta)\, \boldsymbol{c}^T \boldsymbol{V}_K \boldsymbol{c} \sigma^2\}}} - \Phi^{-1}(1-\alpha/2)\right). \tag{3.21}$$

Since the factor $R(K,\alpha,\beta)$ depends on the power $1-\beta$, which we are in the process of calculating, these definitions appear to be somewhat circular. However, it is evident from Tables 2.2, 2.4 and 2.10 that the factors $R_P(K,\alpha,\beta)$, $R_B(K,\alpha,\beta)$ and $R_{WT}(K,\alpha,\beta)$ vary only slightly with β, and it should suffice to work with a factor appropriate to a plausible value of the power, $1-\beta$. Alternatively, the calculation can be repeated a second time, using the factor R appropriate to the power computed in a first iteration.

Table 3.3 shows the Type I error of group sequential t-tests defined in the above manner and their attained power in situations where formula (3.20) gives the value 0.8. Thus, in each example the value of δ is implicitly determined through the non-centrality parameter in (3.20). Of course, the test cannot be designed to attain power precisely without knowledge of σ^2, but the results do demonstrate the accuracy of (3.20) to assess the power that will be attained under plausible values of σ^2. The two values of ν_K for each combination of type of test and number of groups, K, arise when groups are of 3 and 5 observations, respectively, and two degrees of freedom are lost in fitting model parameters at each analysis. It follows from the general results we shall present in Section 11.4 that the null joint distribution of the sequence of t-statistics, $T_1, \ldots, T_K$, is the same for all tests of H_0: $\boldsymbol{c}^T\boldsymbol{\beta} = \gamma$ with the same error degrees of freedom, $\nu_1, \ldots, \nu_K$, and $(\boldsymbol{c}^T \boldsymbol{V}_k \boldsymbol{c})^{-1} \propto k$, $k = 1, \ldots, K$; hence, the tabulated Type I errors apply with the same generality. Further, the joint distribution of $T_1, \ldots, T_K$ at an alternative $\boldsymbol{c}^T\boldsymbol{\beta} - \gamma = \delta$ depends only on the value of $\delta/\sqrt{\{\boldsymbol{c}^T \boldsymbol{V}_K \boldsymbol{c} \sigma^2\}}$, so the attained powers reported in Table 3.3 also apply to a general class of problems.

Departures from the desired Type I error rates are quite minor and most substantial when the degrees of freedom for σ^2 are low. It is to be expected that the greatest discrepancies should occur for the Pocock tests since these afford the most opportunity for stopping at very early analyses when degrees of freedom may be very low. Note that if a precise Type I error probability is required, a test with a particular boundary shape can be constructed using numerically exact computations: see Sections 11.4 and 19.6.2 and Jennison & Turnbull (1991b). Formula (3.20) provides an accurate estimate of power as long as the degrees of freedom are reasonably high but it does over-estimate power when degrees of

Table 3.3 *Properties of group sequential t-tests designed to test H_0: $c^T\beta = \gamma$ with two-sided Type I error rate $\alpha = 0.05$. Degrees of freedom for σ^2 at analysis k are $\nu_k = (\nu_K + 2)(k/K) - 2$ and $Var(c^T\hat{\beta}^{(k)}) = (K/k)Var(c^T\hat{\beta}^{(K)})$, $k = 1, \ldots, K$. The penultimate column shows actual power at the alternative for which the approximation (3.20) gives power 0.8, and the final column shows the power predicted for each test by formula (3.21).*
Type I error and power were estimated by simulation, using 50000 replicates; standard errors are 0.001 for Type I error and 0.002 for power.

Pocock test

K	ν_K	*Type I error*	*Attained power*	*Known σ^2 power*
3	7	0.060	0.741	0.905
3	13	0.054	0.774	0.858
5	13	0.058	0.760	0.858
5	23	0.054	0.780	0.833
8	22	0.058	0.774	0.834
8	38	0.056	0.786	0.820

O'Brien & Fleming test

K	ν_K	*Type I error*	*Attained power*	*Known σ^2 power*
3	7	0.054	0.793	0.905
3	13	0.052	0.798	0.858
5	13	0.055	0.795	0.858
5	23	0.051	0.797	0.833
8	22	0.055	0.799	0.834
8	38	0.052	0.803	0.820

Wang & Tsiatis test, $\Delta = 0.25$

K	ν_K	*Type I error*	*Attained power*	*Known σ^2 power*
3	7	0.057	0.782	0.905
3	13	0.054	0.794	0.858
5	13	0.056	0.791	0.858
5	23	0.051	0.794	0.833
8	22	0.056	0.793	0.834
8	38	0.052	0.796	0.820

freedom are low. This discrepancy is mainly attributable to the use of ν_K in setting the target information levels, whereas t-tests at early analyses have fewer degrees of freedom than this.

The final column of Table 3.3 shows the approximation to the power obtained using formula (3.21). Not surprisingly, this simpler formula gives good results when degrees of freedom are high but is unreliable when the final degrees of freedom are as low as 10 or 20.

3.8.2 Examples

Two-Treatment Comparison

To illustrate the above methods, consider the two-treatment comparison of Chapter 2 but now with σ^2 unknown. Suppose observations $X_{Ai} \sim N(\mu_A, \sigma^2)$ and $X_{Bi} \sim N(\mu_B, \sigma^2)$, $i = 1, 2, \ldots$, and it is required to test H_0: $\mu_A = \mu_B$ against the two-sided alternative $\mu_A \neq \mu_B$ with Type I error probability $\alpha = 0.01$ using an O'Brien & Fleming test with four groups of observations. Supposing each group contains m observations per treatment, the t-statistics at successive analyses are

$$T_k = \frac{\sum_{i=1}^{mk} X_{Ai} - \sum_{i=1}^{mk} X_{Bi}}{\sqrt{2mks_k^2}}, \quad k = 1, \ldots, 4,$$

where

$$s_k^2 = \frac{\sum_{i=1}^{mk}(X_{Ai} - \bar{X}_A^{(k)})^2 + \sum_{i=1}^{mk}(X_{Bi} - \bar{X}_B^{(k)})^2}{2(mk-1)},$$

$\bar{X}_A^{(k)}$ and $\bar{X}_B^{(k)}$ denoting the means of $X_{A1}, \ldots, X_{A,mk}$ and $X_{B1}, \ldots, X_{B,mk}$, respectively. From Table 2.3, $C_B(4, 0.01) = 2.609$, so $c_k = 2.609\sqrt{(4/k)} = 5.218/\sqrt{k}$, $k = 1, \ldots, 4$. Thus, the O'Brien & Fleming test applies two-sided significance levels $2\{1 - \Phi(5.218/\sqrt{k})\}$ at analyses $k = 1, \ldots, 4$, and the group sequential t-test rejects H_0 at analysis k if

$$|T_k| \geq t_{2mk-2, 1-\Phi(5.218\, k^{-1/2})}, \quad k = 1, \ldots, 4,$$

and accepts H_0 if it has not been rejected by the fourth analysis.

By design, this test's Type I error probability will be close to 0.01, but its power depends on m and the unknown σ^2. Suppose our experimental resources make a total of 64 observations a convenient sample size so we could take $m = 8$ observations per treatment in each group, giving a total of 32 observations on each treatment at the final analysis when the variance of $\hat{\mu}_A - \hat{\mu}_B$ would be $\sigma^2/16$. In using the approximation (3.20), $\delta = \mu_A - \mu_B$ but σ^2 is unknown, so we can only evaluate power at given values of the ratio $(\mu_A - \mu_B)/\sigma$. For instance, power is approximately

$$Pr\{T(62; \sqrt{\{16/1.01\}}) \geq t_{62, 0.995}\} = 0.903$$

when $\mu_A - \mu_B = \pm\sigma$. Here, we have used $R_B(4, 0.01, 0.1) = 1.010$ since an initial calculation with $R = 1$ showed power to be approximately 0.9. Simulations show these approximate error probabilities to be highly accurate: based on one million simulations, estimates of Type I error and power at $\theta = \sigma$ are 0.0101 and 0.9021, respectively, with standard errors 0.0001 and 0.0003. In judging whether power close to 0.9 when $\mu_A - \mu_B = \pm\sigma$ is acceptable we have to consider likely values of σ^2 or, if acting cautiously, an upper bound for σ^2. If we do regard this power as acceptable, the experiment can be conducted with $m = 8$. If not, power should be re-evaluated under other values of m until a suitable group size is found.

A more direct approach to sample size calculation is possible if a reliable initial estimate of σ^2, σ_0^2 say, is available. Formula (3.21) provides a good approximation to the sample size required to meet the stipulated power condition when $\sigma^2 = \sigma_0^2$ and the adequacy of this sample size can then be checked using the more accurate formula (3.20) and adjustments made if necessary. The calculation based on (3.21) is really just the sample size calculation for a Z-test when σ^2 is known to be equal to σ_0^2 and reduces to the condition

$$\begin{aligned}(\boldsymbol{c}^T \boldsymbol{V}_k \boldsymbol{c}\sigma_0^2)^{-1} &= R(K,\alpha,\beta)\,\{\Phi^{-1}(1-\alpha/2)+\Phi^{-1}(1-\beta)\}^2/\delta^2 \\ &= R(K,\alpha,\beta)\,\mathcal{I}_{f,2}.\end{aligned}$$

Two-Treatment Comparison Adjusted for Covariates

We are now able to re-visit the second example of Section 3.4.2, where previously we assumed σ^2 to be known. Continuing in our earlier notation, the goal in this example is to test the null hypothesis of no treatment effect, H_0: $\beta_1 = 0$, with Type I error $\alpha = 0.05$ using an O'Brien & Fleming test with six analyses; it is also desired that the test should have power 0.8 to reject H_0 if $\beta_1 = \pm 0.5$. Estimates

$$\hat{\beta}_1^{(k)} \sim N(\beta_1, \{(\boldsymbol{D}^{(k)T}\boldsymbol{D}^{(k)})^{-1}\}_{11}\sigma^2)$$

are available and the t-statistics at successive analyses are

$$T_k = \frac{\hat{\beta}_1^{(k)}}{\surd[\{(\boldsymbol{D}^{(k)T}\boldsymbol{D}^{(k)})^{-1}\}_{11}s_k^2]}, \quad k = 1,\ldots,6,$$

where

$$\begin{aligned}s_k^2 &= (\boldsymbol{X}^{(k)} - \boldsymbol{D}^{(k)}\widehat{\boldsymbol{\beta}}^{(k)})^T(\boldsymbol{X}^{(k)} - \boldsymbol{D}^{(k)}\widehat{\boldsymbol{\beta}}^{(k)})/(n_k - p) \\ &\sim \sigma^2\chi^2_{n_k-p}/(n_k - p), \quad k = 1,\ldots,6.\end{aligned}$$

Table 2.3 gives $C_B(6, 0.05) = 2.503$. Hence,

$$c_k = 2.503\surd(6/k) = 6.131/\surd k, \quad k = 1,\ldots,6,$$

so the O'Brien & Fleming test applies the two-sided significance levels $2(1 - \Phi(6.131/\surd k))$ at analyses $k = 1,\ldots,6$. Comparing the sequence of t-statistics against these significance levels gives the rule for the group sequential t-test: reject H_0 at analysis k if

$$|T_k| \geq t_{n_k-p,1-\Phi(6.131\,k^{-1/2})}, \quad k = 1,\ldots,6,$$

and accept H_0 if it has not been rejected by the sixth analysis.

The power of this test depends primarily on the sequence of values of $Var(\hat{\beta}_1^{(k)})$, which in turn depend on the unknown variance σ^2. If, as before, we believe 1.2 to be a plausible value for σ^2, we can use the sample size that satisfies the power condition in a known variance test for $\sigma^2 = 1.2$ as a starting point for designing a group sequential t-test. We noted in Section 3.4.2 that, if treatment allocation is well balanced with respect to covariates,

$$Var(\hat{\beta}_1^{(k)}) \approx 4\sigma^2/n_k, \quad k = 1, \ldots, 6,$$

where n_k is the number of patients, divided equally between treatments A and B, at analysis k. Under this assumption, the known variance test for $\sigma^2 = 1.2$ requires

$$\begin{aligned} \left(\frac{4 \times 1.2}{n_6}\right)^{-1} &= R_B(6, 0.05, 0.2) \{\Phi^{-1}(0.975) + \Phi^{-1}(0.8)\}^2/0.5^2 \\ &= 1.032 \times (1.960 + 0.842)^2/0.5^2 = 32.41, \end{aligned}$$

which is achieved by setting $n_k = 26k$, $k = 1, \ldots, 6$, to give a final sample size $n_6 = 156$. In this case,

$$Var(\hat{\beta}_1^{(6)}) \approx 4\sigma^2/156 = \sigma^2/39.$$

Suppose also that $p = 6$, representing one parameter for the treatment effect and five for covariate terms. Then, using $R_B(6, 0.05, 0.2) = 1.032$ for the sample size factor in formula (3.20), we obtain the approximate power at $\beta_1 = \pm 0.5$:

$$Pr\{T(156 - 6; 0.5/\sqrt{\{1.032\sigma^2/39\}}) \geq t_{156-6,0.975}\}.$$

With $\sigma^2 = 1.2$, this expression is 0.796, admirably close to the target of 0.8. However, the power varies steadily with σ^2, the same formula giving power 0.86 for $\sigma^2 = 1.0$ but only 0.70 if $\sigma^2 = 1.5$. Thus, if σ^2 is unknown, one should consider power under a range of plausible values of σ^2 when choosing sample size, and bear in mind that only the power under the largest plausible value of σ^2 is guaranteed with any certainty.

One way to try and achieve specified power at a given alternative when σ^2 is unknown is to re-compute sample size as the study progresses, using current variance estimates. In Chapter 14 we shall discuss methods of this type for producing a single test on termination or a concurrent group sequential test.

CHAPTER 4

One-Sided Tests

4.1 Introduction

The name *one-sided test* is given to a test of a hypothesis against a one-sided alternative, for example, a test of the null hypothesis H_0: $\theta = 0$ against the alternative H_A: $\theta > 0$. If a fixed sample test based on a statistic Z rejects H_0 when $Z > c$, for some constant c, the test's Type I error probability is

$$Pr_{\theta=0}\{Z > c\},$$

and its power is the probability of rejecting H_0 under values of θ in the alternative hypothesis, i.e., $Pr_\theta\{Z > c\}$ for values $\theta > 0$.

In some problems, a one-sided alternative is appropriate because departures from H_0 in the other direction are either implausible or impossible. In other cases, θ may lie on either side of H_0 but the alternative is chosen in the one direction in which departures from H_0 are of interest. Suppose θ measures the improvement in response achieved by a new treatment over a standard, and the new treatment will only be deemed acceptable if it produces superior responses; then the main aim of a study will be to distinguish between the cases $\theta \leq 0$ and $\theta > 0$. However, the probability of deciding in favor of the new treatment when $\theta \leq 0$ is greatest at $\theta = 0$, so it suffices to specify the Type I error at $\theta = 0$. It matters little whether one regards the null hypothesis in such a study as $\theta \leq 0$ or $\theta = 0$. We adopt the latter formulation and so discuss tests of H_0: $\theta = 0$ against H_A: $\theta > 0$ designed to achieve Type I error probability α when $\theta = 0$ and power $1 - \beta$ at a specified alternative value $\theta = \delta$ where $\delta > 0$.

We shall present group sequential one-sided tests for a parameter θ when standardized statistics $Z_1, \ldots, Z_K$ available at analyses $k = 1, \ldots, K$ follow the canonical joint distribution (3.1). In particular $Z_k \sim N(\theta\sqrt{\mathcal{I}_k}, 1)$, where $\mathcal{I}_k$ is the information for θ at analysis k. As explained in Chapter 3, this joint distribution arises, sometimes approximately, in a great many applications. The group sequential one-sided tests we shall define are directly applicable to all these situations.

A fixed sample test based on a statistic Z distributed as $N(\theta\sqrt{\mathcal{I}}, 1)$ attains Type I error probability α by rejecting H_0 if $Z > \Phi^{-1}(1-\alpha)$. Hence, in order to attain power $1 - \beta$ when $\theta = \delta$, the sample size must be chosen to give an information level

$$\mathcal{I}_{f,1} = \{\Phi^{-1}(1-\alpha) + \Phi^{-1}(1-\beta)\}^2/\delta^2, \tag{4.1}$$

the subscript 1 in $\mathcal{I}_{f,1}$ denoting a one-sided test. As before, Φ denotes the standard normal cdf. As for two-sided tests, we shall express the maximum and expected information levels of group sequential one-sided tests as multiples of the fixed sample information level, $\mathcal{I}_{f,1}$.

After the impact of the two-sided group sequential tests of Pocock (1977) and of O'Brien & Fleming (1979), proposals for one-sided group sequential tests soon followed. DeMets & Ware (1980 and 1982) presented tests adapted from Pocock and O'Brien & Fleming two-sided tests and from Wald's (1947) sequential probability ratio test. Subsequently, Jennison (1987) and Eales & Jennison (1992) explored the extent of possible reductions in expected sample size by searching for optimal group sequential one-sided tests. We shall concentrate in this chapter on two types of group sequential one-sided test, the first a family of tests with boundaries of a certain parametric form and the second an adaptation, due to Whitehead & Stratton (1983), of a fully sequential test referred to by Lorden (1976) as a "2-SPRT".

In Section 4.2 we describe the parametric family of tests proposed by Emerson & Fleming (1989) and extended by Pampallona & Tsiatis (1994) to include asymmetric tests with unequal Type I and Type II error probabilities. Tests in the family are indexed by a parameter Δ that appears as a power in the formulae for their stopping boundaries, and we shall refer to this as the *power family* of group sequential one-sided tests. As Δ is increased, tests allow greater opportunity for early stopping, resulting in lower expected sample size, but the maximum sample size also increases. We provide tables of properties of a range of tests in the power family to guide selection of an appropriate test, bearing in mind the effort of more frequent monitoring or the increase in maximum sample size that accompanies reductions in expected study length.

Although they are designed for a specific sequence of information levels, the power family tests can still be used when observed information levels differ from their planned values. In Section 4.3 we present a way of doing this which maintains Type I error rates quite accurately. Similar reasoning enables us to construct group sequential, one-sided t-tests from the power family tests, and we describe this construction in Section 4.4. The group sequential t-tests maintain a specified Type I error probability to a high degree of accuracy; just as for the two-sided tests of Section 3.8, power at a given value of θ depends on the actual value of σ^2 and thus, for this form of test, power should be assessed under a range of plausible values of σ^2 when determining an appropriate sample size.

Returning to the case of known variance, in Section 4.5 we describe the method proposed by Whitehead & Stratton (1983) and developed further by Whitehead (1997, Chapter 4). This easily implemented test maintains specified Type I error and power to quite a high accuracy for general sequences of observed information levels. The mathematical approximation which underlies these results applies only to tests with straight line boundaries on the score statistic scale and so cannot be used to adapt the power family of one-sided tests to general sequences of information levels. Later, in Section 7.3, we shall see an alternative strategy based on "error spending" functions which does provide a family of group sequential tests qualitatively similar to the power family but able to handle general information sequences.

4.2 The Power Family of One-Sided Group Sequential Tests

4.2.1 *Definition of the Tests*

Consider a group sequential study in which statistics Z_k observed at analyses $k = 1, \dots, K$ follow the canonical joint distribution (3.1). Suppose we wish to test H_0: $\theta = 0$ against H_A: $\theta > 0$ with Type I error probability α and power $1 - \beta$ at $\theta = \delta$. A general one-sided group sequential test is defined by pairs of constants (a_k, b_k) with $a_k < b_k$ for $k = 1, \dots, K-1$ and $a_K = b_K$. It takes the form:

$$\begin{array}{lll} \text{After group } k = 1, \dots, K-1 & & \\ & \text{if } Z_k \geq b_k & \text{stop, reject } H_0 \\ & \text{if } Z_k \leq a_k & \text{stop, accept } H_0 \\ & \text{otherwise} & \text{continue to group } k+1, \\ \text{after group } K & & \\ & \text{if } Z_K \geq b_K & \text{stop, reject } H_0 \\ & \text{if } Z_K < a_K & \text{stop, accept } H_0. \end{array} \tag{4.2}$$

Here, $a_K = b_K$ ensures that the test terminates at analysis K.

Tests in the power family are designed for equally spaced increments in information, i.e., $\mathcal{I}_k = (k/K)\mathcal{I}_K$, $k = 1, \dots, K$. For the test with parameter Δ, critical values are

$$\begin{aligned} b_k &= \tilde{C}_1(K, \alpha, \beta, \Delta)(k/K)^{\Delta - 1/2} \quad \text{and} \\ a_k &= \delta\sqrt{\mathcal{I}_k} - \tilde{C}_2(K, \alpha, \beta, \Delta)(k/K)^{\Delta - 1/2}, \quad k = 1, \dots, K. \end{aligned} \tag{4.3}$$

In order that $a_K = b_K$, the final information level must be

$$\mathcal{I}_K = \frac{\{\tilde{C}_1(K, \alpha, \beta, \Delta) + \tilde{C}_2(K, \alpha, \beta, \Delta)\}^2}{\delta^2}. \tag{4.4}$$

The constants $\tilde{C}_1(K, \alpha, \beta, \Delta)$ and $\tilde{C}_2(K, \alpha, \beta, \Delta)$, which do not depend on δ, are chosen to ensure the Type I error and power conditions.

There is a similarity between these tests and the Wang & Tsiatis tests presented in Section 2.7.1. The upper boundary can be viewed as a repeated significance test of $\theta = 0$ with critical values for the Z_k proportional to $k^{\Delta - 1/2}$, $k = 1, \dots, K$, while the lower boundary arises as a repeated significance test of $\theta = \delta$, this hypothesis being rejected if $Z_k - \delta\sqrt{\mathcal{I}_k}$, the standardized statistic with mean zero if $\theta = \delta$, is negative and less than a critical value proportional to $k^{\Delta - 1/2}$.

From equations (4.1) and (4.4), we see that the ratio of the test's maximum information level to that required for a fixed sample test is

$$\tilde{R}(K, \alpha, \beta, \Delta) = \frac{\mathcal{I}_K}{\mathcal{I}_{f,1}} = \frac{\{\tilde{C}_1(K, \alpha, \beta, \Delta) + \tilde{C}_2(K, \alpha, \beta, \Delta)\}^2}{\{\Phi^{-1}(1-\alpha) + \Phi^{-1}(1-\beta)\}^2}.$$

Values of $\tilde{C}_1(K, \alpha, \beta, \Delta)$, $\tilde{C}_2(K, \alpha, \beta, \Delta)$ and $\tilde{R}(K, \alpha, \beta, \Delta)$, and certain properties of the tests are provided in Tables 4.1, 4.2 and 4.3 for $\Delta = -0.5, -0.25$, 0 and 0.25, $\alpha = 0.05$ and $\beta = 0.8$, 0.9 and 0.95. Entries in these tables were computed numerically using the methods described in Chapter 19. Interpolation

Table 4.1 *Constants* $\tilde{C}_1(K, \alpha, \beta, \Delta)$, $\tilde{C}_2(K, \alpha, \beta, \Delta)$ *and* $\tilde{R}(K, \alpha, \beta, \Delta)$ *for power family one-sided tests with shape parameter* Δ. *Also shown are expected sample sizes at* $\theta = 0$, $\delta/2$ *and* δ *expressed as percentages of the corresponding fixed sample size. Tests are for K groups of observations, Type I error probability* $\alpha = 0.05$ *at* $\theta = 0$ *and power* $1 - \beta = 0.8$ *at* $\theta = \delta$.

	K	$\tilde{C}_1$	$\tilde{C}_2$	$\tilde{R}$	*Expected sample size, as percentage of fixed sample size, at* $\theta=0$	$\theta=\delta/2$	$\theta=\delta$
$\Delta = -0.5$							
	1	1.645	0.842	1.000	100.0	100.0	100.0
	2	1.632	0.870	1.012	75.3	90.9	95.7
	3	1.622	0.899	1.028	72.8	86.4	87.5
	4	1.621	0.916	1.041	69.0	83.5	84.9
	5	1.622	0.927	1.051	67.0	82.0	83.0
	10	1.628	0.956	1.080	63.8	78.9	79.6
	15	1.632	0.970	1.095	62.8	78.0	78.5
	20	1.635	0.978	1.104	62.4	77.5	78.0
$\Delta = -0.25$							
	1	1.645	0.842	1.000	100.0	100.0	100.0
	2	1.623	0.901	1.031	71.7	87.7	90.9
	3	1.625	0.928	1.055	67.7	83.3	84.7
	4	1.629	0.947	1.073	65.4	80.9	81.6
	5	1.633	0.960	1.087	63.5	79.3	79.9
	10	1.646	0.993	1.127	60.1	76.2	76.5
	15	1.653	1.009	1.146	59.0	75.2	75.5
	20	1.658	1.018	1.158	58.5	74.8	74.9
$\Delta = 0.0$							
	1	1.645	0.842	1.000	100.0	100.0	100.0
	2	1.634	0.942	1.073	69.9	84.9	85.6
	3	1.645	0.978	1.113	63.4	80.2	80.9
	4	1.656	0.999	1.140	60.8	77.8	78.0
	5	1.664	1.015	1.161	59.2	76.3	76.2
	10	1.688	1.057	1.219	55.8	73.2	72.8
	15	1.700	1.076	1.247	54.7	72.1	71.7
	20	1.708	1.088	1.264	54.1	71.6	71.1
$\Delta = 0.25$							
	1	1.645	0.842	1.000	100.0	100.0	100.0
	2	1.688	0.990	1.160	70.5	83.9	82.7
	3	1.720	1.054	1.245	61.9	78.5	77.2
	4	1.741	1.093	1.299	58.0	75.8	74.4
	5	1.757	1.119	1.338	55.9	74.1	72.6
	10	1.802	1.185	1.443	51.7	70.6	68.8
	15	1.823	1.215	1.493	50.3	69.3	67.5
	20	1.837	1.233	1.524	49.5	68.7	66.8

Table 4.2 *Constants* $\tilde{C}_1(K, \alpha, \beta, \Delta)$, $\tilde{C}_2(K, \alpha, \beta, \Delta)$ *and* $\tilde{R}(K, \alpha, \beta, \Delta)$ *for power family one-sided tests with shape parameter* Δ. *Also shown are expected sample sizes at* $\theta = 0$, $\delta/2$ *and* δ *expressed as percentages of the corresponding fixed sample size. Tests are for K groups of observations, Type I error probability* $\alpha = 0.05$ *at* $\theta = 0$ *and power* $1 - \beta = 0.9$ *at* $\theta = \delta$.

	K	$\tilde{C}_1$	$\tilde{C}_2$	$\tilde{R}$	*Expected sample size, as percentage of fixed sample size, at* $\theta=0$	$\theta=\delta/2$	$\theta=\delta$
$\Delta = -0.5$							
	1	1.645	1.282	1.000	100.0	100.0	100.0
	2	1.643	1.286	1.002	84.7	96.4	94.3
	3	1.643	1.302	1.012	77.8	90.1	84.3
	4	1.645	1.312	1.021	73.9	87.5	81.6
	5	1.648	1.320	1.029	72.3	85.9	79.6
	10	1.660	1.342	1.052	68.7	82.7	76.0
	15	1.667	1.353	1.065	67.6	81.7	74.9
	20	1.671	1.360	1.073	67.1	81.2	74.3
$\Delta = -0.25$							
	1	1.645	1.282	1.000	100.0	100.0	100.0
	2	1.643	1.300	1.011	77.8	92.6	87.9
	3	1.650	1.320	1.030	73.9	87.5	81.3
	4	1.656	1.334	1.044	70.2	84.7	77.7
	5	1.662	1.344	1.055	68.2	83.2	76.0
	10	1.681	1.371	1.087	64.8	80.1	72.5
	15	1.690	1.384	1.104	63.7	79.1	71.4
	20	1.696	1.392	1.114	63.2	78.6	70.9
$\Delta = 0.0$							
	1	1.645	1.282	1.000	100.0	100.0	100.0
	2	1.657	1.332	1.043	73.0	88.5	81.4
	3	1.673	1.357	1.072	68.2	84.2	76.7
	4	1.686	1.375	1.094	65.6	81.7	73.7
	5	1.696	1.389	1.111	63.8	80.1	71.8
	10	1.725	1.425	1.158	60.1	77.0	68.2
	15	1.739	1.442	1.181	59.0	75.9	67.1
	20	1.747	1.452	1.195	58.4	75.4	66.5
$\Delta = 0.25$							
	1	1.645	1.282	1.000	100.0	100.0	100.0
	2	1.710	1.389	1.121	71.4	86.2	77.8
	3	1.746	1.438	1.184	64.2	81.4	72.0
	4	1.770	1.469	1.225	61.0	79.0	69.1
	5	1.788	1.490	1.255	59.1	77.4	67.3
	10	1.836	1.546	1.336	55.2	74.1	63.5
	15	1.860	1.572	1.375	53.9	72.9	62.2
	20	1.874	1.588	1.400	53.2	72.3	61.5

Table 4.3 *Constants* $\tilde{C}_1(K, \alpha, \beta, \Delta)$, $\tilde{C}_2(K, \alpha, \beta, \Delta)$ *and* $\tilde{R}(K, \alpha, \beta, \Delta)$ *for power family one-sided tests with shape parameter* Δ. *Also shown are expected sample sizes at* $\theta = 0$, $\delta/2$ *and* δ *expressed as percentages of the corresponding fixed sample size. Tests are for K groups of observations, Type I error probability* $\alpha = 0.05$ *at* $\theta = 0$ *and power* $1 - \beta = 0.95$ *at* $\theta = \delta$.

	K	$\tilde{C}_1$	$\tilde{C}_2$	$\tilde{R}$	*Expected sample size, as percentage of fixed sample size, at*		
					$\theta=0$	$\theta=\delta/2$	$\theta=\delta$
$\Delta = -0.5$							
	1	1.645	1.645	1.000	100.0	100.0	100.0
	2	1.645	1.645	1.000	91.6	98.4	91.6
	3	1.650	1.650	1.006	80.7	91.9	80.7
	4	1.656	1.656	1.013	77.9	89.4	77.9
	5	1.661	1.661	1.019	75.8	87.7	75.8
	10	1.676	1.676	1.039	72.0	84.4	72.0
	15	1.685	1.685	1.049	70.9	83.3	70.9
	20	1.690	1.690	1.056	70.3	82.8	70.3
$\Delta = -0.25$							
	1	1.645	1.645	1.000	100.0	100.0	100.0
	2	1.649	1.649	1.005	83.8	95.1	83.8
	3	1.661	1.661	1.020	77.5	89.2	77.5
	4	1.670	1.670	1.031	73.5	86.6	73.5
	5	1.677	1.677	1.040	71.7	85.0	71.7
	10	1.699	1.699	1.067	68.1	81.8	68.1
	15	1.710	1.710	1.081	67.0	80.8	67.0
	20	1.717	1.717	1.090	66.4	80.3	66.4
$\Delta = 0.0$							
	1	1.645	1.645	1.000	100.0	100.0	100.0
	2	1.668	1.668	1.028	76.6	90.5	76.6
	3	1.687	1.687	1.052	72.2	86.0	72.2
	4	1.702	1.702	1.071	69.0	83.4	69.0
	5	1.713	1.713	1.085	67.0	81.8	67.0
	10	1.745	1.745	1.125	63.3	78.7	63.3
	15	1.760	1.760	1.145	62.2	77.6	62.2
	20	1.770	1.770	1.158	61.6	77.1	61.6
$\Delta = 0.25$							
	1	1.645	1.645	1.000	100.0	100.0	100.0
	2	1.722	1.722	1.097	72.9	87.4	72.9
	3	1.762	1.762	1.147	66.6	82.9	66.6
	4	1.787	1.787	1.181	63.6	80.4	63.6
	5	1.806	1.806	1.206	61.8	78.9	61.8
	10	1.857	1.857	1.274	58.0	75.6	58.0
	15	1.881	1.881	1.307	56.6	74.4	56.6
	20	1.896	1.896	1.328	56.0	73.9	56.0

may be used to obtain constants for values of $K < 20$ not present in these tables. Constants for other cases can be found in Emerson & Fleming (1989) for $\Delta = 0$, 0.1, 0.2, 0.3, 0.4 and 0.5 and $\alpha = \beta = 0.05$ and 0.01, and in Pampallona & Tsiatis (1994) for the same Δ and α values and $\beta = 0.8$, 0.9 and 0.95.

We have defined tests in terms of the standardized statistics $Z_1, \ldots, Z_K$. Emerson & Fleming and Pampallona & Tsiatis define the same tests in terms of the score statistics $S_k = Z_k\sqrt{\mathcal{I}_k}$, $k = 1, \ldots, K$, (see Section 3.5.3) and their $C_j(K, \alpha, \beta, \Delta)$ are, therefore, $K^{1/2-\Delta}$ times our $\tilde{C}_j(K, \alpha, \beta, \Delta)$, $j = 1$ and 2. We have expressed tests in terms of the Z_k for several reasons. First, the $\tilde{C}_j(K, \alpha, \beta, \Delta)$ vary slowly with K, facilitating the use of interpolation for values of K omitted from our tables. Second, the $\tilde{C}_j(K, \alpha, \beta, \Delta)$ play a specific role in the final analysis if the test reaches that stage: H_0 is rejected if Z_K, a standard normal variable under $\theta = 0$, exceeds $\tilde{C}_1(K, \alpha, \beta, \Delta)$ and H_0 is accepted if $Z_K - \delta\sqrt{\mathcal{I}_K}$, a standard normal variable under $\theta = \delta$, is less than $-\tilde{C}_2(K, \alpha, \beta, \Delta)$. Third, our definition of the test is easily adapted to give the method we recommend for dealing with departures from planned sequences of information levels.

Figure 4.1 shows boundaries of two power family tests with four groups of observations, expressed on both the Z_k and S_k scales. Both tests have Type I error probability $\alpha = 0.05$ under the null hypothesis, $\theta = 0$, and power $1 - \beta = 0.9$ at $\theta = \delta = 0.2$. The tests have parameter values $\Delta = 0.0$ and $\Delta = -0.5$ and, since $\tilde{R}(K, \alpha, \beta, \Delta)$ increases with Δ, the required information levels are greater for the test with $\Delta = 0.0$. For comparison, the corresponding fixed sample test requires information $\mathcal{I}_{f,1} = \{(1.282 + 1.645)/0.2\}^2 = 214.1$.

4.2.2 Properties of Power Family Tests

We have calculated the maximum information level and the expected amount of information on termination for a number of power family tests. As we saw for two-sided tests in Chapters 2 and 3, the ratios of these quantities to the information required for a fixed sample test with the same error probabilities are invariant to the value of δ. When information is proportional to the number of subjects observed, these ratios also represent a group sequential test's maximum and expected sample sizes expressed as fractions of the corresponding fixed sample size. We shall follow the practice of other authors and refer to sample size when discussing properties of group sequential tests. We note, however, that our results really concern information rather than sample size when the two are not directly proportional.

It is evident from Tables 4.1, 4.2 and 4.3 that, for a fixed Δ, the maximum sample size of a group sequential test, determined by $\tilde{R}(K, \alpha, \beta, \Delta)$, increases with the number of analyses, while its expected sample sizes at $\theta = 0$, $\delta/2$ and δ decrease. Only minor reductions in expected sample size are gained by increasing the number of analyses, K, beyond 5 or 10, and we would expect these values of K to be sufficient in most instances.

Larger values of Δ also increase the maximum sample size and decrease expected sample sizes. We commented in Section 2.6.3 on the significance of

Figure 4.1 *Two power family one-sided tests for four groups of observations*

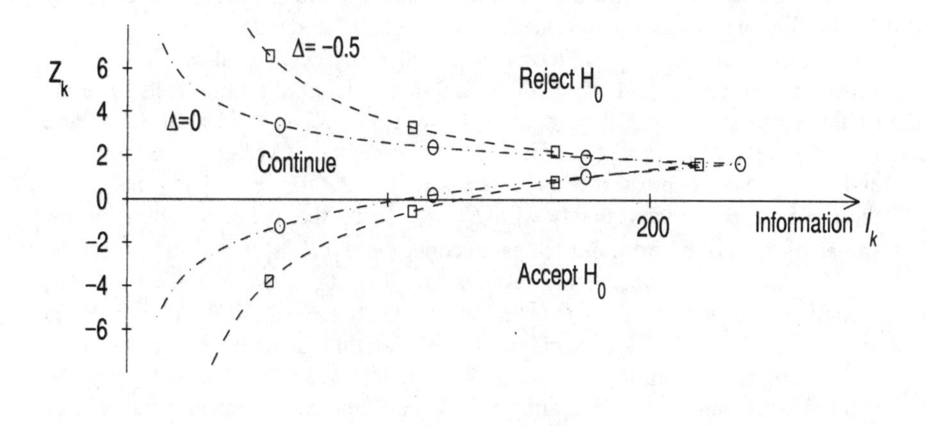

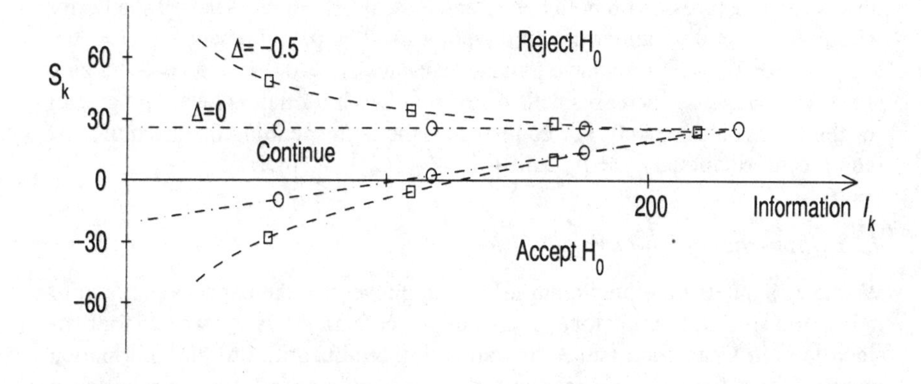

maximum sample size, noting that an experimenter might be deterred by a group sequential design that could require substantially more observations than a fixed sample experiment. The four values of Δ in our tables offer a range of options for balancing savings in expected sample size against higher maximum sample sizes. Although Emerson & Fleming and Pampallona & Tsiatis did not consider tests with negative values of Δ, our results show that such tests offer substantial reductions in expected sample size with maximum sample size just a little greater than that of the fixed sample test. Maximum sample size increases rapidly if Δ is increased beyond 0.25, with only minor reductions, if that, in expected sample sizes: as an example, for $\alpha = 0.05$, $1 - \beta = 0.8$, $K = 10$ and $\Delta = 0.5$, the maximum sample size is 2.13 times the fixed sample size while expected sample sizes at $\theta = 0$, $\delta/2$ and δ are 50.9%, 73.1% and 68.5%, respectively, of the fixed sample size.

It is useful to know just how small the expected sample size of a group

Table 4.4 *Minimum possible expected sample sizes for group sequential one-sided tests with error probabilities* $\alpha = 0.05$ *at* $\theta = 0$ *and* $\theta = \delta$*,* K *equally sized groups, and maximum sample size equal to* t *times the corresponding fixed sample size. Tabulated values are the minimum expected sample sizes at the stated* θ *expressed as a percentage of the fixed sample size. Tests are symmetric about* $\theta = \delta/2$*, so expected sample sizes at* $\theta = 0$ *and* δ *are equal. Note that different tests are used to minimise* $E_{\theta=\delta/2}(N)$ *and* $E_{\theta=0}(N) = E_{\theta=\delta}(N)$.

$E_{\theta=0}(N)$ or $E_{\theta=\delta}E(N)$

				t			
K	1.01	1.05	1.1	1.15	1.2	1.3	*minimum over t*
2	80.9	74.5	72.8	72.7	73.2	75.3	72.7 at $t = 1.15$
5	72.2	65.2	62.2	60.7	59.8	59.0	58.7 at $t = 1.4$
10	69.1	62.1	59.0	57.4	56.3	55.2	54.3 at $t = 1.6$
20	67.6	60.5	57.4	55.7	54.6	53.3	52.0 at $t = 1.6$

$E_{\theta=\delta/2}(N)$

				t			
K	1.01	1.05	1.1	1.15	1.2	1.3	*minimum over t*
2	93.4	88.9	87.3	87.0	87.2	88.3	87.0 at $t = 1.15$
5	87.9	82.5	80.2	79.1	78.6	78.4	78.4 at $t = 1.3$
10	85.7	80.0	77.5	76.2	75.6	75.0	74.9 at $t = 1.4$
20	84.5	78.7	76.1	74.8	74.0	73.3	73.1 at $t = 1.4$

sequential test can be. Table 4.4 gives a summary of the results of Eales & Jennison (1992) concerning optimal group sequential tests. In our notation, these results are for group sequential one-sided tests with Type I and Type II error probabilities $\alpha = \beta = 0.05$ at $\theta = 0$ and $\theta = \delta$, respectively. The table shows the minimum possible expected sample sizes at the stated θ values subject to a fixed number, K, of equally spaced analyses and a fixed maximum sample size equal to t times the corresponding fixed sample size. In view of the problem's symmetry, this minimization is over tests which are symmetric about $\theta = \delta/2$. A different testing boundary is used to minimize $E_\theta(N)$ at each value of θ, so one should not necessarily expect a single test to be close to optimal at several θ values. In each row of the table, minimum values decrease initially as t increases and then, eventually, increase again. The final column shows the smallest minimum expected sample size for each row over the eleven values of t appearing in Eales & Jennison's Table 1.

It is clear from Table 4.4 that substantial reductions in expected sample size can be achieved by tests with maximum sample size only a little greater than the fixed sample size. It is for this reason that we investigated power family tests with the negative values of Δ that lead to lower maximum sample sizes. Direct comparisons can be made between Table 4.4 and the results in Table 4.3 for power family tests with $\alpha = \beta = 0.05$. The power family tests are seen to be quite efficient, for their maximum sample sizes, in reducing expected sample size both at $\theta = 0$ or δ and at $\theta = \delta/2$, although they do fall a few percentage points short of optimality. As an example, the test with $K = 10$ and $\Delta = 0.0$ has maximum sample size a little above $t = 1.1$ times the fixed sample size, and its expected sample sizes at $\theta = 0$ or δ and at $\theta = \delta/2$ are, respectively, 4.3 and 1.2 greater (in the units of the table) than the lowest possible values for $t = 1.1$. We shall see in Section 7.3 and Tables 7.7 to 7.9 that some improvement on power family tests is obtained by another family of group sequential one-sided tests defined through an error spending function.

At first sight, these remarks appear to be at odds with the comment of Emerson & Fleming (1989, p. 913) that the power family tests are 99% efficient at $\theta = 0$ or δ relative to the set of all possible symmetric group sequential tests. The explanation is that Emerson & Fleming's remark refers to the minimum expected sample size at $\theta = 0$ or δ over *all* values of the parameter Δ with no constraint on the maximum sample size, whereas we have drawn comparisons between tests with (roughly) equal maximum sample sizes.

Notwithstanding these comparisons with "optimal" benchmarks and error spending tests, the power family provides a selection of easily implemented, group sequential designs within which an experimenter should have no trouble in finding a suitable test for a particular problem.

4.3 Adapting Power Family Tests to Unequal Increments in Information

4.3.1 *A Method Which Protects Type I Error*

Although the power family tests are designed for the specific sequence of information levels $\mathcal{I}_k = (k/K)\,\tilde{R}(K, \alpha, \beta, \Delta)\,\mathcal{I}_{f,1}$, $k = 1, \ldots, K$, they may still be applied for other observed information levels, but error probabilities will then differ from their intended values. One could simply apply the stopping rule (4.2) with critical values a_k and b_k obtained by substituting the observed information levels $\mathcal{I}_1, \ldots, \mathcal{I}_K$ into (4.3). However, we recommend the following alternative approach which is more successful in maintaining the specified Type I error rate, α.

Note that if equal increments in information occur between analyses, a_k and b_k can be written without explicit mention of $\mathcal{I}_k$ as

$$\begin{aligned} b_k &= \tilde{C}_1(K, \alpha, \beta, \Delta)(k/K)^{\Delta - 1/2} \quad \text{and} \\ a_k &= \{\tilde{C}_1(K, \alpha, \beta, \Delta) + \tilde{C}_2(K, \alpha, \beta, \Delta)\}(k/K)^{1/2} \\ &\quad - \tilde{C}_2(K, \alpha, \beta, \Delta)(k/K)^{\Delta - 1/2}, \quad k = 1, \ldots, K. \end{aligned} \tag{4.5}$$

In adapting the power family tests, we apply the stopping rule (4.2) with a_k and b_k as defined by (4.5). Thus, the sequence of standardized statistics, $Z_1, \ldots, Z_K$, is compared with a fixed sequence of critical values which do not depend on $\mathcal{I}_1, \ldots, \mathcal{I}_K$. Since the joint distribution of $\{Z_1, \ldots, Z_K\}$ under H_0 depends only on the *ratios* between observed information levels, the Type I error probability is exactly α provided only that information levels, $\mathcal{I}_1, \ldots, \mathcal{I}_K$, are equally spaced, just as for two-sided tests in Section 3.3. Unequal spacing will cause minor perturbations in the Type I error rate. Attained power is subject to greater variability, depending primarily on the final information level, $\mathcal{I}_K$, with a subsidiary dependence on the spacing of information levels.

Table 4.5 shows the results of applying our rule with information sequences following the patterns considered for two-sided tests in Table 3.2. Target information levels are $\mathcal{I}_k = (k/K)\mathcal{I}_{max}$, $k = 1, \ldots, K$, where $\mathcal{I}_{max} = \tilde{R}(K, \alpha, \beta, \Delta)\mathcal{I}_{f,1}$, and observed information levels are $\mathcal{I}_k = \pi(k/K)^r \mathcal{I}_{max}$, $k = 1, \ldots, K$, the factor π controlling the final information level and the power r the spacing between levels. The Type I error probability remains within 0.001 of $\alpha = 0.05$ in all cases. The attained power is affected primarily by the overall scale of information and is low for $\pi = 0.9$ and high for $\pi = 1.1$. For comparison, a fixed sample test with 0.9 times the required information, $\mathcal{I}_{f,1}$, has power 0.871 and a fixed sample test with information $1.1 \times \mathcal{I}_{f,1}$ has power 0.923. In all cases where $\pi = 1.0$, so $\mathcal{I}_K$ exactly equals its target $\mathcal{I}_{max}$, power is within 0.022 of its nominal value, and it is often much closer. If, instead, we had obtained values a_k and b_k by substituting observed values of $\mathcal{I}_k$ into (4.3), we would have had to resolve the problem of $a_K \neq b_K$ when $\mathcal{I}_K \neq \mathcal{I}_{max}$; using b_K as the critical value to protect the Type I error still leads to variations in attained Type I error from 0.043 to 0.059 in the examples of Table 4.5.

The preceding proposal and its extension to group sequential t-tests is described by Jennison & Turnbull (2000a). Emerson & Fleming (1989) propose an alternative treatment of general information sequences using boundary values on the score statistic scale, but this approach maintains the Type I error rate less accurately. Emerson & Fleming also suggest using their approach to apply a test when the number of analyses differs from that planned: this can lead to quite large discrepancies in Type I error (their Table 7 shows Type I error probabilities ranging from 0.029 to 0.074, when the intended value is 0.05) and we would recommend use of tests defined through error spending functions (see Section 7.3), which preserve the Type I error rate exactly in such situations.

4.3.2 An Example

We illustrate the design and analysis of a group sequential one-sided test from the power family in a paired two-treatment comparison. With the notation of Section 3.1.3, responses in pair i are denoted X_{Ai} and X_{Bi} for subjects receiving treatments A and B, respectively. We suppose $X_{Ai} - X_{Bi} \sim N(\mu_A - \mu_B, \tilde{\sigma}^2)$, $i = 1, 2, \ldots$, and assume $\tilde{\sigma}^2$ is known to be equal to 200. We shall design a power family test with $\Delta = 0.0$ and four groups of observations to test the null hypothesis H_0: $\mu_A = \mu_B$ against the one-sided alternative $\mu_A > \mu_B$ with Type I error probability $\alpha = 0.05$ and power $1 - \beta = 0.9$ at $\mu_A - \mu_B = \delta = 5.0$. A fixed sample test requires information

$$\mathcal{I}_{f,1} = \{\Phi^{-1}(0.95) + \Phi^{-1}(0.9)\}^2/5.0^2 = 0.3426$$

Table 4.5 *Properties of power family one-sided tests designed for information levels* $\mathcal{I}_k = (k/K)\mathcal{I}_{max}$, $k = 1, \ldots, K$, *but applied with* $\mathcal{I}_k = \pi(k/K)^r\mathcal{I}_{max}$, $k = 1, \ldots, K$. *Attained Type I error probabilities and power are shown for tests with shape parameter* Δ *and* K *analyses, designed to achieve Type I error probability* $\alpha = 0.05$ *and power* $1-\beta = 0.9$ *at* $\theta = \delta$.

	r	π	$\Delta = -0.5$ Type I error	$\Delta = -0.5$ Power	$\Delta = 0$ Type I error	$\Delta = 0$ Power
$K = 2$						
	0.80	0.9	0.050	0.872	0.050	0.877
		1.0	0.050	0.901	0.050	0.905
		1.1	0.050	0.923	0.050	0.927
	1.00	0.9	0.050	0.871	0.050	0.871
		1.0	0.050	0.900	0.050	0.900
		1.1	0.050	0.923	0.050	0.923
	1.25	0.9	0.050	0.870	0.049	0.860
		1.0	0.050	0.899	0.049	0.890
		1.1	0.050	0.922	0.049	0.913
$K = 5$						
	0.80	0.9	0.050	0.875	0.050	0.883
		1.0	0.050	0.904	0.050	0.910
		1.1	0.050	0.926	0.050	0.931
	1.00	0.9	0.050	0.871	0.050	0.871
		1.0	0.050	0.900	0.050	0.900
		1.1	0.050	0.923	0.050	0.923
	1.25	0.9	0.049	0.864	0.050	0.852
		1.0	0.049	0.893	0.050	0.882
		1.1	0.049	0.917	0.050	0.906
$K = 10$						
	0.80	0.9	0.050	0.877	0.050	0.886
		1.0	0.050	0.905	0.050	0.913
		1.1	0.050	0.927	0.050	0.934
	1.00	0.9	0.050	0.871	0.050	0.871
		1.0	0.050	0.900	0.050	0.900
		1.1	0.050	0.923	0.050	0.923
	1.25	0.9	0.050	0.861	0.050	0.847
		1.0	0.050	0.891	0.050	0.878
		1.1	0.050	0.914	0.050	0.902

for $\theta = \mu_A - \mu_B$. Since the estimate of $\mu_A - \mu_B$ from n pairs of subjects has variance $\tilde{\sigma}^2/n = 200/n$, information is $n/200$ and the fixed sample test needs $n = 200 \times 0.3426 = 68.5$, which rounds up to 69 pairs of subjects.

The group sequential experiment should be designed to achieve a final information level $\mathcal{I}_4 = \tilde{R}(4, 0.05, 0.1, 0.0)\,\mathcal{I}_{f,1} = 1.094 \times 0.3426 = 0.3748$, which requires $n = 200 \times 0.3748 = 75.0$ pairs of observations. This can be achieved with four equally sized groups, each of 19 pairs of subjects.

Denoting the total number of pairs observed at analysis k by n_k, the standardized test statistics at the four analyses are

$$Z_k = \frac{1}{\sqrt{(n_k \tilde{\sigma}^2)}} \sum_{i=1}^{n_k} (X_{Ai} - X_{Bi}), \quad k = 1, \ldots, 4,$$

and observed information levels are

$$\mathcal{I}_k = n_k/\tilde{\sigma}^2 = n_k/200, \quad k = 1, \ldots, 4.$$

We use critical values as defined in (4.5) and take values of $\tilde{C}_1(4, 0.05, 0.9, 0.0)$ and $\tilde{C}_2(4, 0.05, 0.9, 0.0)$ from Table 4.2. At analyses $k = 1, 2$ and 3, the test stops to reject H_0 if

$$Z_k \geq \tilde{C}_1(4, 0.05, 0.9, 0.0)\,(k/4)^{-1/2} = 1.686\,(k/4)^{-1/2},$$

stops to accept H_0 if

$$\begin{aligned} Z_k &\leq (\tilde{C}_1(4, 0.05, 0.9, 0.0) + \tilde{C}_2(4, 0.05, 0.9, 0.0))(k/4)^{1/2} \\ &\quad -\tilde{C}_2(4, 0.05, 0.9, 0.0)\,(k/4)^{-1/2} \\ &= 3.061\,(k/4)^{1/2} - 1.375\,(k/4)^{-1/2}, \end{aligned}$$

and otherwise continues to the next group of observations. The test terminates at the fourth analysis if it reaches this stage, rejecting H_0 if $Z_4 \geq 1.686$ and accepting H_0 otherwise. This boundary is shown in Figure 4.2.

Suppose that when the experiment is conducted, the cumulative numbers of pairs of responses available at each analysis are $n_1 = 13$, $n_2 = 31$, $n_3 = 52$ and $n_4 = 75$. The stopping rule is as we have just described even though the n_k are not exactly as planned although, of course, the observed values of $n_1, \ldots, n_4$ are used in defining the Z_ks. Calculations show that the attained Type I error rate in this case is 0.049 and power at $\mu_A - \mu_B = 5.0$ is 0.882. Although the group sizes are unequal, the final sample size is equal to the target for analysis 4 and, in view of earlier evidence of robustness to variations in group sizes, it is no surprise that both error probabilities are close to their nominal values.

4.4 Group Sequential One-Sided t-Tests

We now consider the situation described in Section 3.4 where observations follow a normal linear model with parameter vector $\boldsymbol{\beta}$ and variances depend on a scale factor σ^2. We suppose estimates $\widehat{\boldsymbol{\beta}}^{(1)}, \ldots, \widehat{\boldsymbol{\beta}}^{(K)}$ are obtained at analyses 1 to K, $Var(\widehat{\boldsymbol{\beta}}^{(K)}) = \boldsymbol{V}_k \sigma^2$ and s_k^2 is the usual unbiased estimate of σ^2 at analysis k based on $n_k - p$ degrees of freedom. In this section we shall define group

Figure 4.2 *One-sided test with four groups of observations for paired sample example of Section* 4.3.2

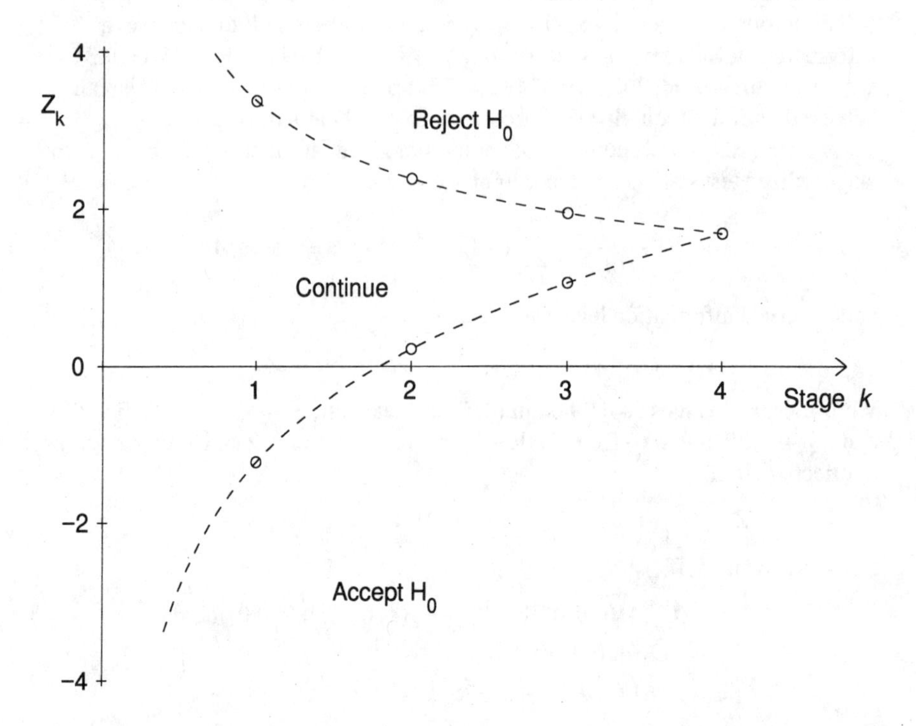

sequential t-tests of a hypothesis of the form H_0: $\boldsymbol{c}^T\boldsymbol{\beta} = \gamma$ against the one-sided alternative $\boldsymbol{c}^T\boldsymbol{\beta} > \gamma$. Our aim is to create tests with Type I error probability α and to assess power at an alternative where $\boldsymbol{c}^T\boldsymbol{\beta}$ exceeds γ by a specified amount δ.

As for the group sequential two-sided t-tests described in Section 3.8,

$$\boldsymbol{c}^T\widehat{\boldsymbol{\beta}}^{(k)} \sim N(\boldsymbol{c}^T\boldsymbol{\beta},\, \boldsymbol{c}^T\boldsymbol{V}_k\boldsymbol{c}\sigma^2),$$

the Z-statistic for testing H_0: $\boldsymbol{c}^T\boldsymbol{\beta} = \gamma$ if σ^2 is known is

$$Z_k = \frac{\boldsymbol{c}^T\widehat{\boldsymbol{\beta}}^{(k)} - \gamma}{\sqrt{\{\boldsymbol{c}^T\boldsymbol{V}_k\boldsymbol{c}\sigma^2\}}},$$

and the t-statistic for testing H_0 is

$$T_k = \frac{\boldsymbol{c}^T\widehat{\boldsymbol{\beta}}^{(k)} - \gamma}{\sqrt{\{\boldsymbol{c}^T\boldsymbol{V}_k\boldsymbol{c}s_k^2\}}}.$$

We shall adapt tests constructed for known σ^2 for use when σ^2 is unknown. However, since observed information is proportional to $1/\sigma^2$, it will not be possible to guarantee both Type I and II error probabilities using pre-specified group sizes, and we shall give priority to maintaining the Type I error rate close to its target value. We follow a similar strategy to that applied in Section 4.3 in dealing with unequally spaced information levels when σ^2 is known. Our starting point is the stopping rule (4.2) with critical values a_k and b_k, $k = 1, \dots, K$, defined without explicit reference to $\mathcal{I}_k$ by equation (4.5). We replace Z_k in (4.2) by T_k and set critical values for T_k to maintain the same marginal probability under H_0 (ignoring the effect of possible earlier stopping) of being above or below the boundary at each analysis. This gives the rule:

$$\begin{array}{lll} \text{After group } k = 1, \dots, K-1 & & \\ \quad \text{if } T_k \geq t_{n_k - p, 1-\Phi(b_k)} & \text{stop, reject } H_0 & \\ \quad \text{if } T_k \leq t_{n_k - p, 1-\Phi(a_k)} & \text{stop, accept } H_0 & \\ \quad \text{otherwise} & \text{continue to group } k+1, & (4.6) \\ \text{after group } K & & \\ \quad \text{if } T_K \geq t_{n_k - p, 1-\Phi(b_K)} & \text{stop, reject } H_0 & \\ \quad \text{if } T_K < t_{n_k - p, 1-\Phi(a_K)} & \text{stop, accept } H_0. & \end{array}$$

Here, $t_{\nu,q}$ is the upper q tail-point of a t-distribution on ν degrees of freedom, i.e., $Pr\{T > t_{\nu,q}\} = q$ when $T \sim t_\nu$.

The same "significance levels" are applied to the T_k in rule (4.6) as to the Z_k in rule (4.2). Thus, our proposed group sequential t-test can be regarded as the "repeated significance test" analogue of the original Z-test. The comparison is a little forced here since the lower boundary does not necessarily lie at extreme values of the null distribution of Z_k. Nevertheless, there are good reasons why this construction should produce a test with Type I error probability close to the target value. First, if the degrees of freedom of the T_k are high, there is little difference between our group sequential t-test and the Z-test proposed in Section 4.3 for handling unpredictable information levels; hence, the Type I error rate will be close to its intended value as long as information levels are close to equally spaced. This is a key property as it overcomes the problem that information levels depend on the unknown σ^2. Second, if the degrees of freedom are low, there is strong empirical evidence that matching the marginal probabilities under H_0 of being above and below each boundary point to those of the original Z-test will maintain the Type I error to considerable accuracy.

We note in passing that there is another way in which the "significance approach" can be used to create a group sequential one-sided t-test from a test for known σ^2. When introducing power family tests in Section 4.2, we observed that the upper and lower boundaries could be viewed as repeated significance tests of $\theta = 0$ and $\theta = \delta$, respectively, tests being applied to Z_k to create the upper boundary and to $Z_k - \delta\sqrt{\mathcal{I}_k}$, the standardized statistic for testing $\theta = \delta$, to create the lower boundary. (In our current problem, $\boldsymbol{c}^T\boldsymbol{\beta} - \gamma$ takes the place of θ and $\mathcal{I}_k$ is $(\boldsymbol{c}^T\boldsymbol{V}_k\boldsymbol{c}\sigma^2)^{-1}$.) A group sequential t-test can be created by applying significance tests at the same sequences of levels to the T_k to obtain the upper boundary, and to the t-statistics for testing $\boldsymbol{c}^T\boldsymbol{\beta} - \gamma = \delta$,

$$T_k' = \frac{\boldsymbol{c}^T\widehat{\boldsymbol{\beta}}^{(k)} - \gamma - \delta}{\sqrt{\{\boldsymbol{c}^T\boldsymbol{V}_k\boldsymbol{c}\, s_k^2\}}}, \quad k = 1, \dots, K,$$

to produce the lower boundary. In some ways, this may appear a more natural analogue of the original Z-test. However, there are difficulties with this approach: there is no guarantee that the boundaries will meet up at the last analysis, and both Type I and Type II error rates vary substantially with the observed sequence of information levels. For these reasons, we shall not pursue this approach further.

Returning to our proposed test, we can repeat the arguments of Section 3.8 to find an approximation to the test's power at a specified alternative and value of σ^2. By analogy with the case of known σ^2, for given $\boldsymbol{V}_1, \ldots, \boldsymbol{V}_K$ we expect the group sequential t-test's power at a certain alternative to be approximately that of a fixed sample t-test with $1/\tilde{R}(K, \alpha, \beta, \Delta)$ times the maximal information. Thus, we need to find the power of a fixed sample test with estimator $\widehat{\boldsymbol{\beta}}$ for which $Var(\boldsymbol{c}^T\widehat{\boldsymbol{\beta}}) = \tilde{R}(K, \alpha, \beta, \Delta)\, \boldsymbol{c}^T \boldsymbol{V}_K \boldsymbol{c} \sigma^2$. The approximation to the power when $\boldsymbol{c}^T\boldsymbol{\beta} - \gamma = \delta$, corresponding to formula (3.20) for a two-sided test, is

$$Pr\{T(n_K - p;\ \delta/\sqrt{\{\tilde{R}(K, \alpha, \beta, \Delta)\, \boldsymbol{c}^T \boldsymbol{V}_K \boldsymbol{c} \sigma^2\}}) \geq t_{n_K - p, 1-\alpha}\}, \qquad (4.7)$$

where $T(\nu; \xi)$ denotes a non-central t random variable with ν degrees of freedom and non-centrality parameter ξ. The simpler but cruder approximation for use when $n_K - p$ is large is

$$\Phi\left(\frac{\delta}{\sqrt{\{\tilde{R}(K, \alpha, \beta, \Delta)\, \boldsymbol{c}^T \boldsymbol{V}_K \boldsymbol{c} \sigma^2\}}} - \Phi^{-1}(1 - \alpha)\right). \qquad (4.8)$$

Table 4.6 shows the Type I error probabilities of our group sequential one-sided t-tests and the power they attain in situations where formula (4.7) gives the value 0.8. As in Table 3.3, the degrees of freedom are those which arise when groups consist of three or five observations and two degrees of freedom are used in fitting the linear model at each analysis. Departures from the intended Type I error rates are minor and decrease as the degrees of freedom increase. Formula (4.7) is seen to provide a good estimate of power, especially when degrees of freedom are high. Because tests with $\Delta = -0.5$ have less opportunity for early stopping than those with $\Delta = 0.0$, the slightly higher discrepancies in error rates in the second case are as one might expect.

Since our definition of group sequential t-tests does not rely on equally spaced information levels, these tests may also be used with unequal group sizes or information increments. We have simulated tests with sequences of information levels of the form

$$\mathcal{I}_k = (k/K)^r \mathcal{I}_{max}, \quad k = 1, \ldots, K, \qquad (4.9)$$

to investigate the effects of such unequal spacing. Our findings are similar to those reported in Section 4.3 for the known variance problem. With $r = 0.8$ and 1.25 in (4.9), the Type I error and power of a test differ only slightly from those of the same test with $r = 1$, i.e., with equally spaced information levels and $\mathcal{I}_K = \mathcal{I}_{max}$. Thus, there is no difficulty and no serious loss of accuracy in applying these tests with both an unknown variance and unequal information increments.

Table 4.6 *Properties of group sequential one-sided t-tests designed to test* H_0: $c^T\beta = \gamma$ *with Type I error* $\alpha = 0.05$*, based on power family tests for known variance with* $\Delta = -0.5$ *and* 0.0*. Degrees of freedom for* σ^2 *are* $\nu_k = (\nu_K+2)(k/K)-2$ *and* $Var(c^T\hat{\beta}^{(k)}) = (K/k)Var(c^T\hat{\beta}^{(K)})$*, at analyses* $k = 1, \ldots, K$*. Actual power at the alternative for which the approximation* (4.7) *gives power* 0.8 *is shown in the penultimate column. The final column gives the power predicted by formula* (4.8).
Type I error and power were estimated by simulation using 50000 *replicates; standard errors are* 0.001 *for Type I error and* 0.002 *for power.*

$\Delta = -0.5$

K	ν_K	*Type I error*	*Attained power*	*Known* σ^2 *power*
3	7	0.055	0.817	0.869
3	13	0.050	0.811	0.837
5	13	0.055	0.814	0.837
5	23	0.053	0.810	0.821
8	22	0.054	0.811	0.822
8	38	0.052	0.804	0.813

$\Delta = 0.0$

K	ν_K	*Type I error*	*Attained power*	*Known* σ^2 *power*
3	7	0.057	0.823	0.869
3	13	0.054	0.814	0.837
5	13	0.056	0.814	0.837
5	23	0.054	0.810	0.821
8	22	0.056	0.810	0.822
8	38	0.053	0.806	0.813

4.4.1 Example: A Paired Two-Treatment Comparison

To illustrate the above methods, we revisit the paired comparison of Section 4.3.2 but now suppose $\tilde{\sigma}^2$ is unknown. Responses in pair i are denoted X_{Ai} and X_{Bi} and we suppose $X_{Ai} - X_{Bi} \sim N(\mu_A - \mu_B, \tilde{\sigma}^2)$, $i = 1, 2, \ldots$. Our aim is to design a power family test with $\Delta = 0.0$ and four groups of observations to test H_0: $\mu_A = \mu_B$ against the one-sided alternative $\mu_A > \mu_B$ with Type I error probability $\alpha = 0.05$. We further suppose there is evidence that $\tilde{\sigma}^2$ is likely to be in the region of 200 and, in so far as it is possible, we would like to achieve power of about 0.9 at $\mu_A - \mu_B = 5.0$.

If each group contains m pairs of observations, the t-statistics for testing H_0 at successive analyses are

$$T_k = \frac{\sum_{i=1}^{mk}(X_{Ai} - X_{Bi})}{\sqrt{\{mks_k^2\}}}, \quad k = 1, \ldots, 4,$$

where

$$s_k^2 = \frac{\sum_{i=1}^{mk}\{X_{Ai} - X_{Bi} - (\bar{X}_A^{(k)} - \bar{X}_B^{(k)})\}^2}{mk - 1},$$

with $\bar{X}_A^{(k)}$ denoting the mean of $X_{A1}, \ldots, X_{A,mk}$ and $\bar{X}_B^{(k)}$ the mean of $X_{B1}, \ldots, X_{B,mk}$.

Table 4.2 gives $\tilde{C}_1(4, 0.05, 0.1, 0.0) = 1.686$, $\tilde{C}_2(4, 0.05, 0.1, 0.0) = 1.375$ and $\tilde{R}(4, 0.05, 0.1, 0.0) = 1.094$. Thus, for $k = 1, \ldots, 4$, the test stops to reject H_0 at analysis k if

$$T_k \geq t_{mk-1, 1-\Phi(b_k)}$$

and to accept H_0 at analysis k if

$$T_k \leq t_{mk-1, 1-\Phi(a_k)},$$

where, from (4.5),

$$b_k = 1.686 \times (k/4)^{-1/2}$$

and

$$a_k = (1.686 + 1.375) \times (k/4)^{1/2} - 1.375 \times (k/4)^{-1/2}.$$

This test will have Type I error probability close to 0.05, but its power depends on m and the unknown $\tilde{\sigma}^2$. In the known variance case, a group size of $m = 19$ produced power 0.9 at $\mu_A - \mu_B = 5.0$ when $\tilde{\sigma}^2 = 200$. The expression (4.7) gives approximate power

$$Pr\{T(76 - 1;\ 5.0/\sqrt{\{1.094 \times (\tilde{\sigma}^2/76)\}}) \geq t_{76-1, 0.95}\}$$

for the group sequential t-test with the same group size, and this is equal to 0.899 when $\tilde{\sigma}^2 = 200$. Simulations show the test's actual Type I error rate rate is 0.051 and its power at $\mu_A - \mu_B = 5.0$ when $\tilde{\sigma}^2 = 200$ is 0.900 (standard errors of these estimates are less than 0.0005). If these properties are regarded as satisfactory, the group size $m = 19$ can be used. Evaluating the upper boundary values as given above, we find $b_1, \ldots, b_4 = 3.372, 2.384, 1.947$ and 1.686 and the lower boundary values are $a_1, \ldots, a_4 = -1.220, 0.220, 1.063$ and 1.686. The degrees of freedom for $T_1, \ldots, T_4$ are 18, 37, 56 and 75; hence, the test has upper boundary 4.053, 2.497, 1.989, 1.708 and lower boundary −1.263, 0.221, 1.073, 1.708 for the T_k. A plot of these boundary values for $T_1, \ldots, T_4$ reveals a continuation region similar in shape to that for $Z_1, \ldots, Z_4$ in Figure 4.2, but somewhat wider.

If, however, the experimenter suspects the estimated value of 200 for $\tilde{\sigma}^2$ may be inaccurate, a larger group size can be chosen to safeguard power. If, for example, it is thought that $\tilde{\sigma}^2$ could be as high as 250, a group size of $m = 24$ would be appropriate since (4.7) then gives

$$Pr\{T(96 - 1;\ 5.0/\sqrt{\{1.094 \times (250/96)\}}) \geq t_{96-1, 0.95}\} = 0.903$$

as an approximation to the power at $\mu_A - \mu_B = 5.0$ if $\tilde{\sigma}^2 = 250$.

4.5 Whitehead's Triangular Test

4.5.1 Definition

This test is more naturally explained in terms of the score statistics $S_1, \ldots, S_K$. Recall from Section 3.5.3 that $S_k = Z_k\sqrt{\mathcal{I}_k}$, and the score statistics are multivariate normal with $S_k \sim N(\theta\mathcal{I}_k, \mathcal{I}_k)$, $k = 1, \ldots, K$, and independent increments $S_1, S_2-S_1, \ldots, S_K-S_{K-1}$. This joint distribution is that of a Brownian motion with drift θ, $\{S(\mathcal{I}), \mathcal{I} > 0\}$, observed at times $\mathcal{I} = \mathcal{I}_1, \ldots, \mathcal{I}_K$; here $S(\mathcal{I}) \sim N(\theta\mathcal{I}, \mathcal{I})$, $\mathcal{I} > 0$, and the continuous S process has independent increments.

The origins of Whitehead's test lie in a sequential test of H_0: $\theta = 0$ against $\theta > 0$ in which the S process is monitored continuously. This continuous test has upper and lower boundaries

$$d(\mathcal{I}) = \frac{2}{\delta}\log\left(\frac{1}{2\alpha}\right) + \frac{\delta}{4}\mathcal{I} \quad \text{and} \quad c(\mathcal{I}) = -\frac{2}{\delta}\log\left(\frac{1}{2\alpha}\right) + \frac{3\delta}{4}\mathcal{I}$$

for $\mathcal{I}$ in the range

$$0 < \mathcal{I} \le \frac{8}{\delta^2}\log\left(\frac{1}{2\alpha}\right).$$

Termination occurs the first time $S(\mathcal{I}) \ge d(\mathcal{I})$ or $S(\mathcal{I}) \le c(\mathcal{I})$, although, since the process is continuous, the relevant condition is always met with equality. The test rejects H_0 if $S(\mathcal{I}) = d(\mathcal{I})$ at termination and accepts H_0 if $S(\mathcal{I}) = c(\mathcal{I})$. Lorden (1976) introduced this test, calling it a 2-SPRT, and gave a likelihood ratio argument to show that the Type I error probability is exactly equal to α and power at $\theta = \delta$ is exactly $1 - \alpha$ under continuous monitoring.

Whitehead & Stratton (1983) adapt the continuous test to discrete monitoring using a result of Siegmund (1979) concerning the expected overshoot of a straight line boundary by a discretely monitored Brownian motion. They subtract the expected overshoot from the continuous boundary to obtain a discrete boundary with approximately the same exit probabilities. If information levels are equally spaced and $\mathcal{I}_K = \mathcal{I}_{max}$, so $\mathcal{I}_k = (k/K)\mathcal{I}_{max}$ at analyses $k = 1, \ldots, K$, the upper and lower boundaries for S_k are, respectively,

$$d_k = \frac{2}{\delta}\log\left(\frac{1}{2\alpha}\right) - 0.583\sqrt{\frac{\mathcal{I}_{max}}{K}} + \frac{\delta}{4}\frac{k}{K}\mathcal{I}_{max} \tag{4.10}$$

and

$$c_k = -\frac{2}{\delta}\log\left(\frac{1}{2\alpha}\right) + 0.583\sqrt{\frac{\mathcal{I}_{max}}{K}} + \frac{3\delta}{4}\frac{k}{K}\mathcal{I}_{max}. \tag{4.11}$$

If the boundaries are to meet with $d_K = c_K$ at the final analysis, we find, by solving a quadratic equation, that $\mathcal{I}_K$ must take the value

$$\mathcal{I}_{max} = \left[\sqrt{\frac{4 \times 0.583^2}{K} + 8\log\left(\frac{1}{2\alpha}\right)} - \frac{2 \times 0.583}{\sqrt{K}}\right]^2 \frac{1}{\delta^2}. \tag{4.12}$$

For given K and α, taking $\mathcal{I}_{max}$ from (4.12) and boundary values from (4.10) and (4.11) gives a group sequential one-sided test of H_0: $\theta = 0$ with K analyses, achieving a Type I error rate approximately equal to α and power approximately $1 - \alpha$ at $\theta = \delta$. The formulae for c_k and d_k indicate that the boundary values $(c_1, d_1), \ldots, (c_K, d_K)$ define a triangular continuation region in the $(S, \mathcal{I})$ plane.

Whitehead & Stratton (1983) also explain how to create a test with, approximately, Type I error probability α at $\theta = 0$ and power $1 - \beta$ at $\theta = \delta$ when $\alpha \neq \beta$. They first note that a fixed sample test with Type I error α and power $1 - \beta$ at $\theta = \delta$ has power $1 - \alpha$ at $\theta = \xi\delta$ where

$$\xi = \frac{2\Phi^{-1}(1-\alpha)}{\Phi^{-1}(1-\alpha) + \Phi^{-1}(1-\beta)}.$$

The group sequential test is then conducted as defined above, but with $\tilde{\delta} = \xi\delta$ in place of δ in the formulae for $\mathcal{I}_{max}$ and the boundary values. Since the power curves of the group sequential test and fixed sample test follow each other closely, the group sequential test also has power close to $1 - \beta$ at $\theta = \delta$.

If the power family tests of Section 4.2 are expressed in terms of the score statistics $\{S_1, \ldots, S_K\}$, boundary values a_k and b_k for Z_k become $c_k = a_k\sqrt{\mathcal{I}_k}$ and $d_k = b_k\sqrt{\mathcal{I}_k}$ for S_k. The power family test with $\Delta = 0$ also has a triangular continuation region in the $(S, \mathcal{I})$ plane, but this is not the same as Whitehead's triangular test: the boundary of the power family test is wider early on and slopes to a point more rapidly, ending at a lower maximum information level. This can be seen by considering again the example at the end of Section 4.2.1. Suppose we wish to construct a one-sided test with $K = 4$ stages, Type I error rate $\alpha = 0.05$ and power $1 - \beta = 0.9$ at $\theta = \delta = 0.2$. Figure 4.1 showed the boundary for two power family tests with these specifications. Because the triangular tests here require $\alpha = \beta$, we replace δ by $\xi\delta = 2 \times 1.645(1.645 + 1.282)^{-1}0.2 = 0.2248$, as the alternative hypothesis value for θ for which the power is to be $1-\alpha = 0.95$. For fully sequential or continuous monitoring, the 2-SPRT with maximum information $-8\log(2\alpha)/0.2248^2 = 364.51$ guarantees the Type I and II error probability requirements. Using 0.2248 for δ in (4.12), the maximum information for the test of Whitehead & Stratton (1983) with four stages is 278.03. The boundaries (using the S scale) for both tests are shown in Figure 4.3. For comparison, the triangular test in the power family ($\Delta = 0$), which has $\mathcal{I}_{max} = 234.31$, is also displayed; it is the same as that shown in Figure 4.1.

4.5.2 *Properties of Whitehead's Triangular Test for Equally Spaced Information Levels*

Table 4.7 shows properties of Whitehead's test when information levels are equally spaced and boundaries meet at the final analysis. The first two columns show the actual Type I error rate and power, which differ slightly from the specified values due to the approximations used in deriving the tests. However, we see that all entries are extremely close to their intended values. The results for small numbers of groups are surprisingly good since there is little reason to expect Siegmund's boundary crossing result to apply accurately in these cases. Results for $K = 1$ are for the extreme case where, after a rather large initial group, the

Figure 4.3 *One-sided triangular tests for four groups of observations*

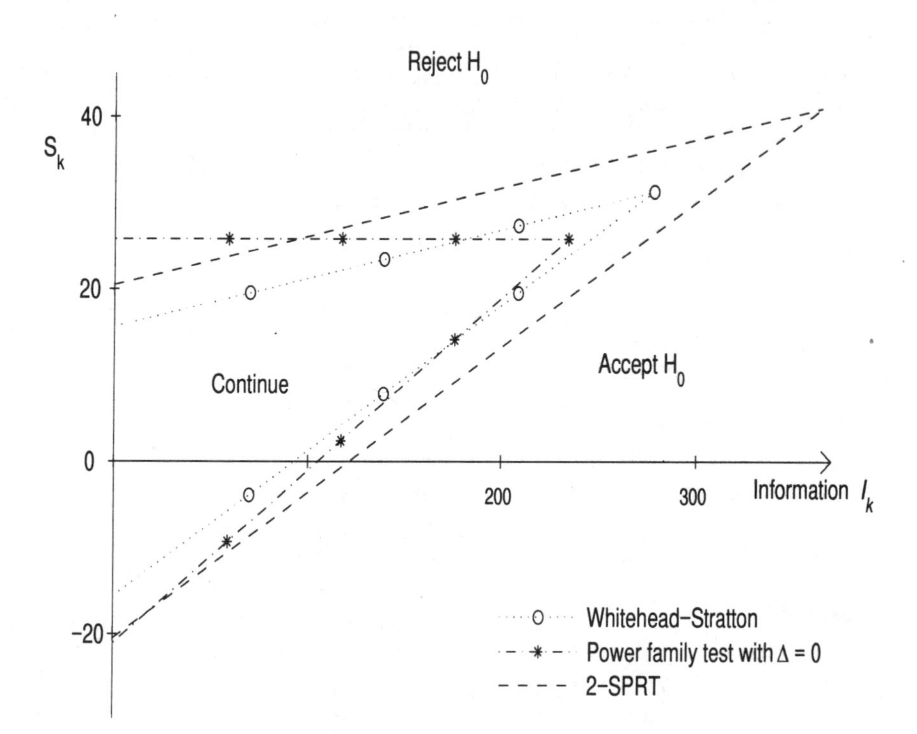

boundaries defined by (4.10) and (4.11) meet up and, thus, the test terminates. The information level at which this occurs is not quite equal to that required by a fixed sample test, and hence the attained error probabilities are not exactly equal to their target values. However, the differences are surprisingly small and the results show that (4.12) gives a value of $\mathcal{I}_{max}$ within half a percent of the fixed sample size and Type I error and power are in fact very close to their nominal values. As Whitehead remarks (1997, p. 133), the accuracy of the approximation under the two extremes of continuous monitoring and a single analysis gives strong support for its adequacy in intermediate cases.

The third column of Table 4.7 contains values of $R_{Wh}(K, \alpha, \beta)$, the ratio between each group sequential test's maximum information level and the information, $\mathcal{I}_{f,1}$, required by a fixed sample test with the same error probabilities. (Although $R_{Wh}(K, \alpha, \beta)$ depends on K and α but not on β, we have retained the more general notation.) Expected sample sizes on termination under $\theta = 0, \delta/2$ and δ are shown in the remaining columns.

The results follow the standard pattern, expected sample sizes decreasing and maximum sample size increasing as the number of analyses grows. In general, the maximum sample sizes tend to be high for the expected sample sizes achieved.

Table 4.7 *Properties of Whitehead's triangular tests with equal group sizes. Constants $R_{Wh}(K, \alpha, \beta)$ are ratios of the maximum sample size to that of a fixed sample test with the same error probabilities. Expected sample sizes at $\theta = 0$, $\delta/2$ and δ are expressed as percentages of the corresponding fixed sample size. Tests are for K groups of observations, and designed to have Type I error probability $\alpha = 0.05$ at $\theta = 0$ and power $1 - \beta = 0.8$, 0.9 and 0.95 at $\theta = \delta$.*

K	*Type I error*	*Power at* $\theta = \delta$	R_{Wh}	*Expected sample size, as percentage of fixed sample size, at* $\theta=0$	$\theta=\delta/2$	$\theta=\delta$
$1-\beta=0.8$						
1	0.050	0.799	0.995	99.5	99.5	99.5
2	0.052	0.800	1.162	71.8	84.3	80.9
3	0.051	0.802	1.245	65.1	80.1	76.1
4	0.051	0.802	1.298	62.6	78.1	73.9
5	0.050	0.803	1.336	61.1	76.9	72.6
10	0.050	0.803	1.434	57.5	73.8	69.3
15	0.050	0.803	1.479	56.2	72.6	68.1
20	0.050	0.803	1.508	55.5	71.9	67.4
$1-\beta=0.9$						
1	0.050	0.899	0.995	99.5	99.5	99.5
2	0.052	0.899	1.162	71.8	85.1	76.0
3	0.051	0.900	1.245	65.1	81.1	70.3
4	0.051	0.901	1.298	62.6	79.2	67.9
5	0.050	0.901	1.336	61.1	78.0	66.5
10	0.050	0.902	1.434	57.5	74.9	63.1
15	0.050	0.902	1.479	56.2	73.7	61.8
20	0.050	0.902	1.508	55.5	73.1	61.1
$1-\beta=0.95$						
1	0.050	0.950	0.995	99.5	99.5	99.5
2	0.052	0.948	1.162	71.8	85.4	71.8
3	0.051	0.949	1.245	65.1	81.4	65.1
4	0.051	0.949	1.298	62.6	79.5	62.6
5	0.050	0.950	1.336	61.1	78.3	61.1
10	0.050	0.950	1.434	57.5	75.2	57.5
15	0.050	0.950	1.479	56.2	74.0	56.2
20	0.050	0.950	1.508	55.5	73.4	55.5

For example, comparing Table 4.7 with Tables 4.1, 4.2 and 4.3, we see that in many cases the corresponding power family one-sided tests either have a similar maximum sample size and lower expected sample sizes or comparable expected sample sizes and a lower maximum sample size.

4.5.3 Applying Whitehead's Triangular Test with Unequal Increments in Information

Whitehead (1997, Chapter 4) makes further use of Siegmund's expected overshoot result to adapt the triangular test to general information sequences. At analysis k, the boundaries of the original continuous test are brought in by an amount $0.583\sqrt{(\mathcal{I}_k - \mathcal{I}_{k-1})}$. Thus, for a general sequence $\{\mathcal{I}_1, \ldots, \mathcal{I}_K\}$, at analysis k the test stops to reject H_0 if

$$S_k \geq d_k = \frac{2}{\delta}\log\left(\frac{1}{2\alpha}\right) - 0.583\sqrt{(\mathcal{I}_k - \mathcal{I}_{k-1})} + \frac{\delta}{4}\mathcal{I}_k,$$

stops to accept H_0 if

$$S_k \leq c_k = -\frac{2}{\delta}\log\left(\frac{1}{2\alpha}\right) + 0.583\sqrt{(\mathcal{I}_k - \mathcal{I}_{k-1})} + \frac{3\delta}{4}\mathcal{I}_k$$

and continues to stage $k+1$ otherwise. At stage 1, $\mathcal{I}_0$ is taken to be zero. If S_k continues to fall in the continuation region, a stage will eventually be reached at which $c_K \geq d_K$ and the test must then terminate. Clarification of the decision rule at this final stage is needed. We suggest retaining the condition $S_K \geq d_K$ for rejecting H_0 and accepting H_0 if $S_K < d_K$, thereby gaining as much power as possible while still protecting the Type I error probability. Because of the appearance of a plot of the resulting boundary, Whitehead refers to this as the "Christmas tree" adjustment.

Table 4.8 shows the Type I error probability and power attained by Whitehead's triangular test under a variety of information sequences. This test differs from others previously discussed in that it can be applied without any initial estimate of the maximum number of analyses, K, or of the information levels which will arise at each analysis. For comparison with earlier results, we have investigated attained error rates under observed information sequences of the form used in Sections 3.3 and 4.3, i.e., $\mathcal{I}_k = \pi(k/K)^r \mathcal{I}_{max}$, $k = 1, \ldots, K$, where now $\mathcal{I}_{max}$ is given by (4.12). If $\pi = r = 1$, the boundaries meet up exactly at analysis K and the test is sure to terminate at this point. For some combinations of π and r, the test has $c_K < d_K$ and we enforce termination at analysis K by rejecting H_0 if $S_K \geq d_K$ and accepting H_0 otherwise. Such a modification might be necessary if the number of analyses is limited due, for example, to budgetary restrictions; in other circumstances, it may be possible to continue sampling as long as is necessary for the boundaries to meet and terminate the test automatically. For certain other combinations of π and r, the test terminates at analysis $K-1$ since $c_{K-1} > d_{K-1}$ and, following our stated rule, we reject H_0 in such situations if and only if $S_{K-1} \geq d_{K-1}$.

Table 4.8 *Properties of Whitehead's triangular test applied with information levels* $\mathcal{I}_k = \pi(k/K)^r \mathcal{I}_{max}$, $k = 1, \ldots, K$, *where* $\mathcal{I}_{max}$ *is such that boundaries meet up exactly at analysis* K *for information levels* $\mathcal{I}_k = (k/K)\mathcal{I}_{max}$, $k = 1, \ldots, K$. *Attained Type I error probabilities and power are shown for tests designed to achieve Type I error* $\alpha = 0.05$ *and power* $1 - \beta = 0.9$ *at* $\theta = \delta$.

		$K = 2$		$K = 5$		$K = 10$	
r	π	*Type I error*	*Power*	*Type I error*	*Power*	*Type I error*	*Power*
0.80	0.9	0.049	0.874	0.050	0.890	0.050	0.897
	1.0	0.052	0.895	0.052	0.899	0.051	0.901
	1.1	0.053	0.904	0.052	0.900	0.051	0.901
1.00	0.9	0.049	0.878	0.049	0.893	0.049	0.898
	1.0	0.052	0.899	0.050	0.901	0.050	0.902
	1.1	0.053	0.910	0.051	0.902	0.050	0.902
1.25	0.9	0.048	0.883	0.048	0.894	0.049	0.898
	1.0	0.051	0.906	0.050	0.903	0.050	0.902
	1.1	0.053	0.918	0.050	0.905	0.050	0.902

It is clear from Table 4.8 that the attained Type I error and power are very close to their nominal values in all the situations considered. Results for tests with power 0.8 and 0.95 are not shown here but these were equally impressive. Interestingly, power is not adversely affected by the lower information levels that arise when $\pi = 0.9$, possibly because there is relatively little probability of continuing to the final stage and so truncation of the final sample size has only a limited effect.

A key feature of Whitehead's triangular test is that only elementary calculations are needed to determine boundary values, and yet the test satisfies error probability requirements accurately under quite general information sequences. Application of the alternative, error spending approach, which we shall present in Chapter 7, involves the numerical computation of successive boundary points. Against this, the triangular test does not manage to achieve the best possible reductions in expected sample size given its rather high maximum sample size. (The sample size at which boundaries meet up depends on the observed pattern of group sizes, but the maximum sample sizes for equally sized groups are already quite high.) Although the probability that the test proceeds to its maximum sample size may be small, this eventuality does have to be allowed for when designing a study and it is difficult not to favor a test with similar properties but a smaller maximum sample size.

CHAPTER 5

Two-Sided Tests with Early Stopping Under the Null Hypothesis

5.1 Introduction

We return to the two-sided testing problem of Chapters 2 and 3 but now consider tests which allow early stopping to accept, as well as to reject, the null hypothesis. Following the general treatment of normal data described in Chapter 3, we suppose standardized statistics $Z_1, \ldots, Z_K$ available at analyses $k = 1, \ldots, K$, follow the canonical joint distribution (3.1), in particular, $Z_k \sim N(\theta\sqrt{\mathcal{I}_k}, 1)$ where $\mathcal{I}_k$ is the information for θ available at analysis k. Our objective is to test, group sequentially, the null hypothesis H_0: $\theta = 0$ with Type I error probability α and power $1 - \beta$ at some specified alternative $\theta = \pm\delta$.

A general group sequential test with possible early stopping to accept H_0 is defined by pairs of constants (a_k, b_k) with $0 \leq a_k < b_k$ for $k = 1, \ldots, K - 1$ and $a_K = b_K$. It has the form

$$
\begin{array}{lll}
\text{After group } k = 1, \ldots, K-1 & & \\
\quad \text{if } |Z_k| \geq b_k & \text{stop, reject } H_0 & \\
\quad \text{if } |Z_k| < a_k & \text{stop, accept } H_0 & \\
\quad \text{otherwise} & \text{continue to group } k+1, & \quad (5.1) \\
\text{after group } K & & \\
\quad \text{if } |Z_K| \geq b_K & \text{stop, reject } H_0 & \\
\quad \text{if } |Z_k| < a_K & \text{stop, accept } H_0. &
\end{array}
$$

Since $a_K = b_K$, termination at analysis K is ensured. At analysis k, the set of values $\{Z_k; |Z_k| < a_k\}$ forms an "inner wedge" within the continuation region $\{Z_k; |Z_k| < b_k\}$ where early stopping to accept H_0 occurs. It may be that such early stopping is not deemed appropriate at the first few analyses, in which case one can set $a_1 = 0$, $a_2 = 0$, etc., to preclude this possibility.

The tests introduced in Chapter 2 have no inner wedges at all and, if $\theta = 0$, sampling must continue up to analysis K with probability at least $1-\alpha$ in order to satisfy the Type I error requirement. Consequently, the expected sample sizes of these tests at $\theta = 0$ show no reduction below the corresponding fixed sample size. In fact, we see from Tables 2.7 and 2.8 that expected sample sizes under $\theta = \delta/2$ are also above the fixed sample size for the Pocock test and only a little below the fixed sample size in the case of the O'Brien & Fleming test. We shall see that early stopping to accept H_0 can lead to reductions in expected sample size at all values of θ, including $\theta = 0$. Although the ethical motivation for stopping a clinical trial early is greatest when a treatment difference is found and randomization of patients to an inferior treatment can be avoided, there are sound financial reasons to curtail a study when it is evident that there is no treatment difference to detect. Moreover, such curtailment can benefit future patients by releasing experimental resources for the earlier exploration of further promising treatments.

Gould & Pecore (1982) note the importance of early stopping to accept the null hypothesis, and Gould (1983) proposes a method of "abandoning lost causes" in which early termination occurs *only* to accept H_0. In Gould & Pecore's inner wedge design, the stopping rule has the form (5.1) with $a_k = a$ and $b_k = b$, $k = 1, \ldots, K$, where a and b are selected constants. Thus, early stopping to accept H_0 occurs at any analysis where the two-sided significance level of a test of H_0 is greater than $2\Phi(-a)$, irrespective of how much data this test is based on. Calculations show the Gould & Pecore tests have rather high maximum sample sizes, especially when there are five or more analyses, and they are not as effective in reducing expected sample size under H_0 as the family of tests we shall present in Section 5.2.

We shall focus on the tests described by Pampallona & Tsiatis (1994) which are indexed by a parameter Δ, occurring as a power in formulae for the boundary points a_k and b_k, $k = 1, \ldots, K$. (Emerson & Fleming (1989) proposed similar tests which achieve the power condition conservatively.) We shall refer to this family of tests as the *power family* of two-sided inner wedge tests. In Sections 5.2.1 and 5.2.2 we define the tests and present their properties. Jennison & Turnbull (2000a) show how the "significance level" approach can be used to apply these tests when observed information levels depart from their planned values and to create group sequential t-tests for normal data with unknown variance; we describe these extensions in Sections 5.2.3 and 5.2.4, respectively.

An alternative way to construct two-sided tests with early stopping to accept H_0 is to combine two one-sided tests. We present the group sequential test of this form described by Whitehead & Stratton (1983) and Whitehead (1997) in Section 5.3.

5.2 The Power Family of Two-Sided Inner Wedge Tests

5.2.1 *Definition of the Tests*

Consider a group sequential study in which statistics Z_k observed at analyses $k = 1, \ldots, K$ follow the canonical joint distribution (3.1) and suppose we wish to test $H_0\colon \theta = 0$ against $H_A\colon \theta \neq 0$ with Type I error probability α and power $1 - \beta$ at $\theta = \pm\delta$. A fixed sample test based on a statistic Z distributed as $N(\theta\sqrt{\mathcal{I}}, 1)$ can attain these requirements if $\mathcal{I}$ is equal to the value $\mathcal{I}_{f,2}$ given by (3.6). The power family inner wedge tests are group sequential and designed for equally spaced information levels, $\mathcal{I}_k = (k/K)\mathcal{I}_K$, $k = 1, \ldots, K$. For the test with parameter Δ, the critical values a_k and b_k to be used in (5.1) are

$$\begin{aligned} b_k &= \tilde{C}_{W1}(K, \alpha, \beta, \Delta)(k/K)^{\Delta - 1/2} \quad \text{and} \\ a_k &= \delta\sqrt{\mathcal{I}_k} - \tilde{C}_{W2}(K, \alpha, \beta, \Delta)(k/K)^{\Delta - 1/2}, \quad k = 1, \ldots, K. \end{aligned} \tag{5.2}$$

A final information level

$$\mathcal{I}_K = \frac{\{\tilde{C}_{W1}(K, \alpha, \beta, \Delta) + \tilde{C}_{W2}(K, \alpha, \beta, \Delta)\}^2}{\delta^2}$$

ensures that $a_K = b_K$ and the test terminates properly.

The constants $\tilde{C}_{W1}(K, \alpha, \beta, \Delta)$ and $\tilde{C}_{W2}(K, \alpha, \beta, \Delta)$ do not depend on δ and are chosen to ensure the Type I error and power conditions. These constants determine $\mathcal{I}_K$ and, hence, the ratio of the test's maximum information level to that required for a fixed sample test,

$$\tilde{R}_W(K, \alpha, \beta, \Delta) = \frac{\mathcal{I}_K}{\mathcal{I}_{f,2}} = \frac{\{\tilde{C}_{W1}(K, \alpha, \beta, \Delta) + \tilde{C}_{W2}(K, \alpha, \beta, \Delta)\}^2}{\{\Phi^{-1}(1 - \alpha/2) + \Phi^{-1}(1 - \beta)\}^2}.$$

Values of $\tilde{C}_{W1}(K, \alpha, \beta, \Delta)$, $\tilde{C}_{W2}(K, \alpha, \beta, \Delta)$ and $\tilde{R}_W(K, \alpha, \beta, \Delta)$ and some properties of these tests are provided in Tables 5.1, 5.2 and 5.3 for $\Delta = -0.5$, -0.25, 0 and 0.25, $\alpha = 0.05$ and $\beta = 0.8$, 0.9 and 0.95; interpolation may be used to obtain constants for values of $K < 20$ not present in the tables. For many of the tabulated tests, the first few values of a_k are negative, which we interpret as indicating there is no opportunity to stop and accept H_0 at these analyses, a reasonable feature since acceptance of H_0 requires evidence that θ is both less than δ and greater than $-\delta$ and insufficient information may be available at early analyses to limit θ to such a narrow range. In the tables, the value k^* indicates the first analysis at which the test can stop to accept H_0.

As in Chapter 4, we have defined tests in terms of the standardized statistics $Z_1, \ldots, Z_K$, whereas Pampallona & Tsiatis defined the same tests in terms of the score statistics $S_k = Z_k\sqrt{\mathcal{I}_k}$, $k = 1, \ldots, K$, and their $C_j(K, \alpha, \beta, \Delta)$ are $K^{1/2-\Delta}$ times our $\tilde{C}_{Wj}(K, \alpha, \beta, \Delta)$, $j = 1$ and 2. Constants for other cases with $\alpha = 0.05$ and 0.01, $\beta = 0.8$, 0.9 and 0.95, and $\Delta = 0$, 0.1, 0.2, 0.3, 0.4 and 0.5 can be found in Pampallona & Tsiatis (1994). Also, as in Chapter 4, we follow the standard practice of referring to expected and maximum sample size when discussing properties of group sequential tests, although it would be more correct to talk of information when the two are not directly proportional.

Figure 5.1 shows the boundary of the power family inner wedge test with $\Delta = 0$ and five groups of observations, expressed on both the Z_k and S_k scales. The test has Type I error probability $\alpha = 0.05$ and power $1 - \beta = 0.9$ at $\theta = \pm 0.2$.

5.2.2 Properties of Power Family Inner Wedge Tests

It is clear from Tables 5.1 to 5.3 that the inner wedge is successful in allowing early stopping to accept H_0, and expected sample sizes under $\theta = 0$ of around 70% to 75% of the corresponding fixed sample size can be obtained in tests with 5 or 10 analyses. These reductions in expected sample size are broadly comparable with those at the alternative $\theta = \pm\delta$. In view of the savings that can be achieved in experimental costs and time, we would recommend that early stopping to accept the null hypothesis be considered in any group sequential two-sided test.

The ratio $\tilde{R}_W(K, \alpha, \beta, \Delta)$ of the maximum sample size to the fixed sample size increases with Δ. We have added negative values of Δ, not considered by

Table 5.1 *Constants* $\tilde{C}_{W1}(K, \alpha, \beta, \Delta)$, $\tilde{C}_{W2}(K, \alpha, \beta, \Delta)$ *and* $\tilde{R}_W(K, \alpha, \beta, \Delta)$ *for power family two-sided inner wedge tests with shape parameter* Δ. *The first opportunity for early stopping to accept* H_0 *occurs at analysis* k^*. *Also shown are expected sample sizes at* $\theta = 0$, $\pm\delta/2$ *and* $\pm\delta$ *expressed as percentages of the corresponding fixed sample size. Tests are for K groups of observations, Type I error probability* $\alpha = 0.05$ *at* $\theta = 0$ *and power* $1 - \beta = 0.8$ *at* $\theta = \pm\delta$.

K	$\tilde{C}_{W1}$	$\tilde{C}_{W2}$	$\tilde{R}_W$	k^*	*Expected sample size, as percentage of fixed sample size, at* $\theta=0$	$\theta=\pm\delta/2$	$\theta=\pm\delta$
$\Delta = -0.5$							
1	1.960	0.842	1.000	1	100.0	100.0	100.0
2	1.949	0.867	1.010	1	90.7	94.6	98.1
3	1.933	0.901	1.023	2	79.6	87.1	89.8
4	1.929	0.919	1.033	2	79.0	85.7	87.2
5	1.927	0.932	1.041	3	75.9	83.4	85.1
10	1.928	0.964	1.066	5	73.2	80.6	81.6
15	1.931	0.979	1.078	8	72.2	79.6	80.5
20	1.932	0.988	1.087	10	71.8	79.1	80.0
$\Delta = -0.25$							
1	1.960	0.842	1.000	1	100.0	100.0	100.0
2	1.936	0.902	1.026	1	83.3	89.9	94.2
3	1.932	0.925	1.040	2	78.8	85.8	86.9
4	1.930	0.953	1.059	2	74.7	82.4	83.8
5	1.934	0.958	1.066	3	74.8	82.0	82.2
10	1.942	0.999	1.102	5	70.8	78.4	78.7
15	1.948	1.017	1.120	7	69.7	77.4	77.6
20	1.952	1.027	1.131	9	69.2	76.9	77.1
$\Delta = 0.0$							
1	1.960	0.842	1.000	1	100.0	100.0	100.0
2	1.935	0.948	1.058	1	78.3	86.0	88.4
3	1.950	0.955	1.075	1	78.5	84.7	83.6
4	1.953	0.995	1.107	2	72.2	80.2	80.2
5	1.958	1.017	1.128	2	71.0	78.8	78.4
10	1.980	1.057	1.175	4	67.9	75.9	75.0
15	1.991	1.075	1.198	6	67.0	74.9	73.9
20	1.998	1.087	1.212	8	66.6	74.5	73.4
$\Delta = 0.25$							
1	1.960	0.842	1.000	1	100.0	100.0	100.0
2	1.982	1.000	1.133	1	75.9	83.9	84.0
3	2.009	1.059	1.199	1	73.2	80.9	79.0
4	2.034	1.059	1.219	1	71.8	79.3	76.5
5	2.048	1.088	1.252	2	68.8	76.9	74.6
10	2.088	1.156	1.341	3	65.3	73.7	71.0
15	2.109	1.180	1.379	4	64.3	72.6	69.7
20	2.122	1.195	1.402	6	63.7	72.1	69.1

Table 5.2 *Constants* $\tilde{C}_{W1}(K, \alpha, \beta, \Delta)$, $\tilde{C}_{W2}(K, \alpha, \beta, \Delta)$ *and* $\tilde{R}_W(K, \alpha, \beta, \Delta)$ *for power family two-sided inner wedge tests with shape parameter* Δ. *The first opportunity for early stopping to accept* H_0 *occurs at analysis* k^*. *Also shown are expected sample sizes at* $\theta = 0, \pm\delta/2$ *and* $\pm\delta$ *expressed as percentages of the corresponding fixed sample size. Tests are for K groups of observations, Type I error probability* $\alpha = 0.05$ *at* $\theta = 0$ *and power* $1 - \beta = 0.9$ *at* $\theta = \pm\delta$.

K	$\tilde{C}_{W1}$	$\tilde{C}_{W2}$	$\tilde{R}_W$	k^*	*Expected sample size, as percentage of fixed sample size, at* $\theta=0$	$\theta=\pm\delta/2$	$\theta=\pm\delta$
$\Delta = -0.5$							
1	1.960	1.282	1.000	1	100.0	100.0	100.0
2	1.960	1.282	1.000	2	100.0	99.9	97.4
3	1.952	1.305	1.010	2	83.4	90.9	86.9
4	1.952	1.316	1.016	3	83.1	89.4	84.2
5	1.952	1.326	1.023	3	80.3	87.2	82.0
10	1.958	1.351	1.042	6	76.9	84.1	78.2
15	1.963	1.363	1.053	9	76.0	83.1	77.1
20	1.967	1.370	1.060	12	75.7	82.7	76.5
$\Delta = -0.25$							
1	1.960	1.282	1.000	1	100.0	100.0	100.0
2	1.957	1.294	1.006	1	95.6	97.2	92.2
3	1.954	1.325	1.023	2	80.8	88.5	83.5
4	1.958	1.337	1.033	2	81.3	87.4	80.4
5	1.960	1.351	1.043	3	77.2	84.8	78.5
10	1.975	1.379	1.071	5	74.7	82.0	74.8
15	1.982	1.394	1.085	8	73.4	80.9	73.7
20	1.988	1.403	1.094	10	73.0	80.4	73.1
$\Delta = 0.0$							
1	1.960	1.282	1.000	1	100.0	100.0	100.0
2	1.958	1.336	1.032	1	85.4	91.2	84.8
3	1.971	1.353	1.051	2	79.7	86.7	79.4
4	1.979	1.381	1.075	2	75.8	83.6	76.0
5	1.990	1.385	1.084	3	75.8	82.9	74.1
10	2.013	1.428	1.127	5	71.6	79.4	70.6
15	2.026	1.447	1.148	7	70.5	78.3	69.4
20	2.034	1.458	1.160	9	69.9	77.8	68.9
$\Delta = 0.25$							
1	1.960	1.282	1.000	1	100.0	100.0	100.0
2	2.003	1.398	1.100	1	79.3	87.1	79.4
3	2.037	1.422	1.139	1	78.5	85.0	74.1
4	2.058	1.443	1.167	2	73.5	81.4	71.1
5	2.073	1.477	1.199	2	71.4	79.7	69.3
10	2.119	1.521	1.261	4	68.6	76.8	65.6
15	2.140	1.551	1.297	5	67.3	75.7	64.3
20	2.154	1.565	1.316	7	66.7	75.1	63.7

Table 5.3 *Constants* $\tilde{C}_{W1}(K, \alpha, \beta, \Delta)$, $\tilde{C}_{W2}(K, \alpha, \beta, \Delta)$ *and* $\tilde{R}_W(K, \alpha, \beta, \Delta)$ *for power family two-sided inner wedge tests with shape parameter* Δ. *The first opportunity for early stopping to accept* H_0 *occurs at analysis* k^*. *Also shown are expected sample sizes at* $\theta = 0$, $\pm\delta/2$ *and* $\pm\delta$ *expressed as percentages of the corresponding fixed sample size. Tests are for K groups of observations, Type I error probability* $\alpha = 0.05$ *at* $\theta = 0$ *and power* $1 - \beta = 0.95$ *at* $\theta = \pm\delta$.

K	$\tilde{C}_{W1}$	$\tilde{C}_{W2}$	$\tilde{R}_W$	k^*	*Expected sample size, as percentage of fixed sample size, at* $\theta=0$	$\theta=\pm\delta/2$	$\theta=\pm\delta$
$\Delta = -0.5$							
1	1.960	1.645	1.000	1	100.0	100.0	100.0
2	1.960	1.645	1.000	2	100.0	99.8	95.7
3	1.959	1.653	1.004	2	88.2	93.6	83.3
4	1.961	1.661	1.010	3	84.5	90.7	80.8
5	1.964	1.666	1.014	3	85.2	89.9	78.4
10	1.974	1.685	1.030	6	80.2	86.1	74.5
15	1.981	1.695	1.040	9	78.8	85.0	73.3
20	1.985	1.702	1.046	12	78.2	84.4	72.8
$\Delta = -0.25$							
1	1.960	1.645	1.000	1	100.0	100.0	100.0
2	1.962	1.644	1.001	2	100.0	99.0	88.7
3	1.964	1.666	1.014	2	83.6	90.5	79.8
4	1.970	1.674	1.022	3	83.4	88.9	76.4
5	1.975	1.685	1.031	3	80.2	86.7	74.5
10	1.992	1.709	1.054	6	76.9	83.6	70.6
15	2.002	1.721	1.066	9	76.1	82.7	69.5
20	2.008	1.729	1.075	11	75.5	82.2	68.9
$\Delta = 0.0$							
1	1.960	1.645	1.000	1	100.0	100.0	100.0
2	1.970	1.667	1.018	1	92.9	94.6	80.3
3	1.983	1.691	1.039	2	80.9	87.9	75.1
4	1.995	1.708	1.055	2	79.8	85.9	71.5
5	2.004	1.718	1.066	3	77.1	84.0	69.5
10	2.032	1.753	1.102	5	73.8	80.9	65.8
15	2.046	1.767	1.119	7	73.1	80.0	64.7
20	2.055	1.778	1.131	10	72.4	79.5	64.1
$\Delta = 0.25$							
1	1.960	1.645	1.000	1	100.0	100.0	100.0
2	2.015	1.730	1.079	1	83.0	89.2	74.5
3	2.052	1.729	1.100	2	80.9	86.2	68.6
4	2.072	1.776	1.140	2	75.1	82.6	65.8
5	2.088	1.799	1.163	2	74.3	81.5	64.0
10	2.136	1.845	1.220	4	70.5	78.2	60.2
15	2.159	1.867	1.247	6	69.5	77.1	58.9
20	2.173	1.880	1.264	8	69.0	76.6	58.2

Figure 5.1 *A power family inner wedge test for five groups of observations*

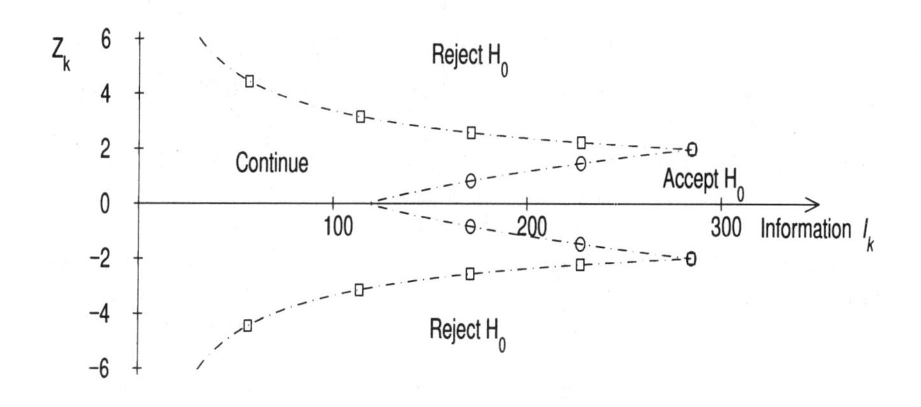

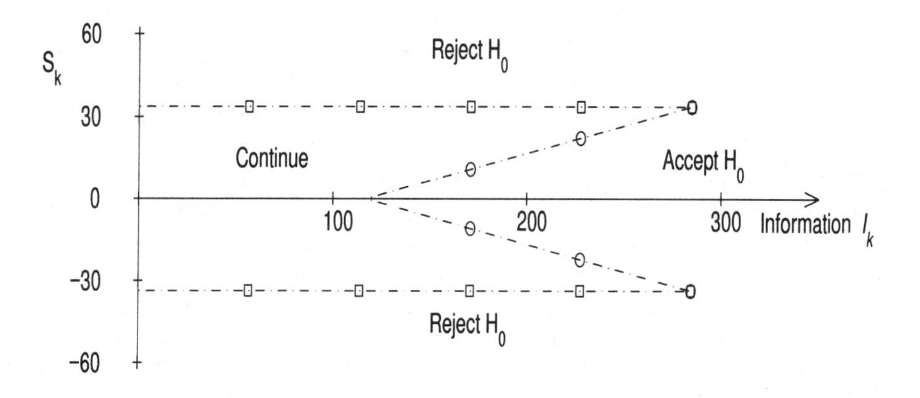

Pampallona & Tsiatis, to allow a choice of tests with lower maximum sample sizes, but we have stopped at an upper limit of $\Delta = 0.25$ since higher values require substantial increases in maximum sample size and yield little reduction, or sometimes even an increase, in expected sample size.

As the number of analyses K increases, the maximum sample size increases and expected sample sizes decrease. As for other types of test, there is little additional benefit to be gained in planning more than about 5 or 10 analyses.

5.2.3 *Adapting Power Family Inner Wedge Tests to Unequal Increments in Information*

The power family inner wedge tests are easily adapted for use with unpredictable sequences of information levels. Our adaptation follows similar lines to that of the power family, one-sided tests of Chapter 4. We first note that the a_k and b_k defined by (5.2) for the case of equally spaced information levels can be rewritten as

$$\begin{aligned} b_k &= \tilde{C}_{W1}(K, \alpha, \beta, \Delta)(k/K)^{\Delta-1/2} \text{ and} \\ a_k &= \{\tilde{C}_{W1}(K, \alpha, \beta, \Delta) + \tilde{C}_{W2}(K, \alpha, \beta, \Delta)\}(k/K)^{1/2} \\ &\quad -\tilde{C}_{W2}(K, \alpha, \beta, \Delta)(k/K)^{\Delta-1/2}, \quad k = 1, \ldots, K. \end{aligned} \tag{5.3}$$

This alternative definition has the advantage that the information levels $\mathcal{I}_k$ do not appear explicitly, and we shall use this in adapting the tests to general information sequences. Note that this definition automatically implies $a_K = b_K$.

Suppose a study gives rise to the sequence of standardized statistics $\{Z_1, \ldots, Z_K\}$ and observed information levels $\{\mathcal{I}_1, \ldots, \mathcal{I}_K\}$ for θ. In our adaptation of the inner wedge test, we apply the original stopping rule (5.1) but with a_k and b_k, $k = 1, \ldots, K$, defined by (5.3). Since $Z_1, \ldots, Z_K$ follow the canonical joint distribution (3.1), the joint distribution of the Z_ks under H_0: $\theta = 0$ depends only on the ratios between the observed $\mathcal{I}_k$s, and hence the Type I error probability remains at precisely α if observed information levels are equally spaced. Unequal spacing causes minor variations in Type I error. We have chosen this adaptation to preserve the Type I error probability as closely as possible, and it is only to be expected that variations in power will be greater. The attained power depends primarily on the final information level, $\mathcal{I}_K$, with additional dependence on the spacing of earlier information levels.

Table 5.4 shows the Type I error probability and power obtained when our rule is applied with information levels departing from their planned values. The target information levels are $\mathcal{I}_k = (k/K)\mathcal{I}_{max}$, $k = 1, \ldots, K$, where $\mathcal{I}_{max} = \tilde{R}_W(K, \alpha, \beta, \Delta)\mathcal{I}_{f,2}$ and observed information levels are $\mathcal{I}_k = \pi(k/K)^r\mathcal{I}_{max}$, $k = 1, \ldots, K$. Here, π controls the final information level and r the spacing between successive information levels. The Type I error probability remains within 0.001 of $\alpha = 0.05$ in all cases. Power is affected most by the overall scale of information. For the low information levels arising when $\pi = 0.9$, power is low and varies around the value 0.868 achieved in a fixed sample test with 0.9 times the required information, $\mathcal{I}_{f,2}$. Conversely, $\pi = 1.1$ gives rise to higher information levels and higher attained powers, varying around the power 0.925 of a fixed sample test with information $1.1 \times \mathcal{I}_{f,2}$.

Unequal increments in information can also be handled using an "error spending" approach. We shall present such methods for two-sided tests with an inner wedge in Section 7.2.5.

In "equivalence testing" problems where one hopes to show that a treatment difference, θ, is close to zero, it is important to limit the probability of concluding $\theta = 0$ when, really, θ differs from zero by a clinically significant amount, δ. Thus, in adapting a test of H_0: $\theta = 0$ to unpredictable information levels, the priority is to preserve a stated power at $\theta = \pm\delta$. This can be achieved by applying the "significance level" approach to Z-statistics for testing $\theta = \delta$ and $\theta = -\delta$, namely $Z_k - \delta\sqrt{\mathcal{I}_k}$ and $Z_k + \delta\sqrt{\mathcal{I}_k}$ where $Z_k \sim N(\theta\sqrt{\mathcal{I}_k}, 1)$. We shall discuss such methods in detail, and also related group sequential t-tests, in Chapter 6.

Table 5.4 *Properties of power family inner wedge tests designed for information levels* $\mathcal{I}_k = (k/K)\mathcal{I}_{max}$, $k = 1, \ldots, K$, *applied with* $\mathcal{I}_k = \pi(k/K)^r\mathcal{I}_{max}$, $k = 1, \ldots, K$. *Attained Type I error probabilities and power are shown for tests with shape parameter* Δ *and* K *analyses, designed to achieve two-sided Type I error* $\alpha = 0.05$ *and power* $1 - \beta = 0.9$ *at* $\theta = \pm\delta$.

			$\Delta = -0.5$		$\Delta = 0.0$	
	r	π	*Type I error*	*Power*	*Type I error*	*Power*
$K = 2$						
	0.80	0.9	0.050	0.868	0.051	0.874
		1.0	0.050	0.900	0.051	0.905
		1.1	0.050	0.925	0.051	0.930
	1.00	0.9	0.050	0.868	0.050	0.868
		1.0	0.050	0.900	0.050	0.900
		1.1	0.050	0.925	0.050	0.925
	1.25	0.9	0.050	0.868	0.049	0.857
		1.0	0.050	0.900	0.049	0.890
		1.1	0.050	0.925	0.049	0.915
$K = 5$						
	0.80	0.9	0.051	0.872	0.050	0.878
		1.0	0.051	0.904	0.050	0.909
		1.1	0.051	0.928	0.050	0.932
	1.00	0.9	0.050	0.868	0.050	0.868
		1.0	0.050	0.900	0.050	0.900
		1.1	0.050	0.925	0.050	0.925
	1.25	0.9	0.049	0.860	0.049	0.851
		1.0	0.049	0.893	0.049	0.885
		1.1	0.049	0.919	0.049	0.911
$K = 10$						
	0.80	0.9	0.051	0.874	0.050	0.882
		1.0	0.051	0.906	0.050	0.912
		1.1	0.051	0.930	0.050	0.935
	1.00	0.9	0.050	0.868	0.050	0.868
		1.0	0.050	0.900	0.050	0.900
		1.1	0.050	0.925	0.050	0.925
	1.25	0.9	0.049	0.857	0.050	0.845
		1.0	0.049	0.890	0.050	0.879
		1.1	0.049	0.916	0.050	0.907

5.2.4 Applying Power Family Inner Wedge Tests When Variance Is Unknown

Consider the setting of Section 3.4 in which observations follow a normal linear model with parameter vector $\boldsymbol{\beta}$ and variances depend on a scale factor σ^2. Group sequential estimates $\widehat{\boldsymbol{\beta}}^{(1)}, \ldots, \widehat{\boldsymbol{\beta}}^{(K)}$ are obtained at analyses 1 to K, $Var(\widehat{\boldsymbol{\beta}}^{(K)}) = \boldsymbol{V}_k\sigma^2$ and s_k^2 is the usual unbiased estimate of σ^2 at analysis k on $n_k - p$ degrees of freedom. We shall define group sequential two-sided t-tests of a null hypothesis H_0: $\boldsymbol{c}^T\boldsymbol{\beta} = \gamma$. Our main aim is for tests to have Type I error probability α, but we also wish to assess power at alternatives of the form $\boldsymbol{c}^T\boldsymbol{\beta} - \gamma = \pm\delta$.

As before, we have

$$\boldsymbol{c}^T\widehat{\boldsymbol{\beta}}^{(k)} \sim N(\boldsymbol{c}^T\boldsymbol{\beta}, \boldsymbol{c}^T\boldsymbol{V}_k\boldsymbol{c}\sigma^2)$$

and the t-statistic for testing H_0 is

$$T_k = \frac{\boldsymbol{c}^T\widehat{\boldsymbol{\beta}}^{(k)} - \gamma}{\sqrt{\{\boldsymbol{c}^T\boldsymbol{V}_k\boldsymbol{c}\, s_k^2\}}}.$$

The group sequential inner wedge tests already introduced in this chapter are for known σ^2. In adapting these tests to an unknown variance we begin with the stopping rule (5.1) and constants a_k and b_k, $k = 1, \ldots, K$, defined by (5.3). We replace Z_k in (5.1) by T_k and choose critical values for T_k to preserve the marginal probability under H_0 of being above or below each boundary point at analysis k. The new stopping rule is therefore:

After group $k = 1, \ldots, K-1$

if $\lvert T_k\rvert \geq t_{n_k-p,1-\Phi(b_k)}$	stop, reject H_0
if $\lvert T_k\rvert < t_{n_k-p,1-\Phi(a_k)}$	stop, accept H_0
otherwise	continue to group $k+1$,

after group K

if $\lvert T_K\rvert \geq t_{n_K-p,1-\Phi(b_K)}$	stop, reject H_0
if $\lvert T_K\rvert < t_{n_K-p,1-\Phi(a_K)}$	stop, accept H_0,

where $a_K = b_K$. Here, $t_{\nu,q}$ is such that $Pr\{T > t_{\nu,q}\} = q$ when $T \sim t_\nu$.

This construction is closely related to that used in Section 4.4 to create group sequential one-sided t-tests. Essentially the same arguments imply that the resulting tests have Type I error probability close to the target value α, especially if information levels are approximately equally spaced and the degrees of freedom for each s_k^2 are not too low. Also, a similar approach can be taken to estimate a test's power. The approximation analogous to (4.7) gives

$$Pr\{T(n_K - p; \delta/\sqrt{[\tilde{R}_W(K, \alpha, \beta, \Delta)\, \boldsymbol{c}^T\boldsymbol{V}_K\boldsymbol{c}\sigma^2]}) \geq t_{n_K-p,1-\alpha/2}\} \tag{5.4}$$

as an estimate of the power at $\boldsymbol{c}^T\boldsymbol{\beta} - \gamma = \pm\delta$ for a given value of σ^2. The cruder approximation for large $n_K - p$ is

$$\Phi\left(\frac{\delta}{\sqrt{\{\tilde{R}_W(K, \alpha, \beta, \Delta)\, \boldsymbol{c}^T\boldsymbol{V}_K\boldsymbol{c}\sigma^2\}}} - \Phi^{-1}(1 - \alpha/2)\right). \tag{5.5}$$

Table 5.5 *Properties of power family inner wedge t-tests designed to test* H_0*:* $c^T\beta = \gamma$ *with two-sided Type I error* $\alpha = 0.05$*, based on tests for known variance with* $\Delta = -0.5$ *and* 0.0. *Degrees of freedom for* σ^2 *are* $\nu_k = (\nu_K + 2)(k/K) - 2$ *and* $Var(c^T\hat{\beta}^{(k)}) = (K/k)Var(c^T\hat{\beta}^{(K)})$*, at analyses* $k = 1, \ldots, K$*. Actual power at the alternatives for which the approximation* (5.4) *gives power* 0.8 *is shown in the penultimate column. The final column gives the power predicted by formula* (5.5).
Type I error and power were estimated by simulation using 50000 *replicates; standard errors are* 0.001 *for Type I error and* 0.002 *for power.*

	K	ν_K	*Type I error*	*Attained power*	*Known* σ^2 *power*
$\Delta = -0.5$					
	3	7	0.054	0.820	0.905
	3	13	0.052	0.814	0.858
	5	13	0.057	0.816	0.858
	5	23	0.054	0.813	0.833
	8	22	0.056	0.813	0.834
	8	38	0.053	0.806	0.820
$\Delta = 0.0$					
	3	7	0.059	0.822	0.905
	3	13	0.055	0.814	0.858
	5	13	0.058	0.821	0.858
	5	23	0.056	0.814	0.833
	8	22	0.056	0.816	0.834
	8	38	0.053	0.809	0.820

Table 5.5 shows the Type I error probability of our group sequential inner wedge t-tests and the power they attain in situations where (5.4) gives the value 0.8. The degrees of freedom are those which arise when each group contains three or five observations and two degrees of freedom are used in fitting the linear model at each analysis. Results follow the pattern previously seen for group sequential t-tests. There are only minor departures from the target Type I error rates and formula (5.4) gives a reliable approximation to attained power, particularly when the degrees of freedom are fairly high. Once again, the definition of group sequential t-tests does not rely on equally spaced information levels and these tests may also be used with unequal group sizes or information increments.

5.2.5 *Example: Two-Treatment Comparison*

We illustrate the above methods with an example of a parallel two-treatment comparison conducted group sequentially with five groups of observations. Suppose observations $X_{Ai} \sim N(\mu_A, \sigma^2)$ and $X_{Bi} \sim N(\mu_B, \sigma^2)$, $i = 1, 2, \ldots,$

and we wish to test H_0: $\mu_A = \mu_B$ against the two-sided alternative $\mu_A \neq \mu_B$ with Type I error probability $\alpha = 0.05$ using a power family inner wedge test with $\Delta = 0.25$. We further suppose there is reason to believe σ^2 is in the region of 1.0, and we would like the test to have power of about 0.95 to detect a difference of $\mu_A - \mu_B = \pm 0.6$, bearing in mind our uncertainty about σ^2. If groups contain m observations per treatment, the sequence of t-statistics is

$$T_k = \frac{\sum_{i=1}^{mk} X_{Ai} - \sum_{i=1}^{mk} X_{Bi}}{\sqrt{\{2mks_k^2\}}}, \quad k = 1, \ldots, 5,$$

where

$$s_k^2 = \frac{\sum_{i=1}^{mk}(X_{Ai} - \bar{X}_A^{(k)})^2 + \sum_{i=1}^{mk}(X_{Bi} - \bar{X}_B^{(k)})^2}{2(mk-1)}.$$

The constants defining this inner wedge test, taken from Table 5.3, are $\tilde{C}_{W1}(5, 0.05, 0.05, 0.25) = 2.088$, $\tilde{C}_{W2}(5, 0.05, 0.05, 0.25) = 1.799$ and $\tilde{R}_W(5, 0.05, 0.05, 0.25) = 1.163$. For $k = 1, \ldots, 5$, the test stops to reject H_0 at analysis k if

$$|T_k| \geq t_{2mk-2, 1-\Phi(b_k)}$$

and to accept H_0 at analysis k if

$$|T_k| < t_{2mk-2, 1-\Phi(a_k)},$$

where, from (5.3), $b_k = 2.088 \times (k/5)^{-0.25}$ and

$$a_k = (2.088 + 1.799) \times (k/5)^{0.5} - 1.799 \times (k/5)^{-0.25}.$$

We expect the Type I error probability of this test to be close to 0.05, but its power will depend on m and the unknown σ^2. If σ^2 were known to be equal to 1.0, the corresponding five-group test for known variance would need a final information level $\tilde{R}_W(5, 0.05, 0.05, 0.25) \times \mathcal{I}_{f,2}$, i.e.,

$$1.163 \times \{\Phi^{-1}(0.975) + \Phi^{-1}(0.95)\}^2 / 0.6^2 = 41.98.$$

Five groups of m observations on each treatment give an estimate of $\mu_A - \mu_B$ with variance $2\sigma^2/(5m)$ and, therefore, information $5m/(2\sigma^2)$ for $\mu_A - \mu_B$. Equating this to 41.98 when $\sigma^2 = 1.0$ gives the value $m = 16.8$. We know the corresponding group sequential t-test will require a slightly higher sample size, but rounding up to the next integer, $m = 17$, is evidently sufficient since (5.4) then gives 0.950 as the approximate power at $|\mu_A - \mu_B| = 0.6$ if $\sigma^2 = 1.0$. Simulations with one million replications show this test's actual Type I error rate to be 0.051 and its power at $|\mu_A - \mu_B| = 0.6$ when $\sigma^2 = 1.0$ to be 0.951 (standard errors of these estimates are less than 0.0005).

The above power calculation relies on σ^2 being equal to its predicted value of 1.0. If the experimenter desires greater confidence that the power condition will actually be met, the sample size should be calculated using an upper bound on plausible values of σ^2. Suppose, for example, it is thought that σ^2 could be as high as 1.4; the analogous calculation to that shown above gives the value $m = 23.5$

and the rounded value $m = 24$ appears adequate since formula (5.4) then gives 0.952 as the approximate power at $|\mu_A - \mu_B| = 0.6$ if $\sigma^2 = 1.4$ (the estimated power from one million simulations is 0.953, again with a standard error of less than 0.0005).

5.3 Whitehead's Double Triangular Test

Sobel & Wald (1949) describe a way of combining two one-sided sequential probability ratio tests to create a two-sided test with early stopping to accept the null hypothesis. Whitehead & Stratton (1983) and Whitehead (1997) have used this technique to combine two triangular tests, producing a "double triangular" test.

Suppose standardized statistics $Z_1, \ldots, Z_K$ at analyses $k = 1, \ldots, K$ follow the canonical joint distribution (3.1), and we require a test of H_0: $\theta = 0$ with Type I error probability α and power $1 - \beta$ at $\theta = \pm\delta$. The double triangular test is formed from two of Whitehead's one-sided triangular boundaries for testing the null hypothesis $\theta = 0$ with Type I error rate $\alpha/2$ and power $1 - \beta$ at $\theta = \delta$ and $\theta = -\delta$, respectively. Sampling continues until both tests have reached a conclusion, then H_0 is rejected if either of the tests has rejected $\theta = 0$ and accepted otherwise.

The test is most naturally described in terms of the score statistics $S_k = Z_k\sqrt{\mathcal{I}_k}$, $k = 1, \ldots, K$. For equally spaced information levels, the one-sided triangular test of $\theta = 0$ versus $\theta > 0$ has upper and lower boundaries for S_k at analysis k given by

$$d_k = \frac{2}{\tilde{\delta}} \log\left(\frac{1}{\alpha}\right) - 0.583\sqrt{\frac{\mathcal{I}_{max}}{K}} + \frac{\tilde{\delta}}{4}\frac{k}{K}\mathcal{I}_{max} \tag{5.6}$$

and

$$c_k = -\frac{2}{\tilde{\delta}} \log\left(\frac{1}{\alpha}\right) + 0.583\sqrt{\frac{\mathcal{I}_{max}}{K}} + \frac{3\tilde{\delta}}{4}\frac{k}{K}\mathcal{I}_{max}\,, \tag{5.7}$$

where

$$\tilde{\delta} = \frac{2\Phi^{-1}(1-\alpha/2)\,\delta}{\Phi^{-1}(1-\alpha/2) + \Phi^{-1}(1-\beta)}$$

and

$$\mathcal{I}_{max} = \left[\sqrt{\frac{4 \times 0.583^2}{K} + 8\log\left(\frac{1}{\alpha}\right)} - \frac{2 \times 0.583}{\sqrt{K}}\right]^2 \frac{1}{\tilde{\delta}^2}.$$

The upper and lower boundaries of the test of $\theta = 0$ versus $\theta < 0$ are $c'_k = -c_k$ and $d'_k = -d_k$, respectively. Combining these tests in the specified manner gives the formal stopping rule:

$$
\begin{array}{lll}
\text{After group } k = 1, \ldots, K-1 & & \\
\quad \text{if } |Z_k| \geq d_k & \text{stop, reject } H_0 & \\
\quad \text{if } Z_j \leq c_j \text{ for some } j \leq k \text{ and} & & \\
\quad\quad Z_j \geq -c_j \text{ for some } j \leq k & \text{stop, accept } H_0 & \\
\quad \text{otherwise} & \text{continue to group } k+1, & \quad (5.8) \\
\text{after group } K & & \\
\quad \text{if } |Z_K| \geq d_K & \text{stop, reject } H_0 & \\
\quad \text{otherwise} & \text{stop, accept } H_0. &
\end{array}
$$

For more general information sequences, $\mathcal{I}_{max}/K$ is replaced by $\mathcal{I}_k - \mathcal{I}_{k-1}$ in the second terms of equations (5.6) and (5.7) and $(k/K)\mathcal{I}_{max}$ is replaced by $\mathcal{I}_k$ in the third terms. The first part of rule (5.8) defines the test until a stage K is reached where $c_K \geq d_K$; in keeping with our suggestion in Section 4.5.3 for the one-sided test, we recommend that H_0 be rejected at this final stage if $|Z_K| \geq d_K$ and accepted otherwise.

Table 5.6 shows properties of the double triangular test when information levels are equally spaced and boundaries meet at the final analysis. The Sobel-Wald construction guarantees Type I error probability equal to the sum of the Type I error probabilities of the two one-sided tests, and power at $\theta = \pm\delta$ is that of the relevant one-sided test in each case. Thus, the slight inaccuracies in Type I error rate and power in the first two columns of Table 5.6 are due only to approximations made in the original one-sided tests. The third column of the table contains values of $R_{DT}(K, \alpha, \beta)$, the ratio between each group sequential test's maximum information level and the information, $\mathcal{I}_{f,2}$, required by a fixed sample test with error probabilities α and β. The final three columns show expected information levels on termination under $\theta = 0$, $\pm\delta/2$ and $\pm\delta$. As for the single triangular test of Section 4.5, results for $K = 1$ represent the case where a large first information level $\mathcal{I}_1$ leads to $d_1 = c_1$ and termination of the test. This time, the value of $\mathcal{I}_1$ is not quite so close to the information level needed for a fixed sample test with error probabilities exactly α and β, but it is still fairly close, and the results for this case testify to the robustness of Whitehead & Stratton's scheme for converting a continuous boundary to discrete monitoring.

A comparison with Tables 5.1 to 5.3 shows the double triangular tests' maximum sample sizes to be similar to those of power family tests with $\Delta = 0.25$ in the case $1 - \beta = 0.8$ and higher for $1 - \beta = 0.9$ and 0.95. Apart from some instances when only two analyses are performed, the power family tests with $\Delta = 0.25$ yield lower or roughly equal expected sample sizes across the range of θ values for $1 - \beta = 0.8$ and 0.9 and similar expected sample sizes for $1 - \beta = 0.95$, when their maximum sample sizes are lower.

Figure 5.1 at the end of Section 5.2.1 showed the boundary of a power family inner wedge test with $\Delta = 0$, five groups of observations, Type I error rate $\alpha = 0.05$ and power $1 - \beta = 0.9$ at $\delta = 0.2$. Figure 5.2 compares this boundary with that of Whitehead's double triangular test meeting the same specifications.

Table 5.6 *Properties of Whitehead's double triangular tests with equal group sizes. Constants $R_{DT}(K, \alpha, \beta)$ are ratios of the maximum sample size to that of a fixed sample test with the same error probabilities. Expected sample sizes at $\theta = 0$, $\delta/2$ and δ are expressed as percentages of the corresponding fixed sample size. Tests are for K groups of observations, and designed to have Type I error probability $\alpha = 0.05$ at $\theta = 0$ and power $1 - \beta = 0.8$, 0.9 and 0.95 at $\theta = \pm\delta$.*

K	*Type I error*	*Power at* $\theta = \pm\delta$	R_{DT}	*Expected sample size, as percentage of fixed sample size, at* $\theta=0$	$\theta=\pm\delta/2$	$\theta=\pm\delta$
$1-\beta=0.8$						
1	0.053	0.797	0.973	97.3	97.3	97.3
2	0.053	0.800	1.115	80.1	85.6	81.2
3	0.052	0.802	1.186	84.3	87.8	78.8
4	0.051	0.803	1.230	75.9	82.1	75.9
5	0.051	0.803	1.261	74.2	80.5	74.4
10	0.050	0.804	1.342	71.1	77.7	71.2
15	0.050	0.804	1.379	70.1	76.6	70.1
20	0.050	0.804	1.402	69.2	75.9	69.5
$1-\beta=0.9$						
1	0.053	0.897	0.973	97.3	97.3	97.3
2	0.053	0.899	1.115	80.1	86.3	76.2
3	0.052	0.901	1.186	84.3	87.8	72.4
4	0.051	0.902	1.230	75.9	82.7	69.8
5	0.051	0.902	1.261	74.2	81.2	68.2
10	0.050	0.902	1.342	71.1	78.4	64.8
15	0.050	0.902	1.379	70.1	77.4	63.6
20	0.050	0.902	1.402	69.2	76.7	63.0
$1-\beta=0.95$						
1	0.053	0.948	0.973	97.3	97.3	97.3
2	0.053	0.949	1.115	80.1	86.5	71.7
3	0.052	0.950	1.186	84.3	87.5	66.8
4	0.051	0.950	1.230	75.9	82.9	64.3
5	0.051	0.951	1.261	74.2	81.4	62.8
10	0.050	0.951	1.342	71.1	78.6	59.2
15	0.050	0.951	1.379	70.1	77.5	58.0
20	0.050	0.951	1.402	69.2	76.9	57.3

Figure 5.2 *Comparison of two inner wedge tests with five groups of observations*

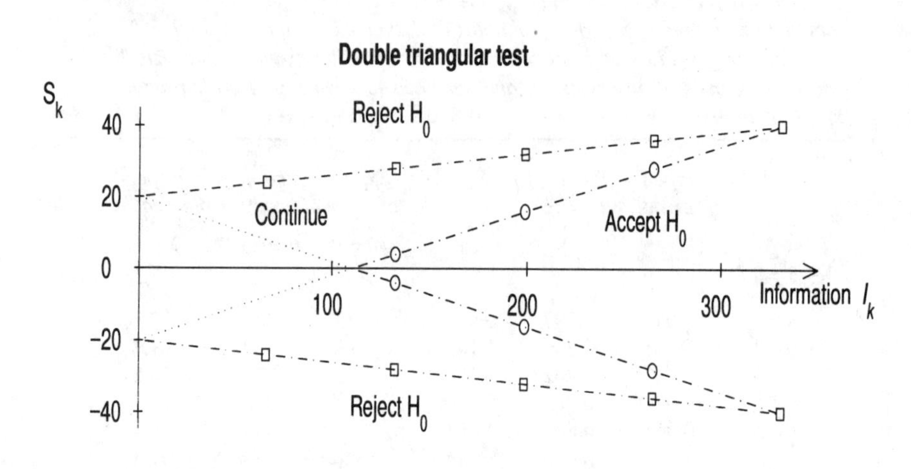

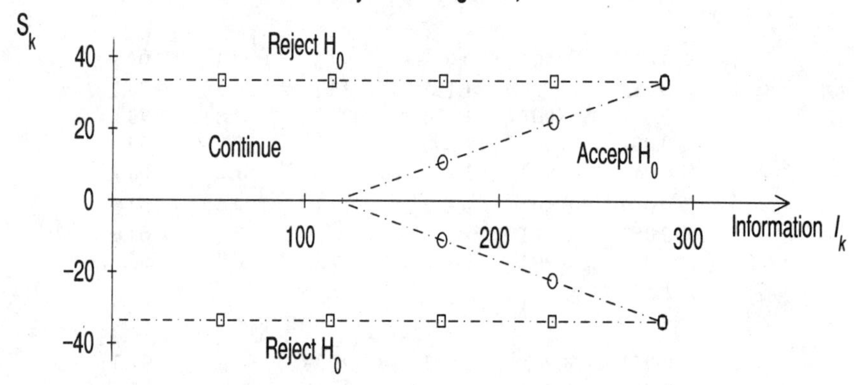

In constructing the double triangular test we set power $1 - \alpha = 0.95$ at $\theta = \tilde{\delta} = 2 \times 1.960 \times 0.2/(1.960 + 1.282) = 0.2418$. The double triangular test has $\mathcal{I}_{max} = R_{DT}(5, 0.05, 0.1)\,\mathcal{I}_{f,2} = 1.261 \times 262.76 = 331.3$, somewhat higher than the value $\tilde{R}_W(5, 0.05, 0.1, 0)\,\mathcal{I}_{f,2} = 1.084 \times 262.76 = 284.8$ for the power family inner wedge test with $\Delta = 0$. These values of $\tilde{R}_W(5, 0.05, 0.1, 0)$ and $R_{DT}(5, 0.05, 0.1)$ are taken from Tables 5.2 and 5.6, respectively.

The Sobel-Wald construction is unusual in that the stopping rule produced is not a function of a sufficient statistic for θ. Suppose, for example, Z_k lies below the lower boundary of the one-sided test of $\theta = 0$ versus $\theta > 0$ but in the continuation region of the test of $\theta = 0$ versus $\theta < 0$. Then, early stopping to accept H_0 occurs if the upper boundary of the test of $\theta = 0$ *vs* $\theta < 0$ was crossed previously, i.e., if $Z_j \geq -c_j$ for some $j < k$. However, given the value of Z_k, the conditional distribution of $Z_1, \ldots, Z_{k-1}$ is independent of θ, so it is difficult to justify why a conclusion should depend on the values of $Z_1, \ldots, Z_{k-1}$ once Z_k is known. The double triangular test can be simplified by ignoring the inner boundary until c_k becomes positive, in which case the test has the form (5.1) with $a_k = d_k$ and $b_k = c_k$, $k = 1, \ldots, K$. Calculations show this modification has almost no effect on the Type I error probability, the only change to values in Table 5.6 being an increase from 0.052 to 0.053 for $K = 3$. There are small increases in power, the largest being 0.009, 0.007 and 0.005 for $K = 3$ and $1 - \beta = 0.8$, 0.9 and 0.95, respectively. In view of the sound theoretical reasons for defining statistical procedures in terms of sufficient statistics, we recommend making this modification in applying Whitehead's double triangular test .

CHAPTER 6

Equivalence Tests

6.1 Introduction

Sometimes the goal of a clinical trial is to establish *equivalence* between two treatments rather than the superiority in efficacy of one over the other. For example, if a new therapy is less toxic or less expensive than the standard, it may not be necessary to prove it is also more effective; instead, it can suffice to demonstrate that it is equally effective or that it is less effective than the standard by at most a small amount. Dunnett & Gent (1977) give an example of a trial in which an objective was to determine whether certain aspects of health care could be delivered equally well by a system involving a triage process by nurse-practitioners as by conventional primary physician care methods. Other examples include: lumpectomy versus radical mastectomy for breast cancer treatment, a local rice-based beverage versus WHO oral rehydration solution for diarrhea in infants in Mexico, and low-dose AZT treatment versus standard dose during pregnancy and delivery to prevent mother-to-child HIV transmission in a developing country. We call these "one-sided equivalence" problems.

A "two-sided equivalence" problem can arise in the area of bioequivalence testing. Here, a pharmaceutical manufacturer hopes to demonstrate that a new preparation of a drug has the same bioavailability properties as a standard, within a small tolerance limit, as a step toward proving that the new and standard preparations have equal therapeutic effects. Demonstrating "bioequivalence" in this way can greatly reduce the amount of experimentation required for approval of a new drug.

Chinchilli (1996) classifies equivalence problems into the following categories:

Population equivalence: the responses for both treatments have the same probability distribution;

Average equivalence: the responses have the same mean;

Individual equivalence: the responses are "approximately" the same for a large proportion of subjects when they receive either treatment.

In Sections 6.2 and 6.3 we shall be concerned principally with average bioequivalence; we consider tests of individual equivalence in Section 6.4.

Of course, to conclude equivalence, it is not sufficient that the data fail to reject a null hypothesis of equality. This might simply be due to a lack of power of the study, and a *practically significant* difference could still exist despite the lack of *statistically significant* evidence. Thus, if a hypothesis test of equality is to be employed as a means of establishing equivalence, this test's Type II error probability, representing the probability of wrongly declaring equivalence when a practically significant difference exists, must be restricted to an acceptable level. An alternative approach is to test a specific hypothesis of non-equality or "inequivalence" and conclude equivalence if this hypothesis is rejected. In this case, the error requirements have a more familiar form since priority is given to the test's Type I error rate, i.e., the probability of rejecting the hypothesis of inequivalence when this hypothesis is true. We shall illustrate both these approaches: in the following section we adopt the second method, creating a hypothesis of inequivalence in order to test for one-sided equivalence, and in Section 6.3 we take the first approach, basing a test for two-sided equivalence on a test of a null hypothesis of no treatment difference.

6.2 One-Sided Tests of Equivalence

Let μ_A and μ_B denote the true means of the primary response variable for a new and standard treatment, respectively, where higher responses are more favorable. Suppose previous studies have shown that the new treatment has less toxic side effects than the standard. In view of this known advantage of the new treatment, we can define a hypothesis of inequivalence as H_I: $\mu_A - \mu_B \le -\delta$, where δ is a positive constant and a decrease in mean response up to δ is deemed acceptable for the new treatment in view of its reduced toxicity. The hypothesis of equivalence is then H_E: $\mu_A - \mu_B > -\delta$, and it is appropriate to conduct a one-sided equivalence test to choose between H_I and H_E. Note that H_E includes instances where μ_A is considerably greater than μ_B since in this one-sided case we intend "equivalence" of the two treatments to mean that the new treatment is at least as good, overall, as the standard.

In essence, this problem is the same as the one-sided hypothesis testing problem of Chapter 4, and if we define $\theta = \mu_A - \mu_B + \delta$, the methods of Chapter 4 can be applied directly. Then, H_0: $\theta = 0$ occurs at the upper limit of H_I, $\mu_A - \mu_B = -\delta$, and so the Type I error rate of the test of H_0 becomes the maximum probability of wrongly declaring equivalence. The power at $\theta = \delta$ is of particular interest as this represents the probability of declaring equivalence when μ_A and μ_B are exactly equal. Since the new treatment has other advantages over the standard, a high power to decide in favor of the new treatment is desirable when both treatments are equal with regard to the primary response .

6.3 Two-Sided Tests of Equivalence: Application to Comparative Bioavailability Studies

6.3.1 The Testing Problem

As mentioned above, two-sided equivalence tests arise most frequently in bioequivalence studies, so we shall frame our discussion here in that context. Westlake (1979) reviews comparative bioavailability trials for testing the bioequivalence of two competing formulations of a drug. In a typical trial, a single dose is administered to a subject and blood samples are drawn at various times over the next 24, 36 or 48 hours. This leads to a sequence of drug concentration levels in the blood, or "drug profile", in which the drug level usually rises to a peak during the initial absorption phase and then decays. A univariate statistic summarizing this response might be the "area under the curve" (AUC) or the peak concentration level (C_{max}). It is often reasonable to assume these quantities are log-normally distributed. The experimental design may utilize two parallel patient samples, as in Section 3.1.1 but it is more usual to employ a two-period crossover design as described in Section 3.1.4. The crossover design has the advantage of removing the between-subject component of variability, resulting in a much more sensitive test, and this in turn permits use of smaller sample sizes. A "washout" interval between the administrations of the two drugs in a given patient should be of sufficient length to eliminate any carry-over effect of the drug given first. In some cases it is possible to ascertain the presence of carry-over effects by measuring concentration levels during the washout period. Another possible complication is the existence of treatment-by-period interactions. More sophisticated designs have been proposed which need to be analyzed by more complex linear models incorporating such carry-over and interaction effects — see, for example, Jones & Kenward (1989, Section 1.6). In general, group sequential versions of these designs can be adapted from those proposed in this section using techniques for normal linear models described in Section 3.4 and Chapter 11. Here we shall confine ourselves to the standard 2×2 crossover design of Section 3.1.4.

Consider the design of a group sequential two-treatment, two-period crossover trial. For $i = 1, 2, \dots$, let X_i denote the natural logarithm of the ratio of response on treatment A to response on treatment B for the ith subject receiving treatment A first. Similarly, define Y_i to be the logarithm of the same ratio for the ith subject receiving treatment B first. Response here may be defined as the AUC, C_{max}, or other summary feature of the drug profile. The usual model treats the responses as log-normally distributed with

$$X_i \sim N(\theta + \phi, \sigma^2) \text{ and } Y_i \sim N(\theta - \phi, \sigma^2), \quad i = 1, 2, \dots, \tag{6.1}$$

where θ is the treatment difference and ϕ a period effect.

In a two-sided test of equivalence, the treatments A and B are to be considered equivalent if $|\theta| < \delta$. Here, δ should be "determined from the practical aspects of the problem in such a way that the treatments can be considered for all practical purposes to be equivalent if their true difference is unlikely to exceed the specified δ" (Dunnett & Gent, 1977, p. 594). Let us impose the error probability requirements

$$Pr_{\theta=\pm\delta}\{\text{Declare equivalence}\} \leq \beta \tag{6.2}$$

and

$$Pr_{\theta=0}\{\text{Do not declare equivalence}\} \leq \alpha. \tag{6.3}$$

Some authors would interchange the symbols α and β here, but we use the above choice for consistency with the notation for two-sided tests in Chapter 5. The important point is that β in (6.2) represents the "consumer's risk" since wrongly declaring equivalence may lead to an unsuitable preparation being allowed onto the market. Values of β and δ must be chosen to satisfy the appropriate regulatory agency. Recommended choices are often $\beta = 0.05$ and $\delta = \log(1.25)$ so that

$|\theta| < \delta$ implies that, on the antilog scale, the treatment effect ratio lies in the range 0.8 to 1.25. The probability α in (6.3) is the "manufacturer's risk" and, since the benefits of proving equivalence are so great, one would expect a small value of α to be chosen in order to ensure a high probability of a positive conclusion when two treatments really are equivalent.

6.3.2 *Using the Power Family of Inner Wedge Tests*

If σ^2 is known, we may directly utilize the techniques of Chapter 5 to design a group sequential crossover trial to test for two-sided equivalence. The number of analyses, K, and the shape parameter Δ of the power family test must be chosen. Suppose for now that the study can be organized so that equal numbers of observations following each treatment sequence accrue between successive analyses. The factor $\tilde{R}_W(K, \alpha, \beta, \Delta)$, taken from Table 5.1, 5.2 or 5.3 is used to determine the required sample size. Constants $\tilde{C}_{W1}(K, \alpha, \beta, \Delta)$ and $\tilde{C}_{W2}(K, \alpha, \beta, \Delta)$ are also read from the table and used to determine critical values a_k and b_k for $k = 1, \ldots, K$. The stopping rule (5.1) is then applied with the modification that the decision "accept H_0" is replaced by "declare equivalence" and "reject H_0" is replaced by "declare non-equivalence".

As an example, suppose we specify $\alpha = \beta = 0.05$, $\delta = \log(1.25) = 0.223$, $\Delta = 0$ and a balanced design with $K = 4$ equally sized groups. Suppose also that the within-subject coefficient of variation (CV) of the responses on the original antilog scale is known to be 24% — Hauck, Preston & Bois (1997, p. 91) suggest this as a "moderate range" value for a CV for AUC. It follows that $\sigma^2 \approx 2 \times 0.24^2 = 0.115$.

After n_k observations on each treatment sequence, the estimate

$$\hat{\theta}^{(k)} = (\bar{X}^{(k)} + \bar{Y}^{(k)})/2$$

has variance $\sigma^2/(2n_k)$, so the information for θ is $\mathcal{I}_k = 2n_k/\sigma^2$. From (3.6), the information needed for a fixed sample size test is

$$\mathcal{I}_{f,2} = (1.960 + 1.645)^2/0.223^2 = 261.3,$$

which requires $261.3\,\sigma^2/2 = 261.3 \times 0.115/2 = 15.0$ subjects on each treatment sequence. For our sequential test we multiply $\mathcal{I}_{f,2}$ by $\tilde{R}_W(4, 0.05, 0.05, 0) = 1.055$ to obtain the maximum information level 275.7, and solving $2n_4/0.115 = 275.7$ gives the final sample size per treatment sequence $n_4 = 15.9$. Rounding this value of n_4 up to 16, we see the study should be designed with four subjects on each treatment sequence in each of the four groups. The test is implemented by applying rule (5.1) to the standardized statistics

$$Z_k = \hat{\theta}^{(k)}\sqrt{\mathcal{I}_k} = (\bar{X}^{(k)} + \bar{Y}^{(k)})\sqrt{\{n_k/(2\sigma^2)\}}, \quad k = 1, \ldots, 4,$$

taking acceptance of H_0 to indicate declaration of equivalence. The critical values a_k and b_k are obtained from (5.2) using $\tilde{C}_{W1}(4, 0.05, 0.05, 0) = 1.995$ and $\tilde{C}_{W2}(4, 0.05, 0.05, 0) = 1.708$ from Table 5.3. With $\delta = 0.223$ this gives

$$(a_1, a_2, a_3, a_4) = (-1.56, 0.21, 1.25, 2.01)$$

and

$$(b_1, b_2, b_3, b_4) = (3.99, 2.82, 2.30, 1.995).$$

Since a_1 is negative, it is not possible to stop and declare equivalence at the first analysis. Due to the rounding of n_4 to an integer sample size, the values of a_4 and b_4 are not exactly equal; although the difference is slight, one could choose to use the lower value, b_4, as the critical value for $|Z_4|$ in order to protect against the key error of wrongly declaring equivalence. (This minor difficulty can be avoided altogether by following the method for dealing with unequal group sizes explained in the next section.) The result of applying this test is a noticeable saving in expected total sample size across the range of θ values: expected samples sizes are 24.1, 26.0 and 21.6 under $\theta = 0, \pm\delta/2$ and $\pm\delta$, respectively, compared to the 30 subjects required by a fixed sample procedure.

6.3.3 Adapting to Unequal Group Sizes and Unknown Variance

To satisfy real practical needs, methods must be able to handle unequal numbers on each treatment at any stage in a parallel design or unequal numbers on each sequence (AB or BA) during a crossover design. Later, in Section 7.2.5, we shall discuss how unequal increments in information can be handled using an "error spending" approach to create two-sided tests with an inner wedge. Here, we describe an approximate approach using power family inner wedge tests.

It is also important to deal with normal responses of unknown variance and power family inner wedge tests can also be adapted to this problem too. In dealing with either unequal increments in information or unknown variance, special modifications are needed to ensure the probability of wrongly declaring equivalence remains within a specified limit. In Chapters 4 and 5 we adapted power family tests in a way which preserved the Type I error rate by expressing the stopping boundary in terms of significance levels under H_0: $\theta = 0$. We shall follow a similar approach, working with significance levels against the hypotheses $\theta = \delta$ and $\theta = -\delta$ in order to preserve the *power* of the original test. Our development here parallels that of Jennison & Turnbull (2000a).

Suppose we wish to construct a two-sided equivalence test satisfying

$$Pr_{\theta=\pm\delta}\{\text{Declare equivalence}\} \leq \beta$$

for specified δ and β, using a group sequential design with K analyses based on a power family inner wedge test with shape parameter Δ. Supposing, for now, that σ^2 is known, we can also plan to satisfy a second error condition

$$Pr_{\theta=0}\{\text{Do not declare equivalence}\} \leq \alpha,$$

noting that this condition will not be met precisely if actual information levels differ from their design values.

We take as our starting point the two-sided test of H_0: $\theta = 0$ with Type I error probability α and power $1 - \beta$ at $\theta = \pm\delta$. Thus, we plan to achieve information levels

$$\mathcal{I}_k = (k/K)\,\tilde{R}_W(K, \alpha, \beta, \Delta)\,\mathcal{I}_{f,2}$$

at analyses 1 to K. If these information levels arise exactly, the test defined by rule (5.1) with a_k and b_k, $k = 1, \ldots, K$, given by (5.2) will have Type I error probability α and power $1 - \beta$ at $\theta = \pm\delta$ and the equivalence test will have exactly the desired error probabilities.

When observed information levels differ from their planned values, we use the significance level approach to maintain properties under $\theta = \pm\delta$. Consider first the case $\theta = \delta$: since $Z_k - \delta\sqrt{\mathcal{I}_k}$ has a standard normal distribution under $\theta = \delta$, we can proceed by expressing the boundary as a sequence of critical values for $Z_k - \delta\sqrt{\mathcal{I}_k}$ in a form which does not explicitly involve the information levels $\mathcal{I}_1, \ldots, \mathcal{I}_K$. However, we must simultaneously treat the case $\theta = -\delta$. Fortunately, a typical test generates little probability of crossing the lower boundary arms if $\theta = \delta$ or the upper arms if $\theta = -\delta$, and there is no serious loss of accuracy in defining the upper section by considering $\theta = \delta$ and the lower section by considering $\theta = -\delta$.

To simplify notation, we shall omit the arguments of $\tilde{C}_{W1}$ and $\tilde{C}_{W2}$ in the following derivation. For $\theta = \delta$, the upper part of the stopping boundary defined by (5.1) with a_k and b_k as specified in (5.2) is based on comparing

$$Z_k \quad \text{versus} \quad \begin{cases} \tilde{C}_{W1}(k/K)^{\Delta-1/2} & \text{and} \\ \delta\sqrt{\mathcal{I}_k} - \tilde{C}_{W2}(k/K)^{\Delta-1/2}, & \end{cases}$$

i.e., comparing

$$Z_k - \delta\sqrt{\mathcal{I}_k} \quad \text{versus} \quad \begin{cases} -\delta\sqrt{\mathcal{I}_k} + \tilde{C}_{W1}(k/K)^{\Delta-1/2} & \text{and} \\ -\tilde{C}_{W2}(k/K)^{\Delta-1/2}, & \end{cases}$$

at each analysis $k = 1, \ldots, K$. Under the planned sequence of information levels, $\mathcal{I}_k = (k/K)\{\tilde{C}_{W1} + \tilde{C}_{W2}\}^2/\delta^2$ and we can write this comparison as

$$Z_k - \delta\sqrt{\mathcal{I}_k} \quad \text{versus} \quad h_k \text{ and } g_k,$$

where

$$h_k = -\{\tilde{C}_{W1} + \tilde{C}_{W2}\}(k/K)^{1/2} + \tilde{C}_{W1}(k/K)^{\Delta-1/2}$$

and

$$g_k = -\tilde{C}_{W2}(k/K)^{\Delta-1/2}, \quad k = 1, \ldots, K.$$

These formulae for g_k and h_k avoid explicit mention of $\mathcal{I}_k$. Also, g_K is automatically equal to h_K. By symmetry, the lower section of the stopping boundary arises from comparing $Z_k + \delta\sqrt{\mathcal{I}_k}$ with $-g_k$ and $-h_k$ at analyses $k = 1, \ldots, K$. Incorporating the additional feature that stopping to accept H_0 should not occur before analysis k^*, the first stage at which g_k is positive, we obtain the full stopping rule:

$$
\begin{array}{lll}
\text{After group } k = 1, \dots, k^* - 1 & & \\
\quad \text{if } Z_k - \delta\sqrt{\mathcal{I}_k} \ge h_k \text{ or} & & \\
\quad\quad Z_k + \delta\sqrt{\mathcal{I}_k} \le -h_k & \text{stop, reject equivalence} & \\
\quad \text{otherwise} & \text{continue to group } k+1, & \\
\text{after group } k = k^*, \dots, K - 1 & & \\
\quad \text{if } Z_k - \delta\sqrt{\mathcal{I}_k} \ge h_k \text{ or} & & \\
\quad\quad Z_k + \delta\sqrt{\mathcal{I}_k} \le -h_k & \text{stop, reject equivalence} & \\
\quad \text{if } Z_k - \delta\sqrt{\mathcal{I}_k} < g_k \text{ and} & & (6.4) \\
\quad\quad Z_k + \delta\sqrt{\mathcal{I}_k} > -g_k & \text{stop, declare equivalence} & \\
\quad \text{otherwise} & \text{continue to group } k+1, & \\
\text{after group } K & & \\
\quad \text{if } Z_K - \delta\sqrt{\mathcal{I}_K} \ge h_K \text{ or} & & \\
\quad\quad Z_K + \delta\sqrt{\mathcal{I}_K} \le -h_K & \text{stop, reject equivalence} & \\
\quad \text{otherwise} & \text{stop, declare equivalence.} &
\end{array}
$$

The condition to stop and reject equivalence at analysis k can be re-expressed as

$$
\begin{aligned}
|Z_k| \ \ge \ h_k + \delta\sqrt{\mathcal{I}_k} \ &= \ \tilde{C}_{W1}(k/K)^{\Delta-1/2} + \delta\sqrt{\mathcal{I}_k} \\
&\quad -\{\tilde{C}_{W1} + \tilde{C}_{W2}\}(k/K)^{1/2}
\end{aligned}
$$

and that to declare equivalence as

$$
|Z_k| \ < \ g_k + \delta\sqrt{\mathcal{I}_k} \ = \ \delta\sqrt{\mathcal{I}_k} - \tilde{C}_{W2}(k/K)^{\Delta-1/2}.
$$

The above test can now be applied using the information levels $\mathcal{I}_1, \dots, \mathcal{I}_K$ actually observed. Table 6.1 shows the Type I error probability and power achieved by such tests with $K = 2, 5$ and 10 analyses and shape parameter $\Delta = -0.5$ and 0, under sequences of information levels of the form $\mathcal{I}_k = \pi(k/K)^r \mathcal{I}_{max}$, where $\mathcal{I}_{max} = \tilde{R}_W(K, \alpha, \beta, \Delta)\,\mathcal{I}_{f,2}$. It is clear from the table that, as intended, power remains close to its nominal value, 0.95, in all cases. Although the same two-sided tests were originally planned in the examples of Table 5.4 in Section 5.2.3 and the same information sequences were observed, we have worked toward a different objective in adapting these tests to unequal group sizes and the resulting tests have quite different properties. Whereas the tests in Table 5.4 maintain a fixed Type I error probability and have variable power at $\theta = \pm\delta$, our new equivalence tests closely control power, the probability of correctly rejecting equivalence when $\theta = \pm\delta$, and channel variability into the Type I error rate, the probability of wrongly rejecting equivalence when $\theta = 0$.

It remains to consider adaptation of power family equivalence tests to the case of unknown variance in a way which maintains power at $\theta = \pm\delta$ as closely as possible. We shall illustrate this in the context of a crossover trial where we suppose data follow the normal linear model (6.1). If observations $X_1, \dots, X_{n_{Xk}}$ and $Y_1, \dots, Y_{n_{Yk}}$ are available at analysis k, the estimate of θ is

$$
\hat{\theta}^{(k)} = (\bar{X}^{(k)} + \bar{Y}^{(k)})/2
$$

Table 6.1 *Properties of power family two-sided equivalence tests designed for information levels* $\mathcal{I}_k = (k/K)\mathcal{I}_{max}$ *applied with* $\mathcal{I}_k = \pi(k/K)^r\mathcal{I}_{max}$, $k = 1, \ldots, K$, *in a manner which preserves power, i.e., the probability of correctly rejecting equivalence when* $\theta = \pm\delta$. *Attained Type I error probabilities and power are shown for tests with shape parameter* Δ *and K analyses, designed to achieve Type I error probability* $\alpha = 0.05$ *and power* $1 - \beta = 0.95$ *at* $\theta = \pm\delta$.

			$\Delta = -0.5$		$\Delta = 0.0$	
	r	π	*Type I error*	*Power*	*Type I error*	*Power*
$K = 2$						
	0.80	0.9	0.076	0.950	0.074	0.950
		1.0	0.050	0.950	0.049	0.950
		1.1	0.033	0.950	0.032	0.950
	1.00	0.9	0.076	0.950	0.077	0.951
		1.0	0.050	0.950	0.050	0.950
		1.1	0.033	0.950	0.033	0.950
	1.25	0.9	0.076	0.950	0.082	0.953
		1.0	0.050	0.950	0.054	0.953
		1.1	0.033	0.950	0.036	0.951
$K = 5$						
	0.80	0.9	0.075	0.950	0.070	0.951
		1.0	0.049	0.950	0.046	0.951
		1.1	0.032	0.950	0.030	0.951
	1.00	0.9	0.076	0.950	0.076	0.950
		1.0	0.050	0.950	0.050	0.950
		1.1	0.033	0.950	0.033	0.950
	1.25	0.9	0.079	0.950	0.087	0.950
		1.0	0.052	0.950	0.059	0.950
		1.1	0.034	0.950	0.040	0.950
$K = 10$						
	0.80	0.9	0.073	0.951	0.068	0.951
		1.0	0.048	0.950	0.044	0.951
		1.1	0.031	0.950	0.028	0.951
	1.00	0.9	0.076	0.950	0.076	0.950
		1.0	0.050	0.950	0.050	0.950
		1.1	0.033	0.950	0.033	0.950
	1.25	0.9	0.081	0.950	0.091	0.950
		1.0	0.054	0.950	0.062	0.950
		1.1	0.036	0.950	0.042	0.950

where

$$\bar{X}^{(k)} = \sum_{i=1}^{n_{Xk}} X_i / n_{Xk} \text{ and } \bar{Y}^{(k)} = \sum_{i=1}^{n_{Yk}} Y_i / n_{Yk}, \quad k = 1, \ldots, K.$$

The sequence of estimates $\{\hat{\theta}^{(1)}, \ldots, \hat{\theta}^{(K)}\}$ is multivariate normal with

$$Var(\hat{\theta}^{(k)}) = \sigma^2 (n_{Xk}^{-1} + n_{Yk}^{-1})/4, \quad k = 1, \ldots, K,$$

and

$$Cov(\hat{\theta}^{(k_1)}, \hat{\theta}^{(k_2)}) = Var(\hat{\theta}^{(k_2)}), \quad 1 \le k_1 \le k_2 \le K.$$

The usual estimate of σ^2 at analysis k is

$$s_k^2 = \{\sum_{i=1}^{n_{Xk}} (X_i - \bar{X}_k)^2 + \sum_{i=1}^{n_{Yk}} (Y_i - \bar{Y}_k)^2\} / (n_{Xk} + n_{Yk} - 2)$$

on $\nu_k = n_{Xk} + n_{Yk} - 2$ degrees of freedom.

In the known variance problem, the Z-statistics $Z_k - \delta\sqrt{\mathcal{I}_k}$ and $Z_k + \delta\sqrt{\mathcal{I}_k}$ had standard normal distributions under the hypotheses $\theta = \delta$ and $\theta = -\delta$, respectively. With σ^2 unknown, we now use the t-statistics

$$T_k^+ = \frac{\hat{\theta}^{(k)} - \delta}{\sqrt{\{s_k^2 (n_{Xk}^{-1} + n_{Yk}^{-1})/4\}}} \quad \text{and} \quad T_k^- = \frac{\hat{\theta}^{(k)} + \delta}{\sqrt{\{s_k^2 (n_{Xk}^{-1} + n_{Yk}^{-1})/4\}}}$$

which have t_{ν_k} distributions under the same two hypotheses. To create a group sequential t-test, we replace $Z_k - \delta\sqrt{\mathcal{I}_k}$ by T_k^+ and $Z_k + \delta\sqrt{\mathcal{I}_k}$ by T_k^- in rule (6.4) and convert the g_k and h_k into percentiles of the t_{ν_k} distribution rather than the standard normal distribution. The test is then:

After group $k = 1, \ldots, k^* - 1$

if $T_k^+ \ge t_{\nu_k, 1-\Phi(h_k)}$ or

$T_k^- \le -t_{\nu_k, 1-\Phi(h_k)}$ — stop, reject equivalence

otherwise — continue to group $k+1$,

after group $k = k^*, \ldots, K - 1$

if $T_k^+ \ge t_{\nu_k, 1-\Phi(h_k)}$ or

$T_k^- \le -t_{\nu_k, 1-\Phi(h_k)}$ — stop, reject equivalence

if $T_k^+ < t_{\nu_k, 1-\Phi(g_k)}$ and (6.5)

$T_k^- > -t_{\nu_k, 1-\Phi(g_k)}$ — stop, declare equivalence

otherwise — continue to group $k+1$,

after group K

if $T_K^+ \ge t_{\nu_K, 1-\Phi(h_K)}$ or

$T_K^- \le -t_{\nu_K, 1-\Phi(h_K)}$ — stop, reject equivalence

otherwise — stop, declare equivalence.

Here, $t_{\nu,q}$ is the value such that $Pr\{T > t_{\nu,q}\} = q$ when $T \sim t_\nu$. Recall also that Φ denotes the standard normal cdf.

The prime objective of this construction is to achieve power close to $1-\beta$ at $\theta = \pm\delta$. A target for the Type I error rate is implicit in the design since a value of α is needed to determine the constants $\tilde{C}_{W1}(K,\alpha,\beta,\Delta)$ and $\tilde{C}_{W2}(K,\alpha,\beta,\Delta)$ on which g_k and h_k depend. However, the test's actual Type I error probability will depend strongly on the observed sample sizes $n_{X1},\ldots,n_{XK}$ and $n_{Y1},\ldots,n_{YK}$ and the unknown value of σ^2.

The following approximation to the Type I error probability under a given σ^2 is useful as it allows one to check that this error rate is acceptably low over a plausible range of σ^2 values. We note that a fixed sample test based on estimates $\hat{\theta} \sim N(\theta,\, V\sigma^2)$ and $s^2 \sim \sigma^2\chi^2_\nu/\nu$ achieves power $1-\beta$ at $\theta = \pm\delta$ by rejecting equivalence if

$$\frac{\hat{\theta}-\delta}{\surd\{Vs^2\}} \geq -t_{\nu,\beta} \quad \text{or} \quad \frac{\hat{\theta}+\delta}{\surd\{Vs^2\}} \leq t_{\nu,\beta},$$

and has Type I error probability equal to

$$2 \times Pr\{T(\nu\,;\,\delta/\surd\{V\sigma^2\}) \leq t_{\nu,\beta}\}.$$

Here, as before, $T(\nu;\xi)$ denotes a non-central t random variable with ν degrees of freedom and non-centrality parameter ξ. Setting $\nu = \nu_K$ in this expression and, by analogy with the known variance case, replacing $V\sigma^2$ by $\tilde{R}_W(K,\alpha,\beta,\Delta)$ times the variance of $\hat{\theta}^{(K)}$, we obtain the approximation

$$2\, Pr\{T(\nu_K;\, \delta/\surd\{\tilde{R}_W(K,\alpha,\beta,\Delta)\,\sigma^2(n_{XK}^{-1}+n_{YK}^{-1})/4\}) \leq t_{\nu_K,\beta}\} \qquad (6.6)$$

to the group sequential t-test's Type I error probability.

Table 6.2 shows the power at $\theta = \pm\delta$ and attained Type I error probability of group sequential t-tests for equivalence when groups are equally sized and consist of four or six subjects on each treatment sequence. The degrees of freedom ν_k are the numbers of observations at each analysis minus two for fitting the linear model. In each example, the value of σ^2 is chosen such that the approximation (6.6) gives a value of 0.05. It is clear from the table that power and Type I error both agree well with their predicted values.

In further simulations conducted with other values of σ^2 and different sequences of information levels, we found power at $\theta = \pm\delta$ to remain remarkably close to $1-\beta = 0.95$. Increasing or decreasing σ^2 by a factor of two changed the power by at most 0.004 (usually by much less) and perturbations in group size produced the same scale of effects as seen in Table 6.1. As one would expect, these changes had considerable effects on the Type I error rate. We conclude that these designs are robust in satisfying constraints on the probability of wrongly declaring equivalence. Furthermore, they provide a framework within which the producers of a new drug formulation can design and conduct a study with suitably high probability of finding equivalence when it is present.

6.3.4 An Example

Chow & Liu (1992, Section 3.6) present an example of a comparison of bioavailability between two formulations of a drug product using a 2×2 crossover design with 24 subjects, 12 on each treatment sequence. Responses are AUC

Table 6.2 *Properties of power family two-sided t-tests designed to test for equivalence, $\theta \approx 0$, with power $1 - \beta = 0.95$ to reject equivalence when $\theta = \pm\delta$. Tests are based on power family tests for known variance with $\Delta = -0.5$ and 0. Degrees of freedom for σ^2 are $\nu_k = (\nu_K + 2)(k/K) - 2$ and $Var(\hat{\theta}^{(k)}) = (K/k)Var(\hat{\theta}^{(K)})$ at analyses $k = 1, \ldots, K$. Values of σ^2 are chosen such that the approximation (6.6) gives the value 0.05 for the Type I error probability, i.e., the probability of failing to declare equivalence when $\theta = 0$.*
Power and Type I error probability were estimated by simulation using 50000 replicates; standard errors for both are 0.001.

	K	ν_K	*Power at* $\theta = \pm\delta$	*Type I error*
$\Delta = -0.5$				
	3	10	0.948	0.049
	3	16	0.949	0.049
	5	18	0.947	0.049
	5	28	0.949	0.048
	8	30	0.948	0.049
	8	46	0.948	0.050
$\Delta = 0.0$				
	3	10	0.948	0.048
	3	16	0.948	0.048
	5	18	0.945	0.047
	5	28	0.947	0.048
	8	30	0.947	0.048
	8	46	0.949	0.047

values calculated from blood samples taken at a sequence of times in a 32-hour period after dosing. We label the test formulation "treatment A" and the reference formulation "treatment B". The original experiment was not designed sequentially, but for the purpose of illustration we shall analyze the data as if they had been obtained in a two-stage group sequential study. Table 6.3 shows the AUC values for the 24 subjects where we have supposed that, due to unpredictable circumstances, results from 13 subjects were available after the first stage, 8 receiving the sequence AB and 5 the sequence BA.

In our analysis, we define X_i, $i = 1, \ldots, 12$, to be the logarithm of the ratio of the response on treatment A to the response on treatment B for the ith subject receiving treatment A first. Similarly Y_i, $i = 1, \ldots, 12$, is defined to be the logarithm of the same ratio for the ith subject receiving treatment B first. We suppose these variables follow the model (6.1) and that a test is required to satisfy the power condition specified in (6.2) with $\delta = \log(1.25) = 0.223$ and $\beta = 0.05$. We shall construct a group sequential test of equivalence from the power family two-sided inner wedge test with $K = 2$ and $\Delta = 0$. Using the

Table 6.3 *AUC equivalence test data, adapted from Chow & Liu* (1992)

	Sequence *AB*			Sequence *BA*		
		Period			Period	
Group	Subject	I	II	Subject	I	II
1	2	74.825	37.350	1	74.675	73.675
	3	86.875	51.925	4	96.400	93.250
	7	81.865	72.175	5	101.950	102.125
	8	92.700	77.500	6	79.050	69.450
	9	50.450	71.875	11	79.050	69.025
	10	66.125	94.025			
	13	122.450	124.975			
	14	99.075	85.225			
2	17	86.350	95.925	12	85.950	68.700
	18	49.925	67.100	15	69.725	59.425
	21	42.700	59.425	16	86.275	76.125
	22	91.725	114.050	19	112.675	114.875
				20	99.525	116.250
				23	89.425	64.175
				24	55.175	74.575

constant $\tilde{R}_W(2, 0.05, 0.05, 0) = 1.018$ from Table 5.3, we see that formula (6.6) gives an approximate Type I error probability of 0.05 if the coefficient of variation of the original data is 20.5%, so that the observations X_i and Y_i have variance $\sigma^2 \approx 0.084$. Of course, the CV is unknown initially, but this value could have been used as a prior estimate of the CV in constructing the design.

Taking $\tilde{C}_{W1}(2, 0.05, 0.05, 0) = 1.970$ and $\tilde{C}_{W2}(2, 0.05, 0.05, 0) = 1.667$ from Table 5.3, we find

$$h_1 = -(1.970 + 1.667)\, 0.5^{0.5} + 1.970 \times 0.5^{-0.5} = 0.214,$$

$$g_1 = -1.667 \times 0.5^{-0.5} = -2.357$$

and

$$h_2 = g_2 = -1.667.$$

Thus, after stage 1, rule (6.5) allows stopping to reject equivalence if $T_1^+ \geq t_{11,1-\Phi(0.214)} = 0.219$ or if $T_1^- \leq -0.219$ and stopping to accept equivalence if both $T_1^+ < t_{11,1-\Phi(-2.357)} = -2.764$ and $T_1^- > 2.764$. From the data, we find $\hat{\theta}^{(1)} = 0.028$, $s_1^2 = 0.0886$, $T_1^+ = -2.302$ and $T_1^- = 2.954$. The large value of T_1^- indicates that $\theta \leq -\delta$ is implausible but T_1^+ is not sufficiently negative to preclude the possibility $\theta \geq +\delta$ and the test continues to the second stage. At stage 2, the rule is simply to reject equivalence if either $T_2^+ \geq t_{22,1-\Phi(-1.667)} = -1.742$ or $T_2^- \leq 1.742$ and to accept equivalence otherwise. The final data set gives $\hat{\theta}^{(2)} = -0.029$, $s_2^2 = 0.0745$, $T_2^+ = -4.516$ and $T_2^- = 3.491$, strong evidence of $\theta < \delta$ and $\theta > -\delta$, respectively, and the decision is to accept equivalence at this stage. It is of interest to note that the final estimate of σ^2 corresponds to a CV of $\surd(0.0745/2) = 0.193$, close to the value of 20.5% for which we supposed the study to be designed.

The finding of bioequivalence agrees with that found by Chow & Liu (1992, pp. 76–90) using various other methods. Since this test compares the overall distributions of responses under the two treatments pooled over patients, the conclusion is of "average bioequivalence", not as strong a statement as "individual bioequivalence", which we examine in the next section.

6.4 Individual Bioequivalence: A One-Sided Test for Proportions

Suppose we wish to compare a test formulation and a reference formulation, which we label A and B, respectively, with respect to a continuous response variable Y. In the procedure for testing individual equivalence ratios or "TIER" (Anderson & Hauck, 1990), the two treatments should be declared equivalent if the probability of the within-subject similarity of response given by

$$p = Pr\{C_L < (Y_A/Y_B) < C_U\} \tag{6.7}$$

exceeds a given critical fraction, p_0 say. Here Y_A and Y_B represent the responses to test and reference formulations *in the same patient*, and C_L and C_U are pre-specified limits. For example, the "75/75" rule proposed by Purich (1980) would use $C_L = 0.75$, $C_U = 1.25$ and $p_0 = 0.75$. Another common choice is $C_L = 0.8$ and $C_U = 1.25$. Suppose we have data from a two-period crossover design, so that each patient i provides responses Y_{Ai} and Y_{Bi} under the two treatments. We assume there are no period effects. For the ith patient, define the binary variable

$$X_i = \begin{cases} 1 & \text{if } C_L < (Y_{Ai}/Y_{Bi}) < C_U, \\ 0 & \text{otherwise.} \end{cases}$$

We may consider the patients' binary responses $X_1, X_2, \ldots$ as a sequence of independent Bernoulli observations with success probability p; we denote this distribution $B(p)$. Two-sided group sequential tests for a proportion, p, based on the normal approximation were described in Section 3.6.1. Here, we require a one-sided test between the hypotheses

$$H_0\colon p \le p_0 \quad \text{and} \quad H_1\colon p > p_0,$$

where, as in Section 6.2, we set up the null hypothesis to denote inequivalence. Proceeding as in Section 3.6.1, we define

$$\hat{p}^{(k)} = \frac{1}{n_k}\sum_{i=1}^{n_k} X_i, \quad k = 1, \ldots, K,$$

to be the cumulative proportion of patients with responses in the equivalence range among those available up to stage k. Defining $\theta = p - p_0$, the information for θ at analysis k is $\mathcal{I}_k = n_k/\{p_0(1-p_0)\}$, and the sequence of standardized statistics $Z_k = (\hat{p}^{(k)} - p_0)\sqrt{\mathcal{I}_k}$, $k = 1, \ldots, K$, has approximately the canonical joint distribution (3.1) when p is close to p_0. Hence, the methods of Chapter 4 can be applied directly to construct a group sequential one-sided test of H_0 versus H_1.

As an example, suppose we take $p_0 = 0.75$ and wish to test H_0: $p = 0.75$ against a one-sided alternative $p > 0.75$ with Type I error probability $\alpha = 0.05$ and power $1 - \beta = 0.8$ at $p = 0.98$. We shall do this using a power family test with $\Delta = 0$ and $K = 2$ stages, as defined in Section 4.2. We obtain the values $\tilde{C}_1(2, 0.05, 0.2, 0) = 1.634$ and $\tilde{C}_2(2, 0.05, 0.2, 0) = 0.942$ from Table 4.1 and, using these in (4.4), we see that the test's final information level should be

$$\mathcal{I}_2 = (1.634 + 0.942)^2/(0.98 - 0.75)^2 = 125.4.$$

Setting $n_2/\{p_0(1-p_0)\} = 125.4$ with $p_0 = 0.75$, we find that a maximum sample size of 23.5 is required and round this up to $n_2 = 24$, so 12 observations are required in each of the two stages. From (4.5), the critical values for

$$Z_1 = \frac{\hat{p}^{(1)} - 0.75}{\sqrt{\{(0.75 \times 0.25)/12\}}}$$

at the first analysis are $a_1 = 0.489$ and $b_1 = 2.311$. Thus, with $n_1 = 12$, the test continues to stage 2 if

$$0.489 < \left(\frac{1}{12}\sum_{i=1}^{12} X_i - 0.75\right)\left(\frac{12}{0.75 \times 0.25}\right)^{1/2} < 2.311,$$

i.e., if

$$9.73 < \sum_{i=1}^{12} X_i < 12.47,$$

which occurs if 10, 11 or 12 patient responses fall in the equivalence range. With 9 such responses or fewer, the procedure stops and accepts the hypothesis H_0, of inequivalence, and it is not possible to stop early at stage 1 to declare equivalence. At stage 2, the critical value for Z_2 is $a_2 = b_2 = 1.634$, and equivalence is accepted if and only if

$$\left(\frac{1}{24}\sum_{i=1}^{24} X_i - 0.75)\right)\left(\frac{24}{0.75 \times 0.25}\right)^{1/2} > 1.634$$

i.e., if

$$\sum_{i=1}^{24} X_i > 21.47,$$

which requires at least 22 out of the 24 patients to have responses in the equivalence range; otherwise equivalence is rejected.

In this example, it is easy to see that the exact probability of accepting equivalence is simply $Pr\{B(24, p) \geq 22\}$, where $B(24, p)$ denotes a binomial random variable with parameter $n = 24$ and success probability p. Thus, when $p = 0.75$ the test's exact Type I error probability is 0.040 and its exact power when $p = 0.98$ is 0.988. In fact, using exact calculation, we see that the specified power of 80% is actually attained at $p = 0.935$, rather than at $p = 0.98$. Clearly, the initial approximation to the power is poor here, which is not surprising since the variances of $\hat{p}^{(1)}$ and $\hat{p}^{(2)}$ change substantially as p moves from 0.75 to 0.98 but the approximation assumes the variance under $p = 0.75$ to apply in all these cases. We shall discuss exact procedures for binary data in greater detail in Chapter 12.

Returning to our pedagogic example of the AUC equivalence data given in Table 6.3, suppose we use the 75/75 rule so that $C_L = 0.75$ and $C_U = 1.25$ with $p_0 = 0.75$. Suppose also that the two-stage plan of the preceding paragraph is specified, but it turns out that results from $n_1 = 13$ rather than 12 patients are available at analysis 1. We must adapt the test to account for the unequal group sizes using the method described in Section 4.3. We see from Table 6.3 that of the 13 patients in stage 1, the response ratios of four, namely patients 2, 3, 9 and 10, fall outside the critical range. Thus $\hat{p}^{(1)} = 9/13$ and $Z_1 = -0.480$. Since $Z_1 < a_1 = 0.489$, the test terminates at stage 1 with H_0 accepted and equivalence rejected. (Had the test continued to stage 2, the proportion $\hat{p}^{(2)}$ would have been 16/24 corresponding to $Z_2 = -0.943$, again below the critical value $a_2 = b_2 = 1.634$.) The property of individual equivalence is more restrictive than that of average equivalence, so we should not be surprised that a hypothesis of individual equivalence fails to be accepted here even though the weaker hypothesis of average bioequivalence was accepted in the analysis of Section 6.3.4.

Methods and concepts relating to individual bioequivalence have been developed further by several authors including Schall (1995) and Ju (1997). Although the 75/75 rule gained some popularity, it is no longer formally used by the FDA; for an assessment of this rule, see Dobbins & Thiyagarajan (1992).

6.5 Bibliography and Notes

The reversal of the roles of null and alternative hypotheses in equivalence testing has been the cause of some confusion. Given the unusual uses of familiar concepts, there is much to be said for making a clean start, defining requirements of a test operationally, i.e., in terms of the probabilities of particular decisions under particular θ values, and constructing a suitable test from first principles.

In the fixed sample case, a number of authors have proposed basing the decision to accept or reject equivalence on whether or not a confidence interval for the treatment difference lies in an "equivalence region"; see, for example, Westlake (1972, 1976 and 1981), Metzler (1974), Kirkwood (1981) and Rocke (1984). The paper by Rocke also contains a compelling example, using data from Selwyn, Dempster & Hall (1981), in which equivalence is declared between two drugs and yet a simple hypothesis test would clearly reject the (inappropriate) null hypothesis of no difference between the two drugs: the large sample sizes show that there is a small difference between the drugs, but it is also clear that this difference is not large enough to be of practical importance.

Use of confidence intervals can also be adopted in the sequential setting. Durrleman & Simon (1990) and Jennison & Turnbull (1993a) define group sequential one-sided equivalence tests in terms of repeated confidence intervals (see Chapter 9). The two-sided tests based on RCIs proposed by Jennison & Turnbull (1993b) are discussed in Section 9.3.4. As a consequence of the flexibility of repeated confidence intervals to cope with non-adherence to a formal stopping rule, the related tests attain their nominal error probabilities conservatively.

If problems in implementing the stopping rule are not envisaged, conventional group sequential tests will usually be preferred to test based on RCIs. In addition to those described in this chapter, Hauck, Preston & Bois (1997) have proposed tests with early stopping just to accept equivalence so there are no outer boundaries at interim analyses and equivalence can only be rejected at the final analysis. These tests might be considered the complement of the two-sided tests described in Chapters 2 and 3 in which there is no early stopping to accept equality. Other forms of testing boundary, primarily with two stages and with opportunity to accept or reject equivalence at each stage, are presented by Gould (1995b).

CHAPTER 7

Flexible Monitoring: The Error Spending Approach

7.1 Unpredictable Information Sequences

The tests described in Chapters 2 to 6 are all originally designed for a fixed number, K, of equally sized groups of observations which give rise to equally spaced information levels $\{\mathcal{I}_1, \ldots, \mathcal{I}_K\}$. We have explained how the "significance level approach" can be used to adapt these tests to unequal information sequences in a way which maintains the Type I error rate close to its nominal value. However, this method breaks down as information increments become more and more uneven. Also, the significance level approach requires the maximum possible number of analyses, K, to be fixed at the design stage. In this chapter we shall describe a more flexible way of dealing with unpredictable information sequences which guarantees Type I error exactly equal to α for any observed information sequence. This method has the further advantage of not requiring the maximum number of analyses to be fixed in advance.

There are sound practical reasons why observed information levels may be unpredictable. Administratively, it is convenient to schedule interim analyses at fixed calendar times, but if patients are recruited at an uneven rate, the number of new observations between analyses will vary. When testing a parameter in a linear model, as discussed in Section 3.4, increments in information depend on covariate values of the new subjects. In the group sequential log-rank test of Section 3.7, the information $\mathcal{I}_k$ is approximately one quarter of the total number of deaths recorded by analysis k. Clearly, methods for handling unpredictable information sequences are an important part of the statistical methodology for such trials.

In the following, we shall suppose a group sequential test concerns a parameter θ, and estimates $\hat{\theta}^{(k)}$ and information levels $\mathcal{I}_k = \{Var(\hat{\theta}^{(k)})\}^{-1}$, $k = 1, 2, \ldots$, arise at successive analyses. The maximum possible number of analyses may not be completely determined at the start of the study; for example, sampling may continue until $\mathcal{I}_k$ reaches some pre-specified value if the stopping rule does not imply earlier termination. Nevertheless, it is convenient to refer to the maximum number of analyses that would arise in a particular realization if there were no early stopping, and we denote this number by K.

We assume the sequence of estimates of θ and associated test statistics follow the joint distributions presented in Chapter 3 conditionally on the observed information sequence $\{\mathcal{I}_1, \ldots, \mathcal{I}_K\}$. In particular, the sequence of standardized statistics $\{Z_1, \ldots, Z_K\}$ for testing $\theta = 0$ has the joint distribution (3.1), either exactly for data following a normal linear model with known variance or approximately for other data types, the basis of this assumption lying in the general theory we shall present in Chapter 11. However, there is a new subtlety that must be noted as we broaden the range of experimental designs. The desired conditional distribution of $\{Z_1, \ldots, Z_K\}$ given $\{\mathcal{I}_1, \ldots, \mathcal{I}_K\}$ will fail to hold if, in the course of a study, future information levels are allowed to depend on current or previous estimates of θ; therefore, for the methods of this chapter, we shall require $\mathcal{I}_{k+1}$ to be conditionally independent of $\{\hat{\theta}^{(1)}, \ldots, \hat{\theta}^{(k)}\}$ given $\{\mathcal{I}_1, \ldots, \mathcal{I}_k\}$. This has the practical implication that a monitoring committee should not be influenced by estimates of the parameter under investigation, or related test statistics, when planning further patient accrual or the times of future analyses. It is however permissible, and indeed desirable, to respond to observed information levels and to be aware of factors which are liable to affect future information levels, such as the overall failure rate in a survival study.

Our aim in this chapter is to describe group sequential "error spending" tests which attain a stated Type I error rate exactly, despite unpredictable information levels. We present methods for two-sided tests in Section 7.2 and for one-sided tests in Section 7.3. In each case, we describe "maximum information" study designs in which a target for the maximum information level is chosen to satisfy a power condition. This power will be attained to a high accuracy as long as the specified maximum information level is reached eventually. In practice, if information levels are lower than anticipated, it may be necessary to increase patient accrual or follow-up to achieve this target and so maintain power. For two-sided tests, we also describe "maximum duration" trials which do not impose such strong constraints on information levels but, in consequence, do not guarantee a pre-specified power. Both maximum information and maximum duration trials attain their stated Type I error probabilities exactly, provided observed information levels are not influenced by previous estimates of θ: in Section 7.4 we present examples to illustrate how the Type I error rate can be inflated by allowing future analysis times to depend on a current estimate of θ. We conclude the chapter in Section 7.5 with details of the numerical computations needed to construct error spending group sequential tests.

7.2 Two-Sided Tests

7.2.1 Spending Type I Error

We introduce the idea of error spending in the context of a two-sided test of the hypothesis H_0: $\theta = 0$, using the exact method for guaranteeing Type I error suggested by Slud & Wei (1982). In this case, the maximum number of analyses, K, is fixed before the study commences, and the Type I error is partitioned into probabilities $\pi_1, \ldots, \pi_K$, which sum to α. As information levels $\mathcal{I}_1, \ldots, \mathcal{I}_K$ are observed, critical values c_k for the standardized statistics Z_k, $k = 1, \ldots, K$, are calculated such that conditionally on $\mathcal{I}_1, \ldots, \mathcal{I}_k$

$$Pr_{\theta=0}\{|Z_1| < c_1, \ldots, |Z_{k-1}| < c_{k-1}, |Z_k| \geq c_k\} = \pi_k. \tag{7.1}$$

The test proceeds according to the familiar stopping rule (3.9), rejecting H_0 at analysis k if $|Z_k| \geq c_k$, $k = 1, \ldots, K$, or stopping to accept H_0 if it has not been rejected by analysis K. Thus, π_k represents the probability of stopping at analysis k to reject H_0 when this hypothesis is true, also termed the "error spent at stage k". (This should not be confused with the nominal significance level $2\{1 - \Phi(c_k)\}$ applied at analysis k in the significance level approach to unequal group sizes.) Since $\pi_1 + \ldots + \pi_K = \alpha$, the overall Type I error rate is exactly α, as required.

The condition $Pr\{|Z_1| \geq c_1\} = \pi_1$ when $\theta = 0$ implies that the first critical value is simply

$$c_1 = \Phi^{-1}(1 - \frac{\pi_1}{2}).$$

Computation of subsequent critical values necessitates solving (7.1) for $k = 2, \ldots, K$ in turn. Note that at the kth stage, c_k depends on $\mathcal{I}_1, \ldots, \mathcal{I}_k$ but not on the as yet unobserved $\mathcal{I}_{k+1}, \ldots, \mathcal{I}_K$. We describe the calculation of c_k, which involves the joint distribution of $\{Z_1, \ldots, Z_k\}$, in Section 7.5 and in the more general discussion of numerical methods in Chapter 19. Proschan (1999) discusses several mathematical properties of the critical values, c_k, and presents reassuring results on their behavior when successive information levels are very close.

Although Slud & Wei's method contains the key idea of error spending, it has certain limitations. Since the maximum number of analyses is fixed, it is difficult to adapt to unexpectedly high or low rates of accrual of information and, hence, to meet a desired power requirement. Also, one may prefer to vary the amount of error spent at analyses in response to the observed information levels; for example, if little information is available at the first analysis due to slow recruitment or delayed patient response, very little power will be gained from Type I error used up at this stage and it would seem reasonable to reduce π_1, saving Type I error for later, more informative analyses. The method introduced by Lan & DeMets (1983) has the potential to overcome these problems. In their original paper, Lan & DeMets propose spending Type I error as a function of the observed information levels and, combined with a sampling rule which aims to continue to a pre-specified maximum information level, this approach can satisfy a power condition quite accurately. We describe this form of maximum information trial in Section 7.2.2. If sampling to a maximum information level is not feasible, it may still be desirable to adapt to irregularities in the calendar times of analyses. Lan & DeMets (1989b) present a group sequential test in which Type I error is spent as a function of calendar time, and we describe tests of this form in Section 7.2.3.

7.2.2 Maximum Information Trials

In the paradigm of a maximum information trial, the Type I error is partitioned according to an error spending function, $f(t)$, which is non-decreasing and satisfies $f(0) = 0$ and $f(t) = \alpha$ for $t \geq 1$. The value $f(t)$ indicates the cumulative Type I error that is to be spent when a fraction t of the maximum anticipated information has been obtained. Thus, in implementing this approach, it is necessary to specify a target for the maximum information, $\mathcal{I}_{max}$. Once this target has been reached, the procedure will terminate, either rejecting or accepting H_0, if it has not stopped already. It is implicitly assumed that the target $\mathcal{I}_{max}$ will eventually be reached if the trial does not terminate with an early decision. Thus if, for example, patients enter a study at a lower rate than anticipated, organizers must take steps to extend the study's duration. In a survival study, where information depends primarily on the number of observed deaths, it may be necessary to recruit more subjects, extend the follow-up period, or both.

The error spending function $f(t)$ and the target information level $\mathcal{I}_{max}$ must be selected before the study commences. Then, the Type I errors allocated to each analysis are

$$\begin{aligned} \pi_1 &= f(\mathcal{I}_1/\mathcal{I}_{max}), \\ \pi_k &= f(\mathcal{I}_k/\mathcal{I}_{max}) - f(\mathcal{I}_{k-1}/\mathcal{I}_{max}), \quad k = 2, 3, \dots, \end{aligned} \tag{7.2}$$

and critical values c_k are computed successively to satisfy (7.1), exactly as in Slud & Wei's method. Note that c_k does not depend on the as yet unobserved $\mathcal{I}_{k+1}, \mathcal{I}_{k+2}, \dots$. The stopping rule has the form (3.9), only now the maximum possible number of analyses, K, depends on the observed values $\mathcal{I}_1, \mathcal{I}_2, \dots$. Specifically, K is the smallest value k for which $\mathcal{I}_k \geq \mathcal{I}_{max}$. Since by definition $f(\mathcal{I}_K/\mathcal{I}_{max}) = \alpha$, we have $\pi_1 + \ldots + \pi_K = \alpha$ and the overall Type I error rate is exactly α, as required.

There have been a number of suggestions for the form of the error spending function $f(t)$. Lan & DeMets (1983) show that the function

$$f(t) = \min\{2 - 2\Phi(z_{\alpha/2}/\sqrt{t}),\ \alpha\} \tag{7.3}$$

yields critical values close to those of the O'Brien & Fleming test when group sizes are equal. (Here, $z_{\alpha/2}$ denotes $\Phi^{-1}(1 - \alpha/2)$.) For a close analogue of the Pocock boundary, Lan & DeMets (1983) suggest

$$f(t) = \min\{\alpha \log[\,1 + (e - 1)\,t\,],\ \alpha\}. \tag{7.4}$$

Hwang, Shih & DeCani (1990) introduce a family of error spending functions indexed by a parameter γ:

$$f(t) = \begin{cases} \alpha(1 - e^{-\gamma t})/(1 - e^{-\gamma}) & \text{for } \gamma \neq 0 \\ \alpha t & \text{for } \gamma = 0, \end{cases}$$

where γ may be positive, negative or equal to zero.

A useful family of error spending functions, indexed by the parameter $\rho > 0$, is given by

$$f(t) = \min\{\alpha t^{\rho},\ \alpha\}. \tag{7.5}$$

The cases $\rho = 1$, 1.5 and 2 are studied by Kim & DeMets (1987a). Jennison & Turnbull (1989, 1990) note that tests using certain values of ρ produce boundaries similar to those of Pocock and O'Brien & Fleming tests. We shall concentrate on tests in this family for the remainder of this section.

Achieving a Specified Power

The joint distribution under $\theta = 0$ of $Z_1, \dots, Z_K$, conditional on $\mathcal{I}_1, \dots, \mathcal{I}_K$, depends only on the ratios $\mathcal{I}_1/\mathcal{I}_{max}, \dots, \mathcal{I}_K/\mathcal{I}_{max}$. Hence, the critical values $c_1, \dots, c_K$ are functions of these ratios. The distribution of $Z_1, \dots, Z_K$ under $\theta \neq 0$ depends on the absolute information levels $\mathcal{I}_1, \dots, \mathcal{I}_K$. The value of

$\mathcal{I}_{max}$ is the major factor in determining power, but there is also some dependence on the actual sequence of observed information levels. For design purposes, it is convenient to anticipate a maximum number of analyses, K, and to suppose information levels will be equally spaced up to the final value $\mathcal{I}_{max}$, i.e.,

$$\mathcal{I}_k = \frac{k}{K}\,\mathcal{I}_{max}, \quad k = 1, \ldots, K. \tag{7.6}$$

Although the test will be implemented using the sequence of information levels actually observed, we shall see that variations in these levels affect the achieved power only slightly. Under assumption (7.6), the value of $\mathcal{I}_{max}$ can be chosen to meet a given power requirement. Alternatively, if the maximum possible information level is fixed by feasibility and cost considerations, the methods we describe can be used to evaluate the study's approximate power.

Under (7.6) the value of $\mathcal{I}_{max}$ needed to achieve power $1-\beta$ at $\theta = \pm\delta$ is proportional to $1/\delta^2$ and can be expressed as a constant times $\mathcal{I}_{f,2}$, given by (3.6), the information required by a fixed sample test with two-sided Type I error probability α and power $1-\beta$ at $\theta = \pm\delta$. We denote this constant $R_{LD}(K, \alpha, \beta, \rho)$ for a Lan & DeMets test defined by the error spending function (7.5) with parameter ρ. Values of $R_{LD}(K, \alpha, \beta, \rho)$ are listed in Table 7.1 for selected K, $\alpha = 0.05$, $\beta = 0.8$ and 0.9, and $\rho = 1, 2$ and 3. Values for other combinations of parameters can be computed using the numerical methods described in Section 7.5 and Chapter 19. Since the maximum possible number of analyses may not be known *a priori*, an estimated value should be used in determining $\mathcal{I}_{max}$. As values of $R_{LD}(K, \alpha, \beta, \rho)$ increase with K, one may wish to use an upper bound for the maximum number of analyses as a conservative choice.

Properties of Tests with $f(t) = \min\{\alpha t^\rho, \alpha\}$

Tables 7.2 and 7.3 show properties of selected maximum information tests based on error spending functions of the form (7.5). As in previous chapters, we follow other authors in referring to the tests' maximum and expected sample sizes but note that our results really concern information levels and this is the interpretation that should be made in situations where information and sample size are not directly proportional. The tabulated tests are designed for equally spaced information levels, and results are for the case where these information levels are actually observed. In practice, one would expect variations about the planned information sequence, leading to a larger final information level since, by definition, this must be greater than or equal to $\mathcal{I}_{max}$, and this will perturb the actual power of the test (sometimes termed the "attained" or "post-hoc" power) and expected sample sizes. Nevertheless, results for this idealized situation give a good indication of the properties of the error spending tests and guidance in the choice of error spending function and frequency of analyses.

Comparisons with Tables 2.7 and 2.8 show that the parameter values $\rho = 1$ and 3 in the error spending function (7.5) yield tests with similar properties to Pocock and O'Brien & Fleming tests, respectively. In fact, these error spending tests have some advantages: setting $\rho = 1$ gives tests with smaller maximum sample sizes than Pocock's tests and roughly the same or sometimes lower expected sample

Table 7.1 *Constants* $R_{LD}(K, \alpha, \beta, \rho)$ *for Lan & DeMets "maximum information" tests using Type I error spending functions* $f(t) = \min\{\alpha t^{\rho}, \alpha\}$. *Implementation with K equally spaced information levels leading to* $\mathcal{I}_{max} = R_{LD}(K, \alpha, \beta, \rho)\mathcal{I}_{f,2}$ *will attain Type I error probability* $\alpha = 0.05$ *and power* $1 - \beta = 0.8$ *or* 0.9 *at* $\theta = \pm\delta$.

	$R_{LD}(K, \alpha, \beta, \rho)$					
		$1-\beta = 0.8$			$1-\beta = 0.9$	
K	$\rho = 1$	$\rho = 2$	$\rho = 3$	$\rho = 1$	$\rho = 2$	$\rho = 3$
1	1.000	1.000	1.000	1.000	1.000	1.000
2	1.082	1.028	1.010	1.075	1.025	1.009
3	1.117	1.045	1.020	1.107	1.041	1.018
4	1.137	1.056	1.027	1.124	1.051	1.025
5	1.150	1.063	1.032	1.136	1.058	1.030
6	1.159	1.069	1.036	1.144	1.063	1.033
7	1.165	1.073	1.039	1.150	1.067	1.036
8	1.170	1.076	1.041	1.155	1.070	1.039
9	1.174	1.079	1.043	1.159	1.073	1.040
10	1.178	1.081	1.045	1.162	1.075	1.042
11	1.180	1.083	1.046	1.164	1.077	1.043
12	1.183	1.085	1.048	1.166	1.078	1.044
15	1.188	1.088	1.050	1.171	1.082	1.047
20	1.193	1.092	1.054	1.176	1.085	1.050

sizes, and $\rho = 3$ achieves useful reductions in expected sample size over the O'Brien & Fleming tests, especially at $\theta = \pm 1.5\delta$. Thus, there is little reason to opt for the more complicated error spending functions (7.3) and (7.4) designed to mimic O'Brien & Fleming and Pocock tests more closely.

The family of tests defined by (7.5) parallels the Wang & Tsiatis (1987) family of two-sided tests when observed information levels are equally spaced. We have noted the relation between the error spending tests with $\rho = 1$ and 3 and Pocock and O'Brien & Fleming tests, both of which belong to the Wang & Tsiatis family. As an intermediate example, the error spending test with $\rho = 2$ behaves very similarly to the Wang & Tsiatis tests with $\Delta = 0.25$, whose properties are shown in Tables 2.11 and 2.12.

An Example

Consider the parallel two-treatment comparison of Section 3.1.1 where responses $X_{Ai} \sim N(\mu_A, \sigma_A^2)$ and $X_{Bi} \sim N(\mu_B, \sigma_B^2)$, $i = 1, 2, \ldots$, are recorded on subjects receiving treatments A and B, respectively. Suppose we wish to test H_0: $\mu_A = \mu_B$ with Type I error probability $\alpha = 0.05$ and power $1 - \beta = 0.9$ at $\mu_A - \mu_B = \pm 1$ when it is known that $\sigma_A^2 = \sigma_B^2 = 4$. If we have n_A and n_B observations from

Table 7.2 *Properties of maximum information tests with Type I error spending functions* $f(t) = \min\{\alpha t^{\rho}, \alpha\}$ *applied with K equally spaced information levels, culminating in* $\mathcal{I}_K = \mathcal{I}_{max} = R_{LD}(K, \alpha, \beta, \rho)\mathcal{I}_{f,2}$. *Maximum and expected sample sizes are expressed as percentages of the corresponding fixed sample size. All tests attain Type I error probability* $\alpha = 0.05$ *and power* $1 - \beta = 0.8$ *at* $\theta = \pm\delta$.

		Sample size as percentage of fixed sample size				
	K	*Maximum*	*Expected sample size at* $\theta =$			
		sample size	0	$\pm 0.5\delta$	$\pm\delta$	$\pm 1.5\delta$
$\rho = 1$	1	100.0	100.0	100.0	100.0	100.0
	2	108.2	106.9	102.1	85.0	64.8
	3	111.7	109.9	103.4	81.2	56.5
	4	113.7	111.6	104.2	79.5	53.0
	5	115.0	112.7	104.8	78.5	51.0
	10	117.8	115.1	106.1	76.6	47.4
	15	118.8	116.0	106.6	76.1	46.3
	20	119.3	116.5	106.9	75.8	45.8
$\rho = 2$	1	100.0	100.0	100.0	100.0	100.0
	2	102.8	102.1	99.3	86.7	67.0
	3	104.5	103.5	99.2	82.3	60.4
	4	105.6	104.4	99.2	80.1	57.1
	5	106.3	105.1	99.3	78.8	55.0
	10	108.1	106.6	99.7	76.2	51.0
	15	108.8	107.2	99.9	75.4	49.7
	20	109.2	107.5	100.0	75.1	49.1
$\rho = 3$	1	100.0	100.0	100.0	100.0	100.0
	2	101.0	100.7	98.9	89.5	70.7
	3	102.0	101.4	98.3	84.6	64.7
	4	102.7	102.0	98.0	82.1	61.0
	5	103.2	102.4	97.9	80.6	58.8
	10	104.5	103.4	97.9	77.8	54.6
	15	105.0	103.9	98.0	76.9	53.3
	20	105.4	104.2	98.0	76.5	52.7

subjects on treatments A and B respectively, the estimate

$$\hat{\mu}_A - \hat{\mu}_B = \bar{X}_A - \bar{X}_B$$

has variance $4\,(n_A^{-1} + n_B^{-1})$ and the information for $\mu_A - \mu_B$ is the reciprocal of this variance, $(n_A^{-1} + n_B^{-1})^{-1}/4$. From (3.6), a fixed sample test with the desired error probabilities needs information

$$\{\Phi^{-1}(0.975) + \Phi^{-1}(0.9)\}^2 = 10.51,$$

Table 7.3 *Properties of maximum information tests with Type I error spending functions* $f(t) = \min\{\alpha t^\rho, \alpha\}$ *applied with K equally spaced information levels, culminating in* $\mathcal{I}_K = \mathcal{I}_{max} = R_{LD}(K, \alpha, \beta, \rho)\,\mathcal{I}_{f,2}$. *Maximum and expected sample sizes are expressed as percentages of the corresponding fixed sample size. All tests attain Type I error probability* $\alpha = 0.05$ *and power* $1 - \beta = 0.9$ *at* $\theta = \pm\delta$.

		Sample size as percentage of fixed sample size				
	K	*Maximum sample size*	*Expected sample size at* $\theta =$ 0	$\pm 0.5\delta$	$\pm\delta$	$\pm 1.5\delta$
$\rho = 1$						
	1	100.0	100.0	100.0	100.0	100.0
	2	107.5	106.1	99.6	77.7	58.7
	3	110.7	108.8	100.1	72.2	48.5
	4	112.4	110.3	100.5	69.8	44.5
	5	113.6	111.3	100.7	68.4	42.3
	10	116.2	113.6	101.5	65.7	38.4
	15	117.1	114.4	101.8	64.9	37.3
	20	117.6	114.8	102.0	64.5	36.7
$\rho = 2$						
	1	100.0	100.0	100.0	100.0	100.0
	2	102.5	101.9	97.9	80.5	59.6
	3	104.1	103.2	97.1	75.0	52.3
	4	105.1	104.0	96.8	72.2	48.9
	5	105.8	104.6	96.7	70.5	46.8
	10	107.5	106.0	96.6	67.2	42.6
	15	108.2	106.5	96.6	66.2	41.3
	20	108.5	106.8	96.6	65.7	40.7
$\rho = 3$						
	1	100.0	100.0	100.0	100.0	100.0
	2	100.9	100.6	98.1	84.1	62.4
	3	101.8	101.3	96.8	78.2	56.7
	4	102.5	101.8	96.2	75.1	53.2
	5	103.0	102.1	95.9	73.3	50.9
	10	104.2	103.1	95.4	69.8	46.5
	15	104.7	103.6	95.4	68.7	45.1
	20	105.0	103.8	95.3	68.2	44.5

which can be achieved with 85 subjects on each treatment.

Suppose we decide to conduct this test group sequentially with error spending function $f(t) = \min\{\alpha t^2, \alpha\}$, i.e., the member of family (7.5) with $\rho = 2$, and we wish to have a maximum of 10 analyses. From Table 7.1, $R_{LD}(10, 0.05, 0.1, 2) = 1.075$. Hence, we set

$$\mathcal{I}_{max} = 1.075 \times 10.51 = 11.30$$

as our target for the final information level. This value can be achieved with 91 observations per treatment arm, and the study should be planned accordingly. For example, we could aim to collect responses from 10 subjects on each treatment per stage, and then $\mathcal{I}_{max}$ would be reached after 10 groups, even if slightly fewer responses were obtained in practice. If, for some reason, we obtain more observations per group, a maximum of eight or nine groups could suffice. Although the power actually achieved at $\mu_A - \mu_B = \pm 1$ will depend on the precise sequence of information levels obtained when the study is conducted, it is a defining property of the error spending test that the Type I error probability will be precisely $\alpha = 0.05$, whatever the observed information sequence.

We can also evaluate the likely power in situations where the maximum possible sample size is determined by external constraints. Suppose, in the above example, the same error spending function is used to apportion a Type I error of $\alpha = 0.05$ but financial costs limit the total number of observations to 160. If it is anticipated that these observations will arise in 10 groups of 8 per treatment arm, the final information level will be

$$\mathcal{I}_{10} = \frac{80}{2 \times 4} = 10.0,$$

so the test should be implemented with $\mathcal{I}_{max} = 10.0$. To find where power 0.9 is achieved by this test we simply calculate the value of δ for which Equation (3.6) gives $\mathcal{I}_{f,2} = 10.0/1.075 = 9.30$. This value is $\delta = 1.06$, so the error spending test has power 0.9 at $\mu_A - \mu_B = \pm 1.06$. A similar calculation using $R_{LD}(10, 0.05, 0.2, 2) = 1.081$ in place of 1.075 shows that the error spending test has power 0.8 at $\mu_A - \mu_B = \pm 0.92$. Once again, any departure from the assumed sequence of information levels will affect the power actually achieved, but the Type I error probability of $\alpha = 0.05$ will be maintained exactly in all cases.

Variations on the Maximum Information Design

A change in the definition of the maximum information design is required to handle one important eventuality. Suppose in the preceding example external constraints impose a limit of 10 groups of observations and we expect 9 patients on each treatment arm in each group, leading to a final information level

$$\mathcal{I}_{10} = \frac{90}{2 \times 4} = 11.25.$$

We set $\mathcal{I}_{max} = 11.25$ and anticipate power close to 0.9 at $\mu_A - \mu_B = \pm 1$, as our previous calculations showed this is achieved by 10 equal groups with $\mathcal{I}_{max} = 11.30$. Now suppose fewer subjects than expected are actually recruited and the study ends at the 10th analysis with $\mathcal{I}_{10} < 11.25$. The error spending procedure was originally defined on the assumption that $\mathcal{I}_{max}$ would eventually be reached and, as that is not the case here, a modification is needed if the full Type I error is to be spent.

We refer to the problem of reaching the last possible analysis with information less than $\mathcal{I}_{max}$ as "under-running". In order for the overall Type I error to equal α, the final boundary value, c_K, is obtained by solving (7.1) for $k = K$ with $\pi_K = \alpha - f(\mathcal{I}_{K-1}/\mathcal{I}_{max})$. Of course, the low final information level will result in reduced power. For instance, if, in our example, patient numbers fluctuate between

8 and 9 per treatment arm in the 10 groups with a total of 85 per treatment and $\mathcal{I}_{10} = 10.59$, power at $\mu_A - \mu_B = \pm 1$ will be reduced to 0.88.

By definition, $f(t) = \alpha$ for $t \geq 1$, and so the analogous problem of "over-running" is handled automatically, the procedure necessarily terminating at any stage when $\mathcal{I}_k > \mathcal{I}_{max}$. In this case, the power will usually be greater than the design value. In our example, if there are 12 patients per treatment arm in each group, the test will terminate by analysis 8, where $\mathcal{I}_8 = 12.0$, attaining power of 0.92 at $\mu_A - \mu_B = \pm 1$.

Another practical difficulty arises when the $\mathcal{I}_k$ depend on an unknown nuisance parameter which can only be estimated as the trial proceeds. For instance, in the comparison of two Bernoulli distributions discussed in Section 3.6.2, under H_0: $p_A = p_B$ the information levels depend on the common success probability. The error spending approach can be applied with information levels calculated using estimates of the nuisance parameter. If these estimates change greatly during the study, it is even possible (although usually unlikely) for the resulting information levels to decrease between successive analyses; in this case we recommend setting the boundary at infinity and continuing to sample the next group of observations.

In some instances, it may be necessary to modify a study's recruitment or follow-up period if information is to approach its target, $\mathcal{I}_{max}$. If it is feasible to make such adjustments, the study's course can be re-considered at appropriate points in the light of current predictions of future information levels. Scharfstein, Tsiatis & Robins (1997) and Scharfstein & Tsiatis (1998) describe a general approach to "information-based design and monitoring" in which simulation is used to assess the range of plausible information levels at future analyses and they illustrate its application to a Phase III clinical trial studying the effects of drug treatments on HIV patients' CD4+ cell counts.

A Systematic Study of Attained Power

Although differences between actual information levels and those used in design calculations affect the power of error spending group sequential tests, the effects are often small. The results in Table 7.4 are for studies planned assuming $\tilde{K}$ analyses at equally spaced information levels but conducted with $\mathcal{I}_k = \pi(k/\tilde{K})^r \mathcal{I}_{max}$, $k = 1, \ldots, \tilde{K}$. These information sequences are of the form considered in previous chapters, the factor π controlling the final information level and r the spacing between successive information levels. In most cases the maximum possible number of analyses, K, is equal to the planned number $\tilde{K}$, but there are a few exceptions: for $\tilde{K} = 10$, $\pi = 1.1$ and $r = 0.8$, we find $\mathcal{I}_9 > \mathcal{I}_{max}$ and so the test terminates after only $K = 9$ analyses; similarly, for $\tilde{K} = 15$, $\pi = 1.1$ and all three values of r, $\mathcal{I}_{14} > \mathcal{I}_{max}$ and at most $K = 14$ analyses are possible. The error spending tests maintain their nominal Type I error rates exactly in all cases, in contrast to tests defined by the significance level approach which attained Type I error rates only approximately (see Table 3.2). The attained power remains within 0.002 of its target value, 0.9, in all cases where $\pi = 1$, i.e., when the test concludes with $\mathcal{I}_K = \mathcal{I}_{max}$. If $\pi = 0.9$ under-running occurs, the test concludes with $\mathcal{I}_K < \mathcal{I}_{max}$ and, not surprisingly, power falls below 0.9. However,

Table 7.4 *Power attained by maximum information tests using Type I error spending functions* $f(t) = \min\{\alpha t^{\rho}, \alpha\}$, *with* $\rho = 1$, 2 *and* 3. *Tests are designed to achieve power* 0.9 *under information levels* $\mathcal{I}_k = (k/\tilde{K})\mathcal{I}_{max}$ *but levels* $\mathcal{I}_k = \pi(k/\tilde{K})^r\mathcal{I}_{max}$, $k = 1, \ldots, \tilde{K}$, *are actually observed.*

			$\tilde{K}$			
	r	π	2	5	10	15
$\rho = 1$						
	0.80	0.9	0.870	0.875	0.878	0.879
		1.0	0.899	0.899	0.899	0.900
		1.1	0.921	0.914	0.902	0.904
	1.00	0.9	0.871	0.875	0.878	0.879
		1.0	0.900	0.900	0.900	0.900
		1.1	0.923	0.917	0.907	0.904
	1.25	0.9	0.872	0.876	0.878	0.879
		1.0	0.902	0.901	0.901	0.901
		1.1	0.925	0.920	0.912	0.902
$\rho = 2$						
	0.80	0.9	0.869	0.873	0.876	0.877
		1.0	0.899	0.899	0.899	0.899
		1.1	0.922	0.915	0.902	0.904
	1.00	0.9	0.870	0.874	0.876	0.877
		1.0	0.900	0.900	0.900	0.900
		1.1	0.923	0.918	0.907	0.904
	1.25	0.9	0.871	0.874	0.877	0.878
		1.0	0.902	0.901	0.901	0.901
		1.1	0.925	0.921	0.913	0.903
$\rho = 3$						
	0.80	0.9	0.868	0.871	0.874	0.875
		1.0	0.899	0.899	0.899	0.899
		1.1	0.923	0.916	0.902	0.904
	1.00	0.9	0.869	0.872	0.874	0.875
		1.0	0.900	0.900	0.900	0.900
		1.1	0.924	0.919	0.908	0.904
	1.25	0.9	0.869	0.872	0.875	0.876
		1.0	0.901	0.901	0.901	0.901
		1.1	0.925	0.921	0.914	0.903

Table 7.5 *Power attained by maximum information tests using Type I error spending functions* $f(t) = \min\{\alpha t^{\rho},\ \alpha\}$, *with* $\rho = 1$, *2 and 3. Tests are designed to achieve power* 0.9 *under* $\tilde{K}$ *equally spaced information levels* $\mathcal{I}_k = (k/\tilde{K})\mathcal{I}_{max}$, *but K analyses with equally spaced information levels reaching* $\mathcal{I}_K = \mathcal{I}_{max}$ *actually occur.*

			$\tilde{K}$			
			2	5	10	15
$\rho = 1$						
	K	2	0.900	0.915	0.921	0.923
		5	0.883	0.900	0.906	0.909
		10	0.875	0.893	0.900	0.902
		15	0.873	0.891	0.898	0.900
$\rho = 2$						
	K	2	0.900	0.909	0.913	0.915
		5	0.891	0.900	0.904	0.906
		10	0.886	0.895	0.900	0.902
		15	0.884	0.894	0.898	0.900
$\rho = 3$						
	K	2	0.900	0.906	0.909	0.910
		5	0.894	0.900	0.903	0.905
		10	0.891	0.897	0.900	0.901
		15	0.889	0.895	0.899	0.900

since analyses occur at lower information levels, less cumulative Type I error is spent at all analyses other than the final one and the loss of power is smaller than that seen in Table 3.2 for significance level tests, especially for the larger values of K. Conversely, $\pi = 1.1$ leads to over-running with $\mathcal{I}_K > \mathcal{I}_{max}$ and attained power in excess of 0.9 but, again, the deviations from 0.9 are smaller than those for significance level tests.

An important feature of the error spending method is its ability to vary the maximum possible number of analyses in response to observed information levels. The effects of applying a test with observed information levels considerably greater or smaller than anticipated are shown in Table 7.5. Here, tests are designed for $\tilde{K}$ equally space information levels but the target $\mathcal{I}_{max}$ is reached at analysis K. Again, the Type I error remains exactly equal to its specified value. Variations do occur in the attained power, and this lies above its target value when there are fewer analyses than anticipated and below its target when increments in information are small and more analyses are required. The effects on attained power are smaller for the error spending functions with $\rho = 2$ and 3, which spend relatively small amounts of power at early analyses. In a typical study, one would also expect to see unequal increments in information. However, comparisons between cases in Table 7.4 with the same π and $\tilde{K}$ and different values of r

show that once the number of analyses and final information level are fixed, the additional effects on attained power due to the spacing of observed information levels are liable to be quite small.

Overall, the variations in attained power seen in Tables 7.4 and 7.5 are quite modest. It is this insensitivity of the attained power to the number of analyses and observed information levels that allows us to design a trial as if information levels will be equally spaced, even though we realize increments in information will be unequal and the number of analyses may not be as planned.

7.2.3 Maximum Duration Trials

It is common practice to organize a clinical trial by setting dates for the beginning and end of patient recruitment, for interim analyses and for the ultimate termination of the trial. Thus, the maximum duration of the trial, T_{max} say, is specified, but the information that will have accrued in this time is not known at the outset. If this final information level is highly unpredictable, it may be unrealistic to define a group sequential design in terms of a target information level, $\mathcal{I}_{max}$; such a level may not be approached at all or may be obtained at quite an early stage of the study. It is still appealing to spend error as a function of the ratio of current information to that which will be available at the final planned analysis. Since this final information level, $\mathcal{I}_K$ say, is unknown, at each analysis k an estimated value $\widehat{\mathcal{I}}_K^{(k)}$ must be used in calculating the cumulative error to be spent up to this point,

$$f(\mathcal{I}_k/\widehat{\mathcal{I}}_K^{(k)}), \quad k = 1, \dots, K.$$

Lan & Lachin (1990) and Kim, Boucher & Tsiatis (1995) describe the application of this method to survival studies and demonstrate how to calculate boundaries satisfying (7.1) with increments in Type I error:

$$\begin{aligned} \pi_1 &= f(\mathcal{I}_1/\widehat{\mathcal{I}}_K^{(1)}), \\ \pi_k &= f(\mathcal{I}_k/\widehat{\mathcal{I}}_K^{(k)}) - f(\mathcal{I}_{k-1}/\widehat{\mathcal{I}}_K^{(k-1)}), \quad k = 2, \dots, K. \end{aligned} \tag{7.7}$$

In this approach, the final information level will not usually be controlled very closely, and so only a rough estimate of the power that will be attained can be made before actual information levels are observed.

A simple, practical alternative is to spend Type I error as a function of elapsed *calendar* time. In place of (7.2) or (7.7), we partition the Type I error α into

$$\begin{aligned} \pi_1 &= f(T_1/T_{max}), \\ \pi_k &= f(T_k/T_{max}) - f(T_{k-1}/T_{max}), \quad k = 2, \dots, K, \end{aligned} \tag{7.8}$$

where T_k is the elapsed calendar time from the start of the trial to the kth analysis and f is a non-decreasing function with $f(0) = 0$ and $f(t) = \alpha$ for $t \geq 1$. The use of the quantities T_k/T_{max} in place of information fractions allows Type I error to be spent at a rate which is responsive to the increments in information between analyses, as long as information accrues fairly evenly over time. Even though $\mathcal{I}_K$ is unknown at any interim stage k, the covariances $Cov(Z_{k_1}, Z_{k_2}) = \surd(\mathcal{I}_{k_1}/\mathcal{I}_{k_2})$

for $k_1 < k_2 \leq k$ *are* available at that time, and these are all that is needed to find c_k by solving (7.1) with π_k given by (7.8). If the dates of analyses are fixed at the design stage, this determines the elapsed times $T_1, \ldots, T_K$ and T_{max}, and hence the partition of α into $\pi_1, \ldots, \pi_K$ is actually fixed in advance, just as in Slud & Wei's (1982) method. The power attained in a maximum duration trial is determined by the observed information levels and, if these are unpredictable, only a rough initial estimate of power will be available when the study commences.

As an illustration of a maximum duration trial with error spent as a function of elapsed calendar time, we consider the Beta-Blocker Heart Attack Trial (BHAT) example given by Lan & DeMets (1989b) and also discussed by DeMets et al. (1984), Lan, Rosenberger & Lachin (1993) and Lan, Reboussin & DeMets (1994). BHAT was planned as a trial of 48 months duration, starting in June 1978. In total, 3837 patients were randomized to either placebo or propanolol treatment arms. The data were monitored at approximate six-month intervals, analyses taking place in May 1979, October 1979, March 1980, October 1980, April 1981 and October 1981. No formal stopping rule was established at the start of the study, but the O'Brien & Fleming test with an overall two-sided Type I error probability of 0.05 was selected early in the trial to serve as a guide to the Policy and Data Monitoring Board. The study was terminated in October 1981 due to an observed benefit of propanolol treatment.

The cumulative numbers of deaths at the six interim analyses were 56, 77, 126, 177, 247 and 318. With overall mortality as the primary endpoint, outcomes can be monitored using the log-rank statistic (see Section 3.7). The sequence of standardized log-rank statistics at the interim analyses, as reported by Lan & DeMets (1989b), was (1.68, 2.24, 2.37, 2.30, 2.34, 2.82). As explained in Section 3.7, we can estimate the information level $\mathcal{I}_k$ at analysis k by one quarter of the total number of deaths, d_k, observed by that time.

We shall reconstruct how this trial would have progressed had it been run as a group sequential test using the error spending function $f(t) = \alpha \min(t, 1)$ with $\alpha = 0.05$. At analysis k, we evaluate $f(T_k/T_{max})$ where T_k is the time in months since the start of the trial and $T_{max} = 48$, the trial's maximum planned duration. Hence, $T_1 = 11$, $T_2 = 16$, $T_3 = 21$, $T_4 = 28$, $T_5 = 34$ and $T_6 = 40$, and $\pi_1 = (11/48) \times 0.05$, $\pi_2 = (16/48) \times 0.05$, etc. The boundary used at the first analysis in May 1979 is found by solving

$$Pr\{|Z_1| \geq c_1\} = \pi_1 = \frac{11}{48} \times 0.05 = 0.0115$$

when $Z_1 \sim N(0, 1)$, and we obtain $c_1 = 2.53$ from standard normal tables. As the observed log-rank statistic was 1.68, the trial continues to the next analysis. At the second analysis in October 1979, we find the boundary value c_2 by solving

$$Pr\{|Z_1| < 2.53,\ |Z_2| \geq c_2\} = \pi_2 = (\frac{16}{48} - \frac{11}{48}) \times 0.05 = 0.0052$$

when Z_1 and Z_2 are standard normal variables with correlation $\surd(\mathcal{I}_1/\mathcal{I}_2)$, which we approximate by

$$\surd\{(d_1/4)/(d_2/4)\} = \surd(56/77) = 0.853.$$

Numerical computations using the methods described in Section 7.5 give the solution $c_2 = 2.59$. Again, the observed log-rank statistic is between $-c_2$ and c_2 and the study continues. At the third analysis in March 1980, we find c_3 by solving

$$Pr\{|Z_1| < 2.53,\ |Z_2| < 2.59, |Z_3| \geq c_3\} = \pi_3$$
$$= (\frac{21}{48} - \frac{16}{48}) \times 0.05 = 0.0052$$

when Z_1, Z_2 and Z_3 are standard normal variables with $Corr(Z_1, Z_2) = \surd(56/77) = 0.853$, $Corr(Z_1, Z_3) = \surd(56/126) = 0.667$ and $Corr(Z_2, Z_3) = \surd(77/126) = 0.782$, since the numbers of deaths observed at analyses 1, 2 and 3 were 56, 77 and 127, respectively. This calculation gives $c_3 = 2.64$ and, as the observed log-rank statistic is 2.37, the study continues. Proceeding in this way, we obtain boundary values $c_4 = 2.50$, $c_5 = 2.51$ and $c_6 = 2.47$ and find the boundary is crossed at the sixth analysis when $Z_6 = 2.82$ is observed. Thus, under this scheme the study would have terminated in October 1981 with rejection of the null hypothesis of no treatment difference.

The numerical values $c_1, \ldots, c_6$ in the above example are fairly close, fluctuating in the range 2.47 to 2.64. This is not surprising as we have already noted that the error spending function (7.5) with $\rho = 1$ produces a boundary similar to that of Pocock's repeated significance test for which the c_k are all equal.

7.2.4 A Note on Information Time

We have defined error spending tests in terms of observed information levels $\mathcal{I}_1, \mathcal{I}_2, \ldots$. A number of authors describe the error spending approach in terms of "information time", defined as the ratio of current information to that which will be available at the final possible analysis. For completeness, we shall explain the relation between our exposition and the information time treatment.

In the case of maximum information trials, we have taken the cumulative Type I error spent up to analysis k to be

$$f(\mathcal{I}_k/\mathcal{I}_{max}).$$

This may be interpreted as $f(t_k)$ where $t_k = \mathcal{I}_k/\mathcal{I}_{max}$ is the information time at analysis k — but note that our $\mathcal{I}_{max}$ is a target information level calculated as part of the experimental design rather than an estimate of the final information level.

In the first form of maximum duration trial, we specified the Type I error spent by analysis k to be

$$f(\mathcal{I}_k/\widehat{\mathcal{I}}_K^{(k)}).$$

This can be viewed as $f(\hat{t}_k)$ where $\hat{t}_k$ is an estimate of the true information time $\mathcal{I}_k/\mathcal{I}_K$. In the second form of maximum duration trial, information time is not used, its place being taken by the ratios of calendar times, T_k/T_{max}, $k = 1, \ldots, K$.

Calculation of the error spending boundary at analysis k involves the joint distribution of $Z_1, \ldots, Z_k$, in particular their covariances. Since

$$Cov(Z_{k_1}, Z_{k_2}) = \surd(\mathcal{I}_{k_1}/\mathcal{I}_{k_2}) = \surd\{(\mathcal{I}_{k_1}/\mathcal{I}_K)/(\mathcal{I}_{k_2}/\mathcal{I}_K)\}$$

for $k_1 < k_2$, this calculation can be expressed in terms of information times. On the other hand, it is just as easy to work directly with the raw information levels without introducing information times at all.

7.2.5 Two-Sided Tests With Early Stopping to Accept H_0

The error spending approach can also be used to create two-sided tests with an "inner wedge" to allow early stopping in favor of H_0. Both inner wedge error spending tests and one-sided error spending tests, which we discuss in the next section, are defined through a *pair* of error spending functions and, for this reason, similar issues arise in their implementation. We shall not investigate inner wedge tests in detail but the brief description we present here is complemented by the fuller treatment of one-sided tests which follows. Our description of inner wedge tests assumes a target information level $\mathcal{I}_{max}$ will ultimately be reached and so is appropriate to maximum information, rather than maximum duration, trials.

If it is desired to test H_0: $\theta = 0$ with Type I error probability α and power $1 - \beta$ at $\theta = \pm\delta$, an inner wedge test is defined by a Type I error spending function $f(t)$ and a Type II error spending function $g(t)$, where $f(0) = g(0) = 0$ and f and g increase monotonically to $f(t) = \alpha$ and $g(t) = \beta$ for $t \geq 1$. The Type I error probability is partitioned as

$$\pi_{1,1} = f(\mathcal{I}_1/\mathcal{I}_{max}),$$

$$\pi_{1,k} = f(\mathcal{I}_k/\mathcal{I}_{max}) - f(\mathcal{I}_{k-1}/\mathcal{I}_{max}), \quad k = 2, 3, \ldots,$$

and the Type II error probability as

$$\pi_{2,1} = g(\mathcal{I}_1/\mathcal{I}_{max}),$$

$$\pi_{2,k} = g(\mathcal{I}_k/\mathcal{I}_{max}) - g(\mathcal{I}_{k-1}/\mathcal{I}_{max}), \quad k = 2, 3, \ldots.$$

Supposing standardized statistics $Z_1, \ldots, Z_K$ follow the canonical joint distribution (3.1), given $\mathcal{I}_1, \ldots, \mathcal{I}_K$, the stopping rule is of the form (5.1) with critical values (a_k, b_k) chosen to satisfy

$$Pr_{\theta=0}\{a_1 < |Z_1| < b_1, \ldots, a_{k-1} < |Z_{k-1}| < b_{k-1}, |Z_k| \geq b_k\} = \pi_{1,k}$$

and

$$Pr_{\theta=\delta}\{a_1 < |Z_1| < b_1, \ldots, a_{k-1} < |Z_{k-1}| < b_{k-1}, |Z_k| < a_k\} = \pi_{2,k},$$

for $k = 1, 2, \ldots$. The target information level $\mathcal{I}_{max}$ should be chosen so that the final boundary points coincide under a plausible information sequence assumed for design purposes. If, for example, one anticipates K equally spaced information levels, then a_K should be equal to b_K when $\mathcal{I}_k = (k/K)\mathcal{I}_{max}$, $k = 1, \ldots, K$.

In the inner wedge tests of Chapter 5, it is not usually possible to stop in favor of H_0 at the first few analyses and we commented on the desirability of this feature. This property can be included in an error spending test by choosing a value t^*, of around 0.3 or 0.5 say, and setting $g(t)$ equal to 0 for $t \leq t^*$ before it rises towards β once t passes t^*.

An extreme case of an inner wedge boundary is when the outer boundary is infinite at all interim looks and hence early stopping is only possible to accept H_0.

Gould (1983) considers this situation in the context of "abandoning a lost cause". He argues that in many trials for non-life-threatening conditions, when interim findings suggest a positive outcome, the trial will be carried on to completion to provide adequate information on safety endpoints and on patient subgroups. Only if the new treatment seems ineffective will early termination of the trial be justified. This can be viewed as a special case of the above test, in which the error spending function for Type I error is given by $f(t) = 0$ for $0 < t < 1$ and $f(t) = \alpha$ for $t \geq 1$, and hence $b_1 = \ldots = b_{K-1} = +\infty$.

7.3 One-Sided Tests

7.3.1 The Error Spending Formulation

Although most authors have discussed error spending in the context of two-sided tests, this approach can also be adapted to one-sided problems. Suppose, as usual, we have estimates $\hat{\theta}^{(k)}$ of a scalar parameter θ and information levels $\mathcal{I}_k = \{Var(\hat{\theta}^{(k)})\}^{-1}$ at analyses $k = 1, \ldots, K$, and the standardized statistics

$$Z_k = \hat{\theta}^{(k)}\sqrt{\mathcal{I}_k}, \quad k = 1, \ldots, K,$$

have the canonical joint distribution (3.1) conditionally on the $\{\mathcal{I}_1, \ldots, \mathcal{I}_K\}$. As for other error spending tests, we do not suppose the maximum number of analyses to be completely determined initially and use K to denote the maximum number of analyses that would occur in a particular realization of the study in the absence of early stopping to accept or reject the null hypothesis. We consider the one-sided problem of Chapter 4 in which it is desired to test H_0: $\theta = 0$ against the alternative H_A: $\theta > 0$ with Type I error probability α and power $1 - \beta$ at $\theta = \delta$ where $\delta > 0$.

Just as for two-sided tests with an inner wedge, we shall define the upper and lower group sequential boundaries through error spending functions for both Type I and Type II error probabilities. In doing this, we anticipate meeting the power requirement quite closely, so a maximum duration design in which attained power is allowed to vary widely, depending on observed information levels, is unsuitable and we restrict attention in this section to maximum information trials.

For a maximum information trial, we specify a target information level $\mathcal{I}_{max}$ which we expect to reach eventually if the study does not terminate with an early decision. We also define two error spending functions $f(t)$ and $g(t)$, for Type I and Type II errors, respectively, which are non-decreasing and satisfy $f(0) = 0$, $g(0) = 0$, $f(t) = \alpha$ for $t \geq 1$ and $g(t) = \beta$ for $t \geq 1$. We shall explain in Section 7.3.2 how to choose the target value $\mathcal{I}_{max}$ so that the power requirement will be satisfied under a design assumption of equally spaced information levels terminating at $\mathcal{I}_{max}$. The Type I error probability α is partitioned between analyses as

$$\begin{aligned} \pi_{1,1} &= f(\mathcal{I}_1/\mathcal{I}_{max}), \\ \pi_{1,k} &= f(\mathcal{I}_k/\mathcal{I}_{max}) - f(\mathcal{I}_{k-1}/\mathcal{I}_{max}), \quad k = 2, 3, \ldots, \end{aligned} \tag{7.9}$$

and the Type II error β as

$$\begin{aligned} \pi_{2,1} &= g(\mathcal{I}_1/\mathcal{I}_{max}), \\ \pi_{2,k} &= g(\mathcal{I}_k/\mathcal{I}_{max}) - g(\mathcal{I}_{k-1}/\mathcal{I}_{max}), \quad k = 2, 3, \ldots . \end{aligned} \tag{7.10}$$

The test is defined through critical values $(a_1, b_1), \ldots, (a_K, b_K)$ for the statistics $Z_1, \ldots, Z_K$, and we use these in the standard form of stopping rule (4.2) for a one-sided group sequential test. In place of (7.1) we now have two equations,

$$Pr_{\theta=0}\{a_1 < Z_1 < b_1, \ldots, a_{k-1} < Z_{k-1} < b_{k-1}, Z_k \geq b_k\} = \pi_{1,k} \tag{7.11}$$

and

$$Pr_{\theta=\delta}\{a_1 < Z_1 < b_1, \ldots, a_{k-1} < Z_{k-1} < b_{k-1}, Z_k < a_k\} = \pi_{2,k}, \tag{7.12}$$

to define the stopping boundary. As before, the critical values are calculated successively, starting with a_1 and b_1 at the first analysis.

Our objective when drawing the test to a conclusion at the end of the error spending process is to achieve a Type I error of exactly α, letting the attained power absorb the effects of variations in observed information levels. If neither boundary is crossed, the test continues until an analysis with information level $\mathcal{I}_k \geq \mathcal{I}_{max}$; this becomes the final possible analysis, K, and we solve (7.11) to obtain b_K and set a_K equal to b_K.

Under-running, as discussed in Section 7.2.2, can occur if external constraints impose a limit on the study duration which forces termination at an analysis K with $\mathcal{I}_K < \mathcal{I}_{max}$. If this occurs, the remaining Type I error should be spent by taking b_K to be the solution to (7.11) with

$$\pi_{1,K} = \alpha - f(\mathcal{I}_{K-1}/\mathcal{I}_{max}). \tag{7.13}$$

Then, setting $a_K = b_K$ ensures termination at this analysis.

It is also possible, under some information sequences, that the test can be terminated at an analysis k with $\mathcal{I}_k < \mathcal{I}_{max}$ with Type I and II errors within their permitted bounds. To check if this is the case for a particular analysis k, equations (7.11) and (7.12) should be solved with $\pi_{1,k} = \alpha - f(\mathcal{I}_{k-1}/\mathcal{I}_{max})$ and $\pi_{2,k} = \beta - g(\mathcal{I}_{k-1}/\mathcal{I}_{max})$; then, if $a_k > b_k$, we define this to be the final analysis, K, and set b_K equal to the value b_k just computed and $a_K = b_K$. If this check fails, the test must be allowed to continue past this analysis and values a_k and b_k should be re-calculated using $\pi_{1,k}$ and $\pi_{2,k}$ defined in the usual way by (7.9) and (7.10).

7.3.2 A Family of Tests

There have been just a few proposals for error spending functions in one-sided tests. Jennison (1987) used a four-parameter family of error spending functions to approximate optimal group sequential boundaries. Eales & Jennison (1992) and Pampallona, Tsiatis & Kim (1995) have created error spending functions from group sequential boundaries defined for fixed information sequences by calculating the cumulative error at each analysis and specifying the error to be spent at intermediate information levels by interpolation. Chang, Hwang & Shih

(1998) have proposed tests based on error spending functions proportional to $(\exp\{4\mathcal{I}_k/\mathcal{I}_{max}\} - 1)$.

Here, we shall use the simple functions

$$f(t) = \min\{\alpha t^\rho, \alpha\} \quad \text{and} \quad g(t) = \min\{\beta t^\rho, \beta\}, \tag{7.14}$$

parameterized by the power $\rho > 0$. At the design stage, we assume there will be K equally spaced information levels ending with $\mathcal{I}_K = \mathcal{I}_{max}$, as in (7.6), and choose the value of $\mathcal{I}_{max}$ for which (7.11) and (7.12) give $a_K = b_K$ so that the test terminates properly at analysis K with error rates exactly α and β. Of course, when applying this test with a general sequence of information levels, the upper and lower boundaries will not necessarily meet at analysis K and the rules given in Section 7.3.1 must be followed to conclude the test with its specified Type I error.

With equally spaced information levels as in (7.6), the value of $\mathcal{I}_{max}$ needed to meet Type I error and power requirements is a constant multiple of $\mathcal{I}_{f,1}$, the information required by a fixed sample one-sided test given by (4.1). We denote this constant $R_{OS}(K, \alpha, \beta, \rho)$ for a test defined by the error spending functions (7.14) with parameter ρ. Values of $R_{OS}(K, \alpha, \beta, \rho)$ are listed in Table 7.6 for selected K, $\alpha = 0.05$, $\beta = 0.8$, 0.9 and 0.95, and $\rho = 2$ and 3. Tests using $\rho = 1$ have rather high maximum information levels, around 25% to 30% greater than a fixed sample test when $K = 5$ and 10, respectively. As for two-sided tests, an estimated value of K, the maximum possible number of analyses, should be used in choosing $\mathcal{I}_{max}$ when designing a test.

7.3.3 *Properties of the Tests*

We see from the values of $R_{OS}(K, \alpha, \beta, \rho)$ in Table 7.6 that error spending functions of the form (7.14) with $\rho = 2$ and 3 require only modest increases in maximum sample size over the fixed sample test; for example, if $K = 5$, increases of around 5% and 10% are necessary for $\rho = 3$ and 2, respectively. Tables 7.7, 7.8 and 7.9 show expected sample sizes (more precisely, the expected information on termination) of these tests when information levels coincide with their design values, and it is informative to compare these with the properties of the parametric "power family" tests in Tables 4.1, 4.2 and 4.3. In comparisons between tests with the same number of analyses, K, and approximately equal maximum sample sizes, the error spending tests have some notable advantages; in particular, they offer lower expected sample sizes than comparable parametric tests at $\theta = \delta$ when power is 0.8 or 0.9 and a good performance across all three θ values, 0, $\delta/2$ and δ, when power is 0.95. The comparison of error spending tests with $\rho = 3$ and parametric tests with $\Delta = -0.25$ is particularly telling: for $K \geq 3$, the error spending tests have lower maximum sample sizes and lower expected sample sizes at all three θ values than the parametric tests. Reference to Table 4.4 shows that when power is 0.95, the error spending tests with $K = 5$ have expected sample sizes under $\theta = \delta/2$ that are very close to optimal for their maximum sample sizes.

Table 7.6 *Constants* $R_{OS}(K, \alpha, \beta, \rho)$ *for one-sided maximum information tests using error spending functions* $f(t) = \min\{\alpha t^{\rho}, \alpha\}$ *and* $g(t) = \min\{\beta t^{\rho}, \beta\}$. *Implementation with K equally spaced information levels leading to* $\mathcal{I}_{max} = R_{OS}(K, \alpha, \beta, \rho)\,\mathcal{I}_{f,1}$ *will attain Type I error probability* $\alpha = 0.05$ *and power* $1 - \beta = 0.8$, 0.9 *or* 0.95 *at* $\theta = \delta$.

	$R_{OS}(K, \alpha, \beta, \rho)$					
	$1-\beta=0.8$		$1-\beta=0.9$		$1-\beta=0.95$	
K	$\rho=2$	$\rho=3$	$\rho=2$	$\rho=3$	$\rho=2$	$\rho=3$
1	1.000	1.000	1.000	1.000	1.000	1.000
2	1.043	1.014	1.044	1.015	1.045	1.016
3	1.070	1.028	1.072	1.030	1.073	1.031
4	1.087	1.038	1.089	1.040	1.090	1.042
5	1.098	1.045	1.100	1.048	1.101	1.050
6	1.106	1.050	1.108	1.053	1.109	1.055
7	1.111	1.054	1.114	1.058	1.115	1.060
8	1.116	1.058	1.119	1.061	1.120	1.063
9	1.120	1.060	1.123	1.064	1.124	1.066
10	1.123	1.062	1.126	1.066	1.127	1.069
11	1.125	1.064	1.128	1.068	1.130	1.071
12	1.127	1.066	1.131	1.070	1.132	1.072
15	1.132	1.069	1.135	1.073	1.137	1.076
20	1.137	1.073	1.140	1.077	1.142	1.080

When the error spending tests are implemented with a general information sequence, departures from the planned information levels do not change the Type I error, but the attained power is subject to perturbations similar to those seen for two-sided error spending tests. Suppose tests are designed using error spending functions (7.14) with $\mathcal{I}_{max}$ chosen so that power 0.9 will be achieved if $\mathcal{I}_k = (k/\tilde{K})\mathcal{I}_{max}$, $k = 1, \ldots, \tilde{K}$. Then, for the values of ρ, $\tilde{K}$, r and π appearing in Table 7.4, attained power under actual information sequences $\mathcal{I}_k = \pi(k/\tilde{K})^r\mathcal{I}_{max}$, $k = 1, \ldots, \tilde{K}$, remains within 0.002 of 0.9 whenever $\pi = 1$, and thus the planned information level $\mathcal{I}_{max}$ is met at the final analysis. Attained power falls below or above its target when there is under-running ($\pi = 0.9$) or over-running ($\pi = 1.1$), respectively, but to a lesser extent than in the two-sided case. If, instead, information levels are equally spaced but do not fall at their planned values, almost identical values of attained power arise to those seen in Table 7.5 for two-sided tests with the same K and $\tilde{K}$. Comparisons with Table 4.5 show that, overall, error spending tests control attained power more closely than tests defined by the significance level approach, and, of course, the error spending tests have additional flexibility to handle variable numbers of analyses.

Although one can easily define other forms of error spending function, our investigations have shown (7.14) to be a good choice, producing one-sided group

Table 7.7 *Properties of one-sided maximum information tests with error spending functions* $f(t) = \min\{\alpha t^{\rho}, \alpha\}$ *and* $g(t) = \min\{\beta t^{\rho}, \beta\}$ *applied with* K *equally spaced information levels, culminating in* $\mathcal{I}_K = \mathcal{I}_{max} = R_{OS}(K, \alpha, \beta, \rho)\mathcal{I}_{f,1}$. *Maximum and expected sample sizes are expressed as percentages of the corresponding fixed sample size. All tests attain Type I error probability* $\alpha = 0.05$ *and power* $1 - \beta = 0.8$ *at* $\theta = \delta$.

$\alpha = 0.05,\ 1 - \beta = 0.8$

		Sample size as percentage of fixed sample size			
	K	*Maximum*	*Expected sample size at* $\theta =$		
		sample size	0	0.5δ	δ
$\rho = 2$					
	1	100.0	100.0	100.0	100.0
	2	104.3	74.5	87.8	84.6
	3	107.0	68.0	82.8	79.2
	4	108.7	64.7	80.2	76.4
	5	109.8	62.7	78.5	74.6
	10	112.3	58.7	75.2	71.1
	15	113.2	57.4	74.0	69.9
	20	113.7	56.8	73.5	69.3
$\rho = 3$					
	1	100.0	100.0	100.0	100.0
	2	101.4	79.6	91.6	88.3
	3	102.8	73.1	86.4	82.6
	4	103.8	69.6	83.7	79.6
	5	104.5	67.6	82.0	77.8
	10	106.2	63.5	78.5	74.2
	15	106.9	62.2	77.3	73.0
	20	107.3	61.6	76.8	72.4

sequential tests which are efficient in reducing expected sample size across a range of θ values. As for two-sided error spending tests, robustness of the attained power to the number of analyses and the spacing of information levels enables us to design a study assuming a fixed number of equally spaced information levels, even when the observed information sequence is liable to be quite different. We shall present an example of a one-sided error spending test applied to survival data in Section 13.6.

7.3.4 *Early Stopping Only to Accept* H_0

At the end of Section 7.2.5, we discussed two-sided tests in which there was only early stopping to accept H_0. If interim findings are positive, in some trials it is desirable to carry on to completion in order to provide adequate information on safety endpoints and on patient subgroups. Only if results appear negative, will

Table 7.8 *Properties of one-sided maximum information tests with error spending functions* $f(t) = \min\{\alpha t^{\rho}, \alpha\}$ *and* $g(t) = \min\{\beta t^{\rho}, \beta\}$ *applied with* K *equally spaced information levels, culminating in* $\mathcal{I}_K = \mathcal{I}_{max} = R_{OS}(K, \alpha, \beta, \rho)\mathcal{I}_{f,1}$. *Maximum and expected sample sizes are expressed as percentages of the corresponding fixed sample size. All tests attain Type I error probability* $\alpha = 0.05$ *and power* $1 - \beta = 0.9$ *at* $\theta = \delta$.

$\alpha = 0.05,\ 1 - \beta = 0.9$

		Sample size as percentage of fixed sample size			
	K	*Maximum sample size*	*Expected sample size at* $\theta =$ 0	0.5δ	δ
$\rho = 2$	1	100.0	100.0	100.0	100.0
	2	104.4	74.5	88.7	79.7
	3	107.2	68.1	83.9	73.8
	4	108.9	64.9	81.3	70.7
	5	110.0	62.9	79.7	68.8
	10	112.6	58.9	76.4	65.1
	15	113.5	57.7	75.3	63.8
	20	114.0	57.0	74.8	63.2
$\rho = 3$	1	100.0	100.0	100.0	100.0
	2	101.5	79.0	92.0	83.6
	3	103.0	72.6	86.9	77.5
	4	104.0	69.2	84.2	74.2
	5	104.8	67.1	82.6	72.2
	10	106.6	63.1	79.2	68.4
	15	107.3	61.8	78.0	67.1
	20	107.7	61.1	77.4	66.5

early termination be considered in order to "abandon a lost cause". The same idea can be applied to a one-sided test. Again no Type I error is spent at interim analyses, which corresponds to a choice of error spending function $f(t) = 0$ for $0 < t < 1$ and $f(t) = \alpha$ for $t \geq 1$. From (7.11), this in turn implies that $b_1 = \ldots = b_{K-1} = +\infty$. In a completely different approach, Berry and Ho (1988) assume a utility structure and use dynamic programming to develop an optimal Bayesian sequential decision procedure for this problem.

7.4 Data Dependent Timing of Analyses

The flexible nature of the error spending approach lends itself well to the accommodation of irregular, unpredictable and unplanned interim analysis schedules. However, there are still some restrictions on how a trial may be conducted if the conditional distribution of $\{Z_1, \ldots, Z_K\}$ given the observed

Table 7.9 *Properties of one-sided maximum information tests with error spending functions* $f(t) = \min\{\alpha t^\rho, \alpha\}$ *and* $g(t) = \min\{\beta t^\rho, \beta\}$ *applied with* K *equally spaced information levels, culminating in* $\mathcal{I}_K = \mathcal{I}_{max} = R_{OS}(K, \alpha, \beta, \rho)\mathcal{I}_{f,1}$. *Maximum and expected sample sizes are expressed as percentages of the corresponding fixed sample size. All tests attain Type I error probability* $\alpha = 0.05$ *and power* $1 - \beta = 0.95$ *at* $\theta = \delta$.

		$\alpha = 0.05,\ 1 - \beta = 0.95$			
		Sample size as percentage of fixed sample size			
	K	*Maximum sample size*	*Expected sample size at* $\theta =$ 0	0.5δ	δ
$\rho = 2$	1	100.0	100.0	100.0	100.0
	2	104.5	74.9	89.2	74.9
	3	107.3	68.7	84.5	68.7
	4	109.0	65.4	81.9	65.4
	5	110.1	63.4	80.3	63.4
	10	112.7	59.5	77.1	59.5
	15	113.7	58.3	76.0	58.3
	20	114.2	57.7	75.5	57.7
$\rho = 3$	1	100.0	100.0	100.0	100.0
	2	101.6	79.0	92.2	79.0
	3	103.1	72.7	87.2	72.7
	4	104.2	69.2	84.5	69.2
	5	105.0	67.1	82.8	67.1
	10	106.9	63.1	79.5	63.1
	15	107.6	61.8	78.3	61.8
	20	108.0	61.2	77.8	61.2

information sequence $\{\mathcal{I}_1, \ldots, \mathcal{I}_K\}$ is to have the standard form (3.1), as we have assumed in deriving properties of error spending tests. Allowing the timing or number of future analyses to depend on the current and past responses can introduce additional dependencies between the Z_ks and $\mathcal{I}_k$s, in which case error probabilities may no longer be guaranteed.

The following example, given by Jennison & Turnbull (1991a), illustrates how Type I error can be affected if $\mathcal{I}_k$ is allowed to depend on $Z_1, \ldots, Z_{k-1}$. Suppose observations are taken in three groups, each contributing one unit of information so the statistics $Z_1 \sim N(\theta, 1)$, $Z_2 \sim N(\theta\sqrt{2}, 1)$ and $Z_3 \sim N(\theta\sqrt{3}, 1)$ will become available. A two-sided test with Type I error probability $\alpha = 0.05$ conducted as a maximum information trial with $\mathcal{I}_{max} = 3$ and error spending function $f(t) = \min(\alpha t, \alpha)$ rejects H_0 if $|Z_1| \geq 2.394$, $|Z_2| \geq 2.294$ or $|Z_3| \geq 2.200$. Suppose now that the experimenter decides to omit the second analysis and pool the second and third groups of observations if $|Z_1| < 1.2$, in which case the critical value for $|Z_3|$ is taken to be 2.076, the value arising for the given error spending function when only Z_1 and Z_3 are observed. The overall test is as follows:

If $|Z_1| \geq 2.394$, reject H_0.

If $1.2 \leq |Z_1| < 2.394$, continue and observe Z_2 then

if $|Z_2| \geq 2.294$, reject H_0, otherwise observe Z_3 then
reject H_0 if $|Z_3| \geq 2.200$ or accept H_0 if $|Z_3| < 2.200$.

If $|Z_1| < 1.2$, take both the second and third groups of observations then

reject H_0 if $|Z_3| \geq 2.076$ or accept H_0 if $|Z_3| < 2.076$.

Jennison & Turnbull (1991a) use numerical integration to show that this test has Type I error probability 0.0525, a small increase over the intended value of 0.05. A similar four-stage procedure in which groups 2 and 3 are pooled if $|Z_1| < 1.2$ and groups 3 and 4 are pooled if $|Z_2| < 1.2$ has Type I error probability 0.0522. Although these effects are small, they do demonstrate the possibility of increases in Type I error probability and suggest a need for caution in the application of error spending tests.

Lan & DeMets (1989a) use simulation to investigate the effects of increasing the frequency of future analyses when Z_k starts to approach an error spending boundary. They report no serious distortion of Type I error rate or power, although perturbations similar to those in Jennison & Turnbull's (1991a) examples cannot be ruled out as these are of the same order as the standard errors of Lan & DeMets' simulation results.

Lan & DeMets (1989a) go on to suggest that a monitoring committee may decide to switch from group sequential to continuous monitoring if it appears at an interim analysis that a testing boundary is likely to be crossed soon. Betensky (1998) has addressed the computational problems involved in implementing this suggestion, but the potential benefits of such a strategy have yet to be evaluated. Comparisons with the examples of Jennison & Turnbull (1991a) and Lan & DeMets (1989a) suggest this practice will produce a slightly elevated Type I error and little change in power (one would expect an increase in power to accompany the higher Type I error rate, but this will be offset by the decrease in power due to spending some Type I error earlier). It is not clear that the switch to continuous monitoring will automatically yield useful gains in terms of earlier stopping: such gains diminish as additional analyses are added, and the results of Tables 7.2, 7.3, 7.7, 7.8 and 7.9 show only slight reductions in expected sample size as the number of planned interim analyses is increased beyond 5 or 10.

Proschan, Follman, & Waclawiw (1992) present a thorough study of a variety of group sequential designs when analysis times are allowed to depend on observed responses. They conclude that the Type I errors of error spending tests are robust to departures from the specified protocol, as long as error is spent as a smooth function of information or calendar time. In other situations, they observe that Type I error can be inflated by a factor of two or more when rather devious strategies are followed in implementing tests based on the Slud & Wei (1982) method or tests defined through discontinuous error spending functions!

Fleming & DeMets (1993) note the importance of providing a full and clear description of any form of error spending test in the study protocol in order to ensure credibility of a study's conclusions. They cite the extreme form of misuse in which the error spending function is changed during a study so that all the two-sided Type I error is spent the first time $|Z_k|$ exceeds $z_{\alpha/2}$, leading to a gross inflation of the Type I error rate comparable to that of repeated fixed sample tests at significance level α discussed in Chapters 1 and 2.

Fleming, Harrington & O'Brien (1984) observe that it may be desirable to extend a study if information accrues too slowly and suggest spending fractions of the Type I error at the extra interim analyses. They reiterate the need to keep any decision to change the study duration independent of the observed responses: cautious experimenters might even avoid legitimate changes in design if there is a perceived danger of compromising their study's credibility. Interestingly, the maximum information designs of Section 7.2.2 share the same motivation as Fleming, Harrington & O'Brien's proposal but, since the rules for continuing to a target information level are specified at the outset, the suggestion that the design is being changed as the study progresses does not arise. If one of the usual forms of error spending function is used, such a maximum information design falls into the category of procedures recommended by Proschan et al. (1992) for their robustness to any misuse.

7.5 Computations for Error Spending Tests

We first consider two-sided tests and the computations needed to obtain critical values c_k by solving equation (7.1). Defining

$$G_k(z; \theta) = Pr_\theta\{|Z_1| < c_1, \ldots, |Z_{k-1}| < c_{k-1}, Z_k \geq z\},$$

we need to solve recursively

$$G_k(c_k; 0) = \pi_k/2, \quad k = 1, \ldots, K,$$

where the π_k are pre-specified in the case of a Slud & Wei (1982) test or obtained from (7.2) for an error spending test with spending function f. For $k = 1$ we obtain $c_1 = \Phi^{-1}(1 - \pi_1/2)$, but computation of $G_k(z; \theta)$ for $k > 1$ would appear to involve a difficult multivariate normal integral. Computer routines for general multivariate normal integrals are available, for example, the program MULNOR of Schervish (1984), but such routines make high demands on computer memory and processing time and their use is practical only for small values of K.

Fortunately, the distribution of the sequence $\{Z_1, \ldots, Z_K\}$ specified by (3.1) is Markov, and this allows use of the recursive formulae of Armitage, McPherson & Rowe (1969). Specifically, for $k = 2, \ldots, K$,

$$Z_k\sqrt{\mathcal{I}_k} - Z_{k-1}\sqrt{\mathcal{I}_{k-1}} \sim N(\theta\Delta_k, \Delta_k),$$

where $\Delta_k = \mathcal{I}_k - \mathcal{I}_{k-1}$ is the increment in information between analyses $k - 1$ and k, and this distribution is independent of $Z_1, \ldots, Z_{k-1}$. We define $g_k(z; \theta)$ to be the derivative of $G_k(z;\theta)$ with respect to z; this is also the sub-density of Z_k for realizations which proceed at least up to analysis k (the integral of $g_k(z;\theta)$ is less than one because of the probability of stopping at earlier analyses). Letting $\phi(z)$ denote the standard normal density, $\exp(-z^2/2)/\sqrt{(2\pi)}$, the g_k are given recursively by

$$g_1(z;\theta) = \phi(z - \theta\sqrt{\mathcal{I}_1})$$

and

$$g_k(z;\theta) = \int_{-c_{k-1}}^{c_{k-1}} g_{k-1}(u;\theta) \frac{\sqrt{\mathcal{I}_k}}{\sqrt{\Delta_k}} \phi\left(\frac{z\sqrt{\mathcal{I}_k} - u\sqrt{\mathcal{I}_{k-1}} - \theta\Delta_k}{\sqrt{\Delta_k}}\right) du$$

for $k = 2, \ldots, K$. The critical values $c_1, \ldots, c_K$ are calculated in sequence. When $c_1, \ldots, c_{k-1}$ are known, the above formulae can be used to evaluate g_k numerically by a succession of $k-1$ univariate integrals, and hence one can solve

$$\int_{c_k}^{\infty} g_k(z;0)\,dz = \pi_k/2$$

to obtain c_k. The attained power at θ can also be computed from the densities $g_1, \ldots, g_K$ since it is equal to

$$\pi_1(\theta) + \ldots + \pi_K(\theta)$$

where

$$\pi_k(\theta) = \int_{-\infty}^{-c_k} g_k(z;\theta)\,dz + \int_{c_k}^{\infty} g_k(z;\theta)\,dz, \quad k = 1, \ldots, K.$$

Calculations for one-sided error spending tests follow the same pattern as those for two-sided tests, using recursive formulae for the densities g_k. In this case, the limits $\pm c_k$ in the integral giving g_{k+1} are replaced by the critical values a_k and b_k found as the solutions of

$$\int_{b_k}^{\infty} g_k(z;0)\,dz = \pi_{1,k} \quad \text{and} \quad \int_{\infty}^{a_k} g_k(z;\delta)\,dz = \pi_{2,k}$$

to satisfy equations (7.11) and (7.12).

Clearly, specialized computer programs are needed to calculate error spending boundaries. The report by Reboussin, DeMets, Kim & Lan (1992) contains FORTRAN 77 programs which do this. We provide further details of the numerical methods used in our own programs in Chapter 19, where we also discuss other sources of computer software.

CHAPTER 8

Analysis Following a Sequential Test

8.1 Introduction

So far we have concentrated on hypothesis tests, establishing a framework for *designing* a group sequential study, i.e., for performing a "pre-data" calculation. However, once data have been collected, the hypothesis testing paradigm may no longer be the most useful one for statistical analysis; see, for example, the discussion in Cutler et al. (1966). Whereas in industrial acceptance sampling it may well be that decisions are made and actions taken as soon as a study is terminated, in medical studies a more complete analysis is usually required than the simple "accept" or "reject" decision of a hypothesis test. In this chapter we discuss the construction of point estimates, P-values and confidence intervals. In particular, an interval estimate for the treatment effect θ will allow consideration of the *magnitude* of the treatment difference and indicate its practical importance, irrespective of whether a hypothesis test declares statistical significance (see Simon, 1993 and Braitman, 1993).

There are two situations in which interval estimates might be required in a group sequential study. The first is upon conclusion of the trial after the test statistic has crossed a stopping boundary, as described in previous chapters. This is the case we shall consider in this chapter. Alternatively, one may wish to give an interval estimate of the treatment effect at an interim stage of the study, regardless of whether the design calls for termination or not; this situation calls for a "repeated confidence interval" sequence, the subject of Chapter 9.

In neither situation is it appropriate to compute a "naive" confidence interval, treating the data as if they had been obtained in a fixed sample size experiment. Tsiatis, Rosner & Mehta (1984) investigate naive 90% confidence intervals calculated on termination of a five-stage Pocock test with Type I error probability 0.05 and find their coverage probabilities to vary between 0.846 and 0.929, depending on the true parameter value.

Note that in this chapter we shall be concerned with frequentist properties of interval estimates. The topic of credible intervals in the Bayesian paradigm will be discussed later in Chapter 18.

8.2 Distribution Theory

We saw in Section 3.1 that many common problems produce a sequence of test statistics $Z_1, \ldots, Z_K$ with the canonical joint distribution (3.1), conditional on observed information levels $\mathcal{I}_1, \ldots, \mathcal{I}_K$. We consider problems of this type in this chapter, although it should be evident that the key ideas extend to other situations;

in Chapter 12 we shall develop similar methods for the discrete distributions arising in the analysis of binary data. Let $\Delta_1 = \mathcal{I}_1$ and $\Delta_k = \mathcal{I}_k - \mathcal{I}_{k-1}$, $k = 2, \ldots, K$. Under (3.1), $Z_1, \ldots, Z_K$ have marginal normal distributions with variance one and their joint distribution is the same as that of the sequence $\{(Y_1 + \ldots + Y_k)/\sqrt{\mathcal{I}_k}; k = 1, \ldots, K\}$, where the Y_k are independent and $Y_k \sim N(\Delta_k\theta, \Delta_k)$. As an example, in the one sample problem described in Section 3.1.2, when $\sigma^2 = 1$ the information increment Δ_k is the number of observations in group k and Y_k is the sum of these Δ_k observations.

In the group sequential tests of Chapters 2 to 7, stopping occurs at stage

$$T = \min\{k : Z_k \notin \mathcal{C}_k\},$$

where $\mathcal{C}_k$ is the continuation region at stage k and $\mathcal{C}_K = \emptyset$, the empty set, to ensure termination by stage K. Let $\boldsymbol{Z}^{(k)} = (Z_1, \ldots, Z_k)$ be the vector of the first k standardized statistics and, for $k = 1, \ldots, K$, define

$$\mathcal{A}_k = \{\boldsymbol{z}^{(k)} : z_i \in \mathcal{C}_i, i = 1, \ldots, k-1, \text{ and } z_k \notin \mathcal{C}_k\},$$

the set of sample paths for $Z_1, Z_2, \ldots$ that terminate precisely at stage k. Thus, $\boldsymbol{Z}^{(k)} \in \mathcal{A}_k$ implies $T = k$. In view of the above representation of $Z_1, \ldots, Z_K$ in terms of independent normal variables $Y_1, \ldots, Y_K$, we can write the joint density of $(Z_1, \ldots, Z_k)$ at a point $\boldsymbol{z}^{(k)}$ in $\mathcal{A}_k$ as

$$p_{T,\boldsymbol{Z_T}}(k, \boldsymbol{z}^{(k)}; \theta) = \prod_{i=1}^{k} \frac{1}{\sqrt{\Delta_i}} \phi\left(\frac{y_i - \Delta_i\theta}{\sqrt{\Delta_i}}\right),$$

where $y_1 = z_1\sqrt{\mathcal{I}_1}$, $y_i = z_i\sqrt{\mathcal{I}_i} - z_{i-1}\sqrt{\mathcal{I}_{i-1}}$, $i = 2, \ldots, k$, and $\phi(x) = \exp(-x^2/2)/\sqrt{(2\pi)}$ is the standard normal density. Using the facts $z_k\sqrt{\mathcal{I}_k} = y_i + \ldots + y_k$ and $\mathcal{I}_k = \Delta_1 + \ldots + \Delta_k$, we find

$$p_{T,\boldsymbol{Z_T}}(k, \boldsymbol{z}^{(k)}; \theta) = \prod_{i=1}^{k} \frac{1}{\sqrt{(2\pi\Delta_i)}} \exp\left\{-\sum_{i=1}^{k} \frac{y_i^2 - 2\Delta_i\theta y_i + \Delta_i^2\theta^2}{2\Delta_i}\right\}$$

$$= h(k, \boldsymbol{z}^{(k)}, \mathcal{I}_1, \ldots, \mathcal{I}_k) \exp(\theta z_k\sqrt{\mathcal{I}_k} - \theta^2\mathcal{I}_k/2), \tag{8.1}$$

where

$$h(k, \boldsymbol{z}^{(k)}, \mathcal{I}_1, \ldots, \mathcal{I}_k) = \prod_{i=1}^{k} \frac{\exp\{-y_i^2/(2\Delta_i)\}}{\sqrt{(2\pi\Delta_i)}}.$$

The form of this joint density shows that the pair (T, Z_T) is a sufficient statistic for θ (since T fixes $\mathcal{I}_T$), and hence the maximum likelihood estimator (MLE) of θ, found by maximizing (8.1), is $\hat{\theta} = Z_T/\sqrt{\mathcal{I}_T}$; see Chang (1989, p. 249). In the one-sample problem of Section 3.1.2, the MLE of $\theta = \mu - \mu_0$ is thus $\bar{X}_T - \mu_0$, implying that $\bar{X}_T$ is the MLE of μ. In the two-sample problem of Chapter 2 and Section 3.1.1, the MLE of $\theta = \mu_A - \mu_B$ is $Z_T/\sqrt{\mathcal{I}_T} = \bar{X}_{AT} - \bar{X}_{BT}$.

We denote by $p(k, z; \theta)$, $k = 1, \ldots, K$, the sub-densities of the terminal statistic Z_k when the test stops at analysis k. Thus, $p(k, z; \theta)$ is non-zero only for values of $z \in \mathcal{A}_k$ and its integral over a set $E \in \mathcal{A}_k$ gives the probability of stopping at stage k with $Z_k \in E$. We obtain the kth of these sub-densities by integrating $p_{T,\,\boldsymbol{Z}_T}(k, \boldsymbol{z}^{(k)}; \theta)$ over possible values of $z_1, \ldots, z_{k-1}$. For $z \notin \mathcal{C}_k$, we have

$$p(k, z; \theta) = \int_{\mathcal{B}_k(z)} \cdots \int h(k, \boldsymbol{z}^{(k)}, \mathcal{I}_1, \ldots, \mathcal{I}_k) \times \exp(\theta z \sqrt{\mathcal{I}_k} - \theta^2 \mathcal{I}_k / 2)\, dz_{k-1} \ldots dz_1, \tag{8.2}$$

where $\mathcal{B}_k(z)$ is the set of vectors $\boldsymbol{z}^{(k)} = (z_1, \ldots, z_k) \in \mathcal{A}_k$ for which $z_k = z$. It is evident from (8.2) that

$$p(k, z; \theta) = p(k, z; 0) \exp(\theta z \sqrt{\mathcal{I}_k} - \theta^2 \mathcal{I}_k / 2). \tag{8.3}$$

This is an example of a likelihood ratio identity, see Siegmund (1985, Propositions 2.24 and 3.2). Emerson & Fleming (1990) note the usefulness of this relation in converting a sub-density evaluated under one value of θ for computations at another θ. Such a relation can also be used in simulation studies to obtain properties of a sequential test under several values of θ from simulations performed at a single θ.

Although it might appear from (8.2) that computation of $p(k, z; \theta)$ involves a difficult multivariate normal integral, the recursive formulae of Armitage, McPherson & Rowe (1969) can be used to calculate $p(1, z; \theta)$ to $p(K, z; \theta)$ in turn. These formulae are

$$p(k, z; \theta) = \begin{cases} g_k(z; \theta) & \text{if } z \notin \mathcal{C}_k \\ 0 & \text{if } z \in \mathcal{C}_k, \end{cases} \tag{8.4}$$

where

$$g_1(z; \theta) = \phi(z - \theta \sqrt{\mathcal{I}_1}) \tag{8.5}$$

and for $k = 2, \ldots, K$,

$$g_k(z; \theta) = \int_{\mathcal{C}_{k-1}} g_{k-1}(u; \theta) \frac{\sqrt{\mathcal{I}_k}}{\sqrt{\Delta_k}} \phi\left(\frac{z\sqrt{\mathcal{I}_k} - u\sqrt{\mathcal{I}_{k-1}} - \Delta_k \theta}{\sqrt{\Delta_k}} \right) du. \tag{8.6}$$

Thus, the computation is very much simplified, requiring only a succession of $K - 1$ univariate integrations. In Chapter 19 we shall describe in detail methods for evaluating these integrals numerically.

As an example, consider a two-sided O'Brien & Fleming test with four equally sized groups of observations. For a test with Type I error rate $\alpha = 0.1$, we take $C_B(4, 0.1) = 1.733$ from Table 2.3 and find the continuation regions at stages 1 to 3 to be $\mathcal{C}_1 = (-3.466, 3.466)$, $\mathcal{C}_2 = (-2.451, 2.451)$ and $\mathcal{C}_3 = (-2.001, 2.001)$. The sub-densities $p(k, z; 0)$ for $k = 1, 2, 3$ and 4 under the null hypothesis $\theta = 0$ are plotted in Figure 8.1. The sub-density for $k = 1$ is only barely visible because $Pr\{T = 1\}$ is so small when $\theta = 0$. Continuing this example, suppose the test had been designed to achieve power $1 - \beta = 0.8$ at $\theta = \pm\delta$ for some specified δ. Then the maximum information would have been set as

$$\mathcal{I}_4 = R_B(4, 0.1, 0.2)\{\Phi^{-1}(0.95) + \Phi^{-1}(0.8)\}^2/\delta^2 = 6.40/\delta^2,$$

taking the value of $R_B(4, 0.1, 0.2) = 1.035$ from Table 2.4. Hence, $\mathcal{I}_k = 1.60\,k/\delta^2$ for $k = 1, \ldots, 4$. Substituting these values in (8.5) and (8.6) we obtain

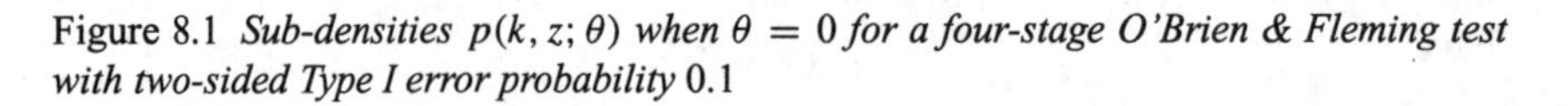

Figure 8.1 *Sub-densities* $p(k, z; \theta)$ *when* $\theta = 0$ *for a four-stage O'Brien & Fleming test with two-sided Type I error probability* 0.1

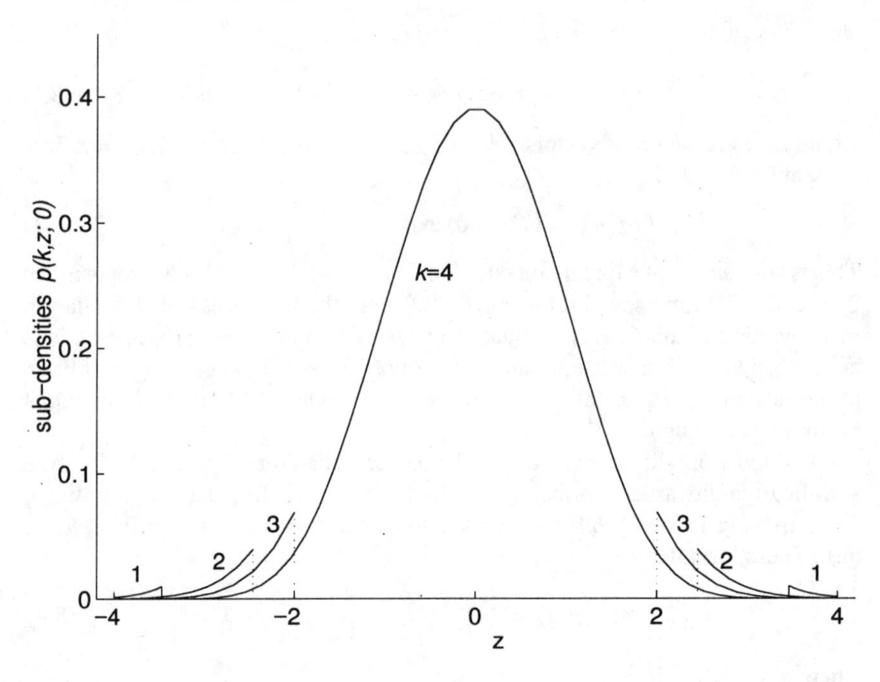

the four sub-densities under $\theta = \delta$, the positive value of θ at which power is 0.8, shown in Figure 8.2.

The area under sub-density k is the probability of stopping at stage k,

$$Pr_\theta\{T = k\} = \int_{z \notin C_k} p(k, z; \theta)\, dz, \quad k = 1, \ldots, K. \tag{8.7}$$

In our example, when $\theta = 0$ these probabilities are 0.0005, 0.0140, 0.0358 and 0.9497 at stages 1 to 4, respectively, and these are the areas under the curves in Figure 8.1. For $\theta = \pm\delta$, the corresponding probabilities are 0.0139, 0.2408, 0.3294 and 0.4159, distributed over z values according to the sub-densities shown in Figure 8.2.

The expected number of groups of observations and the expected final information level are, respectively,

$$E(T) = \sum_{k=1}^{K} k\, Pr_\theta\{T = k\} \quad \text{and} \quad E(\mathcal{I}_T) = \sum_{k=1}^{K} \mathcal{I}_k\, Pr_\theta\{T = k\}.$$

In our four-stage example, calculations show $E(T) = 3.934$ and $E(\mathcal{I}_T) = 6.296/\delta^2$ when $\theta = 0$, whereas $E(T) = 3.147$ and $E(\mathcal{I}_T) = 5.036/\delta^2$ when $\theta = \pm\delta$.

Figure 8.2 *Sub-densities* $p(k, z; \theta)$ *when* $\theta = \delta$ *for a four-stage O'Brien & Fleming test with two-sided Type I error probability* 0.1 *and power* 0.8 *at* $\theta = \delta$

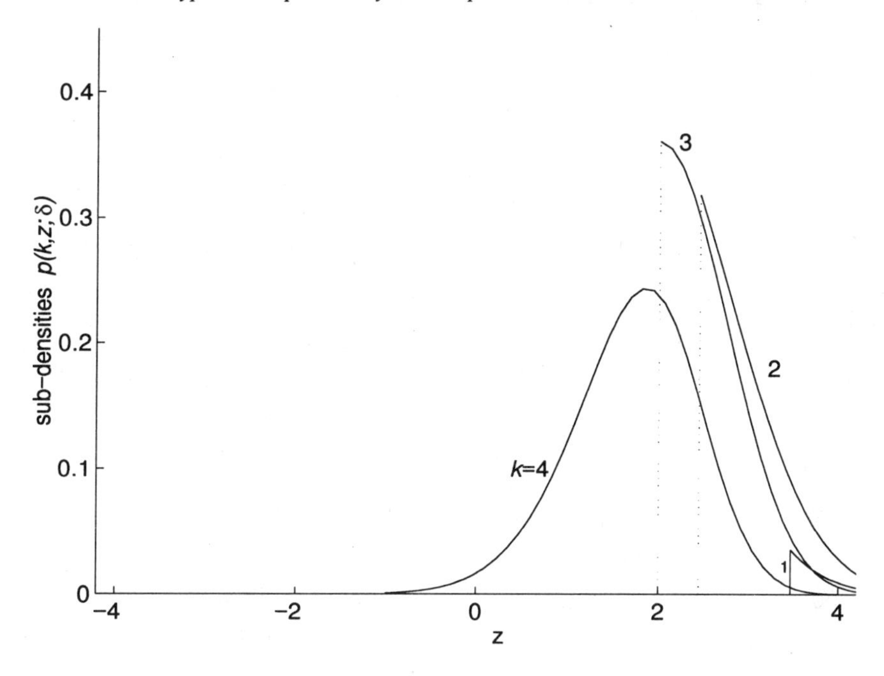

8.3 Point Estimation

We now consider point estimation of the parameter θ. In the previous section we derived the MLE, $\hat{\theta} = Z_T/\sqrt{\mathcal{I}_T}$. Since in the one-sample normal problem $\hat{\theta} = \bar{X}_T$ is the MLE of $\theta = \mu - \mu_0$ and in the two-sample problem $\hat{\theta} = \bar{X}_{AT} - \bar{X}_{BT}$ is the MLE of $\theta = \mu_A - \mu_B$, we can also call $\hat{\theta} = Z_T/\sqrt{\mathcal{I}_T}$ the "sample mean" estimator.

The sampling density of $\hat{\theta}$ at $\hat{\theta} = y$ is given by

$$\sum_{k=1}^{K} p(k, y\sqrt{\mathcal{I}_k}; \theta)\sqrt{\mathcal{I}_k}, \tag{8.8}$$

using the notation of the previous section. We illustrate this in the example of the four-stage, two-sided O'Brien & Fleming test discussed in Section 8.2. The sampling density (8.8) is shown in Figure 8.3 when $\theta = 0$ and in Figure 8.4 when $\theta = \delta = 1$. The components of (8.8) arising from termination at each stage k are indicated in the two figures and these correspond to contributions from the four sub-densities shown in Figures 8.1 and 8.2 respectively.

We can see that the density of $\hat{\theta} = Z_T/\sqrt{\mathcal{I}_T}$ is multi-modal with a peak for each value of $T \in \{1, 2, 3, 4\}$. This density is *not* at all like that of a normal with mean θ and variance $\mathcal{I}_T^{-1}$, as it would be in the analysis of a fixed sample design. In view of the nature of this sampling density, it is not surprising that $\hat{\theta}$ is a biased

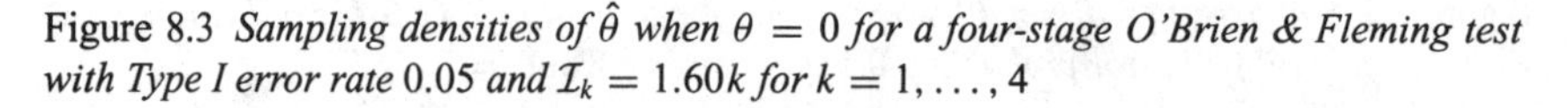

Figure 8.3 *Sampling densities of* $\hat{\theta}$ *when* $\theta = 0$ *for a four-stage O'Brien & Fleming test with Type I error rate* 0.05 *and* $\mathcal{I}_k = 1.60k$ *for* $k = 1, \ldots, 4$

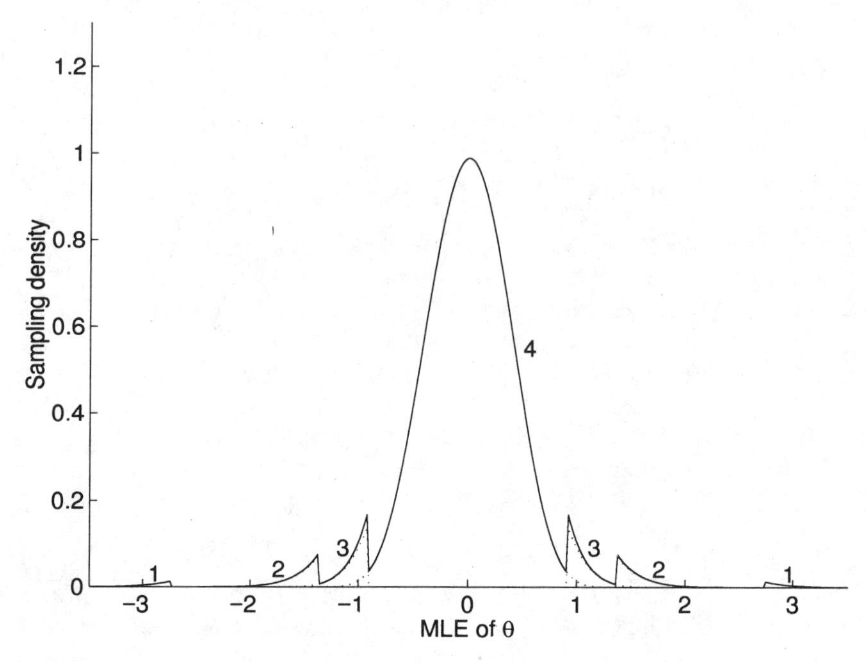

estimator of θ. The expectation of $\hat{\theta}$ can be calculated as

$$E_\theta(\hat{\theta}) = \sum_{k=1}^{K} \int_{z \notin \mathcal{C}_k} \frac{z}{\sqrt{\mathcal{I}_k}}\, p(k, z; \theta)\, dz. \tag{8.9}$$

For the two-sided testing boundaries with no inner wedge presented in Chapters 2 and 3, the MLE typically overestimates the magnitude of θ, giving a positive bias for $\theta > 0$ and a negative bias for $\theta < 0$. To see why this should occur, consider the case $\theta > 0$: if $\hat{\theta}^{(k)}$ is sufficiently larger than θ at an early analysis, the test stops and $\hat{\theta} = \hat{\theta}^{(k)}$; whereas if $\hat{\theta}^{(k)}$ is lower than θ by a similar amount, the test can continue, allowing later data to dilute the effect of early results on the final $\hat{\theta}$. Pinheiro & DeMets (1997, Section 2.2) give an explanation of this phenomenon based on an analytic expression for the bias of the MLE. Whitehead (1986a, Section 9) tabulates the bias of the MLE of θ for the triangular tests of Section 4.5.

For the simple case of a two-stage test with continuation interval $\mathcal{C}_1 = (a, b)$ at stage 1, Emerson (1988) obtains an analytic expression for this bias. From (8.6) and (8.9), we have

$$E_\theta(\hat{\theta}) = \int_{-\infty}^{a} \frac{z_1}{\sqrt{\mathcal{I}_1}} \phi(z_1 - \theta\sqrt{\mathcal{I}_1})\, dz_1 + \int_{b}^{\infty} \frac{z_1}{\sqrt{\mathcal{I}_1}} \phi(z_1 - \theta\sqrt{\mathcal{I}_1})\, dz_1$$

$$+ \int_a^b \int_{-\infty}^{\infty} \frac{z_2}{\sqrt{\Delta_2}} \phi\left(\frac{z_2\sqrt{\mathcal{I}_2} - z_1\sqrt{\mathcal{I}_1} - \Delta_2\theta}{\sqrt{\Delta_2}} \right) \phi(z_1 - \theta\sqrt{\mathcal{I}_1})\, dz_2 dz_1.$$

Figure 8.4 *Sampling densities of* $\hat{\theta}$ *when* $\theta = 1$ *for a four-stage O'Brien & Fleming test with Type I error rate* 0.05 *and* $\mathcal{I}_k = 1.60k$ *for* $k = 1, \ldots, 4$

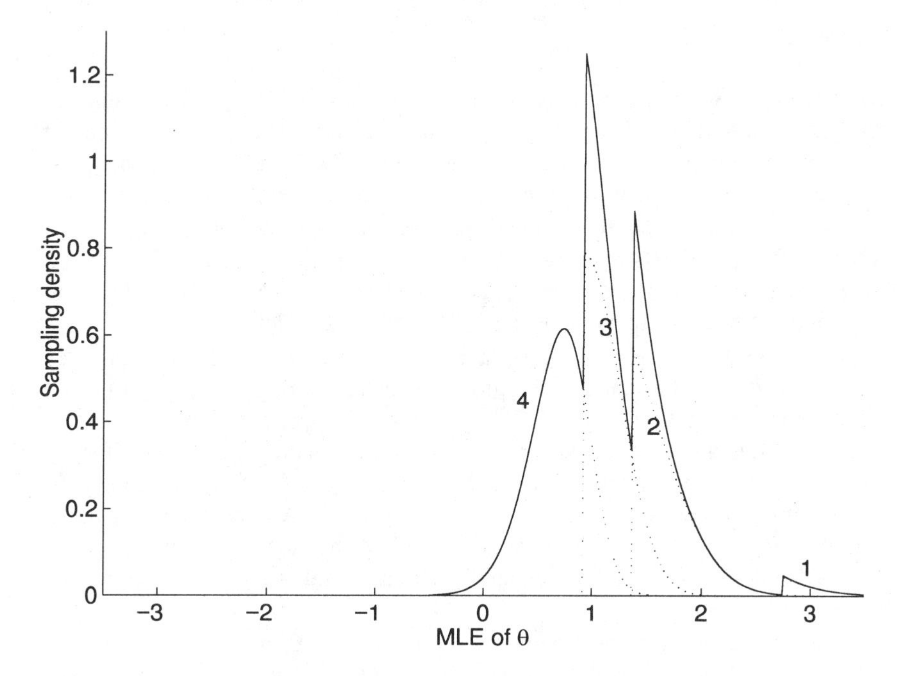

Integrating over z_2, the double integral in the above equation becomes

$$\int_a^b \frac{1}{\mathcal{I}_2}(z_1\sqrt{\mathcal{I}_1} + \Delta_2\theta)\,\phi(z_1 - \theta\sqrt{\mathcal{I}_1})\,dz_1$$

and we can use the fact that

$$\int_{-\infty}^{\infty} z\phi(z - \theta\sqrt{\mathcal{I}})\,dz = \theta\sqrt{\mathcal{I}}$$

to simplify this expression further. It follows that the bias in $\hat{\theta}$ is

$$\begin{aligned} E_\theta(\hat{\theta}) - \theta &= \int_a^b \left(\frac{z_1\sqrt{\mathcal{I}_1}}{\mathcal{I}_2} - \frac{z_1}{\sqrt{\mathcal{I}_1}} + \frac{\Delta_2\theta}{\mathcal{I}_2}\right)\phi(z_1 - \theta\sqrt{\mathcal{I}_1})\,dz_1 \\ &= -\int_a^b \frac{\Delta_2}{\mathcal{I}_2\sqrt{\mathcal{I}_1}}(z_1 - \theta\sqrt{\mathcal{I}_1})\,\phi(z_1 - \theta\sqrt{\mathcal{I}_1})\,dz_1. \end{aligned}$$

Hence, using $\phi'(u) = -u\phi(u)$, we obtain

$$E_\theta(\hat{\theta}) - \theta = \frac{\Delta_2}{\mathcal{I}_2\sqrt{\mathcal{I}_1}}\{\phi(b - \theta\sqrt{\mathcal{I}_1}) - \phi(a - \theta\sqrt{\mathcal{I}_1})\}.$$

For the case of equal group sizes, $\mathcal{I}_2 = 2\mathcal{I}_1$ and $\Delta_2 = \mathcal{I}_1$, so

$$E_\theta(\hat{\theta}) - \theta = \frac{\exp\{-(b - \theta\sqrt{\mathcal{I}_1})^2/2\} - \exp\{-(a - \theta\sqrt{\mathcal{I}_1})^2/2\}}{2\sqrt{(2\pi\mathcal{I}_1)}}.$$

It is straightforward to check that this is only equal to zero when θ happens to equal $(a+b)/(2\sqrt{\mathcal{I}_1})$.

Unbiased Estimators

Whitehead (1986a) suggests adjusting the MLE, $\hat{\theta}$, by subtracting an estimate of the bias of the MLE. Ideally, this bias would be calculated at the true value of θ. Approximating it by the bias at the adjusted MLE leads to the estimator $\breve{\theta}$, for which $E_{\breve{\theta}}(\hat{\theta})$ is equal to the observed value of $\hat{\theta}$. For a given experimental outcome, $\breve{\theta}$ can be found by a numerical search, a task in which formula (8.3) is very useful as it allows the most substantial computations to be performed at a single value of θ. Another approach, suggested by Wang & Leung (1997), is to use parametric bootstrap methods to find bias-adjusted estimators.

It is natural to enquire whether a uniformly minimum variance unbiased estimator of θ can be found in the group sequential setting. Liu & Hall (1999) prove that the sufficient statistic (T, Z_T) is not complete and hence such an estimator does not exist. However, the same authors show there is a uniformly minimum variance unbiased estimator in the class of estimators which do not require knowledge of the number of further analyses and their associated information levels that would have occurred had the study continued past the terminal analysis T. This is a natural restriction and we term this estimator the "UMVUE".

Emerson & Fleming (1990) suggest use of the UMVUE, calculated by applying the familiar Rao-Blackwell technique to the unbiased estimate of θ formed from just the first-stage data, $\hat{\theta}_1 = Z_1/\sqrt{\mathcal{I}_1}$. Emerson (1993) and Emerson & Kittelson (1997) describe the necessary calculations in detail. The UMVUE is $E\{\hat{\theta}_1 \mid (T, Z_T)\}$, and this expectation can be found from the conditional density of Z_1 given $(T, Z_T) = (k, z)$:

$$p(z_1 \mid (T, Z_T) = (k, z); \theta) = \frac{p(1, z_1; \theta)\, p(k, z \mid z_1; \theta)}{p(k, z; \theta)}. \tag{8.10}$$

Here, $p(k, z \mid z_1; \theta)$ denotes the conditional sub-density under θ of outcomes terminating at stage k, given that $Z_1 = z_1$. In Section 8.2 we gave a representation of $Z_1\sqrt{\mathcal{I}_1}, \ldots, Z_K\sqrt{\mathcal{I}_K}$ as partial sums of independent normal variates $Y_1, \ldots, Y_K$. It follows from this representation that $p(k, z \mid z_1; \theta)$ is the same as the sub-density at analysis $k-1$ arising in a "shifted" group sequential test with a maximum of $K-1$ analyses conducted at information levels $\mathcal{I}_2 - \mathcal{I}_1, \ldots, \mathcal{I}_K - \mathcal{I}_1$ and continuation regions $(\mathcal{C}_2\sqrt{\mathcal{I}_2} - z_1\sqrt{\mathcal{I}_1})/\sqrt{(\mathcal{I}_2 - \mathcal{I}_1)}, \ldots, (\mathcal{C}_K\sqrt{\mathcal{I}_K} - z_1\sqrt{\mathcal{I}_1})/\sqrt{(\mathcal{I}_K - \mathcal{I}_1)}$. Hence, $p(k, z \mid z_1; \theta)$ may be calculated using formulae (8.4) to (8.6). Since we are conditioning on the sufficient statistics for θ, the conditional sub-density (8.10) does not depend on θ and may be computed assuming, say, $\theta = 0$.

Emerson & Fleming (1990) compare the UMVUE with several other estimators of θ calculated after four-stage Pocock and O'Brien & Fleming tests. In these examples, the lack of bias of the UMVUE is accompanied by a relatively high variance and Whitehead's bias-adjusted estimator, $\breve{\theta}$, has a noticeably lower mean squared error.

It is important to note that bias may occur in the MLEs of other parameters if these estimators are correlated with the test statistics used in the stopping rule of a group sequential test. Whitehead (1986b) gives examples of this problem and addresses the analysis of secondary endpoints on termination of a group sequential study. In the case of point estimation, his bias correction for a secondary endpoint is a specified multiple of the bias correction for the primary endpoint on which the stopping rule is based.

8.4 P-values

We return to the problem of testing H_0: $\theta = 0$, the null hypothesis of the group sequential tests described in previous chapters. Rather than simply announce acceptance or rejection of H_0, we can enlarge on this by reporting the P-value of the observed data for testing H_0.

Let Ω be the sample space defined by the group sequential design, that is, the set of all pairs (k, z) where $z \notin \mathcal{C}_k$ so that the test can terminate with $(T, Z_T) = (k, z)$. We denote the observed value of (T, Z_T) by (k^*, z^*). The P-value is the minimum significance level under which a test defined on the sample space Ω can reject H_0 on seeing the observed outcome (k^*, z^*), smaller P-values indicating stronger evidence against H_0. For a continuous response distribution, the P-value is uniformly distributed under H_0, i.e., $Pr\{P\text{-value} \le p\} = p$ for all $0 \le p \le 1$.

The P-value for testing H_0 on observing (k^*, z^*) can also be stated as

$$Pr_{\theta=0}\{\text{Obtain } (k, z) \text{ as extreme or more extreme than } (k^*, z^*)\},$$

where "extreme" refers to the ordering of Ω implicit in the construction of tests of H_0 at different significance levels. However, since the number of observations varies between different outcomes, the monotone likelihood ratio property does not hold on Ω. Consequently, there is no single natural way to order possible outcomes and one must choose between a number of orderings of Ω, all of which have intuitive appeal. We write $(k', z') \succ (k, z)$ to denote that (k', z') is above (k, z) in a given ordering. Four orderings which have received attention are

A *Stage-wise ordering.* This was first proposed by Armitage (1957) and later used by Siegmund (1978), Fairbanks & Madsen (1982) and Tsiatis, Rosner & Mehta (1984). It can be used if the continuation regions $\mathcal{C}_1, \ldots, \mathcal{C}_{K-1}$ are intervals, which is true for most of the designs in the previous chapters but not for the "inner wedge" designs of Chapter 5. We define the ordering in a counter-clockwise sense around the continuation region, considering in decreasing order of priority: the boundary crossed, the stage at which stopping occurs, and the value of Z_k on termination. In the resulting ordering $(k', z') \succ (k, z)$ if any one of the following three conditions holds:

$$\begin{aligned} (i) \quad & k' = k \text{ and } z' \geq z, \\ (ii) \quad & k' < k \text{ and } z' \geq b_{k'}, \\ (iii) \quad & k' > k \text{ and } z \leq a_k. \end{aligned}$$

B *MLE ordering.* This was used by Armitage (1958a) in connection with a test for a binomial proportion, and investigated more recently for normal data by Emerson & Fleming (1990). Outcomes are ordered according to the value of the MLE, $\hat{\theta} = z_k/\sqrt{\mathcal{I}_k}$, with

$$(k', z') \succ (k, z) \quad \text{if} \quad z'/\sqrt{\mathcal{I}_{k'}} > z/\sqrt{\mathcal{I}_k}.$$

This is sometimes termed the *sample mean ordering*, because it is equivalent to ordering outcomes by $\bar{X}_T$ in the one-sample problem and by $\bar{X}_{AT} - \bar{X}_{BT}$ in the two-sample problem.

C *Likelihood ratio (LR) ordering.* In this ordering,

$$(k', z') \succ (k, z) \quad \text{if} \quad z' > z.$$

Chang (1989) shows this is the ordering induced by consideration of the signed likelihood ratio statistic for testing H_0: $\theta = 0$ against a general alternative.

D *Score test ordering.* This declares

$$(k', z') \succ (k, z) \quad \text{if} \quad z'\sqrt{\mathcal{I}_{k'}} > z\sqrt{\mathcal{I}_k}.$$

Rosner & Tsiatis (1988) show that this ordering ranks outcomes by values of the score statistic for testing H_0: $\theta = 0$.

For any given ordering, using the formulae given in Section 8.2, we can compute a one-sided upper P-value as

$$Pr_{\theta=0}\{(T, Z_T) \succeq (k^*, z^*)\}$$

and a one-sided lower P-value as

$$Pr_{\theta=0}\{(T, Z_T) \preceq (k^*, z^*)\}.$$

The two-sided P-value is twice the smaller of these two quantities. As an example, suppose we use the stage-wise ordering and the test terminates by exiting the upper boundary or by reaching the last stage K. Then the one-sided P-value is

$$\int_{b_1}^{\infty} p(1, z; 0)dz + \ldots + \int_{b_{k^*-1}}^{\infty} p(k^* - 1, z; 0)dz + \int_{z^*}^{\infty} p(k^*, z; 0)dz,$$

where $p(k, z; \theta)$ is defined in (8.4). This ordering implies that when the test exits the upper boundary, termination at an earlier stage decreases the one-sided upper P-value and, similarly, when the lower boundary is crossed, earlier termination reduces the lower P-value. This is not necessarily the case for the other orderings. Of the four orderings, we prefer (A), the stage-wise ordering. It automatically ensures that

(i) the P-value is less than the significance level α of the group sequential test if and only if H_0 is rejected, an important consideration for internal consistency. Unlike the other orderings, the stage-wise ordering has the property that

(ii) the P-value does not depend on information levels or group sizes beyond the observed stopping stage $T = k^*$.

This is a key feature when increments in information are unpredictable; the P-values based on the other three orderings cannot be computed in such situations. The stage-wise ordering fits naturally with the error spending tests of Chapter 7, and we shall see in the next section that it has similar advantages in relation to confidence intervals computed on termination.

Although it is unfortunate that the definition of a P-value should depend on a choice of ordering on Ω, it should be stressed that different orderings yield very similar P-values for many outcomes. The choice of ordering has the greatest effect when a test stops with a value $Z_k = z_k$ a long way outside the critical region $\mathcal{C}_k$. However, the probability of observing such large "overshoot" is usually small since the sample path is likely to have crossed an earlier boundary on its way to the value z_k at stage k.

8.5 Confidence Intervals

Equal tailed $(1-\alpha)$-level confidence intervals for θ can be derived by inverting a family of hypothesis tests with two-sided Type I error probability α. Consider an ordering of the sample space Ω, as discussed in the previous section, in which we write $(k', z') \succ (k, z)$ to denote that (k', z') is higher in the ordering than (k, z) and higher values of (T, Z_T) are typical of higher values of θ. For any given value θ_0 we can find pairs $(k_u(\theta_0), z_u(\theta_0))$ and $(k_\ell(\theta_0), z_\ell(\theta_0))$ such that

$$Pr_{\theta=\theta_0}\{(T, Z_T) \succeq (k_u(\theta_0), z_u(\theta_0))\} = \alpha/2 \tag{8.11}$$

and

$$Pr_{\theta=\theta_0}\{(T, Z_T) \preceq (k_\ell(\theta_0), z_\ell(\theta_0))\} = \alpha/2. \tag{8.12}$$

Then, the acceptance region

$$A(\theta_0) = \{(k, z)\colon (k_\ell(\theta_0), z_\ell(\theta_0)) \prec (k, z) \prec (k_u(\theta_0), z_u(\theta_0))\} \tag{8.13}$$

defines a two-sided hypothesis test of $H\colon \theta = \theta_0$ with Type I error probability α. Standard arguments imply that the set

$$\{\theta\colon (T, Z_T) \in A(\theta)\} \tag{8.14}$$

obtained by inverting this family of tests is a $(1-\alpha)$-level, equal tailed confidence set for θ. This confidence set contains all values θ_0 for which the hypothesis $H\colon \theta = \theta_0$ is accepted.

If $Pr_\theta\{(T, Z_T) \succeq (k, z)\}$ is an increasing function of θ for each $(k, z) \in \Omega$, we say the distributions on Ω are *stochastically ordered* with respect to θ, and we shall refer to this as the *monotonicity condition.* In this case, $(k_\ell(\theta), z_\ell(\theta))$ and $(k_u(\theta), z_u(\theta))$ increase in the ordering on Ω as θ increases and the set (8.14) is an interval. When the observed value of (T, Z_T) is (k^*, z^*), this interval is (θ_L, θ_U), where

$$Pr_{\theta_L}\{(T, Z_T) \succeq (k^*, z^*)\} = Pr_{\theta_U}\{(T, Z_T) \preceq (k^*, z^*)\} = \alpha/2. \tag{8.15}$$

For a given ordering, the probabilities in (8.15) can be evaluated numerically using the recursive computation of sub-densities described in Section 8.2. Solutions θ_L and θ_U can be found by a search method such as successive bisection. If the monotonicity condition fails to hold, the set (8.14) may not be an interval and must be calculated directly.

Each ordering of Ω discussed in Section 8.4 in the context of P-values can be used to construct confidence intervals. The first two, (A) the stage-wise ordering and (B) the MLE ordering, are the simplest to apply since their definitions do not depend on the hypothesis being tested. The other two orderings are dependent on the hypothesized value of θ, and the order inequalities in (8.11), (8.12) and (8.13) should be treated as being with respect to the ordering for θ_0.

The likelihood ratio ordering, (C), for θ_0 states $(k', z') \succ (k, z)$ if

$$\text{sign}(\hat{\theta}' - \theta_0) \frac{p(k', z'; \hat{\theta}')}{p(k', z'; \theta_0)} > \text{sign}(\hat{\theta}' - \theta_0) \frac{p(k, z; \hat{\theta})}{p(k, z; \theta_0)},$$

where $\hat{\theta}' = z'/\sqrt{\mathcal{I}_{k'}}$ and $\hat{\theta} = z/\sqrt{\mathcal{I}_k}$ are the respective MLEs of θ. Using (8.3), we see that this condition reduces to

$$z' - \theta_0\sqrt{\mathcal{I}_{k'}} > z - \theta_0\sqrt{\mathcal{I}_k}.$$

Finally, the score test ordering, (D), for θ_0 declares $(k', z') \succ (k, z)$ if

$$\left.\frac{\partial}{\partial\theta} \log p(k', z'; \theta)\right|_{\theta=\theta_0} > \left.\frac{\partial}{\partial\theta} \log p(k, z; \theta)\right|_{\theta=\theta_0},$$

which reduces to

$$z'\sqrt{\mathcal{I}_{k'}} - \theta_0\mathcal{I}_{k'} > z\sqrt{\mathcal{I}_k} - \theta_0\mathcal{I}_k$$

or, equivalently,

$$(\hat{\theta}' - \theta_0)\mathcal{I}_{k'} > (\hat{\theta} - \theta_0)\mathcal{I}_k.$$

Each of the orderings (A) to (D) defines a notion of distance of the outcome (T, Z_T) from the hypothesis H: $\theta = \theta_0$. Rosner & Tsiatis (1988) refer to (C) and (D) as the "standardized distance" and "distance" orderings, respectively.

Let us now consider some desiderata for confidence intervals following a group sequential test.

(*i*) *The confidence set given by* (8.14) *should be an interval.* This is guaranteed to occur if the monotonicity condition holds. Computation is simpler in this case and reduces to solving the equations (8.15). If (8.14) is not an interval, we can define θ_L and θ_U to be the infimum and supremum of the set defined in (8.14) but, even so, finding θ_L and θ_U is still more difficult than in the monotone case. Also, the confidence interval (θ_L, θ_U) will be conservative, its coverage probability exceeding $1 - \alpha$ for some values of θ.

(*ii*) *The confidence interval should agree with the original test.* If the original group sequential design is constructed as an α level, two-sided test of the hypothesis H_0: $\theta = \theta_0$ for a certain θ_0, the $1 - \alpha$ confidence interval should exclude θ_0 if and only if H_0 is rejected. Similarly, a $1-\alpha$ confidence interval should exclude the value of θ at the null hypothesis of an $\alpha/2$ level, one-sided test if and only if the test rejects this hypothesis. This corresponds to the consistency property (i) of P-values described towards the end of Section 8.4.

(iii) *The confidence interval should contain the MLE,* $\hat{\theta} = Z_T/\sqrt{\mathcal{I}_T}$. Alternatively, we might ask that one of the other point estimates discussed in Section 8.3 should lie in the confidence interval.

(iv) *Narrower confidence intervals are to be preferred.* A related feature is that the probability of the confidence interval containing particular values of θ other than the true value should be small.

(v) *The confidence interval should be well-defined when information levels are unpredictable.* This ensures that confidence intervals can be obtained when the experimental design follows the error spending approach of Chapter 7.

Confidence intervals based on the four orderings (A) to (D) vary in their performance with respect to these desiderata.

With regard to desideratum (i), note first that it is tacitly assumed in the definition of the stage-wise ordering, (A), that the group sequential test has interval continuation regions: this is not the case for "inner wedge" designs and so ordering (A) cannot be used for such tests. For one-sided or two-sided tests with just an upper and a lower boundary, the stage-wise ordering is well-defined and satisfies the monotonicity condition, so (8.15) does yield an interval. We establish the monotonicity property by a coupling argument which relates outcomes under parameter values θ and θ'. Suppose $\theta' = \theta + \delta$ where $\delta > 0$. Under θ, the joint distribution of $\{Z_1, \ldots, Z_K\}$ is that of the sequence of variables $\{(Y_1 + \ldots + Y_k)/\sqrt{\mathcal{I}_k};\ k = 1, \ldots, K\}$ where the Y_k are independent and $Y_k \sim N(\Delta_k\theta, \Delta_k)$. If we define $Y_k' = Y_k + \Delta_k\delta$ and $Z_k' = (Y_1' + \ldots + Y_k')/\sqrt{\mathcal{I}_k}$, $k = 1, \ldots, K$, the sequence $\{Z_1', \ldots, Z_K'\}$ has the joint distribution appropriate to θ'. Now, by construction, $Z_k' > Z_k$ for all k and hence $(T', Z_{T'}') \succeq (T, Z_T)$ where $T = \min\{k : Z_k \notin \mathcal{C}_k\}$ and $T' = \min\{k : Z_k' \notin \mathcal{C}_k\}$. Since (T, Z_T) and $(T', Z_{T'}')$ have the distributions of the sufficient statistic pair under θ and θ', respectively, we deduce that $Pr_\theta\{(T, Z_T) \succeq (k, z)\}$ increases with θ for any (k, z) and the monotonicity condition is satisfied. This proof is a special case of that used by Bather (1988) to establish monotonicity for the stage-wise ordering applied to response variables in the general exponential family, which includes the normal, binomial and many other distributions.

The same form of argument cannot be used to prove the monotonicity property for the MLE ordering since, in the above coupling, it is possible that $\theta' > \theta$ leads to $T' < T$ but $Z_{T'}'/\sqrt{\mathcal{I}_{T'}} < Z_T/\sqrt{\mathcal{I}_T}$ and so $(T', Z_{T'}') \preceq (T, Z_T)$ in the MLE ordering. This happens when the Z_k sequence crosses a boundary with a particularly large overshoot and the coupled Z_k' sequence stops earlier with little overshoot and a smaller MLE of θ. Nevertheless, Emerson (1988, Section 4.2) has proved that $Pr_\theta\{\hat{\theta} > w\}$ is an increasing function of θ for any fixed w and the monotonicity condition is in fact satisfied for the MLE ordering. This property was shown for binomial responses by Armitage (1958a).

There is no result concerning monotonicity for orderings (C) and (D). Indeed, Emerson & Fleming (1990, p. 880) report numerical studies in which the set (8.14) occasionally fails to be an interval using (C). Rosner & Tsiatis (1988, p. 726) report a similar phenomenon arising with ordering (D). However such occurrences are rare and the occasional extension of a confidence set to a surrounding interval may not be regarded as a serious difficulty.

The consistency property (ii) holds for a one-sided test if every outcome in Ω for which H_0: $\theta = \theta_0$ is rejected is higher in the ordering under θ_0 than every outcome where H_0 is accepted. For two-sided tests, outcomes where H_0 is accepted must be in the middle of the ordering under θ_0, higher than every outcome where H_0 is rejected in favor of $\theta < \theta_0$ and lower than every outcome for which H_0 is rejected in favor of $\theta > \theta_0$.

This consistency property clearly holds for intervals constructed using the stage-wise ordering. To see this in the case of a two-sided test of H_0: $\theta = \theta_0$, suppose a test with interval continuation regions $\mathcal{C}_k = (a_k, b_k)$ terminates at $(T, Z_T) = (k^*, z^*)$, rejecting H_0 after crossing the upper boundary. Then $z^* > b_{k^*}$ and

$$Pr_{\theta_0}\{(T, Z_T) \succeq (k^*, z^*)\} =$$

$$\sum_{k=1}^{k^*-1} \int_{b_k}^{\infty} p(k, u; \theta_0) du + \int_{z^*}^{\infty} p(k^*, u; \theta_0) du$$

$$\leq \sum_{k=1}^{k^*} \int_{b_k}^{\infty} p(k, u; \theta_0) du \leq \sum_{k=1}^{K} \int_{b_k}^{\infty} p(k, u; \theta_0) du = \alpha/2.$$

Similarly, $Pr_{\theta_0}\{(T, Z_T) \preceq (k^*, z^*)\} \leq \alpha/2$ if the lower boundary is crossed and H_0 rejected, and in neither case will θ_0 lie in the interval (θ_L, θ_U) defined by (8.15). Conversely, if the test stops to accept H_0 with $(T, Z_T) = (k^*, z^*)$, then $Pr_{\theta_0}\{(T, Z_T) \succeq (k^*, z^*)\} > \alpha/2$, $Pr_{\theta_0}\{(T, Z_T) \preceq (k^*, z^*)\} > \alpha/2$ and θ_0 does lie in (θ_L, θ_U).

In order for the MLE ordering to satisfy (ii) in a one-sided test of H_0: $\theta = \theta_0$ against $\theta > \theta_0$, values of $\hat{\theta}$ must be larger for all outcomes where H_0 is rejected than for those where it is accepted. For a two-sided test, we require values of $\hat{\theta}$ to be largest for those outcomes where H_0: $\theta = \theta_0$ is rejected in favor of $\theta > \theta_0$ and smallest for outcomes where H_0 is rejected in favor of $\theta < \theta_0$. Since $\hat{\theta} = Z_T/\sqrt{\mathcal{I}_T}$, this implies that a necessary and sufficient condition for a test with interval continuation regions $\mathcal{C}_k = (a_k, b_k)$ is

$$\frac{b_k}{\sqrt{\mathcal{I}_k}} \geq \frac{b_K}{\sqrt{\mathcal{I}_K}} \geq \frac{a_K}{\sqrt{\mathcal{I}_K}} \geq \frac{a_k}{\sqrt{\mathcal{I}_k}} \quad \text{for all } k = 1, \ldots, K-1. \tag{8.16}$$

This condition is satisfied for all the proposed group sequential tests of which we are aware. It is illustrated graphically in Figure 8.5, which shows the boundary of a two-sided test with four analyses plotted on the $(S_k, \mathcal{I}_k)$ scale. In example (a), any ray representing constant $\hat{\theta} = S_k/\mathcal{I}_k = Z_k/\sqrt{\mathcal{I}_k}$ which passes through the upper or lower boundary cannot go through (a_K, b_K) where H_0 is accepted; thus (8.16) holds. In example (b), it *is* possible for a ray to pass through both a rejection and acceptance boundary and (8.16) is violated — but this boundary has a very unnatural shape for a group sequential test.

Figure 8.5 *Stopping boundaries where* (a) *the consistency condition does hold for the MLE ordering and* (b) *this condition does not hold*

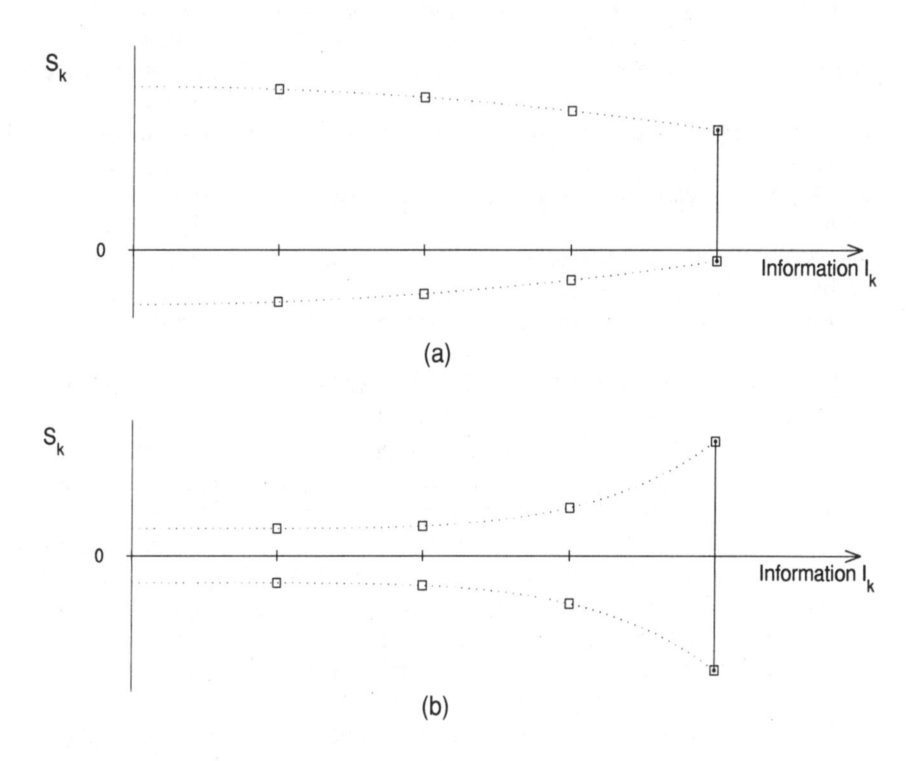

The consistency property (ii) does not necessarily hold for the likelihood ratio (LR) ordering. Emerson & Fleming (1990, Table 1) give an example of a symmetric one-sided test of H_0: $\theta = -0.85$ versus H_1: $\theta = 0.85$ with four analyses and Type I error probability 0.05. If the final result is $(T, Z_T) = (4, \epsilon)$, where ϵ is positive but very small, the test rejects H_0, but the equal tailed 90% confidence interval under the LR ordering is approximately $(-0.89, 0.89)$, and this includes the rejected value of -0.85. Rosner & Tsiatis (1988, p. 726) report numerical studies in which the score test ordering also produces occasional inconsistencies between the confidence interval on termination and the outcome of the group sequential test.

With regard to property (iii), the stage-wise ordering does not always give a confidence interval containing the MLE of θ. Tsiatis, Rosner & Mehta (1984, Table 2) give examples where this can happen even for typical confidence levels such as 0.95. However the MLE is only excluded when the test stops at analysis 2 or later with a large overshoot of the stopping boundary and, typically, this has a very small probability of occurring. Other studies, such as those reported by Rosner & Tsiatis (1988) and Emerson & Fleming (1990), indicate that this phenomenon does not occur under orderings (B), (C) and (D) for standard confidence levels $1 - \alpha$.

The mean length of a confidence interval is obtained by averaging over all possible outcomes in Ω. This mean length depends on the group sequential design used, the confidence level $1-\alpha$ and the true value of θ. Only limited studies based on numerical comparisons have been reported (e.g., Emerson & Fleming, 1990), and these suggest a slight advantage to confidence intervals based on the MLE and LR orderings but only of the order of 1 or 2%. Rosner & Tsiatis (1988, Tables 2 and 3) present a comparison between the stage-wise and score statistic orderings with respect to the probability that confidence intervals contain certain incorrect values of θ. In the one situation investigated, the stage-wise ordering has smaller probabilities of covering an incorrect θ value when θ is close to zero and the score statistic ordering is better for large θ. However, in all cases the differences are small.

As remarked in Section 8.4 in discussing P-values, the stage-wise ordering, (A), is the only one of the four orderings which can be used without knowledge of information levels beyond the observed stopping stage T. Hence this is really the only method available if information levels are unpredictable. Kim & DeMets (1987b) give details of its use in conjunction with designs based on error spending functions. Emerson & Fleming (1990, Section 5) suggest a "patch" to the MLE ordering method in which confidence intervals are calculated assuming that there would have been one more analysis, i.e., $K = T + 1$, with a specified final information level. The authors claim this is a worst case scenario in some sense and present supporting numerical results, but it is not clear that similar results will always be found in other situations.

In summary, we believe confidence interval construction based on the stage-wise ordering to be the preferred method for designs with interval continuation regions. It has the advantages of producing true intervals, consistent with the decision of the group sequential test, and it is the only method available for use with unpredictable information sequences. It has the disadvantage of slightly longer interval lengths, on average, than some other methods. A notable property of this interval is that it reduces to the naive interval $(\hat{\theta} \pm \Phi^{-1}(1 - \alpha/2)/\sqrt{\mathcal{I}_1})$ if the test stops at the first analysis. If $T \geq 2$, the interval is not symmetric about the MLE of θ but shifted towards zero, and in extreme cases it may not even contain the MLE. Although this shift may appear disturbing at first sight, Hughes & Pocock (1988) and Pocock & Hughes (1989) have argued that such shifts may have a desirable effect on bias or effectively incorporate prior information.

For designs with non-interval continuation regions, such as two-sided tests with inner wedges, the stage-wise method is not applicable and we recommend the MLE ordering method. Armitage (1957, p. 25) has suggested a hybrid ordering in which outcomes falling outside the lower and upper boundaries are ordered from each extreme by the stage-wise criterion, while, in between, the points in the inner wedge are ordered by the MLE criterion. We know of no investigations of the properties of this ordering.

Even though normality of the observations is assumed for the construction of the group sequential test, it may be desirable to avoid this assumption when analyzing the results. Chuang & Lai (1998) describe a nonparametric bootstrap procedure for constructing a robust confidence interval which involves resampling the stopped sequence of observations; they consider both the stage-wise and LR orderings of the sample space. Exact methods for inference following a sequential test may be developed for particular response distributions. Examples of this will be seen in Sections 12.1.3 and 12.2.2, where we describe the construction of confidence intervals following tests for binomial probabilities.

In this section we have considered the construction of a confidence interval upon conclusion of a trial conducted using a fixed stopping rule. One may, however, ask what can be done if a rigid stopping rule is not being followed. Or, it may be desirable to report interval estimates at certain interim stages of the trial. These issues will be addressed in the next chapter.

CHAPTER 9

Repeated Confidence Intervals

9.1 Introduction

In Section 8.5 we discussed how a confidence interval for a parameter, θ, could be constructed upon termination of a group sequential procedure. In this chapter we are concerned with the construction of a sequence of interval estimates for θ that we can form at *any* interim look at the data.

The multiple-looks problem affects the construction of confidence intervals just as it affects significance levels of hypothesis tests. Suppose, for example, independent normal observations $X_1, \ldots, X_{mK}$ are available sequentially, each with mean θ and known variance σ^2. Suppose also that after each group k of m observations, $k = 1, \ldots, K$, we form the usual (or "naive") 95% confidence interval $(\bar{X}_{mk} \pm 1.96\sigma/\sqrt{(mk)})$ for θ based on the observations accumulated so far. Then, the probability that all K intervals so formed contain the true value of θ is certainly less than 95%. These probabilities are listed in Table 9.1 for selected values of K and correspond to the probabilities in Table 2 of Armitage, McPherson & Rowe (1969).

Repeated confidence intervals, denoted RCIs, for a parameter θ are defined as a sequence of intervals I_k, $k = 1, \ldots, K$, for which a simultaneous coverage probability is maintained at some level, $1 - \alpha$ say. The defining property of a $(1 - \alpha)$-level sequence of RCIs for θ is

$$Pr_\theta\{\theta \in I_k \text{ for all } k = 1, \ldots, K\} = 1 - \alpha \quad \text{for all } \theta. \tag{9.1}$$

Here, each I_k, $k = 1, \ldots, K$, is an interval computed from the information available at analysis k. We shall use the notation $\mathcal{I}_k = (\underline{\theta}_k, \overline{\theta}_k)$ for these intervals.

The interval I_k provides a statistical summary of the information about the parameter θ at the kth analysis, automatically adjusted to compensate for repeated looks at the accumulating data. As such, it can be presented to a Data and Safety Monitoring Board (DSMB) to be considered with all other relevant information when discussing early termination of a study.

If τ is *any* random stopping time taking values in $\{1, \ldots, K\}$, the guarantee of simultaneous coverage (9.1) implies that the probability I_τ contains θ must be at least $1 - \alpha$, i.e.,

$$Pr_\theta\{\theta \in I_\tau\} \geq 1 - \alpha \quad \text{for all } \theta. \tag{9.2}$$

This property shows that an RCI can be used to summarize information about θ on termination and the confidence level $1 - \alpha$ will be maintained, regardless of how the decision to stop the study was reached. In contrast, the methods of Chapter 8 for constructing confidence intervals on termination all rely on a particular stopping rule being specified at the outset and strictly enforced.

Table 9.1 *Simultaneous coverage probabilities for naive 95% confidence intervals*

Number of looks, K	*Overall probability that all K intervals contain θ*
1	0.95
2	0.92
3	0.89
4	0.87
5	0.86
10	0.81
20	0.75
50	0.68
∞	0

When a study is monitored using RCIs, the intervals computed at interim analyses might also be reported at scientific meetings. The basic property (9.1) ensures that these interim results will not be "over-interpreted". Here, over-interpretation refers to the fact that, when the selection bias or optional sampling bias of reported results is ignored, data may seem more significant than warranted, and this can lead to adverse effects on accrual and drop-out rates, and to pressure to unblind or terminate a study prematurely.

Experience shows that in many medical trials it is unrealistic to expect a designated stopping rule to be enforced under all circumstances, and sometimes there is no planned stopping rule at all. The stopping boundaries of the group sequential designs discussed in earlier chapters are often used only as guidelines, not as strict rules (DeMets, 1984). Other factors, such as side-effects, financial cost, or reports of new scientific developments from outside the trial, will often influence the DSMB in their decision to stop or to continue a trial; see Pocock (1996) for a good discussion of the role external evidence can play in monitoring a clinical trial. As an example, in the NSABP Breast Cancer Prevention Trial (Fisher et al., 1998), the O'Brien & Fleming statistical stopping boundary was crossed in April 1996 but, for very good reasons, the decision to stop the trial was not made until a later interim analysis in March 1998. The opposite happened in a CALGB 3×2 factorial trial reported by Goldhirsch et al. (1998), which examined the use of doxorubicin (adriamycin) and taxol as adjuvant therapy in breast cancer treatment. That trial was unblinded and results reported at the first interim analysis in April 1998 because of strong evidence of benefit of taxol, even though the statistical stopping boundaries had not been crossed. Evidently, the decision to stop a clinical trial is complex and involves many subjective factors, indeed, Meier (1975, p. 526) describes the problem as political, rather than medical, legal or statistical. In such circumstances, the probability statements associated with conventional group sequential tests are of limited value since the stopping rule on which they rely may not be enforced. RCIs do not depend on a particular stopping rule and so remain valid in these situations.

The historical antecedent of repeated confidence intervals is the confidence sequence introduced by Robbins (1970) in his 1969 Wald Lectures. He defined an infinite sequence of intervals $\{I_n;\ n = 1, 2, \ldots\}$, where I_n is calculated from the first n observations and, for a $(1-\alpha)$-level sequence,

$$Pr_\theta\{\theta \in I_n \text{ for all } n = 1, 2, \ldots\} = 1 - \alpha \quad \text{for all } \theta.$$

Initially the theory of confidence sequences had little practical impact, one reason being that the intervals turn out to be extremely wide and unacceptable to investigators accustomed to fixed sample intervals. However, sequences of RCIs are finite in number and much narrower. The development of RCIs is due to Jennison & Turnbull (1984, 1989); similar ideas were introduced by Lai (1984).

Repeated confidence intervals are formed by inverting a family of two-sided group sequential tests with Type I error probability α, of the type described in Chapters 2, 3 and 7. We have seen in Section 3.1 that many common testing problems concerning a parameter θ lead to consideration of a sequence of test statistics $Z_1, \ldots, Z_K$ with the canonical joint distribution (3.1), given observed information levels $\mathcal{I}_1, \ldots, \mathcal{I}_K$. Here, θ might represent a difference, $\mu_A - \mu_B$, in mean response between two treatments as in Section 3.1.1, or a hazard ratio for comparing two survival distributions under the proportional hazards model of Section 3.7. Suppose we define

$$Z_k(\theta_0) = Z_k - \theta_0\sqrt{\mathcal{I}_k}, \quad k = 1, \ldots, K.$$

Then it follows from (3.1) that a two-sided group sequential test of the hypothesis H_0: $\theta = \theta_0$ with Type I error probability α has the form:

$$\text{Reject } H_0 \text{ at stage } k \text{ if } |Z_k(\theta_0)| \geq c_k(\alpha), \quad k = 1, \ldots, K, \tag{9.3}$$

where $c_1(\alpha), \ldots, c_K(\alpha)$ are critical values appropriate to the particular form of test and information sequence $\mathcal{I}_1, \ldots, \mathcal{I}_K$. The argument θ_0 of Z_k is displayed in this notation to signify the explicit dependence on the hypothesized value θ_0, whereas we have previously focused on a single θ_0, typically $\theta_0 = 0$, in any one problem.

The argument θ_0 in (9.3) indexes a family of tests and the RCI sequence $\{I_k;\ k = 1, \ldots, K\}$ is defined from these by

$$I_k = \{\theta_0\colon\ |Z_k(\theta_0)| < c_k(\alpha)\}, \quad k = 1, \ldots, K. \tag{9.4}$$

In inverting a family of group sequential tests to produce a sequence of RCIs, we are using the familiar duality between confidence sets and hypothesis tests. The construction of the test and the critical values $c_1(\alpha), \ldots, c_K(\alpha)$ ensure that

$$Pr_\theta\{|Z_k(\theta)| \geq c_k(\alpha) \text{ for some } k = 1, \ldots, K\} = \alpha.$$

Hence,

$$Pr_\theta\{\theta \in I_k \text{ for all } k = 1, \ldots, K\} = 1 - \alpha$$

and we see that (9.4) does indeed satisfy the RCI property (9.1). This property is satisfied approximately if $Z_1, \ldots, Z_K$ satisfy (3.1) only approximately.

When the information levels $\mathcal{I}_k$ do not depend on θ, as in the case of normally distributed data with a common variance, the RCI at stage k is simply

$$\left(\{Z_k - c_k(\alpha)\}/\sqrt{\mathcal{I}_k},\ \{Z_k + c_k(\alpha)\}/\sqrt{\mathcal{I}_k}\right), \quad k = 1, \ldots, K, \qquad (9.5)$$

or writing $\hat{\theta}^{(k)}$ for $Z_k/\sqrt{\mathcal{I}_k}$, the maximum likelihood estimate of θ at analysis k,

$$\left(\hat{\theta}^{(k)} - c_k(\alpha)/\sqrt{\mathcal{I}_k},\ \hat{\theta}^{(k)} + c_k(\alpha)/\sqrt{\mathcal{I}_k}\right), \quad k = 1, \ldots, K. \qquad (9.6)$$

If the information levels do depend on θ, approximate $(1-\alpha)$-level RCIs may be obtained using $\mathcal{I}_k$ evaluated for the current estimate $\hat{\theta}^{(k)}$ in (9.5) or (9.6). Examples of this are considered for binary and survival data in Chapters 12 and 13, respectively. Direct application of (9.4) when $\mathcal{I}_k$ depends on θ could possibly lead to a confidence set that is not an interval, although this should only happen in rare pathological cases; see Brookmeyer & Crowley (1982) for such an example. If this problem does arise, it can be resolved by defining the RCI, I_k, as the smallest interval containing the set defined in (9.4). In this case, we can always write I_k in the form $(\underline{\theta}_k, \overline{\theta}_k)$ and the RCI property (9.1) becomes

$$Pr_\theta\{\underline{\theta}_k < \theta < \overline{\theta}_k \text{ for all } k = 1, \ldots, K\} = 1 - \alpha. \qquad (9.7)$$

The intervals we shall construct will be symmetric and satisfy

$$Pr_\theta\{\underline{\theta}_k < \theta \text{ for all } k = 1, \ldots, K\} =$$

$$Pr_\theta\{\overline{\theta}_k > \theta \text{ for all } k = 1, \ldots, K\} \approx 1 - \alpha/2 \qquad (9.8)$$

when the Z_k follow (3.1). The second equality here is only approximate because of the possibility that $\underline{\theta}_k > \theta$ for some k and $\overline{\theta}_{k'} < \theta$ at some other analysis k'. However, the probability of this event is negligible and the departure from equality can be ignored in practice; see Proschan (1999, Theorem 1). Later in this chapter, we shall use the notation $\underline{\theta}_k(\alpha/2)$ and $\overline{\theta}_k(\alpha/2)$ to denote $\underline{\theta}_k$ and $\overline{\theta}_k$ satisfying (9.8).

The coverage property (9.1) would still be satisfied if I_k were replaced by the intersection of $I_1, \ldots, I_k$, thereby giving narrower confidence intervals. However, the original sequence (9.4) is to be preferred, because the intervals are then functions of the sufficient statistics for θ at each stage. This also avoids the possibility of obtaining an empty confidence interval, although the probability of this occurring is very small; for a discussion of this point, see Freeman (1989).

The construction of a sequence of RCIs depends on the choice of the group sequential test used in (9.4) and the associated critical values $c_1(\alpha), \ldots, c_K(\alpha)$. One could use a Pocock or O'Brien & Fleming test or one of the other two-sided tests described in Chapters 2 and 3, or a two-sided error spending test from Chapter 7. The test chosen to construct RCIs is called the *parent test* and should be specified in the study protocol. It is not necessary for a stopping rule to be prescribed if RCIs are used to monitor a study. However, if a stopping rule is applied then, for consistency, it should relate to the parent test of the RCIs in a natural manner: we shall describe ways of doing this in Section 9.3. Note that if we adopt the error spending approach, the maximum number of analyses K need not be pre-specified.

Table 9.2 *Ratios of widths of 95% RCIs, $\mathcal{I}_k$, to unadjusted 95% confidence intervals*

	$K = 5$		$K = 10$	
Analysis	*Pocock*	*O'Brien & Fleming*	*Pocock*	*O'Brien & Fleming*
k	$c_k=2.413$	$c_k = 2.040\surd(5/k)$	$c_k=2.555$	$c_k = 2.087\surd(10/k)$
1	1.231	2.328	1.304	3.366
2	1.231	1.646	1.304	2.389
3	1.231	1.344	1.304	1.944
4	1.231	1.164	1.304	1.683
5	1.231	1.041	1.304	1.505
6			1.304	1.374
7			1.304	1.272
8			1.304	1.190
9			1.304	1.122
10			1.304	1.065

9.2 Example: Difference of Normal Means

For illustration, consider the "prototype" problem of Chapter 2. We are interested in constructing RCIs for the difference in means, $\theta = \mu_A - \mu_B$, when comparing two treatments with normal response and common known variance σ^2. Observations are taken in equally sized groups of m on each treatment. The information for θ at analysis k is $\mathcal{I}_k = mk/(2\sigma^2)$ and the standardized statistics for testing $H_0\colon \theta = \theta_0$ are

$$Z_k(\theta_0) = \frac{1}{\surd(2mk\sigma^2)} \left(\sum_{i=1}^{mk} X_{Ai} - \sum_{i=1}^{mk} X_{Bi} - mk\theta_0 \right), \quad k = 1\ldots, K.$$

Thus, at stage k, the interval I_k is obtained from (9.5) as

$$(\bar{X}_{Ak} - \bar{X}_{Bk} \pm c_k(\alpha)\surd\{2\sigma^2/(mk)\}), \tag{9.9}$$

where $\bar{X}_{Ak}$ and $\bar{X}_{Bk}$ denote the cumulative sample means of observations on treatments A and B, respectively. The form of I_k is the same as that of the usual or "unadjusted" interval

$$(\bar{X}_{Ak} - \bar{X}_{Bk} \pm z_{\alpha/2}\surd\{2\sigma^2/(mk)\}),$$

except that the standard normal percentile $z_{\alpha/2} = \Phi^{-1}(1-\alpha/2)$ is replaced by the critical value $c_k(\alpha)$ from the parent group sequential test.

The ratio of the width of interval I_k to that of the unadjusted interval is $c_k(\alpha)/z_{\alpha/2}$, and this varies with the parent test of the RCI sequence. Table 9.2 displays these ratios of widths for RCIs constructed from Pocock (1977) and O'Brien & Fleming (1979) tests using $\alpha = 0.05$ and $K = 5$ and 10 groups of observations. Similar results but for $\alpha = 0.1$ appear in Table 2 of Jennison & Turnbull (1989). The same table could be drawn up just as easily for RCIs with a Wang & Tsiatis test or Haybittle-Peto test as their parent test, using the constants in Tables 2.9 and 2.13, respectively, to determine the $c_k(\alpha)$s. The widths of the RCIs with the Pocock parent test are a constant multiple of those of the unadjusted intervals whereas RCIs based on the O'Brien & Fleming test are very wide at the beginning but narrow rapidly and are quite close to the unadjusted interval at the last analysis. This feature of the O'Brien & Fleming-based RCIs is often quite desirable since the increased width early on may be appropriate in view of uncertainty about validity of model assumptions, and it is advantageous in explaining results that the final RCI, I_K, should be almost the same as the unadjusted interval. The Pocock-based RCIs could be recommended for situations where it is of equal importance to obtain precise estimates of θ at all K analyses.

Suppose now that we desire the final interval I_K to have a specified width δ. On examining (9.9), we see this will occur if we set the group size $m = 8\,\sigma^2 c_K^2(\alpha)/(K\delta^2)$. The ratio of the final sample size to that required for a fixed sample procedure yielding a confidence interval of the same width is $\{c_K(\alpha)/z_{\alpha/2}\}^2$, i.e., the square of the final entry in each column of Table 9.2. For instance, using an O'Brien & Fleming parent test with five analyses, this ratio is $1.041^2 = 1.084$, representing an 8.4% increase in maximum sample size over the fixed sample procedure. This increase in sample size can be viewed as the "cost" of obtaining the benefits of flexible group sequential monitoring and the ability to construct interval estimates for θ at interim analyses, with or without application of a rigid stopping rule.

9.3 Derived Tests: Use of RCIs to Aid Early Stopping Decisions

The most important use that a DSMB might make of RCIs presented at an interim analysis is in reaching a decision for early termination. As stated in Section 9.1, this is often a subjective decision based on many factors but an interval estimate for the primary endpoint, adjusted for optional sampling bias, will clearly play a large role. In this section we describe how RCIs can be employed in the formal construction of one-sided tests, two-sided tests and equivalence tests. We refer to these tests constructed from RCIs as "derived tests". The progression from parent test to derived test is displayed schematically in Figure 9.1.

9.3.1 Two-Sided Derived Tests

Suppose we wish to test a null hypothesis H_0: $\theta = \theta_0$ against the two-sided alternative $\theta \neq \theta_0$ and we are using a sequence of RCIs to monitor the study. Typically, θ_0 might be equal to zero, but we shall continue to discuss a general value θ_0. An obvious way to use the RCIs is to terminate the study early with rejection of H_0 if ever an RCI fails to include θ_0. By definition of the RCIs, this happens exactly when the parent test rejects H_0 and, thus, we recover the original parent test with two-sided Type I error rate α. In this case an RCI can be considered as an adjunct to the test of H_0: $\theta = \theta_0$, indicating which other values of θ are plausible, given the current data.

An RCI can be useful if opinion about an appropriate null hypothesis changes during the course of a study. Suppose we are comparing the efficacy of two treatments A and B, and as the study progresses, there is evidence of some serious

Figure 9.1 *RCIs, parent test and derived tests*

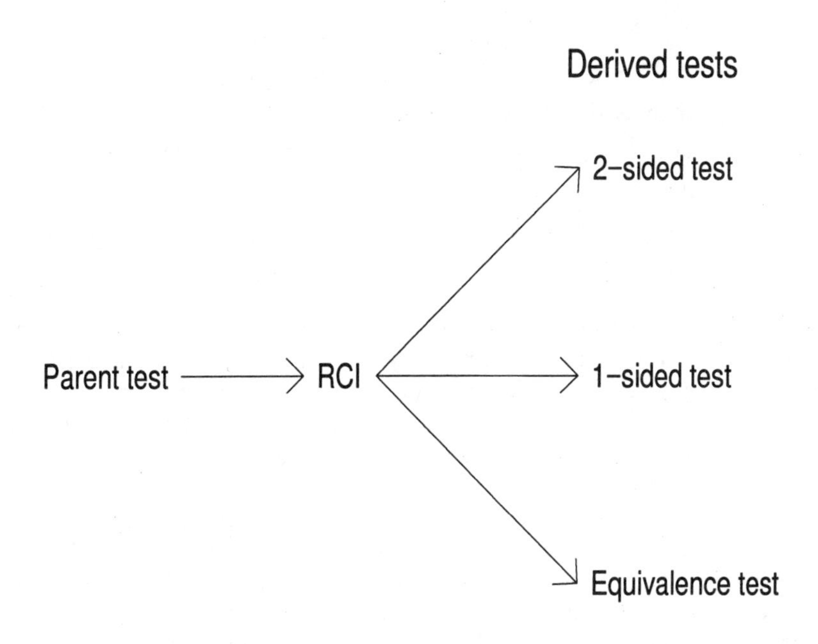

adverse side-effects on treatment B. To compensate for this we might shift H_0 from $\theta_0 = 0$ to a non-zero value, thereby requiring more of an improvement in efficacy of treatment B to offset the extra discomfort or incapacitation caused by the side-effects. The new rule for termination is simply to stop if an RCI fails to include the new value of θ_0.

We would recommend caution in the practice of altering hypotheses during the course of a study, especially if this could cast doubt on the study's credibility. In order to provide protection from possible abuse, blinding should be maintained as much as possible and contingencies should be discussed at the planning stage and written into the protocol. However, it is clear that DSMBs *do* take notice of information from a variety of sources, often unexpected, and this can influence their attitudes to the originally stated goals. RCIs provide flexibility in the monitoring of a trial which can allow external information to be incorporated into the decision making process.

It is possible to derive two-sided tests from RCIs that are not just the parent test but also provide an "inner wedge" in the stopping boundary to allow early stopping in favor of H_0. These tests are similar to those described in Chapter 5. Suppose we desire a group sequential test with Type I error probability α and power $1 - \beta$ at $\theta = \theta_0 \pm \delta$, where $0 < \beta < 0.5$. There are two ways to proceed.

In the first approach, we form a $(1-\alpha)$-level sequence of RCIs, $\{(\underline{\theta}_k, \overline{\theta}_k);\, k = 1, \ldots, K\}$ and define the formal stopping rule:

$$
\begin{array}{lll}
\text{At stage } k = 1, \ldots, K-1 & & \\
& \text{if } \underline{\theta}_k > \theta_0 + \delta \text{ or } \overline{\theta}_k < \theta_0 - \delta & \text{stop, reject } H_0 \\
& \text{if } (\underline{\theta}_k, \overline{\theta}_k) \subset (\theta_0 - \delta, \theta_0 + \delta) & \text{stop, accept } H_0 \\
& \text{otherwise} & \text{continue to group } k+1, \\
\text{at stage } K & & \\
& \text{if } \underline{\theta}_K > \theta_0 + \delta \text{ or } \overline{\theta}_K < \theta_0 - \delta & \text{stop, reject } H_0 \\
& \text{otherwise} & \text{stop, accept } H_0.
\end{array}
$$

It follows from the defining relation (9.1) with $\theta = \theta_0$ that this test's Type I error probability is at most α. Furthermore, by computing the power under different values of m, a group size can be found for which the power requirement is met.

The second procedure involves *two* sequences of RCIs for θ: one of level $(1-\alpha)$ and the other of level $(1-2\beta)$. At each stage, H_0 is rejected if the $(1-\alpha)$ RCI does not contain θ_0, and H_0 is accepted if the current $(1-2\beta)$ RCI lies entirely within the interval $(\theta_0 - \delta, \theta_0 + \delta)$. The group size must be chosen to ensure termination at stage K. This is done by making sure that the sum of the half-widths of the Kth $(1-\alpha)$-level and $(1-2\beta)$-level RCIs is equal to δ, since then precisely one of the conditions for rejecting H_0 or for accepting H_0 is bound to be met. Again, it follows from (9.1) with $\theta = \theta_0$ that this test has a Type I error probability of at most α. To see that the power requirement is satisfied note that, from (9.7) with $\theta = \theta_0 + \delta$,

$$
\begin{aligned}
& Pr_{\theta=\theta_0+\delta}\{\text{Accept } H_0\} \\
& \quad \leq \; Pr_{\theta=\theta_0+\delta}\{\underline{\theta}_k(\beta) > \theta_0 - \delta \text{ and } \overline{\theta}_k(\beta) < \theta_0 + \delta \text{ for some } k\} \\
& \quad \leq \; Pr_{\theta=\theta_0+\delta}\{\overline{\theta}_k(\beta) < \theta_0 + \delta \text{ for some } k\} \\
& \quad = \; 2\beta/2 \; = \; \beta.
\end{aligned}
$$

Here, $\underline{\theta}_k(\beta)$ and $\overline{\theta}_k(\beta)$ denote end points of the kth $(1-2\beta)$-level RCI. A similar argument establishes the power under $\theta = \theta_0 - \delta$.

The first of these procedures maintains the Type I error rate below α for any observed information sequence (as long as the RCI sequence retains its overall coverage probability of $1-\alpha$) but differences from planned information levels will affect the power at $\theta_0 \pm \delta$. In the second procedure, a large value of $\mathcal{I}_K$ may produce a shorter final RCI than anticipated, allowing decisions both to accept H_0 and to reject H_0 according to the stated rule. The justification of this method holds true whichever decision is made in such cases. Intuitively, the data in these situations suggest that θ is between $\theta_0 - \delta$ and θ_0 or between θ_0 and $\theta_0 + \delta$, in which cases neither a Type I error nor a Type II error (at $\theta_0 \pm \delta$) can be made. In order to maximize power subject to a Type I error probability of at most α, one should reject H_0 whenever the formal rule permits, even when acceptance of H_0 is also allowed. If, on the other hand, $\mathcal{I}_K$ is lower than planned, a wide final RCI may contain θ_0 as well as $\theta_0 + \delta$ or $\theta_0 - \delta$. In this case, H_0 should be accepted to keep the Type I error probability at or below α.

9.3.2 One-Sided Derived Tests: Symmetric Case

In Chapter 4, we considered one-sided tests of hypotheses of the form H_0: $\theta = 0$ versus $\theta > 0$ designed to have Type I error probability α and power $1-\beta$ at $\theta = \delta$. We now show how RCIs can be used to monitor a study in a manner which meets these objectives. We first consider the symmetric case, $\alpha = \beta$. We shall allow the study to be terminated at the kth analysis with acceptance of H_0 if $\overline{\theta}_k < \delta$ or with rejection of H_0 if $\underline{\theta}_k > 0$. In order that this test has error probabilities equal to α at $\theta = 0$ and $\theta = \delta$, *we need to use RCIs with confidence level* $1 - 2\alpha$ rather than $1 - \alpha$. Then, by (9.8), the probability of deciding in favor of H_0 if $\theta \geq \delta$ or of rejecting H_0 if $\theta \leq 0$ will be at most α.

To ensure a decision can be made at analysis K, the width of the final RCI must be no more than δ, so that the RCI for θ cannot contain both 0 and δ. Thus, from (9.5), we require $\mathcal{I}_K = 4\, c_K^2(2\alpha)/\delta^2$. In the comparison of two normal means considered in Section 9.2, we had $\mathcal{I}_K = mK/(2\sigma^2)$ and this condition reduces to requiring a group size of $m = 8\,\sigma^2 c_K^2(2\alpha)/(K\delta^2)$. If, in practice, a larger sample is accrued, the width of the final RCI may be less than δ and it it possible that both $\overline{\theta}_k < \delta$ and $\underline{\theta}_k > 0$: as explained for two-sided tests with an inner wedge, either decision is permissible in such a situation and one should choose to reject H_0 in order to maximize power while still satisfying the Type I error condition. If, however, the sample is small and a wide final RCI contains both 0 and δ, H_0 should be accepted to protect the Type I error probability.

We refer to this procedure as a "derived test". This test stands in its own right as a one-sided group sequential test with Type I error probability at most α and power at least $1 - \alpha$ at $\theta = \delta$. Hence, its maximum information level and expected information level under specific values of θ can be compared to those of symmetric tests in Chapter 4. Suppose a study is designed for $K = 5$ stages with error probabilities $\alpha = \beta = 0.05$. We could base RCIs and, hence, derived tests on a Pocock parent test, for which $c_k = C_P(5, 0.05)$, or an O'Brien & Fleming parent test, with $c_k = C_B(5, 0.05)\sqrt{(5/k)}$. Table 9.3 lists properties of these derived tests. The ratio $R = \{c_K(2\alpha)/z_\alpha\}^2$ is the maximum information level, $\mathcal{I}_K$, divided by the information level $\mathcal{I}_{f,1}$ required by the corresponding fixed sample test. The error rate is the attained Type I or Type II error probability (which are equal by symmetry). Also listed are expected information levels on termination when $\theta = 0$, $\delta/2$ and δ, expressed as percentages of $\mathcal{I}_{f,1}$ (the cases $\theta = 0$ and $\theta = \delta$ are identical by symmetry). These ratios and information levels can be compared directly with the analogous results for the power family one-sided tests given in Table 4.3. However, it is more interesting to compare the expected information levels with those of optimal tests with the same maximum information level and the same values of K, α, β and δ, as described in Section 4.2.2. Table 9.3 shows the minimum possible values for the expected information level under $\theta = 0$, or equivalently $\theta = \delta$, under $\theta = \delta/2$, and averaged over several values of θ, first

Table 9.3 *Properties of one-sided derived tests for testing H_0: $\theta = 0$ versus $\theta > 0$ with five analyses and nominal Type I and Type II error rates $\alpha = \beta = 0.05$.*
R denotes the ratio of the maximum information level to that of the corresponding fixed sample test, $\mathcal{I}_{f,1}$. Expected information levels on termination, $E_\theta(\mathcal{I}_\tau)$, are expressed as percentages of $\mathcal{I}_{f,1}$. (Here, τ denotes the analysis at which a group sequential test stops.)

Form of one-sided test	*Maximum inf. ratio* R	*Expected information on termination,* $E_\theta(\mathcal{I}_\tau)$ $\theta = 0$ or δ	$\theta = \delta/2$	*Average*[1]	*Error rate*
Fixed	1	100	100	100	0.050
Pocock RCIs					
Derived test	1.66	63.0	86.1	63.9	0.044
Optimal test with nominal α	1.66	59.5	79.8	60.6	0.050
Optimal test with achieved α	1.66	62.5	85.2	63.8	0.044
O'Brien & Fleming RCIs					
Derived test	1.13	70.0	86.1	69.6	0.046
Optimal test with nominal α	1.13	61.1	79.4	60.7	0.050
Optimal test with achieved α	1.13	65.6	84.9	65.1	0.046

[1] Average expected information on termination =
$\frac{1}{5}\{E_{\theta=\delta/2}(\mathcal{I}_\tau) + E_{\theta=3\delta/4}(\mathcal{I}_\tau) + E_{\theta=\delta}(\mathcal{I}_\tau) + E_{\theta=5\delta/4}(\mathcal{I}_\tau) + E_{\theta=3\delta/2}(\mathcal{I}_\tau)\}$

for tests with error probabilities equal to $\alpha = 0.05$ and then for tests attaining the same error rates as the derived tests.

The derived tests are slightly conservative, having error probabilities below the nominal $\alpha = 0.05$. This conservatism arises because of an inequality in the proof that the error probability conditions are satisfied: in the case of Type I error, for example, if the true value of θ is 0 and $\underline{\theta}_k > 0$ for some k, a Type I error will not be made if $\overline{\theta}_{k'} < \delta$ for some $k' < k$ so that the test has already terminated to accept H_0 before analysis k. Intuitively, since the RCI is designed to accommodate all possible stopping rules, when only a particular one (here the derived test) is being applied, the probability of an incorrect decision being reached is reduced. The derived tests' conservatism is reflected in higher expected information than seen for optimal tests attaining the nominal error probability of 0.05. If, however, the derived tests are compared with one-sided tests achieving the *same* error rates as they do, we see they are close to being fully efficient, particularly when one considers that the optimal results are obtained using a different test for each of the three expected information criteria.

Because the RCIs retain their overall confidence level whether or not a stopping rule is used, the derived test has greater inherent flexibility than the one-sided tests of Chapter 4. If a study continues past an interim analysis at which $\underline{\theta}_k > 0$ or $\overline{\theta}_k < \delta$, later RCIs are still valid and can be used subsequently in reaching decisions. Similarly, the terminal RCI is valid when a trial concludes before the derived test's formal stopping criterion is met. RCIs are designed to "protect" against *all* stopping rules rather than just one. There is a price to pay for this flexibility in terms of sample size but Table 9.3 shows that this price can be remarkably small.

9.3.3 One-Sided Derived Tests: Asymmetric Case

We continue to consider one-sided tests of H_0: $\theta = 0$ versus $\theta > 0$, designed to have Type I error probability α and power $1 - \beta$ at $\theta = \delta$, but now suppose the error rates α and β are unequal. One way to proceed is to force the problem into a symmetric framework by finding a value $\tilde{\delta}$ such that the test of H_0: $\theta = 0$ with Type I error probability α and power $1 - \alpha$ at $\theta = \tilde{\delta}$ will have approximate power $1 - \beta$ at $\theta = \delta$. This method was used by Whitehead & Stratton (1983) and $\tilde{\delta}$ can be found from the formula presented in Section 4.5.1.

A second approach recognizes the essential asymmetry of the formulation. We define $\{\underline{\theta}_k(\alpha);\ k = 1, \ldots, K\}$ to be a $(1-\alpha)$-level lower confidence sequence for θ if

$$Pr_\theta\{\underline{\theta}_k(\alpha) < \theta \text{ for all } k = 1, \ldots, K\} = 1 - \alpha \quad \text{for all } \theta. \qquad (9.10)$$

Similarly, $\{\overline{\theta}_k(\beta);\ k = 1, \ldots, K\}$ is a $(1 - \beta)$-level upper confidence sequence if

$$Pr_\theta\{\overline{\theta}_k(\beta) > \theta \text{ for all } k = 1, \ldots, K\} = 1 - \beta \quad \text{for all } \theta. \qquad (9.11)$$

These definitions imply that

$$Pr_\theta\{\underline{\theta}_k(\alpha) < \theta < \overline{\theta}_k(\beta) \text{ for all } k = 1, \ldots, K\} \geq 1 - \alpha - \beta,$$

with approximate equality if we ignore the very small probability that $\underline{\theta}_k(\alpha) > \theta$ for one value of k and $\overline{\theta}_{k'}(\beta) < \theta$ for some other k', as in (9.8). Consequently, $\{(\underline{\theta}_k(\alpha), \overline{\theta}_k(\beta));\ k = 1, \ldots, K\}$ forms a $(1 - \alpha - \beta)$-level RCI sequence. We can derive a one-sided test from these RCIs which meets the specified error conditions by continuing to sample as long as the interval $(\underline{\theta}_k(\alpha), \overline{\theta}_k(\beta))$ includes *both* $\theta = 0$ and $\theta = \delta$. The study stops at the first analysis k where $(0, \delta)$ is not wholly contained in $(\underline{\theta}_k(\alpha), \overline{\theta}_k(\beta))$ and we accept H_0 if $\overline{\theta}_k(\beta) < \delta$, or reject H_0 if $\underline{\theta}_k(\alpha) > 0$. Termination is ensured if we choose the group size m so that $\overline{\theta}_K(\beta) - \underline{\theta}_K(\alpha) = \delta$. By construction, we have

$$Pr_{\theta=0}\{\text{Reject } H_0\} < Pr_{\theta=0}\{\underline{\theta}_k(\alpha) > 0 \text{ for some } k\} = \alpha$$

and

$$Pr_{\theta=\delta}\{\text{Accept } H_0\} < Pr_{\theta=\delta}\{\overline{\theta}_k(\beta) < \delta \text{ for some } k\} = \beta.$$

Thus, error probabilities at $\theta = 0$ and $\theta = \delta$ are bounded by α and β, respectively.

Returning to the example of Section 9.2 and using the same definitions and notation, upper and lower confidence sequences for $\theta = \mu_A - \mu_B$ are

$$\underline{\theta}_k(\alpha) = \bar{X}_{Ak} - \bar{X}_{Bk} - c_k(2\alpha)\surd\{2\sigma^2/(mk)\}, \quad k = 1, \ldots, K, \tag{9.12}$$

and

$$\overline{\theta}_k(\beta) = \bar{X}_{Ak} - \bar{X}_{Bk} + c_k(2\beta)\surd\{2\sigma^2/(mk)\}, \quad k = 1, \ldots, K. \tag{9.13}$$

Here $c_k(2\alpha)$, $k = 1, \ldots, K$, are critical values of a two-sided group sequential test, for example, a Pocock or O'Brien & Fleming test, *but with Type I error probability equal to* 2α. Similarly, $c_k(2\beta)$, $k = 1, \ldots, K$, are critical values of a two-sided group sequential test with Type I error probability 2β. The sequences (9.12) and (9.13) are constructed to satisfy the conditions (9.10) and (9.11). If a Pocock test is used as the parent test, critical values are

$$c_k(2\alpha) = C_P(K, 2\alpha) \quad \text{and} \quad c_k(2\beta) = C_P(K, 2\beta),$$

where the constants $C_P(K, 2\alpha)$ and $C_P(K, 2\beta)$ can be found in Table 2.1. Using an O'Brien & Fleming parent test, constants $C_B(K, 2\alpha)$ and $C_B(K, 2\beta)$ can be taken from Table 2.3 to give

$$c_k(2\alpha) = C_B(K, 2\alpha)/\surd(K/k) \quad \text{and} \quad c_k(2\beta) = C_B(K, 2\beta)/\surd(K/k).$$

A final sample size of

$$mK = 2\,\{c_K(2\alpha) + c_K(2\beta)\}^2\,\sigma^2/\delta^2 \tag{9.14}$$

on each treatment arm ensures that $\overline{\theta}_K - \underline{\theta}_K = \delta$ and thus the derived test will stop at or before stage K. By comparison, the required sample size for a fixed sample test is obtained by replacing $c_K(2\alpha)$ by z_α and $c_K(2\beta)$ by z_β in (9.14).

When group sizes are liable to be unequal or unpredictable, the error spending approach described in Section 7.2 can be used to obtain the critical values for the parent tests, using separate error spending functions to derive $c_1(2\alpha), \ldots, c_K(2\alpha)$ and $c_1(2\beta), \ldots, c_K(2\beta)$. Once again, a narrow final RCI may permit both acceptance and rejection of H_0, in which case a natural choice is to reject H_0 in order to maximize power while preserving a Type I error rate of at most α. If, instead, the final RCI is wider than planned and contains both 0 and δ, H_0 should be accepted. For more details, see Jennison & Turnbull (1993a).

9.3.4 Equivalence Tests

In Section 6.3, we introduced the problem of a two-sided test of equivalence where it is desired to distinguish between equivalence, when $|\theta|$ is "small", and inequivalence, when $|\theta|$ is "large". In (6.2) and (6.3), the error probability requirements are expressed as

$$Pr_{\theta=\pm\delta}\{\text{Declare equivalence}\} \le \beta \tag{9.15}$$

and

$$Pr_{\theta=0}\{\text{Do not declare equivalence}\} \le \alpha. \tag{9.16}$$

The testing problem is similar to that of the usual two-sided test except that now declaring equivalence when $\theta = \pm\delta$ is treated as the key error and it is of paramount importance to ensure its probability does not exceed β. As noted in Section 6.3, some authors would interchange the symbols α and β but wc use the above choice for consistency with our earlier notation for two-sided tests. In the case of bioequivalence testing, β is the probability of accepting a nonequivalent compound and the values of β and δ must be chosen to satisfy the appropriate regulatory agency. One would expect a manufacturer to choose the value of α to be small since the advantages of establishing equivalence of a new formulation to an existing one are so great.

In a fixed sample experiment, a convenient way to satisfy (9.15) is to conduct two one-sided tests with Type I error rates β (Schuirmann, 1987) and accept equivalence only if both H: $\theta = -\delta$ is rejected in favor of $\theta > -\delta$ and H: $\theta = \delta$ is rejected in favor of $\theta < \delta$. It can be seen that this rule accepts equivalence if and only if the $(1-2\beta)$-level confidence interval $(\underline{\theta}, \overline{\theta})$, for which $Pr_\theta\{\underline{\theta} < \theta\} = Pr_\theta\{\overline{\theta} > \theta\} = 1 - \beta$, is entirely contained within the range $(-\delta, \delta)$; see also Westlake (1981). The condition (9.16) can usually be satisfied by an appropriate choice of sample size or, more generally, information level.

In the group sequential setting, there are two approaches to deriving tests based on repeated confidence intervals. The first is a natural extension of the above idea. Suppose that $\{(\underline{\theta}_k, \overline{\theta}_k);\ k = 1, \ldots, K\}$ is a $(1-2\beta)$-level RCI sequence. Then, we can define the stopping rule:

$$
\begin{array}{lll}
\text{At stage } k = 1, \ldots, K-1 & & \\
 & \text{if } (\underline{\theta}_k, \overline{\theta}_k) \subset (-\delta, \delta) & \text{stop, accept equivalence} \\
 & \text{if } \underline{\theta}_k > \delta \text{ or } \overline{\theta}_k < -\delta & \text{stop, reject equivalence} \\
 & \text{otherwise} & \text{continue to group } k+1, \\
\text{at stage } K & & \\
 & (\underline{\theta}_K, \overline{\theta}_K) \subset (-\delta, \delta) & \text{stop, accept equivalence} \\
 & \text{otherwise} & \text{stop, reject equivalence.}
\end{array}
$$

By construction, the probability of declaring equivalence when $\theta = \pm\delta$ is at most β. However, the sequence of sample sizes or information levels at analyses 1 to K should be planned to ensure that condition (9.16), concerning acceptance of H_0 when $\theta = 0$, is met.

The second approach involves *two* sequences of RCIs: one of level $(1-2\beta)$ and the other of level (1-α). At each stage, equivalence is accepted if the current $(1-2\beta)$-level RCI for θ lies entirely within the interval $(-\delta, \delta)$, and equivalence is rejected if the $(1-\alpha)$-level RCI does not contain 0; otherwise, the procedure continues to the next stage. The sample sizes or information levels must be chosen so that the width of the final RCI is small enough to ensure termination at stage K. It is possible that the stated rule allows both acceptance and rejection of equivalence if the final RCI is narrower than planned. In this case, it is permissible to declare equivalence since the probability of wrongly declaring equivalence under $\theta = \pm\delta$ remains protected. On the other hand, if the final RCI is wide and contains both 0 plus one of δ and $-\delta$, equivalence should be rejected.

Jennison & Turnbull (1993b) describe these procedures more fully, illustrating their implementation and performance characteristics in a comparison of two normal means. In general, the second procedure has a higher maximum sample size and a somewhat higher expected sample size under $\theta = 0$, but a substantially lower expected sample size under $\theta = \pm\delta$ when compared to the first method. Jennison & Turnbull also describe how to employ the error spending function approach when group sizes are unequal or unpredictable. They go on to propose an approximate procedure for handling a nuisance parameter by updating group sizes adaptively as new estimates of the nuisance parameter are obtained. In their example of a comparison between two binomial distributions with success probabilities p_1 and p_2, the parameter of interest is $\theta = p_2 - p_1$ and the average success probability $(p_1 + p_2)/2$ is a nuisance parameter.

9.4 Repeated P-values

A theory of "repeated P-values" can be developed analogously to that of repeated confidence intervals. At the kth analysis, a two-sided repeated P-value for the null hypothesis H_0: $\theta = \theta_0$ is defined as $P_k = \max\{\alpha : \theta_0 \in I_k(\alpha)\}$, where $I_k(\alpha)$ is the current $(1 - \alpha)$-level RCI. In other words, P_k is that value of α for which the kth $(1 - \alpha)$-level RCI contains the null value, θ_0, as one of its endpoints. The construction ensures that, for any $p \in (0, 1)$, the overall probability under H_0 of ever seeing a repeated P-value less than or equal to p is no more than p and this probability is exactly p if all repeated P-values are always observed. Thus, the repeated P-value can be reported with the usual interpretation, yet with protection against the multiple-looks effect. These P-values should not be confused with the significance levels of Section 8.4, which are valid only at termination of a sequential test conducted according to a strictly enforced stopping rule.

9.5 Discussion

Repeated confidence intervals offer a frequentist data summary with the flexibility of application usually needed for interim monitoring of clinical trials. Koepcke (1989, p. 228S) and others have criticized RCIs for being too wide when compared with confidence intervals at termination of a group sequential test of the type described in Section 8.5. However, if the trial continues until the final stage, K, the O'Brien & Fleming based RCI is then only slightly wider than the fixed sample interval; also if stopping occurs earlier, the implication is that the RCI was precise enough to convey the information about θ needed to make that decision. In any case, in the absence of a rigidly followed stopping rule, the methods of Chapter 8 should not really be used to construct a confidence interval on termination.

In summary, RCIs provide interval estimates at each interim analysis "adjusted" for multiple looks. As such, they may be reported as interim estimates of treatment effect at scientific meetings, without the threat of over-interpretation. RCIs can be computed when responses are normally distributed, or follow binary, survival, multivariate, or other distributions, with allowance for covariates if necessary. They can be based on error spending parent tests when group sizes are unequal or unpredictable. At interim analyses, RCIs can serve as an adjunct to a group sequential test enlarging on the simple "stop/continue" decision. On termination, RCIs are valid independently of the stopping rule applied, unlike the terminal confidence intervals of Chapter 8. A sequence of RCIs can be used as a basis for either an informal or formal stopping rule. In the latter case, their flexibility leads to a little conservatism but, with careful choice of parent test, the derived tests are quite efficient in terms of expected sample size. Moreover, RCIs can continue to be used even if a decision is indicated by a formal group sequential test and yet, for some reason, the study continues. The way in which the widths of a sequence of RCIs vary over successive analyses depends on the choice of parent test and this should be selected with a view to how the RCIs are likely to be used. Certainly, the chosen type of RCI should be clearly stated in a study protocol.

Repeated confidence intervals and derived tests are described by Jennison & Turnbull (1989) and debated in the discussion that follows. Jennison & Turnbull describe a number of applications. For accumulating censored survival data, they construct RCIs for the median survival time using the Kaplan-Meier estimate of a survival distribution, and they present RCIs for hazard ratios using log-rank and partial likelihood score statistics. Theory for the median survival time problem is given in Jennison & Turnbull (1985) and will be presented in Section 13.7; RCIs for a hazard ratio will be discussed in Section 13.5 and illustrated in an example in Section 13.6. For discrete data, Jennison & Turnbull (1989) show how to find RCIs for a log odds ratio in a set of 2×2 tables or stratified case-control data, based on the Mantel-Haenszel estimator, and they derive RCIs for the slope coefficient in an odds ratio regression model. A distributional result for group sequential Mantel-Haenszel estimates is proved in Jennison & Turnbull (1991c) and will be reported here in Section 12.3.

Lin & Wei (1991) discuss RCIs for the scale change parameter in a two-sample accelerated failure time model for survival data. Keaney & Wei (1994) show how to construct RCIs for the difference of two median response time distributions based on accumulating survival data. Lin, Wei & DeMets (1991) discuss exact methods for obtaining RCIs for comparing two treatments with dichotomous responses. Coe & Tamhane (1993) also treat exact RCIs for one-sample and two-sample binomial problems. We present methods for these binomial problems in Sections 12.1.4 and 12.2.3. Su & Lachin (1992, p. 1038) describe RCIs based on a multivariate Hodges-Lehmann estimator of group differences with repeated measures data.

In Section 9.3.4 we derived two-sided tests of equivalence from a sequence of RCIs. One-sided equivalence tests, as described in Section 6.2, can also be created from RCIs; for details, see Durrleman & Simon (1990) and Jennison & Turnbull (1993a). Fleming (1992) describes several case studies illustrating the use of repeated confidence intervals in monitoring equivalence trials.

For the two-sided equivalence testing problem, Hsu, Hwang, Liu, & Ruberg (1994) propose alternate forms of RCI in connection with the first approach of Section 9.3.4. They replace the $(1 - 2\beta)$-level RCI as defined in (9.7) by the interval $(\min\{\underline{\theta}_k(\beta), c\}, \max(\overline{\theta}_k\{\beta), c\})$ for a chosen constant c. The usual choice is $c = 0$, or for a more general region of equivalence (δ_1, δ_2), one can take $c = (\delta_1 + \delta_2)/2$. This choice of RCI leads to generally narrower intervals when θ is close to c, the region of most interest, but wider intervals otherwise.

CHAPTER 10

Stochastic Curtailment

10.1 Introduction

This approach to sequential monitoring evolved from the idea of simple curtailment whereby an experiment can be terminated as soon as the ultimate result becomes inevitable. As an example, consider an industrial acceptance sampling scheme in which items are classified as either defective or non-defective. A single-sampling scheme designates a lot as acceptable if fewer than c defectives are found in a random sample of n items taken from the lot. In the curtailed version of this procedure (e.g., Alling, 1966), sampling proceeds sequentially and terminates as soon as the decision is inevitable, that is, when either the number of defectives reaches c or the number of non-defectives reaches $n - c + 1$. Clearly, this curtailed scheme always leads to the same conclusion as the fixed sample procedure. The two methods have identical operating characteristics, but the curtailed procedure has a lower expected sample size. Any fixed sample test with bounded contributions from each new observation, such as the Wilcoxon rank sum test or many other nonparametric tests, can be curtailed in a similar way; see Alling (1963) and Halperin & Ware (1974).

If outcome measures are not bounded, as in the case of normally distributed observations, or if greater savings in expected sample size are desired, then a stochastic form of curtailment may be considered. At any stage we might terminate the procedure if a particular decision, while not inevitable, is highly likely given the current data. We call such a rule a *stochastically curtailed procedure* (SCP). Jennison (1992) reports the success of such rules in a reducing computation in a simulation study conducted to evaluate the actual error rates of a bootstrap test. A form of stochastic curtailment improved greatly on simple curtailment, and computation in this application was reduced, overall, by a factor of as much as 50.

In the following Sections, we describe three approaches to such stochastic curtailment, the conditional power approach, the predictive power approach and a parameter free approach. We illustrate these methods in a case study involving survival data.

10.2 The Conditional Power Approach

Suppose we wish to test a null hypothesis H_0: $\theta = \theta_0$ concerning the parameter θ. First a "reference test", which we shall call $\mathcal{T}$, is designated. This is typically a one-sided or two-sided fixed sample test with specified Type I error probability α under $\theta = \theta_0$ and power $1 - \beta$ at an alternative $\theta = \theta_1$ for a one-sided test or at values θ_1 and θ_2, either side of θ_0, in the case of a two-sided test. However, $\mathcal{T}$ could also be a sequential or group sequential test. At an interim stage, k, during the study, let $D(k)$ denote the data accumulated so far. The conditional power at stage k is defined as

$$p_k(\theta) = Pr_\theta\{\mathcal{T} \text{ will reject } H_0 \mid D(k)\}. \tag{10.1}$$

Initially, when $k = 0$, this is the usual power function. At the planned termination of the study, stage K say, this probability is either zero or one. At an interim stage k, the conditional power can be plotted as a function of θ and its values at $\theta_0, \theta_1, \theta_2$ (for a two-sided test), and $\hat{\theta}^{(k)}$, the current maximum likelihood estimate (MLE) of θ, are of particular interest.

The conditional power function is a useful device for communicating with clinical investigators. For instance, it can be used to illustrate the effects of low accrual or to aid the decision to abandon a study if the conditional power appears poor. The opposite situation, when conditional power is high, will be illustrated in Section 10.5.

A high value of $p_k(\theta_0)$ indicates that the reference test is unlikely to accept H_0 given the accrued data, even if H_0 is true. This led Lan, Simon & Halperin (1982) to suggest a formal rule by which termination occurs at stage k to reject H_0 if $p_k(\theta_0) \geq \gamma$ for a specified constant γ. The value of γ should be between 0.5 and 1 and values 0.8 or 0.9 are recommended. Similarly, early termination may be allowed to accept H_0 if $1 - p_k(\theta_1) \geq \gamma'$ in a one-sided test, or if both $1 - p_k(\theta_1) \geq \gamma'$ and $1 - p_k(\theta_2) \geq \gamma'$ in a two-sided test, where γ' is another constant between 0.5 and 1. The quantity $1 - p_k(\theta_1)$ has been termed the *futility index* by Ware, Muller & Braunwald (1985).

In using the above rules, the error probabilities of the test can be expected to rise since the final decision of the reference test $\mathcal{T}$ will sometimes be incorrectly anticipated. We refer to a formally defined test based on the above rules as a stochastically curtailed procedure (SCP). The error probabilities of an SCP with a given interim analysis schedule can be computed by numerical integration but Lan, Simon & Halperin (1982) use a simple argument to prove that the Type I error probability will not be more than α/γ. It can be shown that $\{p_k(\theta);\ k = 1, 2, \dots\}$ is a martingale with respect to the filtration defined by $\{D(1), D(2), \dots\}$. In fact, it is an example of a Doob's martingale; see Grimmett & Stirzaker (1992, pp. 319 and 456). Let ν denote the stopping time of the reference test $\mathcal{T}$ (allowing the possibility that $\mathcal{T}$ is itself a sequential test). First, suppose $\gamma' = 1$ so there is no early stopping to accept H_0. In this case, the stage at which the SCP stops is

$$\tau = \min(\nu, \min\{k\colon\ p_k(\theta_0) \geq \gamma\}).$$

By the optional stopping theorem (e.g., Grimmett & Stirzaker, 1992, Section 12.5), we have

$$E_{\theta_0}\{p_\tau(\theta_0)\} = E_{\theta_0}\{p_0(\theta_0)\} = p_0(\theta_0) = \alpha.$$

But, from the definition of τ,

$$E_{\theta_0}\{p_\tau(\theta_0)\} \ \geq\ \gamma\ Pr_{\theta_0}\{p_k(\theta_0) \geq \gamma \text{ for some } k \leq \nu\} \ =\ \gamma\ Pr_{\theta_0}\{\text{Reject } H_0\}$$

and hence

$$Pr_{\theta_0}\{\text{Reject } H_0\} \leq \alpha/\gamma.$$

If $\gamma' < 1$, then the actual Type I error probability can only be reduced further and so it is still bounded above by α/γ.

A similar argument shows that the Type II error probability of the SCP is no more than β/γ', where β is the Type II error rate of the reference test. With these results in mind, we could ensure error probabilities of at most α and β for the SCP's Type I and II error probabilities by designing the reference test to have Type I error rate $\alpha\gamma$ and power $1 - \beta\gamma'$ at $\theta = \theta_1$ for a one-sided test, or at $\theta = \theta_1$ and θ_2 for a two-sided test.

We now illustrate the calculation of a conditional power function in the general formulation of Section 3.1. Suppose successive analyses yield a sequence of test statistics $Z_1, \ldots, Z_K$ with the canonical joint distribution (3.1), given information levels $\mathcal{I}_1, \ldots, \mathcal{I}_K$ for θ. Since Z_k is a sufficient statistic for θ at stage k, it can be used in place of $D(k)$ in (10.1). Without loss of generality, let $\theta_0 = 0$ and $\theta_1 = \delta$. Suppose the reference test $\mathcal{T}$ is a one-sided fixed sample test of H_0: $\theta = 0$ with Type I error probability α and power $1 - \beta$ at $\theta = \delta$. The test $\mathcal{T}$ continues to the final stage K where it rejects H_0 if $Z_K \geq z_\alpha$ and accepts H_0 otherwise. Recall $z_\alpha = \Phi^{-1}(1 - \alpha)$, where $\Phi(\cdot)$ is the standard normal cumulative distribution function. Power $1 - \beta$ at $\theta = \delta$ is achieved by choosing the sample size to yield an information level $\mathcal{I}_K = \mathcal{I}_{f,1}$, as given by (4.1). For each $k = 1, \ldots, K - 1$, the conditional distribution of Z_K given Z_k is

$$Z_K \mid Z_k \sim N(Z_k\sqrt{(\mathcal{I}_k/\mathcal{I}_K)} + \{\theta(\mathcal{I}_K - \mathcal{I}_k)/\sqrt{\mathcal{I}_K}\},\ 1 - \mathcal{I}_k/\mathcal{I}_K).$$

Hence, the conditional power at analysis k is

$$p_k(\theta) = \Phi\left\{\frac{Z_k\sqrt{\mathcal{I}_k} - z_\alpha\sqrt{\mathcal{I}_K} + (\mathcal{I}_K - \mathcal{I}_k)\,\theta}{\sqrt{(\mathcal{I}_K - \mathcal{I}_k)}}\right\}, \quad k = 1, \ldots, K - 1. \quad (10.2)$$

The dashed line in Figure 10.1 is a typical conditional power curve (10.2) for a one-sided problem, calculated at an intermediate stage. The solid line shows the original power curve for the reference test $\mathcal{T}$, i.e., $p_k(\theta)$ for $k = 0$. In this example $\alpha = 0.05$ and $\mathcal{I}_K = 214.1$ so that test $\mathcal{T}$ has power 0.9 at $\theta = \delta = 0.2$. The conditional power curve is for a stage k at which half the observations have been taken, so $\mathcal{I}_k = \mathcal{I}_K/2 = 107.1$, and the current MLE of θ is $\hat{\theta}^{(k)} = \delta/2 = 0.1$. This gives a value of $Z_k = 0.1\sqrt{107.1} = 1.035$. We see that under the alternative $\theta = 0.2$, the probability of rejecting H_0 if the experiment goes to completion as planned has been reduced from 0.9 to approximately 0.1.

If we define a formal sequential stopping rule as indicated above, the condition $p_k(\theta_0) \geq \gamma$, with $\theta_0 = 0$, for stopping to reject H_0 becomes

$$Z_k \geq z_\alpha\sqrt{(\mathcal{I}_K/\mathcal{I}_k)} + z_{1-\gamma}\sqrt{\{(\mathcal{I}_K - \mathcal{I}_k)/\mathcal{I}_k\}}. \quad (10.3)$$

Similarly, the condition $p_k(\theta_1) \leq 1 - \gamma'$, with $\theta_1 = \delta$, for stopping to accept H_0 is

$$Z_k \leq z_\alpha\sqrt{(\mathcal{I}_K/\mathcal{I}_k)} - z_{1-\gamma'}\sqrt{\{(\mathcal{I}_K - \mathcal{I}_k)/\mathcal{I}_k\}} - \delta(\mathcal{I}_K - \mathcal{I}_k)/\sqrt{\mathcal{I}_k}. \quad (10.4)$$

This stopping boundary is shown in Figure 10.2 for $\alpha = 0.05$, $1 - \beta = 0.9$, $\delta = 0.2$, $\mathcal{I}_K = 214.1$, and $\gamma = \gamma' = 0.8$. Whatever the interim analysis schedule,

Figure 10.1 *Conditional and unconditional power curves for a one-sided test*

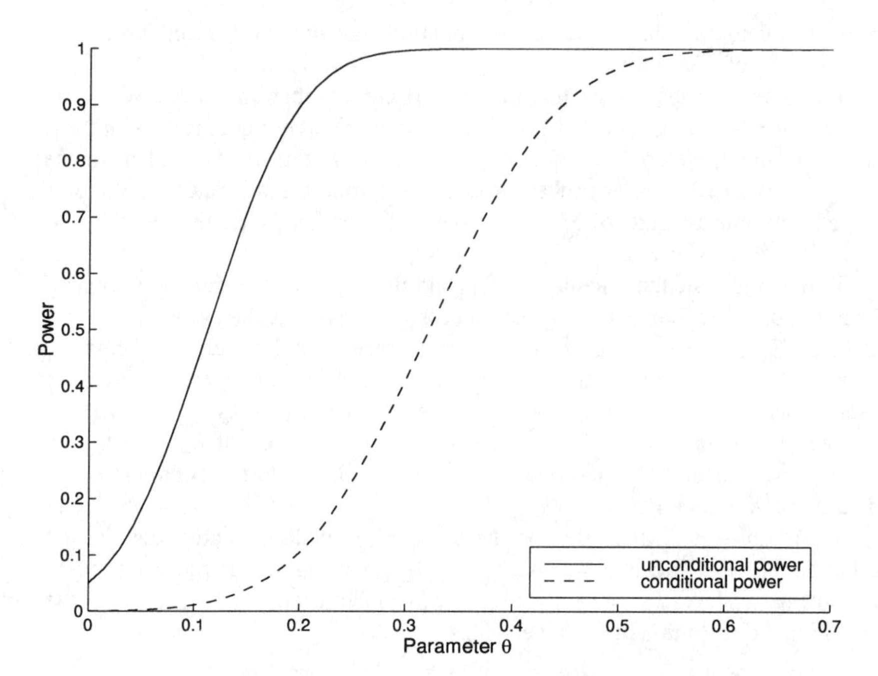

the Type I error probability of this procedure will not exceed $0.05/0.8 = 0.0625$ and the power at $\theta = 0.2$ is guaranteed to be at least $1 - (0.1/0.8) = 0.875$. This boundary can be compared with the continuation regions shown in Figure 4.1 for two power family one-sided tests with $K = 4$ analyses and the same error probability specifications.

Now suppose the reference test $\mathcal{T}$ is a two-sided fixed sample test of H_0: $\theta = 0$ with Type I error probability α and power $1 - \beta$ at $\theta = \pm\delta$. The test $\mathcal{T}$ only makes a decision at the final stage K, rejecting H_0 if $|Z_K| \geq z_{\alpha/2}$ and accepting H_0 otherwise. The sample size should be chosen to yield an information level $\mathcal{I}_K = \mathcal{I}_{f,2}$ as given in (3.6). The conditional power at analysis k is

$$p_k(\theta) = \Phi\left\{\frac{Z_k\sqrt{\mathcal{I}_k} - z_{\alpha/2}\sqrt{\mathcal{I}_K} + (\mathcal{I}_K - \mathcal{I}_k)\,\theta}{\sqrt{(\mathcal{I}_K - \mathcal{I}_k)}}\right\} + \Phi\left\{\frac{-Z_k\sqrt{\mathcal{I}_k} - z_{\alpha/2}\sqrt{\mathcal{I}_K} - (\mathcal{I}_K - \mathcal{I}_k)\,\theta}{\sqrt{(\mathcal{I}_K - \mathcal{I}_k)}}\right\}.$$

Suppose we use stochastic curtailment to define a formal stopping rule which allows early stopping to reject H_0 if $p_k(0) \geq \gamma$. By the standard argument, the Type I error probability of this SCP is at most α/γ. The stopping boundary for

Figure 10.2 *Stopping boundary for a stochastically curtailed one-sided test using the conditional power approach. The reference test is a fixed sample one-sided test with Type I error probability* $\alpha = 0.05$ *and information level* $\mathcal{I}_{f,1} = 214.1$, *set to achieve power* 0.9 *at* $\theta = 0.2$. *The stochastic curtailment parameters are* $\gamma = \gamma' = 0.8$.

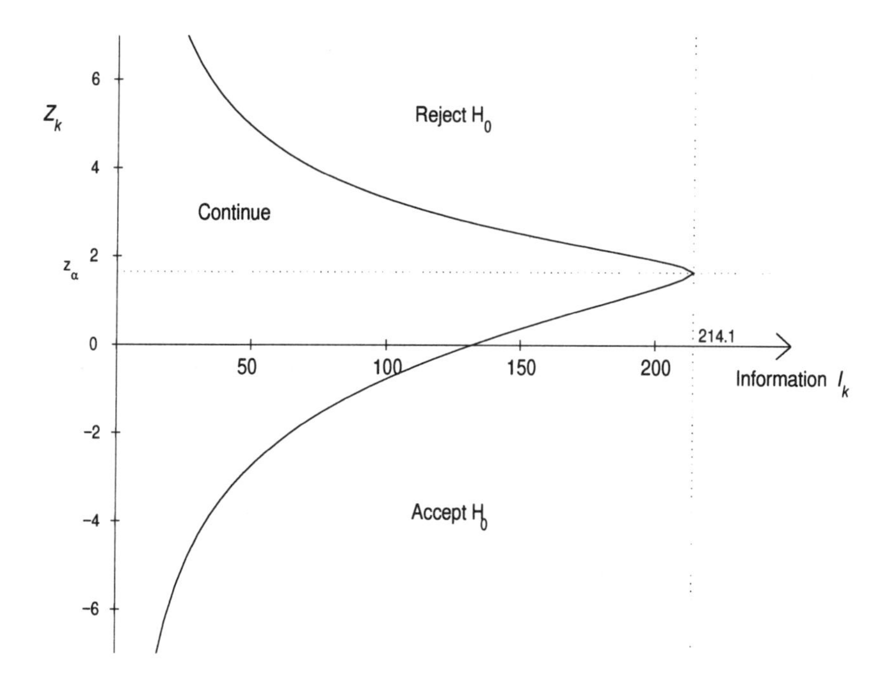

the case $\alpha = 0.05$, $\gamma = 0.8$ and $\mathcal{I}_K = 262.7$ is shown in Figure 10.3. The reference test has power 0.9 when $\theta = \delta = \pm 0.2$ and so is directly comparable with the boundaries of Pocock and O'Brien & Fleming tests with $K = 4$ groups of observations and the same error probability specifications, which were displayed in Figure 3.1. Note that we have not introduced early stopping to accept H_0 based on large values of $1 - p_k(\delta)$ and $1 - p_k(-\delta)$. If we had done this, the SCP would have an inner wedge, and so would resemble the tests of Chapter 5.

In the case of a two-sided SCP defined without an inner wedge, if the reference test is formed with Type I error probability $\alpha\gamma$ instead of α, the SCP has Type I error probability at most α and can be compared directly with the two-sided tests of Chapter 2. Figure 10.3 shows that the boundaries are wide initially and then converge, in a similar manner to the O'Brien & Fleming (1979) boundaries in Figures 2.2 and 3.1. In fact, if $\gamma = 0.5$, the SCP is the continuous-monitoring version of an O'Brien & Fleming procedure. This SCP also coincides with the test suggested by Samuel-Cahn (1980) and is related to proposals of Chatterjee & Sen (1973), Davis (1978) and Koziol & Petkau (1978); see Halperin et al. (1982, p. 322). If the number of analyses K is small, α/γ will be a very conservative

Figure 10.3 *Stopping boundary for a stochastically curtailed two-sided test using the conditional power approach. The reference test is a fixed sample test with two-sided Type I error probability* $\alpha = 0.05$ *and information level* $\mathcal{I}_{f,2} = 262.7$*, set to achieve power* 0.9 *at* $\theta = 0.2$*. The stochastic curtailment parameter is* $\gamma = 0.8$.

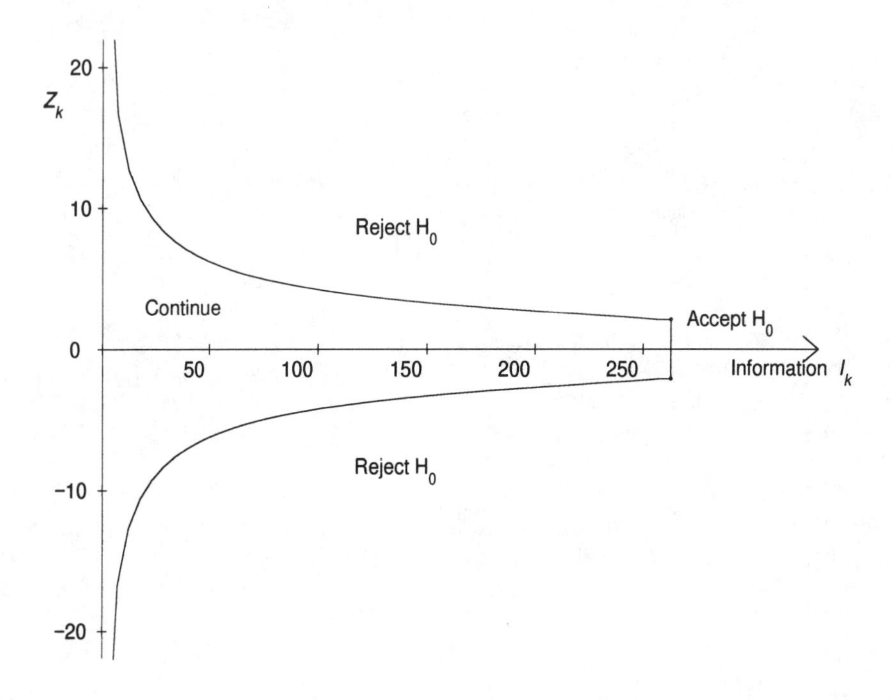

bound on the Type I error probability. What is gained from this conservatism is the ability to do unplanned interim analyses at arbitrary, even data-dependent, times. However, if the timing of analyses is fixed in advance, numerical methods may be used to obtain an exact value of the Type I error probability and less conservative boundaries could be derived.

10.3 The Predictive Power Approach

A criticism of the methods of the previous section is that they are based on conditional power calculated under values of θ which may not be supported by the current data. For instance, the criterion for stopping to reject H_0 involves $p_k(\theta)$ evaluated at $\theta = \theta_0$, a value of θ unlikely to be true if rejection is being considered. We now introduce a procedure which obviates this problem, averaging conditional power over values of θ in a Bayesian calculation, but still with a frequentist test in mind.

As before, we suppose a reference test $\mathcal{T}$ of $H_0\colon \theta = 0$ is designated with Type I error α and power $1 - \beta$ at $\theta = \theta_1$ in the case of a one-sided test or at $\theta = \theta_1$

and θ_2 for a two-sided test. Instead of using the conditional power at particular θ values, we define the "predictive power" at stage k to be a weighted average of the conditional power function,

$$P_k = \int p_k(\theta)\, \pi\{\theta \mid D(k)\}\, d\theta, \tag{10.5}$$

where $p_k(\theta)$ is as defined in (10.1). The weight function π is the posterior density of θ, given a prior distribution for θ and the data $D(k)$ accumulated by analysis k, so π reflects current belief about the value of θ. This approach has been advocated by Herson (1979); Choi, Smith & Becker (1985); and Spiegelhalter, Freedman & Blackburn (1986). The predictive power is again a useful quantity to communicate to applied researchers at an intermediate stage of a trial. As with conditional power, it can be used to define a formal stopping rule by stopping at stage k to reject H_0 if $P_k \geq \gamma$ or to accept H_0 if $P_k \leq 1 - \gamma'$.

Consider again the example of Section 10.2. Standardized statistics $Z_1, \ldots, Z_K$ are assumed to follow the joint distribution (3.1), given $\mathcal{I}_1, \ldots, \mathcal{I}_K$, and $\mathcal{T}$ is a fixed sample one-sided reference test with Type I error probability α and power $1 - \beta$ at $\theta = \delta$, conducted with information level $\mathcal{I}_K = \mathcal{I}_{f,1}$. This test rejects H_0: $\theta = \theta_0$ if and only if $Z_K \geq z_\alpha$. Suppose we use the improper prior, $\pi(\theta) = 1$ for all θ, to represent an initial lack of knowledge about θ. Then, at stage k, when the MLE of θ is $Z_k/\sqrt{\mathcal{I}_k}$, the posterior distribution for θ is

$$\theta \mid Z_K \sim N(Z_k/\sqrt{\mathcal{I}_k},\ 1/\mathcal{I}_k).$$

Substituting this density into (10.5) and carrying out the integration, we obtain

$$P_k = \Phi\left\{\frac{Z_k\sqrt{\mathcal{I}_K} - z_\alpha\sqrt{\mathcal{I}_k}}{\sqrt{(\mathcal{I}_K - \mathcal{I}_k)}}\right\}. \tag{10.6}$$

The argument of Φ in (10.6) is similar to that in (10.2) after θ has been replaced by its MLE but, in fact, it differs by a factor $\sqrt{(\mathcal{I}_k/\mathcal{I}_K)}$. Some such difference is to be expected since θ is fixed for the conditional power calculation whereas the MLE is the center of a posterior distribution in the case of predictive power.

The stopping criteria $P_k \geq \gamma$ and $P_k \leq 1 - \gamma'$ are:

$$\text{Reject } H_0 \text{ if } \ Z_k \geq z_\alpha\sqrt{(\mathcal{I}_k/\mathcal{I}_K)} + z_{1-\gamma}\sqrt{\{(\mathcal{I}_K - \mathcal{I}_k)/\mathcal{I}_K\}}, \tag{10.7}$$

and

$$\text{Accept } H_0 \text{ if } \ Z_k \leq z_\alpha\sqrt{(\mathcal{I}_k/\mathcal{I}_K)} - z_{1-\gamma'}\sqrt{\{(\mathcal{I}_K - \mathcal{I}_k)/\mathcal{I}_K\}}. \tag{10.8}$$

Figure 10.4 displays these boundaries when $\gamma = \gamma' = 0.8$ and the reference test $\mathcal{T}$ is the same one-sided test used in Figure 10.2.

Although the criteria (10.7) and (10.8) are similar in form to those for the conditional power stopping rule in (10.3) and (10.4), a comparison of Figures 10.4 and 10.2 shows that the predictive power approach gives much narrower boundaries for the same γ and γ'. Early stopping is permitted more readily since the conditional probabilities are based on an estimate of θ obtained from the data rather than the hypothesized values $\theta = \theta_0$ and $\theta = \delta$. Although simple analytic results are not available, the effects of this early stopping on Type I

Figure 10.4 *Stopping boundary for a stochastically curtailed one-sided test using the predictive power approach with a uniform prior. The reference test is a fixed sample one-sided test with Type I error probability* $\alpha = 0.05$ *and information level* $\mathcal{I}_{f,1} = 214.1$, *set to achieve power* 0.9 *at* $\theta = 0.2$. *The stochastic curtailment parameters are* $\gamma = \gamma' = 0.8$.

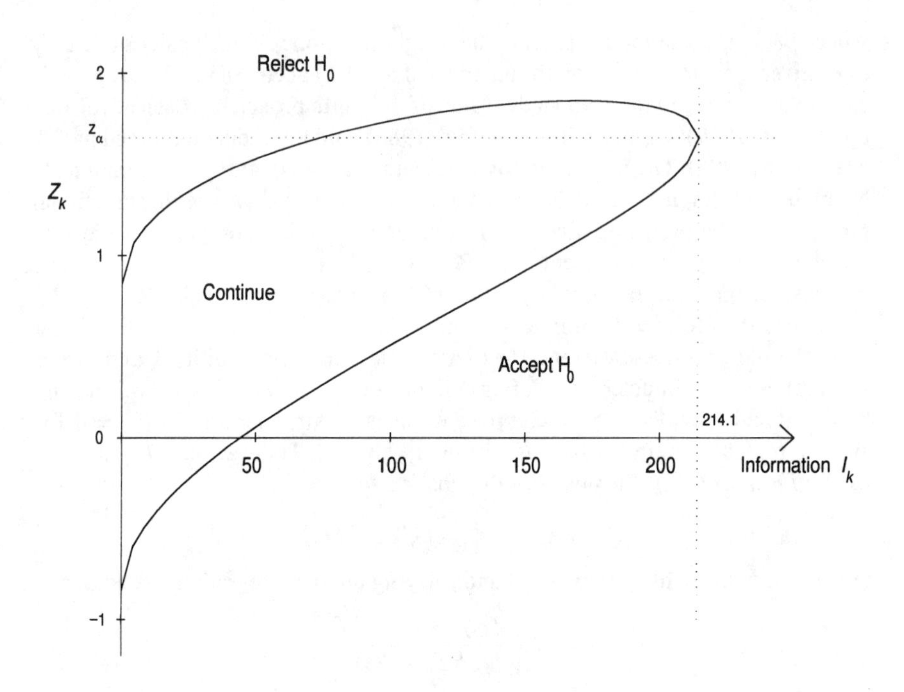

and II error rates can be computed numerically using the methods described in Chapter 19. If these error probabilities are deemed too high, they can be reduced by increasing γ and γ' or, in the case of the Type II error rate, by setting a larger horizon $\mathcal{I}_K$.

In the two-sided testing problem of Section 10.2, the reference test has information level $\mathcal{I}_K = \mathcal{I}_{f,2}$ and rejects H_0: $\theta = 0$ if $|Z_K| \geq z_{\alpha/2}$. The criterion $P_k \geq \gamma$ now calls for a decision to stop and reject H_0 at stage k if

$$\Phi\left\{\frac{|Z_k|\sqrt{\mathcal{I}_K} - z_{\alpha/2}\sqrt{\mathcal{I}_k}}{\sqrt{(\mathcal{I}_K - \mathcal{I}_k)}}\right\} + \Phi\left\{\frac{-|Z_k|\sqrt{\mathcal{I}_K} - z_{\alpha/2}\sqrt{\mathcal{I}_k}}{\sqrt{(\mathcal{I}_K - \mathcal{I}_k)}}\right\} \geq \gamma. \qquad (10.9)$$

The boundary using $\gamma = 0.8$ is shown in Figure 10.5. Here, the reference test has two-sided Type I error probability $\alpha = 0.05$ and $\mathcal{I}_K = 262.7$, set to achieve power $1 - \beta = 0.9$ at $\theta = 0.2$, as in the example used to illustrate the conditional power approach in Figure 10.3.

Once more, the continuation region is narrower earlier on than that of the conditional power approach, permitting early stopping more readily. If a particular

Figure 10.5 *Stopping boundary for a stochastically curtailed two-sided test using the predictive power approach with a uniform prior. The reference test is a fixed sample test with two-sided Type I error probability* $\alpha = 0.05$ *and information level* $\mathcal{I}_{f,2} = 262.7$*, set to achieve power* 0.9 *at* $\theta = 0.2$*. The stochastic curtailment parameter is* $\gamma = 0.8$.

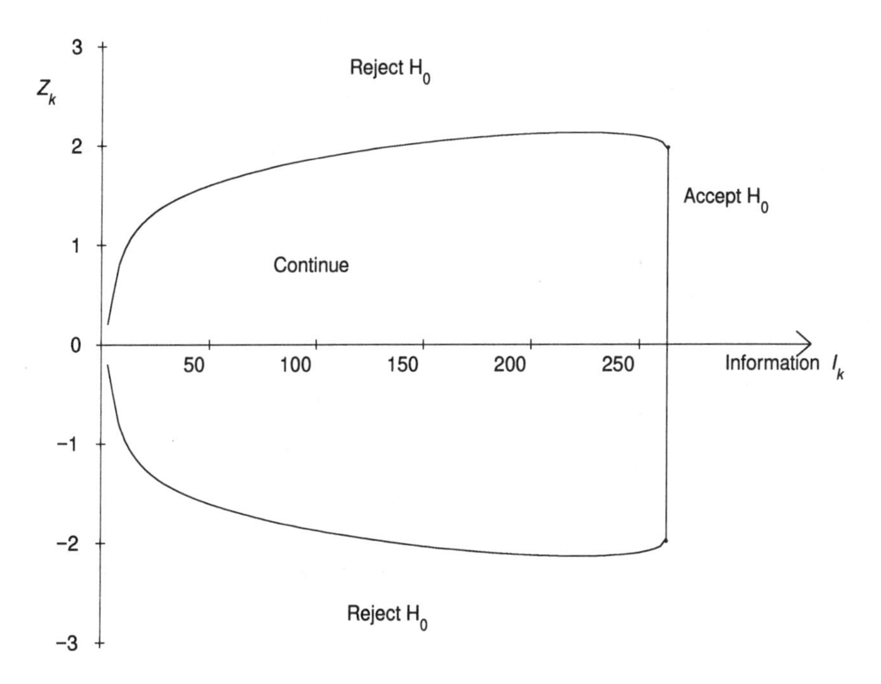

schedule of analyses is planned, the attained error rates could be calculated numerically and γ or $\mathcal{I}_K$ increased if it is desired to reduce these error rates.

We have only used the criterion $P_k \geq \gamma$ for early stopping in this example. An early decision to accept H_0 if $P_k \leq 1 - \gamma'$ could also be permitted, in which case the stopping boundary would contain an inner wedge as in the tests of Chapter 5.

10.4 A Parameter-Free Approach

The two previous approaches to stochastic curtailment require specification of θ, either a particular value at which to evaluate the conditional power, or a prior distribution for θ in the predictive power approach. A third method, proposed by Jennison (1992), dispenses with the need to specify θ at all. This approach has been further developed by Xiong (1995); Tan & Xiong (1996); and Tan, Xiong & Kutner (1998). These authors use the terms "sequential conditional probability ratio test" and "reverse stochastic curtailing" in describing their procedures.

Suppose statistics $Z_1, \ldots, Z_K$ follow the usual joint distribution (3.1), given $\mathcal{I}_1, \ldots, \mathcal{I}_K$, and we have a fixed sample one-sided reference test with Type I error probability α and power $1-\beta$ at $\theta = \delta$, conducted at information level $\mathcal{I}_K = \mathcal{I}_{f,1}$. This test rejects $H_0\colon \theta = \theta_0$ if and only if $Z_K \geq z_\alpha$. Suppose at stage k the information level is $\mathcal{I}_k$ and we observe $Z_k = z$. A pertinent question is "If the reference test will eventually accept H_0, how unusual is it that at stage k we should observe Z_k as large or larger than z?" This leads us to consider

$$\begin{aligned}\sup_{\tilde{z}\leq z_\alpha} Pr\{Z_k \geq z \mid Z_K = \tilde{z}\} &= Pr\{Z_k \geq z \mid Z_K = z_\alpha\} \\ &= 1 - p_k(z), \quad \text{say.}\end{aligned}$$

Similarly, we can ask "If the reference test will eventually reject H_0, how unusual is it to observe Z_k no larger than z at stage k?" This conditional probability is

$$\sup_{\tilde{z}\geq z_\alpha} Pr\{Z_k \leq z \mid Z_K = \tilde{z}\} = Pr\{Z_k \leq z \mid Z_K = z_\alpha\} = p_k(z).$$

Now, if $S_k = Z_k\sqrt{\mathcal{I}_k}$, $k = 1, \ldots, K$, the conditional joint distribution of the process $\{S_k\}$ given $Z_K = z_\alpha$ is that of a Brownian bridge observed at discrete time points. In particular, the conditional distribution of Z_k given $Z_K = z_\alpha$ is

$$Z_k \mid (Z_K = z_\alpha) \sim N(z_\alpha\sqrt{(\mathcal{I}_k/\mathcal{I}_K)},\ (\mathcal{I}_K - \mathcal{I}_k)/\mathcal{I}_K)$$

and, hence,

$$p_k(z) = \Phi\left\{\frac{z\sqrt{\mathcal{I}_K} - z_\alpha\sqrt{\mathcal{I}_k}}{\sqrt{(\mathcal{I}_K - \mathcal{I}_k)}}\right\}, \quad k = 1, \ldots, K. \tag{10.10}$$

As in the previous methods, a formal procedure can be created by stopping at stage k according to the following rules:

Reject H_0 if $p_k(Z_k) \geq \gamma$ and Accept H_0 if $p_k(Z_k) \leq 1 - \gamma'$.

Here γ and γ' are specified constants, greater than 0.5. This procedure stops at stage k to reject H_0 if

$$Z_k \geq z_\alpha\sqrt{(\mathcal{I}_k/\mathcal{I}_K)} + z_{1-\gamma}\sqrt{\{(\mathcal{I}_K - \mathcal{I}_k)/\mathcal{I}_K\}} \tag{10.11}$$

and to accept H_0 if

$$Z_k \leq z_\alpha\sqrt{(\mathcal{I}_k/\mathcal{I}_K)} - z_{1-\gamma'}\sqrt{\{(\mathcal{I}_K - \mathcal{I}_k)/\mathcal{I}_K\}}. \tag{10.12}$$

Comparison with (10.7) and (10.8) shows these are exactly the same boundaries as obtained in the predictive approach using an improper prior! The quantities $p_k(Z_k)$ are identical to the P_k defined in the previous section and the example shown in Figure 10.4 remains the same under the parameter-free treatment.

For the two-sided test, we consider the probability of observing a Z_k with an absolute value as large as that of the observed statistic, z say, given that the reference test eventually accepts H_0. If this conditional probability is low, we can stop to reject H_0. Thus we consider

$$\begin{aligned}\sup_{|\tilde{z}|\leq z_{\alpha/2}} Pr\{|Z_k| \geq |z| \mid |Z_K| = |\tilde{z}|\} &= Pr\{|Z_k| \geq |z| \mid |Z_K| = z_{\alpha/2}\} \\ &= 1 - \tilde{p}_k(z), \quad \text{say.}\end{aligned} \tag{10.13}$$

A formal rule can be defined by stopping to reject H_0 if $1 - \tilde{p}_k(Z_k)$ is less than $1 - \gamma$

Figure 10.6 *Stopping boundary for a stochastically curtailed two-sided test using the parameter-free approach. The reference test is a fixed sample test with two-sided Type I error probability* $\alpha = 0.05$ *and information level* $\mathcal{I}_{f,2} = 262.7$*, set to achieve power* 0.9 *at* $\theta = 0.2$*. The stochastic curtailment parameter is* $\gamma = 0.8$*.*

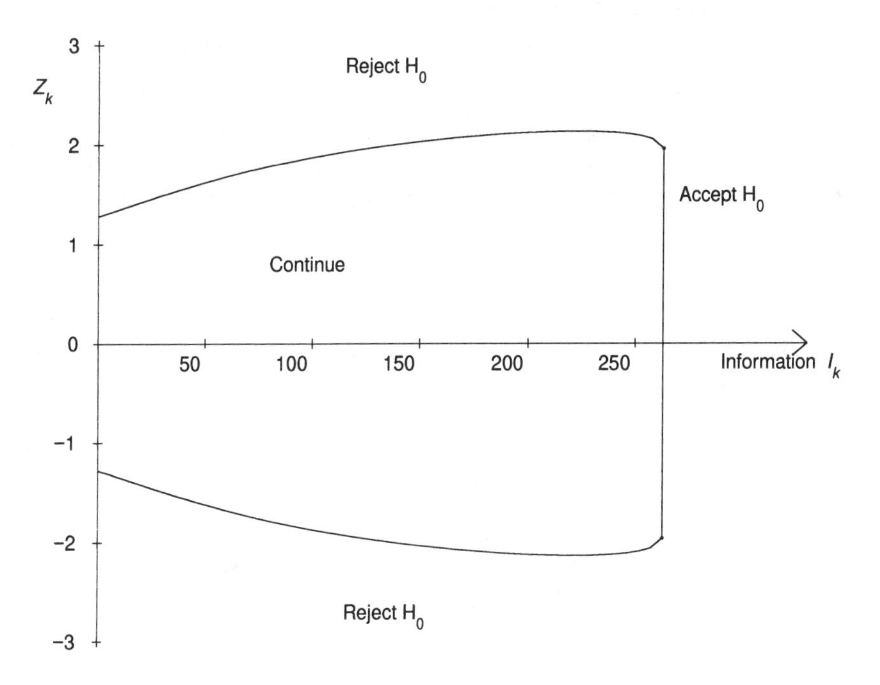

for a chosen constant γ. A calculation analogous to that which produced (10.10) shows that H_0 is rejected if

$$\Phi\left\{\frac{|z|\sqrt{\mathcal{I}_K} - z_{\alpha/2}\sqrt{\mathcal{I}_k}}{\sqrt{(\mathcal{I}_K - \mathcal{I}_k)}}\right\} - \Phi\left\{\frac{-|z|\sqrt{\mathcal{I}_K} - z_{\alpha/2}\sqrt{\mathcal{I}_K}}{\sqrt{(\mathcal{I}_K - \mathcal{I}_k)}}\right\} \geq \gamma. \qquad (10.14)$$

This differs from condition (10.9) of the predictive power approach in the sign of the second term. Typically, this term is small unless $\mathcal{I}_k/\mathcal{I}_K$ is small, hence the parameter-free and predictive power boundaries grow more similar as $\mathcal{I}_k/\mathcal{I}_K$ increases. Figure 10.6 shows the boundary for the two-sided testing problem considered earlier with $\alpha = 0.05$ and $\mathcal{I}_K = 262.7$ using $\gamma = 0.8$. Comparing this with Figure 10.3, we see that the boundary of the parameter-free test is wider initially but soon becomes indistinguishable from the predictive power boundary.

10.5 A Case Study with Survival Data

We shall illustrate conditional power calculations using interim data in a randomized clinical trial designed to compare survival times of subjects on two treatment arms. These calculations are loosely adapted from those requested by the data and safety monitoring board (DSMB) at an interim analysis of the

Nutritional Prevention of Cancer Trial (see Section 1.4.5) and they follow the development of Andersen (1987).

We assume survival times to be exponentially distributed with mean μ_A for patients on treatment A and μ_B for those on treatment B. We let $\lambda_A = 1/\mu_A$ and $\lambda_B = 1/\mu_B$ denote the hazard rates on treatments A and B respectively and define $\psi = \lambda_B/\lambda_A$ to be the hazard ratio or "relative hazard". The null hypothesis to be tested is H_0: $\psi = 1$.

We first describe a fixed sample test of H_0. Let X_A denote the total number of patient-years observed on treatment A, that is the sum of each patient's survival times until failure or censoring, and let N_A be the number of patients observed to fail on treatment A. Similarly, define X_B and N_B for treatment B. We estimate the hazard rates by $\hat{\lambda}_A = N_A/X_A$ and $\hat{\lambda}_B = N_B/X_B$, and the hazard ratio by

$$\hat{\psi} = \hat{\lambda}_B/\hat{\lambda}_A.$$

A test of H_0 can be based on the statistic $W = \log(\hat{\psi})$, which is approximately normally distributed with mean $\log(\psi)$ and variance $N_A^{-1} + N_B^{-1}$. Thus, a two-sided test with Type I error probability approximately equal to α rejects H_0 if

$$|W| \geq z_{\alpha/2}\sqrt{(N_A^{-1} + N_B^{-1})}.$$

In the notation of previous sections, we have information $\mathcal{I} = (N_A^{-1} + N_B^{-1})^{-1}$, a standardized statistic $Z = W\sqrt{\mathcal{I}}$, and canonical parameter $\theta = \log(\psi)$.

Given an initial estimate of λ_A, a Type I error probability α and power $1-\beta$ to be achieved at a specified alternative $\psi = \psi^*$, it is possible to determine the number of person-years that should be observed in the study. The power of the above test, at a given value of ψ, is approximately

$$\Phi\left\{-z_{\alpha/2} + \frac{\log(\psi)}{\sqrt{(N_A^{-1} + N_B^{-1})}}\right\} + \Phi\left\{-z_{\alpha/2} - \frac{\log(\psi)}{\sqrt{(N_A^{-1} + N_B^{-1})}}\right\}. \quad (10.15)$$

If the study accrues a total of T person-years, divided equally between the two treatments, the expected values of N_A and N_B are $\lambda_A T/2$ and $\psi^*\lambda_A T/2$, respectively. Substituting these values for N_A and N_B in (10.15) yields an expression which can be evaluated to find the value of T giving approximate power $1-\beta$ when $\psi = \psi^*$. Knowledge of accrual and dropout rates can then be used to estimate the required sample sizes and study duration to attain this value of T person-years. Various charts, nomograms and programs are available to aid this calculation; see, for example, George & Desu (1974), Schoenfeld & Richter (1982) and Makuch & Simon (1982).

In our example, treatment A was a control group and a failure rate of 3.14% per year was anticipated from previous experience. With time measured in years, this gives $\lambda_A = 0.0314$. A reduction in hazard rate of 25% was considered to be a meaningful improvement and hence we set $\psi^* = 0.75$. For a Type I error rate of $\alpha = 0.05$ and power $1-\beta = 0.8$, we find a total of $T = 14,116$ person-years are needed. Evaluating (10.15) as a function of $\psi > 0$ with $N_A = \lambda_A T/2$ and $N_B = \psi^*\lambda_A T/2$, where $\lambda_A = 0.0314$, $\psi^* = 0.75$ and $T = 14,116$, gives the power function for the original design which is shown as the solid line in Figure 10.7.

Figure 10.7 *Power and conditional power curves for the case study. The power function for the original design is shown by the solid line. The other curves represent conditional power functions under three different scenarios,* (1), (2) *and* (3), *for continuing after an interim analysis*

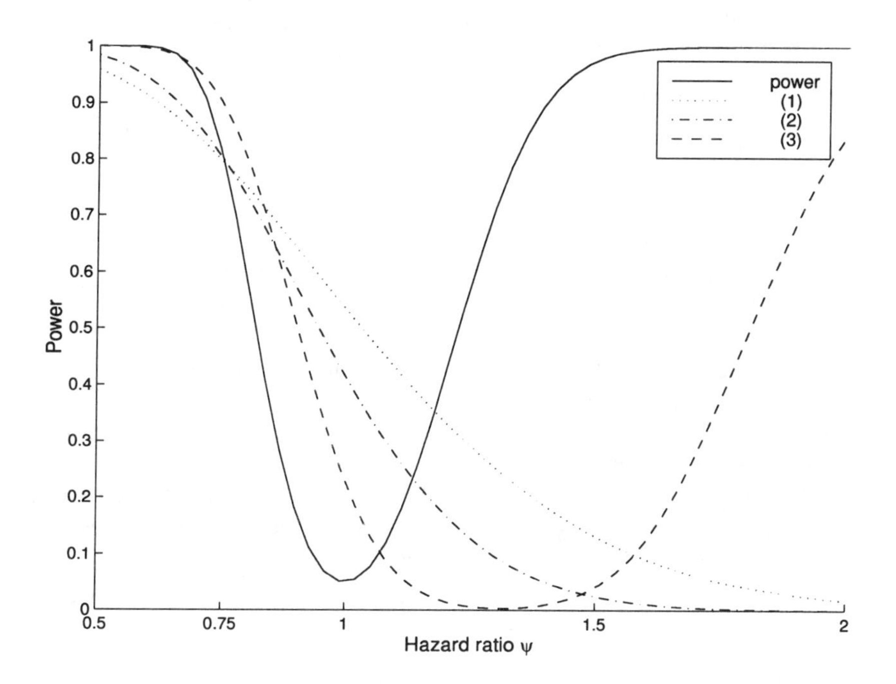

At an interim stage of the trial, we can consider the distribution of the statistic $W = \log(\hat{\psi})$ at termination, given the current data. Let n_A denote the number of patients who have failed so far, x_A the total person-years observed so far, and s_A the projected additional person-years for subjects on treatment A. Define n_B, x_B and s_B similarly for treatment B and let $s = s_A + s_B$. Let the random variables D_A and D_B be the numbers of further deaths that will be observed on treatments A and B, respectively, in the additional follow-up times of s_A and s_B person-years.

At termination, we shall have

$$W = \log(\hat{\psi}) = \log(\hat{\lambda}_B) - \log(\hat{\lambda}_A) = \log\left(\frac{n_B + D_B}{x_B + s_B}\right) - \log\left(\frac{n_A + D_A}{x_A + s_A}\right).$$

The conditional distribution of this statistic given the currently observed values n_A, x_A, n_B and x_B is approximately normal with mean

$$\log\left(\frac{n_B + \psi\,\lambda_A\, s_B}{x_B + s_B}\right) - \log\left(\frac{n_A + \lambda_A\, s_A}{x_A + s_A}\right)$$

Table 10.1 *Interim mortality data for the case study*

Treatment arm	*Deaths*	*Person-years*
A, *Control*	$n_A = 118$	$x_A = 3896$
B, *Active treatment*	$n_B = 89$	$x_B = 3943$
Total	$n = 207$	$x = 7839$

and variance

$$\frac{\psi\,\lambda_A\,s_B}{(\psi\,\lambda_A\,s_B + n_B)^2} + \frac{\lambda_A\,s_A}{(\lambda_A\,s_A + n_A)^2}$$

(see Andersen, 1987). The test on termination will reject H_0 if

$$|W| \geq z_{\alpha/2}\sqrt{\{(n_A + D_A)^{-1} + (n_B + D_B)^{-1}\}}. \tag{10.16}$$

Hence, we can estimate the conditional power from the conditional distribution of W stated above, substituting estimates $s_A\hat{\lambda}$ for D_A and $s_B\hat{\lambda}$ for D_B in the right hand side of (10.16), where $\hat{\lambda} = (n_A + n_B)/(x_A + x_B)$ is the current estimate of the common hazard rate under H_0.

At an interim meeting, the DSMB was faced with the mortality data displayed in Table 10.1. An analysis conducted at this interim point as if it were the final analysis yields an estimate of the hazard ratio

$$\hat{\psi} = \left(\frac{89}{3943}\right) / \left(\frac{118}{3896}\right) = 0.7452,$$

indicating better observed survival on the active treatment. From this, we find $W = \log(0.7452) = -0.2940$, and the standardized test statistic is

$$Z = \frac{W}{\sqrt{\{\frac{1}{118} + \frac{1}{89}\}}} = -2.094,$$

for which the two-sided P-value is 0.036. Of course, this P-value is not adjusted for the effect of multiple looks and, for example, either a Pocock-type or O'Brien & Fleming-type 95% repeated confidence interval for ψ (see Chapter 9) would still contain the null value $\psi = 1$. However, even though the protocol indicated the trial should continue, the DSMB had cause for concern and asked that conditional power curves be calculated for a fixed sample test at termination under the following three scenarios:

(1) One more year of follow-up,

(2) Two more years of follow-up,

(3) Continuation to termination as originally planned.

Table 10.2 shows the additional and total person-years of follow-up estimated under each scenario, using observed accrual and dropout rates and the numbers of subjects currently active. Conditional power curves were then computed using the above formulae. These are plotted in Figure 10.7 for each of the three scenarios

Table 10.2 *Additional person-years under three possible scenarios for continuing the case study*

	Scenario	*Additional person-years*			*Total person-years*		
		s_A	s_B	s	$x_A + s_A$	$x_B + s_B$	$x + s$
(1)	1 *more year*	375	375	750	4271	4318	8589
(2)	2 *more years*	815	815	1630	4711	4758	9469
(3)	*Original plan*	3138	3139	6276	7034	7082	14116

along with the power function for the original design. All three conditional power curves are U-shaped but those for scenarios (1) and (2) do not start to rise on the right until θ reaches higher values, about $\psi = 3$ for (2) and $\psi = 5$ for (1). From these curves we see that, under either $\psi^* = 0.75$ or the current estimate $\hat{\psi} = 0.7452$, there was a high conditional probability of a significant result: 0.79, 0.80 and 0.90 for scenarios (1), (2) and (3), respectively. Even if the null hypothesis were true and $\psi = 1$, the chances of it being rejected were as high as 53%, 41% and 23% under the three scenarios. After much discussion involving many issues, it was decided to continue the trial. In fact, the trial was terminated early at the next interim analysis.

In scenarios (1) and (2), the conditional powers calculated are those of fixed sample tests applied to the terminal set of data. Strictly speaking, such terminal tests are inappropriate since the sample size would have been chosen in the light of earlier data — although it is difficult to make a suitable adjustment when the sampling rule is not clearly defined. The conditional power calculations are also non-standard in that they do not refer to a single, well-defined reference test. In order to avoid such difficulties, it is wise to define a study protocol as unambiguously as possible at the outset. If this is done thoroughly and an interim analysis schedule is also defined, the full range of group sequential tests are available for use and one of these tests may be preferred to stochastic curtailment.

10.6 Bibliography and Notes

The idea of stochastic curtailment was first proposed by Lan, Simon & Halperin (1982). Earlier, Pasternack & Ogawa (1961) developed the related concept of *probability of reversal* of a test in the context of missing observations. This quantity relates to the question of whether the conclusion based on current data could be altered by the data yet to be observed. Pasternack (1984) discusses further the connection with curtailment procedures. Tan & Xiong (1996) describe the similar concept of a "discordant probability" in the context of the parameter-free stochastic curtailment procedure described in Section 10.4.

Details of the conditional power approach for comparing two treatment groups were given by Halperin et al. (1982) for dichotomous outcome variables; by Halperin et al. (1987) for slopes in longitudinal studies; by Andersen (1987) for exponentially distributed survival outcomes; by Pawitan and Hallstrom (1990) for survival data using the log-rank test; and by Lin, Yao and Ying (1999) for survival data using a proportional hazards regression model (see Section 13.4). The construction of repeated confidence intervals based on inverting an SCP is described in Davis & Hardy (1992).

Lan & Wittes (1988) present an application of conditional power but with θ replaced in (10.1) by the current estimate $\hat{\theta}^{(k)}$ or by limits of a confidence interval for θ based on the current data, $D(k)$. Pepe & Anderson (1992) use a similar idea in a one-sided testing procedure with two stages where $\hat{\theta}^{(k)} + \text{s.e.}(\hat{\theta}^{(k)})$ is used in place of θ in (10.1). Ware, Muller & Braunwald (1985) and Pepe & Anderson (1992) describe stochastic curtailment plans with special emphasis on stopping early if a negative result is indicated. Further discussion on the use of conditional power in decisions to stop early under H_0 is contained in Betensky (1997a,b). Applications of the predictive approach with binomial data have been described by Herson (1979), Choi, Smith & Becker (1985), Hilsenbeck (1988) and Johns & Andersen (1999).

CHAPTER 11

General Group Sequential Distribution Theory

11.1 Introduction

In Chapter 3 we showed that a wide variety of situations and data types lead to sequences of statistics with a common form of joint distribution. Consequently, the group sequential methods presented in Chapters 2 to 10 are widely applicable. In this chapter we prove general results which broaden further the applicability of these methods.

If observations follow a normal linear model, the distribution theory for a sequence of estimates is exact. We derive this theory in Section 11.3 and show that it extends to correlated observations, such as repeated measurements on subjects in a longitudinal study, as long as the correlation structure is known. If the covariance matrix in a normal linear model is completely known, Z-statistics can be created and these will have the canonical joint distribution (3.1). In most applications, a variance parameter σ^2 must be estimated from the observed data. Group sequential tests may then be based on a sequence of t-statistics and approximate procedures for doing this have been presented in Chapters 2 to 6. Results presented in Section 11.4 show that the joint distributions of sequences of t-statistics conform to a standard pattern and exact group sequential methods can be based on this joint distribution.

For non-normal data, the theory is asymptotic as sample size increases, but it provides a good approximation in small samples and this can serve as the basis of group sequential tests for parameters in, for example, a generalized linear model. We have already seen such applications in Sections 3.5, 3.6 and 10.5. The theory for general parametric models is presented in Section 11.6. Statistics arising in the group sequential analysis of survival data share similar asymptotic properties. Theory for the log-rank test, which underlies the example in Section 3.7, and for semi-parametric regression models for survival data subject to censoring will be discussed in Chapter 13.

11.2 A Standard Joint Distribution for Successive Estimates of a Parameter Vector

Consider a group sequential study with a maximum of K groups of observations. Let $\widehat{\boldsymbol{\beta}}^{(k)}$, $k = 1, \ldots, K$, denote the estimates of the parameter vector $\boldsymbol{\beta} = (\beta_1, \ldots, \beta_p)^T$ at successive analyses. It is not uncommon to find, at least approximately, that $(\widehat{\boldsymbol{\beta}}^{(1)}, \ldots, \widehat{\boldsymbol{\beta}}^{(K)})$ is multivariate normal with

$$\begin{cases} \widehat{\boldsymbol{\beta}}^{(k)} \sim N(\boldsymbol{\beta}, \mathcal{I}^{-1}(k, \boldsymbol{\beta})), & k = 1, \ldots, K, \\ \mathbf{Cov}(\widehat{\boldsymbol{\beta}}^{(k_1)}, \widehat{\boldsymbol{\beta}}^{(k_2)}) = \mathbf{Var}(\widehat{\boldsymbol{\beta}}^{(k_2)}) = \mathcal{I}^{-1}(k_2, \boldsymbol{\beta}), & k_1 \leq k_2, \end{cases} \tag{11.1}$$

for certain $p \times p$ matrices $\mathcal{I}^{-1}(k, \boldsymbol{\beta})$, $k = 1, \ldots, K$. This is the multi-parameter generalization of the distribution of a sequence of scalar parameter estimates, $\hat{\theta}^{(k)}$, given in (3.15), and this property forms the basis of many group sequential procedures. Suppose, for example, we wish to test the hypothesis H_0: $\boldsymbol{c}^T \boldsymbol{\beta} = \gamma$ for a given p-vector $\boldsymbol{c}$ and scalar constant γ. Define $\theta = \boldsymbol{c}^T \boldsymbol{\beta} - \gamma$ and

$$\mathcal{I}_k = \{Var(\boldsymbol{c}^T \widehat{\boldsymbol{\beta}}^{(k)})\}^{-1} = (\boldsymbol{c}^T \mathcal{I}^{-1}(k, \boldsymbol{\beta})\boldsymbol{c})^{-1},$$

the Fisher information for $\boldsymbol{c}^T \boldsymbol{\beta}$ at analysis k. A group sequential test of H_0 can be based on the score statistics

$$S_k = \mathcal{I}_k(\boldsymbol{c}^T \widehat{\boldsymbol{\beta}}^{(k)} - \gamma), \quad k = 1, \ldots, K,$$

which follow a multivariate normal distribution with

$$\begin{cases} S_k \sim N(\theta\, \mathcal{I}_k, \mathcal{I}_k), & k = 1, \ldots, K, \\ Cov(S_{k_1}, S_{k_2}) = Var(S_{k_1}) = \mathcal{I}_{k_1}, & k_1 \leq k_2, \end{cases} \tag{11.2}$$

as in (3.15). Alternatively, a test can be defined in terms of the Wald statistics,

$$Z_k = (\boldsymbol{c}^T \widehat{\boldsymbol{\beta}}^{(k)} - \gamma)\sqrt{\mathcal{I}_k}, \quad k = 1, \ldots, K,$$

which are are jointly multivariate normal with

$$\begin{cases} Z_k \sim N(\theta \sqrt{\mathcal{I}_k}, 1), & k = 1, \ldots, K, \\ Cov(Z_{k_1}, Z_{k_2}) = \sqrt{(\mathcal{I}_{k_1}/\mathcal{I}_{k_2})}, & k_1 \leq k_2. \end{cases} \tag{11.3}$$

It is evident from (11.2) that the increments $S_1, S_2 - S_1, \ldots, S_K - S_{K-1}$ are independent. Hence, both sequences $S_1, \ldots, S_K$ and $Z_1, \ldots, Z_K$ are Markov. This property greatly simplifies the numerical computations for group sequential tests described in Chapter 19. Without the Markov structure, a general multivariate normal integration routine such as MULNOR (Schervish, 1984) would be needed.

The distribution (11.3) of the standardized statistics Z_k is the canonical joint distribution (3.1). We showed this distribution to apply in the examples of parallel treatment studies and crossover trials in Sections 3.1.1 to 3.1.4. We now prove a theorem that shows these results hold for much more general linear mixed-effects normal models. This theorem helps to explain why the standard pattern occurs so frequently and also indicates when other behavior is liable to be found.

11.3 Normal Linear Models

We suppose univariate observations $X_1, X_2, \ldots$ are normally distributed with means depending linearly on an unknown parameter vector $\boldsymbol{\beta} = (\beta_1, \ldots, \beta_p)^T$. In a group sequential study with a maximum of K groups of observations, we denote the total number of observations in the first k groups by n_k, where $n_1 < \ldots < n_K$, and the vector of observations available at the kth analysis by

$$\boldsymbol{X}^{(k)} = (X_1, \ldots, X_{n_k})^T, \quad k = 1, \ldots, K.$$

We assume the full vector of n_K observations, $\boldsymbol{X}^{(K)}$, has a multivariate normal distribution with design matrix $\boldsymbol{D}^{(K)}$ and non-singular covariance matrix $\boldsymbol{\Sigma}^{(K)}\sigma^2$, where $\boldsymbol{D}^{(K)}$ and $\boldsymbol{\Sigma}^{(K)}$ are known. At each analysis $k = 1, \ldots, K$, we observe

$$\boldsymbol{X}^{(k)} \sim N(\boldsymbol{D}^{(k)}\boldsymbol{\beta},\ \boldsymbol{\Sigma}^{(k)}\sigma^2),$$

where $\boldsymbol{D}^{(k)}$ and $\boldsymbol{\Sigma}^{(k)}$ can be deduced from $\boldsymbol{D}^{(K)}$ and $\boldsymbol{\Sigma}^{(K)}$ by extracting the elements relating to the first n_k components of $\boldsymbol{X}^{(K)}$. We assume $\boldsymbol{\beta}$ is estimable at each stage $k = 1, \ldots, K$. In fact this may not always be true, especially at the earliest stages but we postpone discussion of this case to the end of the section. If $\boldsymbol{\beta}$ is estimable from $\boldsymbol{X}^{(k)}$, the maximum likelihood estimate (MLE) at stage k based on $\boldsymbol{X}^{(k)}$ is the generalized least squares estimate (LSE)

$$\widehat{\boldsymbol{\beta}}^{(k)} = (\boldsymbol{D}^{(k)T}\boldsymbol{\Sigma}^{(k)^{-1}}\boldsymbol{D}^{(k)})^{-1}\boldsymbol{D}^{(k)T}\boldsymbol{\Sigma}^{(k)^{-1}}\boldsymbol{X}^{(k)}, \quad k = 1, \ldots, K. \tag{11.4}$$

Theorem 11.1. Under the above model, the vectors $\widehat{\boldsymbol{\beta}}^{(1)}, \ldots, \widehat{\boldsymbol{\beta}}^{(K)}$ follow the multivariate normal joint distribution given by (11.1) with

$$\mathcal{I}^{-1}(k, \boldsymbol{\beta}) \;=\; \mathbf{Var}(\widehat{\boldsymbol{\beta}}^{(k)}) \;=\; \sigma^2(\boldsymbol{D}^{(k)^T}\boldsymbol{\Sigma}^{(k)^{-1}}\boldsymbol{D}^{(k)})^{-1} \;=\; \sigma^2\boldsymbol{V}_k, \tag{11.5}$$

for $k = 1, \ldots, K$, where $\boldsymbol{V}_k = (\boldsymbol{D}^{(k)^T}\boldsymbol{\Sigma}^{(k)^{-1}}\boldsymbol{D}^{(k)})^{-1}$ does not depend on $\boldsymbol{\beta}$.

Proof. As each $\widehat{\boldsymbol{\beta}}^{(k)}$ is a linear function of $\boldsymbol{X}^{(K)}$, elements of the vectors $\widehat{\boldsymbol{\beta}}^{(1)}, \ldots, \widehat{\boldsymbol{\beta}}^{(K)}$ have a multivariate normal joint distribution. It is well known that the marginal distribution of each $\widehat{\boldsymbol{\beta}}^{(k)}$ is that given in the theorem so it remains to determine the covariances of $\widehat{\boldsymbol{\beta}}^{(1)}, \ldots, \widehat{\boldsymbol{\beta}}^{(K)}$. Now, for $k_1 < k_2$, the data seen at analysis k_1 are a subset of the data at analysis k_2. We can, therefore, write

$$\widehat{\boldsymbol{\beta}}^{(k_1)} = \boldsymbol{A}^T\boldsymbol{X}^{(k_2)}$$

for some $n_{k_2} \times p$ matrix $\boldsymbol{A}$. Since $\widehat{\boldsymbol{\beta}}^{(k_1)}$ is an unbiased estimate of $\boldsymbol{\beta}$,

$$E(\boldsymbol{A}^T\boldsymbol{X}^{(k_2)}) \;=\; \boldsymbol{A}^T\boldsymbol{D}^{(k_2)}\boldsymbol{\beta} \;=\; \boldsymbol{\beta} \quad \text{for all } \boldsymbol{\beta}$$

and it follows that $\boldsymbol{A}^T\boldsymbol{D}^{(k_2)} = \boldsymbol{I}_p$, where $\boldsymbol{I}_p$ is the $p \times p$ identity matrix. Hence,

$$\begin{aligned}
&\mathbf{Cov}(\widehat{\boldsymbol{\beta}}^{(k_1)}, \widehat{\boldsymbol{\beta}}^{(k_2)}) \\
&= \mathbf{Cov}(\,\boldsymbol{A}^T\boldsymbol{X}^{(k_2)},\ (\boldsymbol{D}^{(k_2)^T}\boldsymbol{\Sigma}^{(k_2)^{-1}}\boldsymbol{D}^{(k_2)})^{-1}\boldsymbol{D}^{(k_2)^T}\boldsymbol{\Sigma}^{(k_2)^{-1}}\boldsymbol{X}^{(k_2)}\,) \\
&= \boldsymbol{A}^T\,\mathbf{Var}(\boldsymbol{X}^{(k_2)})\,\boldsymbol{\Sigma}^{(k_2)^{-1}}\boldsymbol{D}^{(k_2)}(\boldsymbol{D}^{(k_2)^T}\boldsymbol{\Sigma}^{(k_2)^{-1}}\boldsymbol{D}^{(k_2)})^{-1} \\
&= (\boldsymbol{D}^{(k_2)^T}\boldsymbol{\Sigma}^{(k_2)^{-1}}\boldsymbol{D}^{(k_2)})^{-1}\sigma^2 \\
&= \mathbf{Var}(\widehat{\boldsymbol{\beta}}^{(k_2)}),
\end{aligned}$$

as required. □

It follows from (11.5) that, for $k \neq k'$,

$$\mathbf{Cov}(\boldsymbol{V}_k^{-1}\widehat{\boldsymbol{\beta}}^{(k)} - \boldsymbol{V}_{k-1}^{-1}\widehat{\boldsymbol{\beta}}^{(k-1)}, \boldsymbol{V}_{k'}^{-1}\widehat{\boldsymbol{\beta}}^{(k')} - \boldsymbol{V}_{k'-1}^{-1}\widehat{\boldsymbol{\beta}}^{(k'-1)}) = \mathbf{0}.$$

Hence, the process $\{\boldsymbol{V}_k^{-1}\widehat{\boldsymbol{\beta}}^{(k)};\ k = 1, \ldots, K\}$ has independent increments and we deduce that $\{\widehat{\boldsymbol{\beta}}^{(k)};\ k = 1, \ldots, K\}$ is a Markov sequence.

Consider the problem of testing the hypothesis H_0: $\boldsymbol{c}^T\boldsymbol{\beta} = \gamma$ for a given p-vector $\boldsymbol{c}$ and scalar constant γ. The standardized test statistic at analysis k is

$$Z_k = (\boldsymbol{c}^T\widehat{\boldsymbol{\beta}}^{(k)} - \gamma)\sqrt{\mathcal{I}_k}, \quad k = 1, \ldots, K, \tag{11.6}$$

where

$$\mathcal{I}_k = \{Var(\boldsymbol{c}^T\widehat{\boldsymbol{\beta}}^{(k)})\}^{-1} = (\sigma^2\boldsymbol{c}^T\boldsymbol{V}_k\boldsymbol{c})^{-1} \tag{11.7}$$

is the Fisher information for $\boldsymbol{c}^T\boldsymbol{\beta}$ at analysis k. Theorem 11.1 shows that $(Z_1, \ldots, Z_K)$ has the canonical joint distribution (3.1) and so can be used with any of the group sequential procedures of Chapters 2 to 10. In particular, this justifies the two-sided tests for normal linear models presented in Section 3.4.

It remains to discuss the case where $\boldsymbol{c}^T\boldsymbol{\beta}$ is estimable but the whole of $\boldsymbol{\beta}$ cannot be estimated at the earliest analyses. This is likely to occur in longitudinal studies when initial analyses take place before accrual is complete and subject effects are not estimable for individuals yet to enter the study. An example was given in Section 3.4.4. In such a case, we can still use the same procedure based on the statistics $Z_1, \ldots, Z_K$ defined in (11.6) to test the hypothesis H_0: $\boldsymbol{c}^T\boldsymbol{\beta} = \gamma$, but now inverse matrices $\boldsymbol{V}_k = (\boldsymbol{D}^{(k)T}\boldsymbol{\Sigma}^{(k)^{-1}}\boldsymbol{D}^{(k)})^{-1}$ in (11.4), (11.5) and (11.7) should be interpreted as generalized inverses. As long as $\boldsymbol{c}^T\boldsymbol{\beta}$ is estimable at each stage k, $\boldsymbol{c}^T\widehat{\boldsymbol{\beta}}^{(k)}$ and Z_k will be uniquely defined even if $\widehat{\boldsymbol{\beta}}^{(k)}$ is not.

Theorem 11.1 covers uncorrelated and correlated normal observations, including as special cases normal linear mixed-effects models with their particular covariance matrices. The covariance properties of estimates derived by Halperin et al. (1987), Reboussin et al. (1992) and Wu & Lan (1992) follow from this result. The restriction of the theorem to the sequence of MLEs, or equivalently generalized LSEs, is critical and explains why the estimates used by Armitage et al. (1985, Section 4) and Geary (1988), which are ordinary LSEs squares rather than generalized LSEs, do not follow the standard pattern (11.1)

11.4 Normal Linear Models with Unknown Variance: Group Sequential *t*-Tests

We consider the same model as in the previous section, but now suppose the scale factor σ^2 in the covariance matrix is unknown. If $\boldsymbol{\beta}$ is estimable from $\boldsymbol{X}^{(k)}$, the MLE at stage k is still the generalized LSE given in (11.4). If $n_k > p$, the standard unbiased estimate of σ^2 based on the residuals at analysis k is

$$s_k^2 = (\boldsymbol{X}^{(k)} - \boldsymbol{D}^{(k)}\widehat{\boldsymbol{\beta}}^{(k)})^T\,\boldsymbol{\Sigma}^{(k)^{-1}}(\boldsymbol{X}^{(k)} - \boldsymbol{D}^{(k)}\widehat{\boldsymbol{\beta}}^{(k)})/(n_k - p), \tag{11.8}$$

which is marginally distributed as $\sigma^2\chi^2_{n_k-p}/(n_k - p)$ for each $k = 1, \ldots, K$. Suppose we are interested again in testing the hypothesis H_0: $\boldsymbol{c}^T\boldsymbol{\beta} = \gamma$ for a given

p-vector $\boldsymbol{c}$ and scalar constant γ. At each analysis $k = 1, \ldots, K$, the estimate of $\boldsymbol{c}^T\boldsymbol{\beta}$ is

$$\boldsymbol{c}^T\widehat{\boldsymbol{\beta}}^{(k)} \sim N(\boldsymbol{c}^T\boldsymbol{\beta},\ \boldsymbol{c}^T\boldsymbol{V}_k\boldsymbol{c}\sigma^2),$$

and the t-statistic for testing H_0 is

$$T_k = \frac{\boldsymbol{c}^T\widehat{\boldsymbol{\beta}}^{(k)} - \gamma}{\sqrt{\{\boldsymbol{c}^T\boldsymbol{V}_k\boldsymbol{c}\, s_k^2\}}}. \tag{11.9}$$

Marginally, T_k has a Student's t-distribution on $n_k - p$ degrees of freedom.

We have described how the significance level approach can be used to construct approximate two-sided tests (Section 3.8), one-sided tests (Section 4.4), tests with inner wedges (Section 5.2.4), and equivalence tests (Section 6.3.3) from a sequence of t-statistics T_k, $k = 1, \ldots, K$. However, to obtain exact properties for such tests we need to derive the exact joint distribution of $T_1, \ldots, T_K$. Unlike $Z_1, \ldots, Z_K$, the sequence of t-statistics is *not* Markov. An argument showing this is given by Jennison and Turnbull (1997b, p. 305). However, the sequence of pairs $\{(\boldsymbol{c}^T\widehat{\boldsymbol{\beta}}^{(k)}, s_k^2);\ k = 1, \ldots, K\}$ *is* Markov and the following theorem establishes its joint distribution. This result can be used to compute exact properties of group sequential t-tests.

Theorem 11.2. Suppose

$$\boldsymbol{X}^{(K)} = (X_1, \ldots, X_{n_K})^T \sim N(\boldsymbol{D}^{(K)}\boldsymbol{\beta},\ \boldsymbol{\Sigma}^{(K)}\sigma^2)$$

where the covariance matrix $\boldsymbol{\Sigma}^{(K)}\sigma^2$ is non-singular and at each analysis $k = 1, \ldots, K$ the first n_k elements of $X^{(K)}$ are available. Suppose also that $\boldsymbol{\beta}$ is estimable from $\boldsymbol{X}^{(1)} = (X_1, \ldots, X_{n_1})^T$ and let $\widehat{\boldsymbol{\beta}}^{(k)}$, $\boldsymbol{V}_k = Var(\widehat{\boldsymbol{\beta}}^{(k)})/\sigma^2$ and s_k^2, $k = 1, \ldots, K$, be as defined by (11.4), (11.5) and (11.8), respectively.

Then, the sequence $\{(\boldsymbol{c}^T\widehat{\boldsymbol{\beta}}^{(k)}, s_k^2);\ k = 1, \ldots, K\}$ is Markov,

$$\boldsymbol{c}^T\widehat{\boldsymbol{\beta}}^{(1)} \sim N(\boldsymbol{c}^T\boldsymbol{\beta}, \boldsymbol{c}^T\boldsymbol{V}_1\boldsymbol{c}\sigma^2), \quad s_1^2 \sim \sigma^2\chi^2_{n_1-p}/(n_1 - p)$$

and, for $k = 1, \ldots, K-1$,

$$\boldsymbol{c}^T\widehat{\boldsymbol{\beta}}^{(k+1)} \mid \boldsymbol{c}^T\widehat{\boldsymbol{\beta}}^{(k)}, s_k^2 \sim$$

$$N\left(\boldsymbol{c}^T\boldsymbol{\beta} + \frac{\boldsymbol{c}^T\boldsymbol{V}_{k+1}\boldsymbol{c}}{\boldsymbol{c}^T\boldsymbol{V}_k\boldsymbol{c}}\,\boldsymbol{c}^T(\widehat{\boldsymbol{\beta}}^{(k)} - \boldsymbol{\beta}),\ \boldsymbol{c}^T\boldsymbol{V}_{k+1}\boldsymbol{c}\sigma^2 - \frac{(\boldsymbol{c}^T\boldsymbol{V}_{k+1}\boldsymbol{c})^2}{\boldsymbol{c}^T\boldsymbol{V}_k\boldsymbol{c}}\,\sigma^2\right)$$

and

$$(n_{k+1}-p)s_{k+1}^2 \mid \boldsymbol{c}^T\widehat{\boldsymbol{\beta}}^{(k+1)}, \boldsymbol{c}^T\widehat{\boldsymbol{\beta}}^{(k)}, s_k^2 \sim (n_k - p)s_k^2 +$$

$$\{\boldsymbol{c}^T(\widehat{\boldsymbol{\beta}}^{(k+1)} - \widehat{\boldsymbol{\beta}}^{(k)})\}^2\{\boldsymbol{c}^T(\boldsymbol{V}_k - \boldsymbol{V}_{k+1})\boldsymbol{c}\}^{-1} + \sigma^2\chi^2_{n_{k+1}-n_k-1}$$

provided $\boldsymbol{c}^T(\widehat{\boldsymbol{\beta}}^{(k+1)} - \widehat{\boldsymbol{\beta}}^{(k)})$ is non-degenerate. If $\boldsymbol{c}^T\boldsymbol{\beta}$ is not estimable from the observations added between analyses k and $k+1$, then $\boldsymbol{c}^T\widehat{\boldsymbol{\beta}}^{(k+1)} = \boldsymbol{c}^T\widehat{\boldsymbol{\beta}}^{(k)}$ and

$$(n_{k+1} - p)s_{k+1}^2 \mid \boldsymbol{c}^T\widehat{\boldsymbol{\beta}}^{(k+1)}, \boldsymbol{c}^T\widehat{\boldsymbol{\beta}}^{(k)}, s_k^2 \sim (n_k - p)s_k^2 + \sigma^2\chi^2_{n_{k+1}-n_k}.$$

The proof of this theorem, which is rather lengthy, can be found in Jennison &

Turnbull (1997b). They also treat the case where $\boldsymbol{c}^T \boldsymbol{\beta}$ is estimable but the whole of $\boldsymbol{\beta}$ is not estimable at early analyses. Note that σ^2 appears as a scale factor in the variance of each $\boldsymbol{c}^T \widehat{\boldsymbol{\beta}}^{(k)}$ and in the distribution of each s_k^2, $k = 1, \ldots, K$. Thus, the distribution of the sequence $\{T_k;\, k = 1, \ldots, K\}$ is independent of σ^2 under H_0: $\boldsymbol{c}^T \boldsymbol{\beta} = \gamma$, and any convenient value of σ^2, such as $\sigma^2 = 1$, can be used in calculating properties of a group sequential t-test under the null hypothesis.

11.5 Example: An Exact One-Sample Group Sequential t-Test

An important special case of the general theory of Section 11.4 occurs when $X_1, X_2, \ldots$ are independent univariate $N(\mu, \sigma^2)$ random variables with scalar parameter μ. This was the situation considered by Jennison & Turnbull (1991b). In order to test the null hypothesis H_0: $\mu = \mu_0$, we use the above results with $\boldsymbol{c}^T \boldsymbol{\beta} = \mu$ and $\gamma = \mu_0$. Then

$$\boldsymbol{c}^T \widehat{\boldsymbol{\beta}} = \bar{X}^{(k)} = \frac{1}{n_k} \sum_{i=1}^{n_k} X_i, \quad s_k^2 = \frac{1}{n_k - 1} \sum_{i=1}^{n_k} (X_i - \bar{X}^{(k)})^2$$

and $\boldsymbol{c}^T \boldsymbol{V}_k \boldsymbol{c}$ is simply n_k^{-1} for $k = 1, \ldots, K$. The statistic (11.9) reduces to the usual one-sample t-statistic,

$$T_k = \frac{\bar{X}^{(k)} - \mu_0}{\sqrt{(s_k^2 / n_k)}}. \tag{11.10}$$

Suppose analyses are conducted after each new group of m observations, so $n_k = m\,k$, $k = 1, \ldots, K$. A general two-sided test of H_0: $\mu = \mu_0$ without early stopping in favor of H_0 stops at stage k to reject H_0 if

$$|T_k| \;\geq\; t_{mk-1,1-\Phi(d_k)}, \quad k = 1, \ldots, K, \tag{11.11}$$

and if H_0 has not been rejected by analysis K, it is accepted. Here, $t_{\nu,q}$ denotes the upper q tail-point of a t-distribution on ν degrees of freedom and Φ is the standard normal cdf. The sequence of constants $d_1, \ldots, d_K$ defines the testing boundary. These constants can be chosen so that the Type I error probability is exactly equal to a desired value α. If we adopt Pocock's approach of applying constant nominal significance levels at each stage, we set

$$d_k = Z_P(K, m, \alpha), \quad k = 1, \ldots, K,$$

whereas for an O'Brien & Fleming-type test, we set

$$d_k = Z_B(K, m, \alpha)\sqrt{(K/k)}, \quad k = 1, \ldots, K.$$

In either case, the constants $Z_P(K, m, \alpha)$ or $Z_B(K, m, \alpha)$ can be computed, using nested numerical integrations described in Chapter 19, so that the Type I error probability is α. The tests described in Section 3.8 have the same general form but their Type I error rates are only approximately equal to α. Since those tests apply the same nominal significance level at each stage to a t-statistic as known variance tests apply to a Z-statistic, they correspond to using the constants $C_P(K, \alpha)$ or $C_B(K, \alpha)$ defined in Chapter 2 in place of $Z_P(K, m, \alpha)$ or $Z_B(K, m, \alpha)$, respectively, in the above definitions.

Table 11.1 *Constants $Z_P(K, m, \alpha)$ and $Z_B(K, m, \alpha)$ for Pocock-type and O'Brien & Fleming-type two-sided repeated t-tests with exact Type I error probability $\alpha = 0.05$. Designs are for K groups of m observations and at each stage $k = 1, \ldots, K$, H_0 is rejected if Student's t-statistic* (11.10) *exceeds $t_{mk-1,1-\Phi(Z_P)}$ in the case of a Pocock-type test or $t_{mk-1,1-\Phi\{Z_B\surd(K/k)\}}$ for an O'Brien & Fleming-type test.*

K	Group size, m					
	1†	2	3	5	10	∞
			$Z_P(K, m, \alpha)$ *for Pocock-type tests*			
1*	—	1.960	1.960	1.960	1.960	1.960
2	1.960	2.220	2.210	2.198	2.188	2.178
3	2.203	2.344	2.329	2.315	2.303	2.289
4	2.323	2.418	2.404	2.389	2.376	2.361
5	2.400	2.472	2.457	2.442	2.428	2.413
6	2.455	2.512	2.498	2.482	2.468	2.453
7	2.495	2.543	2.530	2.514	2.500	2.485
8	2.532	2.570	2.556	2.541	2.527	2.512
9	2.558	2.591	2.579	2.563	2.550	2.535
10	2.582	2.611	2.598	2.583	2.569	2.555
			$Z_B(K, m, \alpha)$ *for O'Brien & Fleming-type tests*			
1*	—	1.960	1.960	1.960	1.960	1.960
2	1.960	1.995	1.993	1.989	1.984	1.977
3	2.047	2.034	2.027	2.019	2.012	2.004
4	2.077	2.058	2.050	2.041	2.033	2.024
5	2.097	2.075	2.065	2.056	2.048	2.040
6	2.112	2.084	2.077	2.068	2.061	2.053
7	2.117	2.094	2.088	2.078	2.071	2.063
8	2.128	2.100	2.096	2.086	2.079	2.072
9	2.133	2.105	2.102	2.093	2.087	2.080
10	2.138	2.109	2.108	2.099	2.093	2.087

* The case $K = 1$ corresponds to a fixed sample t-test on $m - 1$ degrees of freedom.
† If $m = 1$, it is assumed that no analysis is performed at the first stage.

Table 11.1 gives values of $Z_P(K, m, \alpha)$ and $Z_B(K, m, \alpha)$ for $\alpha = 0.05, m = 1$, 2, 3, 5 and 10 and $K = 1$ to 10. The entries in this table are taken from Jennison & Turnbull (1991b, Table 1), where corresponding values for $\alpha = 0.01$ are also listed. If $m = 1$, it is assumed that no analysis is performed at the first stage as s_1^2 would be undefined: this explains the different pattern in the column for $m = 1$. The case $K = 1$ is a fixed sample test in which T_1 is compared with the usual critical value for a two-sided t-test, $t_{m-1,\alpha/2}$, and so $Z_P(1, m, \alpha)$ and $Z_B(1, m, \alpha)$

are both equal to $z_{\alpha/2}$. The final column shows limiting values of $Z_P(K, m, \alpha)$ and $Z_B(K, m, \alpha)$ as m increases to infinity and these are the values $C_P(K, \alpha)$ and $C_B(K, \alpha)$ for known σ^2 in Tables 2.1 and 2.3, respectively. The entries of Table 11.1 were computed using numerical integration and the distributional results of Theorem 11.2 for this special case; for more details, see Chapter 19 and the appendix of Jennison & Turnbull (1991b).

As an example, consider designing a test with Type I error probability $\alpha = 0.05$ and a maximum of $K = 5$ groups of 3 observations each. Suppose we choose a Pocock-type procedure so that $d_k = Z_P(5, 3, 0.05) = 2.457$ for $k = 1, \ldots, 5$, taking $Z_P(5, 3, 0.05)$ from Table 11.1. Since $\Phi(2.457) = 0.993$, the critical value for $|T_1|$ at stage 1 is $t_{2,0.007} = 8.36$. At stage 2, the critical value for $|T_2|$ is $t_{5,0.007} = 3.70$ and critical values at stages 3, 4 and 5 are 3.13, 2.92 and 2.81, respectively. Since the degrees of freedom increase with each stage, the critical values for $|T_k|$ decrease while the nominal significance levels remain constant. The "significance level" approach proposed by Pocock (1977) and described in Section 3.8 would use $d_k = C_P(5, 0.05) = 2.413$ for $k = 1, \ldots, 5$, where $C_P(5, 0.05)$ is taken from Table 2.1, and this yields critical values 7.86, 3.58, 3.05, 2.85 and 2.75 at stages 1 to 5 respectively. These values are smaller than those of the exact test, indicating that the actual Type I error rate of the approximate test is higher than the nominal 0.05. In fact, exact computation shows the Type I error probability to be 0.056. Nevertheless, the approximation has performed quite well in this example, especially in view of the small group sizes.

We can also construct repeated confidence intervals for μ using the statistics given in (11.10). A $(1 - \alpha)$-level sequence of repeated confidence intervals is

$$(\bar{X}^{(k)} - c_k(\alpha)\sqrt{\{s_k^2/n_k\}},\ \bar{X}^{(k)} + c_k(\alpha)\sqrt{\{s_k^2/n_k\}}), \quad k = 1, \ldots, K,$$

where $c_k(\alpha) = t_{mk-1,1-\Phi(d_k)}$ is the critical value for $|T_k|$ stated in (11.11). The use of such intervals has been described in Chapter 9.

11.6 General Parametric Models: Generalized Linear Models

Suppose observations X_i, $i = 1, \ldots, n_K$, are independent and we observe vectors $\boldsymbol{X}^{(k)} = (X_1, \ldots, X_{n_k})^T$ at analyses $k = 1, \ldots, K$. Denote the density or discrete distribution of X_i by $f_i(x_i; \boldsymbol{\beta})$, where $\boldsymbol{\beta}$ is a p-dimensional parameter vector. For example, $f_i(x_i; \boldsymbol{\beta})$ could specify a generalized linear model with linear predictor $d_{i1}\beta_1 + \ldots + d_{ip}\beta_p$. We define the column vector of efficient scores and the information matrix for each observation $i = 1, \ldots, n_K$ as

$$\boldsymbol{U}_i(X_i; \boldsymbol{\beta}) = \frac{\partial}{\partial \boldsymbol{\beta}} \log\{f_i(X_i; \boldsymbol{\beta})\} \quad \text{and} \quad \mathcal{I}_i(\boldsymbol{\beta}) = E\left\{\frac{-\partial}{\partial \boldsymbol{\beta}} \boldsymbol{U}_i^T(X_i; \boldsymbol{\beta})\right\},$$

respectively. The sum of scores and information matrix at analysis k are then

$$\boldsymbol{U}(k, \boldsymbol{\beta}) = \sum_{i=1}^{n_k} \boldsymbol{U}_i(X_i; \boldsymbol{\beta}) \quad \text{and} \quad \mathcal{I}(k, \boldsymbol{\beta}) = \sum_{i=1}^{n_k} \mathcal{I}_i(\boldsymbol{\beta}).$$

We first review standard, fixed sample asymptotic theory applied at a single analysis, k. In the asymptotic setting we index sample sizes by n and suppose

$n_k \to \infty$ and $\mathcal{I}(k, \boldsymbol{\beta}) \to \infty$ with $\mathcal{I}(k, \boldsymbol{\beta})/n$ converging to a fixed limit $\overline{\mathcal{I}}(k, \boldsymbol{\beta})$ as n increases. Under suitable regularity conditions on the $f_i(x_i; \boldsymbol{\beta})$, (see, for example, Cox & Hinkley, 1974, ch. 9)

$$E\{\boldsymbol{U}_i(X_i; \boldsymbol{\beta})\} = \mathbf{0} \quad \text{and} \quad \mathcal{I}_i(\boldsymbol{\beta}) = \mathbf{Var}\{\boldsymbol{U}_i(X_i; \boldsymbol{\beta})\} \tag{11.12}$$

for each $i = 1, \ldots, n_k$. With probability approaching 1 as $n \to \infty$, the MLE of $\boldsymbol{\beta}$ at analysis k satisfies

$$\boldsymbol{U}(k, \widehat{\boldsymbol{\beta}}^{(k)}) = 0. \tag{11.13}$$

Also, $\widehat{\boldsymbol{\beta}}^{(k)}$ is a consistent estimator of $\boldsymbol{\beta}$. Using (11.13) in a Taylor series expansion for each element of $\boldsymbol{U}(k, \boldsymbol{\beta})$ we obtain

$$n^{-1/2}\, U^j(k, \boldsymbol{\beta}) = n^{-1} \sum_{i=1}^{n_k} \left(\frac{-\partial}{\partial \boldsymbol{\beta}}\, U_i^j(X_i; \boldsymbol{\beta}_{jk}^*) \right)^T n^{1/2}\, (\widehat{\boldsymbol{\beta}}^{(k)} - \boldsymbol{\beta}) \tag{11.14}$$

for $j = 1, \ldots, p$. Here, $U^j(k, \boldsymbol{\beta})$ denotes the jth element of $\boldsymbol{U}(k, \boldsymbol{\beta})$, $U_i^j(k, \boldsymbol{\beta})$ is the jth element of $\boldsymbol{U}_i(k, \boldsymbol{\beta})$ and $\boldsymbol{\beta}_{jk}^*$ is a value of $\boldsymbol{\beta}$ on the line segment between $\boldsymbol{\beta}$ and $\widehat{\boldsymbol{\beta}}^{(k)}$. Again with suitable regularity conditions, the weak law of large numbers implies

$$n^{-1} \sum_{i=1}^{n_k} \frac{-\partial}{\partial \boldsymbol{\beta}}\, \boldsymbol{U}_i^T(X_i; \boldsymbol{\beta}) \;\longrightarrow\; \overline{\mathcal{I}}(k, \boldsymbol{\beta}) \tag{11.15}$$

in probability as $n \to \infty$, and a multivariate central limit theorem gives

$$n^{-1/2}\, \boldsymbol{U}(k, \boldsymbol{\beta}) \;\xrightarrow{\mathcal{D}}\; N(0, \overline{\mathcal{I}}(k, \boldsymbol{\beta})), \tag{11.16}$$

where $\xrightarrow{\mathcal{D}}$ denotes convergence in distribution. An important constraint on the experimental design for (11.15) and (11.16) to apply for a general response distribution is that the fraction of the total information contributed by any individual observation should decrease to zero as n increases. The further requirement that $\overline{\mathcal{I}}(k, \boldsymbol{\beta})$ be uniformly continuous in $\boldsymbol{\beta}$ in a neighborhood of the true value of $\boldsymbol{\beta}$ ensures that the difference between $\boldsymbol{\beta}_{jk}^*$ and $\boldsymbol{\beta}_j$ is asymptotically negligible and the standard result

$$n^{1/2}\, (\widehat{\boldsymbol{\beta}}^{(k)} - \boldsymbol{\beta}) \;\xrightarrow{\mathcal{D}}\; N(0, \overline{\mathcal{I}}^{-1}(k, \boldsymbol{\beta})) \quad \text{as } n \to \infty \tag{11.17}$$

follows from (11.14), (11.15) and (11.16).

The following theorem establishes the asymptotic *joint* distribution of $(\widehat{\boldsymbol{\beta}}^{(1)}, \ldots, \widehat{\boldsymbol{\beta}}^{(K)})$ under the regularity conditions used above in deriving the marginal distribution of each $\widehat{\boldsymbol{\beta}}^{(k)}$. Thus, for any particular group sequential experiment, it suffices to check that standard, non-sequential asymptotic methods can be applied to deduce the asymptotic distribution of each individual $\widehat{\boldsymbol{\beta}}^{(k)}$. The sequential theory then follows automatically. In general, the regularity conditions that must be satisfied depend on the type of distribution the data follow and the form of dependence on the parameter vector $\boldsymbol{\beta}$. In the important case of generalized linear models, we refer the reader to McCullagh & Nelder (1989) for an account of asymptotic theory and for further references.

Theorem 11.3. Suppose observations X_i are independent with distributions $f_i(x_i; \boldsymbol{\beta})$, where $\boldsymbol{\beta}$ is p-dimensional, and observations $X_1, \ldots, X_{n_k}$ are available at analyses $k = 1, \ldots, K$. Let $\widehat{\boldsymbol{\beta}}^{(k)}$ denote the MLE of $\boldsymbol{\beta}$ based on $X_1, \ldots, X_{n_k}$ and $\mathcal{I}(k, \boldsymbol{\beta})$ the Fisher information for $\boldsymbol{\beta}$ summed over the first n_k observations. Suppose sample sizes are indexed by n and $n_k \to \infty$ and $\mathcal{I}(k, \boldsymbol{\beta}) \to \infty$ in such a way that

$$\mathcal{I}(k, \boldsymbol{\beta})/n \to \overline{\mathcal{I}}(k, \boldsymbol{\beta})$$

for each $k = 1, \ldots, K$.

Suppose also that the distributions f_i are sufficiently regular that (11.12), (11.14), (11.15) and (11.16) hold, each $\overline{\mathcal{I}}(k, \boldsymbol{\beta})$ is uniformly continuous in $\boldsymbol{\beta}$ in a neighborhood of the true value of $\boldsymbol{\beta}$ and each $\widehat{\boldsymbol{\beta}}^{(k)}$ is consistent for $\boldsymbol{\beta}$ as $n \to \infty$.

Then, the joint distribution of $(\widehat{\boldsymbol{\beta}}^{(1)}, \ldots, \widehat{\boldsymbol{\beta}}^{(K)})$ is asymptotically multivariate normal,

$$n^{1/2}(\widehat{\boldsymbol{\beta}}^{(k)} - \boldsymbol{\beta}) \xrightarrow{\mathcal{D}} N(0, \overline{\mathcal{I}}^{-1}(k, \boldsymbol{\beta})) \quad \text{as } n \to \infty, \quad k = 1, \ldots, K,$$

and

$$\mathbf{Cov}_A(n^{1/2}\widehat{\boldsymbol{\beta}}^{(k_1)}, n^{1/2}\widehat{\boldsymbol{\beta}}^{(k_2)}) = \mathbf{Var}_A(n^{1/2}\widehat{\boldsymbol{\beta}}^{(k_2)}) \quad \text{for } k_1 \le k_2,$$

where $\mathbf{Var}_A$ and $\mathbf{Cov}_A$ denote asymptotic variance and covariance.

Proof. The increments in the score statistic, $n^{-1/2}\boldsymbol{U}(1, \boldsymbol{\beta})$ and

$$n^{-1/2}\{\boldsymbol{U}(k, \boldsymbol{\beta}) - \boldsymbol{U}(k-1, \boldsymbol{\beta})\}, \quad k = 2, \ldots, K,$$

depend on distinct sets of independent variables X_i and, hence, are independent. With (11.16), this implies that the increments have independent, asymptotically normal distributions with mean zero and variances equal to $\overline{\mathcal{I}}(1, \boldsymbol{\beta})$ and

$$\overline{\mathcal{I}}(k, \boldsymbol{\beta}) - \overline{\mathcal{I}}(k-1, \boldsymbol{\beta}), \quad k = 2, \ldots, K.$$

The sequence

$$\{n^{-1/2}\boldsymbol{U}(1, \boldsymbol{\beta}), \ldots, n^{-1/2}\boldsymbol{U}(K, \boldsymbol{\beta})\}$$

is, thus, asymptotically multivariate normal with mean zero,

$$\mathbf{Var}(n^{-1/2}\boldsymbol{U}(k, \boldsymbol{\beta})) = \overline{\mathcal{I}}(k, \boldsymbol{\beta}), \quad k = 1, \ldots, K,$$

and independent increments. This, together with (11.14) and (11.15), the consistency of $\widehat{\boldsymbol{\beta}}^{(k)}$ and the uniform continuity of each $\overline{\mathcal{I}}(k, \boldsymbol{\beta})$, implies that $\{n^{1/2}(\widehat{\boldsymbol{\beta}}^{(k)} - \boldsymbol{\beta}); k = 1, \ldots, K\}$ has the same limiting joint distribution as

$$\{\overline{\mathcal{I}}^{-1}(k, \boldsymbol{\beta})\, n^{-1/2}\boldsymbol{U}(k, \boldsymbol{\beta}); k = 1, \ldots, K\}$$

and the result follows. □

Because the asymptotic distribution of $(\widehat{\boldsymbol{\beta}}^{(1)}, \ldots, \widehat{\boldsymbol{\beta}}^{(K)})$ possesses the standard variance structure (11.1), group sequential tests can be constructed using boundaries computed for the normal case. For instance, a group sequential test of H_0: $\boldsymbol{c}^T\boldsymbol{\beta} = \gamma$ can be based on

$$S_k = \mathcal{I}_k\, n^{1/2}(\boldsymbol{c}^T\widehat{\boldsymbol{\beta}}^{(k)} - \gamma), \quad k = 1, \ldots, K,$$

where $\mathcal{I}_k = (\boldsymbol{c}^T \overline{\mathcal{I}}^{-1}(k, \boldsymbol{\beta})\boldsymbol{c})^{-1}$, and the vector $(S_1, \ldots, S_K)$ is asymptotically multivariate normal with independent increments. Furthermore, under a series of contiguous alternatives $\boldsymbol{\beta}^n$ for which $n^{1/2}(\boldsymbol{c}^T \boldsymbol{\beta}^n - \gamma) \to \theta$, S_k converges in distribution to $N(\theta \mathcal{I}_k, \mathcal{I}_k)$, $k = 1, \ldots, K$, and the standard distribution (11.2) applies. Alternatively, the standardized statistics

$$Z_k = \mathcal{I}_k^{1/2} n^{1/2} (\boldsymbol{c}^T \widehat{\boldsymbol{\beta}}^{(k)} - \gamma), \quad k = 1, \ldots, K,$$

are asymptotically multivariate normal with $Z_k \sim N(\theta\sqrt{\mathcal{I}_k}, 1)$ for each k and $Cov_A(Z_{k_1}, Z_{k_2}) = (\mathcal{I}_{k_1}/\mathcal{I}_{k_2})^{1/2}$ for $k_1 \leq k_2$, under the same series of contiguous alternatives. This is the canonical joint distribution (3.1) for the vector $(Z_1, \ldots, Z_K)$ and hence tests designed for normal observations, as described in the preceding chapters, can be applied without modification.

The asymptotic theory for S_k and Z_k remains the same if $\overline{\mathcal{I}}(k, \boldsymbol{\beta})$ is replaced by a consistent estimate and, since $\overline{\mathcal{I}}^{-1}(k, \boldsymbol{\beta})$ is also the asymptotic variance of $n^{1/2} \widehat{\boldsymbol{\beta}}^{(k)}$, it suffices to have a consistent estimate of this variance. In finite samples we can use

$$(n\overline{\mathcal{I}}_k)^{-1} \simeq Var(\boldsymbol{c}^T \widehat{\boldsymbol{\beta}}^{(k)})$$

to obtain standardized statistics

$$Z_k = \{Var(\boldsymbol{c}^T \widehat{\boldsymbol{\beta}}^{(k)})\}^{-1/2} (\boldsymbol{c}^T \widehat{\boldsymbol{\beta}}^{(k)} - \gamma), \quad k = 1, \ldots, K,$$

which are approximately multivariate normal with

$$Z_k \sim N(\{Var(\boldsymbol{c}^T \widehat{\boldsymbol{\beta}}^{(k)})\}^{-1/2} (\boldsymbol{c}^T \boldsymbol{\beta} - \gamma), 1)$$

and

$$Cov(Z_{k_1}, Z_{k_2}) = \sqrt{\{Var(\boldsymbol{c}^T \widehat{\boldsymbol{\beta}}^{(k_2)}) / Var(\boldsymbol{c}^T \widehat{\boldsymbol{\beta}}^{(k_1)})\}} \quad \text{for } k_1 \leq k_2.$$

Alternatively, we can define score statistics corresponding to $n^{1/2} S_k$,

$$\widetilde{S}_k = \{Var(\boldsymbol{c}^T \widehat{\boldsymbol{\beta}}^{(k)})\}^{-1} (\boldsymbol{c}^T \widehat{\boldsymbol{\beta}}^{(k)} - \gamma), \quad k = 1, \ldots, K,$$

which are approximately multivariate normal with

$$\widetilde{S}_k \sim N(\{Var(\boldsymbol{c}^T \widehat{\boldsymbol{\beta}}^{(k)})\}^{-1} (\boldsymbol{c}^T \boldsymbol{\beta} - \gamma), \{Var(\boldsymbol{c}^T \widehat{\boldsymbol{\beta}}^{(k)})\}^{-1})$$

and independent increments. Note that all we need here to calculate Z_k or $\widetilde{S}_k$ at analysis k is the MLE, $\widehat{\boldsymbol{\beta}}^{(k)}$, and an estimate of its variance at each analysis, both of which are usually provided by computer software programs for statistical model fitting.

Our general theory provides a basis for group sequential testing in a range of important applications, including the whole family of generalized linear models. One interesting application of the theory is to the sequential analysis of logistic regression models for the decay in germination rates of seeds, for which Whitehead (1989) proposed a sequential monitoring scheme based on the assumption that the sequence of score statistics is approximately multivariate normal with independent increments. Our results provide an asymptotic justification of this assumption to supplement the evidence of Whitehead's small sample simulations. In the next chapter we shall apply the theory to binary responses, including the analysis of logistic regression models in Section 12.5.

The general theory can also be extended to studies with correlated observations by replacing the distribution $f_i(x_i; \boldsymbol{\beta})$ by the conditional distribution of X_i given $X_1, \ldots, X_{i-1}$ and defining efficient scores $\boldsymbol{U}_i(X_i; \boldsymbol{\beta})$ in terms of this conditional distribution (see Cox & Hinkley, 1974, p. 299). The conclusion of Theorem 11.3 remains valid if it is permissible to apply a weak law of large numbers to sums of conditional information and a central limit theorem to sums of conditional scores to deduce the conditions required in the statement of Theorem 11.3.

We conclude this section by noting a remarkably simple proof that all asymptotically efficient estimators have the standard covariance structure (11.1). We consider the case $p = 1$ when β is a scalar, although the argument is easily generalized. Suppose the asymptotic covariance between $\hat{\beta}^{(k_2)}$ and $\hat{\beta}^{(k_2)} - \hat{\beta}^{(k_1)}$ is not zero; then a new estimate of the form $\hat{\beta}^{(k_2)} + \epsilon(\hat{\beta}^{(k_2)} - \hat{\beta}^{(k_1)})$, for ϵ close to zero and of the opposite sign to $Cov(\hat{\beta}^{(k_2)}, \hat{\beta}^{(k_2)} - \hat{\beta}^{(k_1)})$, will have lower variance than $\hat{\beta}^{(k_2)}$, contradicting the asymptotic efficiency of $\hat{\beta}^{(k_2)}$. For example, Lai & Ying (1991) have proved that a modified version of the Buckley-James estimator (Buckley & James, 1979) is asymptotically efficient for the regression analysis of censored normal data and so the above argument establishes the asymptotic covariance structure of successive values of their estimate. In cases such as this, it remains to prove the asymptotic joint normality of the sequence of estimates. We note, conversely, that examples such as those described at the end of Section 11.3, in which the "standard distribution" does not apply, involve tests or estimates which are not founded on maximum likelihood methods.

11.7 Bibliography and Notes

The material in this chapter follows closely the development in Jennison & Turnbull (1997a,b). We have presented a general distribution theory for sequences of MLEs of a parameter vector. Examples include normal observations, both uncorrelated and correlated, and general parametric regression models. This theory forms the basis of a unified approach to group sequential analysis and supports the use of existing methods in a wide range of applications.

In fact, this general theory can be extended further. Tsiatis, Boucher & Kim (1995) obtain general results for parametric survival distributions when data are subject to right censoring. Scharfstein, Tsiatis & Robins (1997) show in great generality that score statistics in parametric and semi-parametric models have the independent increments structure (11.2). The asymptotic normality and efficiency of score statistics at individual analyses are required as conditions for Scharfstein et al.'s (1997) key Theorem 1 and, in general, these properties must be verified on a case-by-case basis to confirm that their theorem can be applied. The general theory for semi-parametric models applies to the proportional hazards regression model, where the baseline hazard function is an infinite-dimensional nuisance parameter. Applications to models for survival data will be discussed in Chapter 13.

The history of the use of the standard distribution (11.1) in the group sequential analysis of longitudinal data is interesting. Sequences of estimates have been shown to follow this standard distribution in some, but not all, cases. Armitage, Stratton & Worthington (1985) proved that the differences in mean response of two groups of subjects measured at three successive occasions satisfy (11.1) under a model assuming independent within-subject variation. However, these authors and Geary (1988) found that this property is lost when a within-subject autoregression term is added. Halperin et al. (1987) proved that estimates of the difference in the mean slopes of two groups in a random effects model follow the standard distribution even when subject entry is staggered and patterns of timing of observations for each subject are irregular. Lee & DeMets (1991) proposed a group sequential method for comparing rates of change in different forms of linear mixed-effects model and, subsequently, Reboussin, Lan & DeMets (1992) showed that their estimates follow (11.1). The standard distribution also arises in the asymptotic theory for generalized estimating equation models derived by Gange & DeMets (1996). Wu & Lan (1992) considered a group sequential procedure to compare areas under expected response change curves and showed, in important special cases with non-informative censoring, that the sequence of score statistics follows (11.2) asymptotically; see, for example, their equations (3.9) and (3.12).

There are however important applications where the distributions (11.1) and (11.2) fail to apply even asymptotically. Counter-examples are provided by the linear rank statistics of Lee & DeMets (1992), distribution-free multivariate Hodges-Lehmann estimators (Su & Lachin, 1992) and estimates obtained from "independence estimating equations" (Wei, Su & Lachin, 1990). Jennison & Turnbull (1991c) established conditions under which successive Mantel-Haenszel estimates of the odds ratio in stratified 2×2 tables are asymptotically multivariate normal and satisfy (11.1), but they note that other covariance structures occur if data do not accumulate in a specific manner (see Section 12.3).

In the group sequential analysis of survival data there are certain test statistics that also do not follow the standard distribution even asymptotically. Slud & Wei (1982) derive the asymptotic joint distribution of a sequence of modified-Wilcoxon scores, analogous to our $S_1, \ldots, S_K$, for comparing two sets of censored survival times and show that they can have correlated increments if patient entry is staggered. Lin (1991) notes that sequences of sums of linear rank statistics for analyzing multiple survival endpoints are asymptotically multivariate normal but have independent increments *only* if the limiting weight function is independent of survival time. Gu & Ying (1993, Section 4) consider the asymptotic joint distribution of successive Buckley-James score statistics (Buckley & James, 1979) for accumulating survival data with covariates, staggered entry and right censoring and they show this joint distribution differs from (11.2). The independent increment structure has also been shown not to hold for certain robust score statistics used in semi-parametric multiplicative intensity regression models for recurrent event data in complex situations where there may be frailties or other dependencies present (see Cook & Lawless, 1996, Section 5, and Jiang, 1999).

In Sections 11.3 and 11.4, we discussed group sequential procedures based on successive Z-statistics or t-statistics for testing a hypothesis of the form H_0: $c^T \beta = \gamma$ where c and β are vectors of dimension p. More generally we might consider hypotheses of the form H_0: $C^T \beta = 0$ where C is a $p \times q$

matrix of rank q. This leads to consideration of group sequential procedures based on successive χ^2 or F statistics. These have been considered by Jennison & Turnbull (1997b). Earlier, Jennison & Turnbull (1991b) treated the special case of testing the value of a multivariate normal mean with independent observations. In their Table 2, they provide tables of critical values for use with group sequential χ^2 procedures. This problem will be considered further in Chapters 15 and 16 as it is applicable to analysis of clinical trial data when there are multiple endpoints or more than two competing treatments.

CHAPTER 12

Binary Data

12.1 A Single Bernoulli Probability

12.1.1 Using the Normal Approximation

In this chapter we consider group sequential experiments where the primary outcome is binary. We start by revisiting the one sample problem first considered in Section 3.6.1 and illustrated in an application to individual equivalence studies in Section 6.4. Here, individual responses $X_1, X_2, \ldots$ are independent Bernoulli random variables taking the value one, or "success", with probability p and zero, or "failure", with probability $1 - p$. We shall assume responses are to be observed in up to K stages, with m_k observations in the kth group, $k = 1, \ldots, K$. We denote the cumulative sample size at the kth stage by $n_k = m_1 + \ldots + m_k$ and define $S_k = X_1 + \ldots + X_{n_k}$ to be the total number of successes in the first k groups. The maximum likelihood estimate of p based on data available at stage k is thus

$$\hat{p}^{(k)} = S_k / n_k.$$

Suppose we wish to test H_0: $p = p_0$ against a two-sided alternative. In Section 3.6.1 we explained how the standardized test statistics

$$Z_k = \frac{\hat{p}^{(k)} - p_0}{\sqrt{\{p_0(1 - p_0)/n_k\}}}, \quad k = 1, \ldots, K, \tag{12.1}$$

may be used to construct such a two-sided test. There are, however, two problems with this approximation. First, the normal approximation is inaccurate if sample sizes are small or p is close to zero or one. Second, the variance of $\hat{p}^{(k)}$ is taken to be $p_0(1 - p_0)/n_k$ in both Type I error and power calculations, whereas a variance of $p_A(1 - p_A)/n_k$ should be used to calculate the power under the alternative $p = p_A$. In the example of Section 3.6.1, a test of H_0: $p = p_0 = 0.6$ with Type I error probability $\alpha = 0.05$ and power $1 - \beta = 0.9$ at $p = p_0 \pm 0.2$ has up to four groups of 19 observations each, and H_0 is rejected at analysis k if $|Z_k| \geq C_P(4, 0.05) = 2.361$, $k = 1, \ldots, 4$. Using the normal approximation with $Var(X_i) = p_A(1 - p_A) = 0.16$, the power at $p = p_A = 0.8$ is found to be 0.939, in contrast to the value 0.906 obtained under the assumption $Var(X_i) = p_0(1 - p_0) = 0.24$ which was used to calculate the group size of 19.

The same difficulties arise when using normal approximations to apply the one-sided tests of Chapter 4 to binary data. One common method of handling data whose variance is a function of the mean is to use a variance stabilizing transformation. For binary data, one would work with $\arcsin\sqrt{(\hat{p}^{(k)})}$ in place of $\hat{p}^{(k)}$, but even then this method is still approximate. Fortunately, it is possible to use exact methods for Bernoulli data, and we shall now describe these.

12.1.2 Exact Calculations for Binary Data

Since the cumulative numbers of successes, S_k, take integer values, it is easier to perform calculations in terms of these variables than the standardized statistics, Z_k, used previously. The two-sided and one-sided procedures of Chapters 3 and 4 are then determined by the maximum number of stages K, the numbers of observations to be taken at each stage $(m_1, \ldots, m_K)$ and critical values for the $S_1, \ldots, S_K$. A general two-sided test has the form:

$$
\begin{array}{ll}
\text{After group } k = 1, \ldots, K-1 & \\
\quad \text{if } S_k \le a_k \text{ or } S_k \ge b_k & \text{stop, reject } H_0 \\
\quad \text{otherwise} & \text{continue to group } k+1, \\
\text{after group } K & \\
\quad \text{if } S_K \le a_K \text{ or } S_K \ge b_K & \text{stop, reject } H_0 \\
\quad \text{otherwise} & \text{stop, accept } H_0.
\end{array}
\tag{12.2}
$$

A one-sided test of H_0: $p = p_0$ against $p > p_0$ has the general form:

$$
\begin{array}{ll}
\text{After group } k = 1, \ldots, K-1 & \\
\quad \text{if } S_k \le a_k & \text{stop, accept } H_0 \\
\quad \text{if } S_k \ge b_k & \text{stop, reject } H_0 \\
\quad \text{otherwise} & \text{continue to group } k+1, \\
\text{after group } K & \\
\quad \text{if } S_K \le a_K & \text{stop, accept } H_0 \\
\quad \text{if } S_K \ge b_K & \text{stop, reject } H_0.
\end{array}
\tag{12.3}
$$

In this case a_K must equal $b_K - 1$ to ensure a final decision. One-sided tests against $p < p_0$ are similar but with the inequalities reversed. Note that these boundaries are defined in terms of sample sums and the critical values a_k and b_k are set on the S-scale, not on the Z-scale as before.

Calculations for obtaining the operating characteristic and sample size distribution of a group sequential test for binary data are described by Schultz et al. (1973). Similar calculations appear earlier in the quality control literature on multi-stage acceptance sampling for attributes; see, for example, Wilson & Burgess (1971) and MIL-STD-105E (1989).

The number of successes in stage k has a binomial distribution with parameters m_k and p, which we denote $B_{m_k}(y, p)$. Thus

$$B_{m_k}(y, p) = \binom{m_k}{y} p^y (1-p)^{m_k - y}, \quad 0 \le y \le m_k, \tag{12.4}$$

and $B_{m_k}(y, p) = 0$ otherwise. We define $C_k(y, p)$ to be the probability of reaching stage k with $S_k = y$ when the success probability is p. At stage 1, $C_1(y, p) = B_{m_1}(y, p)$ for $0 \le y \le m_1$ and the following recursive formulae, analogous to (8.6) in the normal case, relate C_k to C_{k-1} for $k = 2, \ldots, K$. Let

$E_k(y) = \max(a_{k-1}+1, y-m_k)$ and $F_k(y) = \min(b_{k-1}-1, y)$; then

$$C_k(y, p) = \sum_{j=E_k(y)}^{F_k(y)} C_{k-1}(j, p) B_{m_k}(y-j, p), \quad y = 0, \ldots, n_k. \tag{12.5}$$

The probabilities of crossing the lower and upper boundaries at stage k are, respectively,

$$r_k^L(p) = \sum_{y=0}^{a_k} C_k(y, p) \quad \text{and} \quad r_k^U(p) = \sum_{y=b_k}^{n_k} C_k(y, p). \tag{12.6}$$

Let $\pi(p)$ denote a test's power function, the probability of rejecting H_0 as a function of p. Then, for a one-sided test,

$$\pi(p) = \sum_{k=1}^{K} r_k^U(p), \tag{12.7}$$

while the power function of a two-sided test is

$$\pi(p) = \sum_{k=1}^{K} \{r_k^U(p) + r_k^L(p)\} = 1 - \sum_{y=a_K+1}^{b_K-1} C_K(y, p). \tag{12.8}$$

For both types of test, the Type I error probability is given by $\pi(p_0)$ and the expected sample size or average sample number (ASN) is

$$ASN(p) = \sum_{k=1}^{K-1} n_k r_k(p) + n_K \{1 - \sum_{k=1}^{K-1} r_k(p)\}, \tag{12.9}$$

where $r_k(p) = r_k^U(p) + r_k^L(p)$ is the probability of stopping at the kth stage, $k = 1, \ldots, K$.

To illustrate these calculations, consider the test with up to four groups of 19 observations described in Section 12.1.1. The procedure specified that sampling should stop with rejection of H_0: $p = 0.6$ if $|Z_k| \geq 2.361$ at any stage $k = 1, 2, 3$ or 4. This criterion corresponds to critical numbers for the S_k of $(a_1, b_1) = (6, 17)$, $(a_2, b_2) = (15, 30)$, $(a_3, b_3) = (25, 43)$ and $(a_4, b_4) = (35, 56)$. Evaluating (12.8), we find the exact Type I error rate of the test to be $\pi(0.6) = 0.0517$, and at 0.6 ± 0.2 it has power $\pi(0.4) = 0.905$ and $\pi(0.8) = 0.946$. From (12.9), the ASNs at $p = 0.4$, 0.6 and 0.8 are 43.97, 74.24 and 42.36, respectively.

In choosing boundary values $\{(a_k, b_k); k = 1, \ldots, K\}$ for a one-sided or two-sided test, a useful strategy is to start with a procedure based on the normal approximation and find the precise error rates for that design by exact calculation. If these are acceptable, the test can be adopted, but if they are not, the design can be modified and its error rates checked again until a satisfactory test is obtained. Fleming (1982) has catalogued a collection of one-sided tests with two and three groups of observations for use in Phase II clinical trials. The procedures are for testing H_0: $p = p_0$ versus $p > p_0$ with particular interest in the power at $p = p_A$ for pairs $(p_0, p_A) = (0.05, 0.2), (0.1, 0.3), (0.2, 0.4)$ and $(0.3, 0.5)$. All tests have Type I error probability of approximately 0.05, their maximum sample sizes range

Table 12.1 *Selected two-stage and three-stage one-sided binomial tests of H_0: $p = p_0$ versus $p \geq p_0$ taken from Fleming (1982). All tests are designed to have Type I error probability approximately equal to $\alpha = 0.05$ and power at $p = p_A$ approximately $1 - \beta = 0.9$. Exact Type I error probabilities and power are as tabulated.*

Two-stage procedures

Plan:	1	2	3	4
(p_0, p_A)	(0.05, 0.2)	(0.1, 0.3)	(0.2, 0.4)	(0.3, 0.5)
n_K	40	35	45	50
Type I error rate	0.052	0.053	0.055	0.048
Power	0.922	0.920	0.909	0.894
(a_1, b_1, m_1)	(0, 4, 20)	(2, 6, 20)	(5, 10, 25)	(7, 14, 25)
(a_2, b_2, m_2)	(4, 5, 20)	(6, 7, 15)	(13, 14, 20)	(20, 21, 25)

Three-stage procedures

Plan:	5	6	7	8
(p_0, p_A)	(0.05, 0.2)	(0.1, 0.3)	(0.2, 0.4)	(0.3, 0.5)
n_K	40	35	45	50
Type I error rate	0.046	0.063	0.057	0.049
Power	0.913	0.929	0.907)	0.887
(a_1, b_1, m_1)	(–, 4, 15)	(0, 5, 15)	(1, 8, 15)	(5, 12, 20)
(a_2, b_2, m_2)	(2, 5, 15)	(3, 6, 10)	(7,11, 15)	(12, 17, 15)
(a_3, b_3, m_3)	(4, 5, 10)	(6, 7, 10)	(13, 14, 15)	(20, 21, 15)

from 15 to 50, and their boundaries are similar in shape to those of the symmetric power family tests with parameter $\Delta = 0$ described in Section 4.2. Fleming (1982, Table 2) lists the exact Type I error probability, power and expected sample sizes under p_0 and p_A. Eight of these plans, all of which have approximate power 90% at $p = p_A$, are shown in Table 12.1.

12.1.3 *Exact Methods for Inference upon Termination*

A P-value or a confidence interval for p upon termination of a group sequential test can be constructed in a fashion analogous to that described in Sections 8.4 and 8.5 for normally distributed outcomes. Inferences are based on the sufficient statistic pair (T, S_T), where $T \in \{1, \ldots, K\}$ is the stage at which the test stops and $S_T = X_1 + \ldots + X_{n_T}$ is the number of successes observed by this point. Suppose we are using a one-sided test or a two-sided test with no inner wedge and we adopt the stage-wise ordering of outcomes (T, Z_T) specified by (A) in Section 8.4. It is straightforward to restate this ordering in terms of S_T rather than the standardized statistic Z_T. For a boundary of the form (12.2) or (12.3) defined through critical values $\{(a_k, b_k); k = 1, \ldots, K\}$ on the S-scale, we say $(k', s') \succ (k, s)$ if any one of the following three conditions holds:

$$\begin{array}{ll} (i) & k' = k \text{ and } s' \geq s, \\ (ii) & k' < k \text{ and } s' \geq b_{k'}, \\ (iii) & k' > k \text{ and } s \leq a_k. \end{array}$$

Let (k^*, s^*) be the observed value of (T, S_T). We can use the formulae developed in Section 12.1.2 to compute a one-sided upper P-value as

$$Pr_{p=p_0}\{(T, S_T) \succeq (k^*, s^*)\}$$

and a one-sided lower P-value as

$$Pr_{p=p_0}\{(T, S_T) \preceq (k^*, s^*)\}.$$

The two-sided P-value is twice the smaller of these two quantities. As an example, suppose the test terminates by exiting the upper boundary or by reaching the final analysis K; then the one-sided upper P-value is

$$Pr_{p=p_0}\{(T, S_T) \succeq (k^*, s^*)\} = \sum_{k=1}^{k^*-1} r_k^U(p_0) + \sum_{y=s^*}^{n_{k^*}} C_{k^*}(y, p_0),$$

where the $r_k^U(p_0)$, $k = 1, \ldots, k^* - 1$, and $C_{k^*}(y, p_0)$ are as defined in Section 12.1.2.

Derivation of a $(1-\alpha)$-level confidence interval for p is analogous to that for a normal mean in Section 8.5. The confidence interval is (p_L, p_U) where the lower and upper limits satisfy

$$Pr_{p=p_L}\{(T, S_T) \succeq (k^*, s^*)\} = \alpha/2 \qquad (12.10)$$

and

$$Pr_{p=p_U}\{(T, S_T) \preceq (k^*, s^*)\} = \alpha/2. \qquad (12.11)$$

Computation of p_L and p_U necessitates calculations similar to those for a one-sided P-value but repeated over a succession of values of p in order to find solutions to (12.10) and (12.11). Further details may be found in Jennison & Turnbull (1983), who list, in their Table 6, 80%, 90% and 95% confidence intervals for p following all possible outcomes of the three-stage designs described in Table 12.1. The same paper also tabulates 90%, 95% and 99% intervals for various multi-stage plans described in MIL-STD-105E (1989).

The 90% confidence intervals for p following three-stage plan number 6 of Table 12.1 are shown in Tables 12.2 and 12.3 in the column headed "Terminal"; these values were taken from Jennison & Turnbull (1983). For comparison, 90% confidence intervals calculated as if the same data had arisen in a fixed sample test are also listed in the column headed "Fixed". These fixed sample intervals, (p_{Lf}, p_{Uf}) say, can be obtained from the formulae

$$p_{Lf} = \frac{S_k}{S_k + (n_k - S_k + 1)\, F_{2(n_k - S_k+1),\, 2S_k}(\alpha/2)}$$

Table 12.2 90% *confidence intervals following a three-stage sampling plan*

Stage k	n_k	S_k	*Action**	*Fixed*	*Terminal*	*RCI*
1	15	0	Acc	(.000, .181)	(.000, .181)	(.000, .239)
1	15	1	Cont	(.003, .279)	‡	(.001, .342)
1	15	2	Cont	(.024, .363)	‡	(.013, .427)
1	15	3	Cont	(.057, .440)	‡	(.037, .503)
1	15	4	Cont	(.097, .511)	‡	(.069, .572)
1	15	5	Rej	(.142, .577)	(.142, .577)	(.107, .636)
1	15	6	Rej	(.191, .640)	(.191, .640)	(.150, .696)
1	15	7	Rej	(.244, .700)	(.244, .700)	(.197, .752)
1	15	8	Rej	(.300, .756)	(.300, .756)	(.248, .803)
1	15	9	Rej	(.360, .809)	(.360, .809)	(.304, .850)
1	15	10	Rej	(.423, .858)	(.423, .858)	(.364, .893)
1	15	11	Rej	(.489, .903)	(.489, .903)	(.428, .931)
1	15	12	Rej	(.560, .943)	(.560, .943)	(.497, .963)
1	15	13	Rej	(.637, .976)	(.637, .976)	(.573, .987)
1	15	14	Rej	(.721, .997)	(.721, .997)	(.658, .999)
1	15	15	Rej	(.819, 1.00)	(.819, 1.00)	(.761, 1.00)
2	25	0	‡	(.000, .113)	‡	(.000, .151)
2	25	1	Acc	(.002, .176)	(.003, .199)	(.001, .219)
2	25	2	Acc	(.014, .231)	(.016, .238)	(.010, .267)
2	25	3	Acc	(.034, .282)	(.034, .284)	(.024, .325)
2	25	4	Cont	(.057, .330)	‡	(.042, .367)
2	25	5	Cont	(.082, .375)	‡	(.069, .419)
2	25	6	Rej	(.110, .420)	(.108, .412)	(.092, .458)
2	25	7	Rej	(.139, .462)	(.127, .445)	(.116, .503)
2	25	8	Rej	(.170, .504)	(.137, .470)	(.150, .543)
2	25	9	Rej	(.202, .544)	(.141, .489)	(.176, .576)
2	25	10	Rej	(.236, .583)	(.142, .501)	(.204, .622)
2	25	11	Rej	(.270, .621)	(.142, .508)	(.243, .654)
2	25	12	Rej	(.305, .659)	(.142, .510)	(.272, .696)
2	25	13	Rej	(.341, .695)	(.142, .511)	(.304, .728)
2	25	14	Rej	(.379, .730)	(.142, .511)	(.346, .757)
2	25	15	‡	(.417, .764)	‡	(.378, .796)
2	25	16	‡	(.456, .798)	‡	(.424, .824)
2	25	17	‡	(.496, .830)	‡	(.457, .850)
2	25	18	‡	(.538, .861)	‡	(.497, .884)
2	25	19	‡	(.580, .890)	‡	(.542, .908)
2	25	20	‡	(.625, .918)	‡	(.581, .931)
2	25	21	‡	(.670, .943)	‡	(.633, .958)
2	25	22	‡	(.718, .966)	‡	(.675, .976)
2	25	23	‡	(.769, .986)	‡	(.733, .990)
2	25	24	‡	(.824, .998)	‡	(.781, .999)
2	25	25	‡	(.887, 1.00)	‡	(.849, 1.00)

* Key: Rej = reject H_0, Acc = accept H_0, Cont = continue to next stage.
‡ Stopping is impossible here under the prescribed plan.

Table 12.3 90% *confidence intervals following a three-stage sampling plan (continued)*

Stage k	n_k	S_k	*Action**	*Fixed*	*Terminal*	*RCI*
3	35	0	‡	(.000, .082)	‡	(.000, .110)
3	35	1	‡	(.001, .129)	‡	(.001, .151)
3	35	2	‡	(.010, .169)	‡	(.008, .200)
3	35	3	‡	(.024, .207)	‡	(.019, .232)
3	35	4	Acc	(.040, .243)	(.057, .286)	(.033, .267)
3	35	5	Acc	(.058, .277)	(.066, .297)	(.047, .307)
3	35	6	Acc	(.077, .311)	(.081, .315)	(.069, .336)
3	35	7	Rej	(.098, .343)	(.095, .335)	(.088, .367)
3	35	8	Rej	(.119, .375)	(.104, .351)	(.107, .404)
3	35	9	Rej	(.141, .406)	(.107, .363)	(.125, .429)
3	35	10	Rej	(.164, .436)	(.108, .369)	(.150, .458)
3	35	11	Rej	(.187, .466)	(.108, .372)	(.173, .496)
3	35	12	Rej	(.211, .496)	(.108, .373)	(.195, .520)
3	35	13	Rej	(.236, .524)	(.108, .374)	(.214, .545)
3	35	14	Rej	(.260, .553)	(.108, .374)	(.243, .576)
3	35	15	Rej	(.286, .581)	(.108, .374)	(.268, .606)
3	35	16	‡	(.312, .608)	‡	(.291, .631)
3	35	17	‡	(.338, .635)	‡	(.312, .654)
3	35	18	‡	(.365, .662)	‡	(.346, .688)
3	35	19	‡	(.392, .688)	‡	(.369, .709)
3	35	20	‡	(.419, .714)	‡	(.394, .732)
3	35	21	‡	(.447, .740)	‡	(.424, .757)
3	35	22	‡	(.476, .764)	‡	(.455, .786)
3	35	23	‡	(.504, .789)	‡	(.480, .805)
3	35	24	‡	(.534, .813)	‡	(.504, .827)
3	35	25	‡	(.564, .836)	‡	(.542, .850)
3	35	26	‡	(.594, .859)	‡	(.571, .875)
3	35	27	‡	(.625, .881)	‡	(.596, .893)
3	35	28	‡	(.657, .902)	‡	(.633, .912)
3	35	29	‡	(.689, .923)	‡	(.664, .931)
3	35	30	‡	(.723, .942)	‡	(.693, .953)
3	35	31	‡	(.757, .960)	‡	(.733, .967)
3	35	32	‡	(.793, .976)	‡	(.768, .981)
3	35	33	‡	(.831, .990)	‡	(.800, .992)
3	35	34	‡	(.871, .999)	‡	(.849, ,999)
3	35	35	‡	(.918, 1.00)	‡	(.890, 1.00)

* Key: Rej = reject H_0, Acc = accept H_0, Cont = continue to next stage.
‡ Stopping is impossible here under the prescribed plan.

and

$$p_{U_f} = \frac{(S_k + 1)\, F_{2(S_k+1),\, 2(n_k - S_k)}(\alpha/2)}{(n_k - S_k) + (S_k + 1)\, F_{2(S_k+1),\, 2(n_k - S_k)}(\alpha/2)}$$

with the adjustment that p_{L_f} is set equal to 0 if $S_k = 0$ and p_{U_f} to 1 if $S_k = n_k$. Here, $F_{\nu_1, \nu_2}(q)$ denotes the value exceeded with probability q by an F-statistic on ν_1 and ν_2 degrees of freedom. The above confidence limits arise from the relation between the binomial, beta and F distributions (see, for example, Bowker & Lieberman, 1972, p. 467), that the p_{L_f} and p_{U_f} so defined satisfy

$$\sum_{i=S_k}^{n_k} \binom{n_k}{i} p_{L_f}^i (1 - p_{L_f})^{n_k - i} = \alpha/2$$

and

$$\sum_{i=0}^{S_k} \binom{n_k}{i} p_{U_f}^i (1 - p_{U_f})^{n_k - i} = \alpha/2.$$

Of course, for tests with $K \geq 2$ stages, (p_{L_f}, p_{U_f}) does not have the correct coverage probability $1 - \alpha$. However, under the sample space ordering (A), which we are using here, if the procedure stops at stage $k = 1$, the fixed sample interval coincides with that constructed taking into account the group sequential design. Rows in Tables 12.2 and 12.3 containing the symbol ‡ represent outcomes that cannot be reached under the prescribed plan, either because the sampling rule specifies continuation to the next stage or because the outcome implies that stopping would have occurred at an earlier stage. The last column, headed "RCI", concerns repeated confidence intervals for p which we shall discuss in Section 12.1.4.

In the above construction of confidence intervals for p on termination of a group sequential test, equal error probabilities, $\alpha/2$, are allocated to each tail of the interval. In a fixed sample analysis, this approach is referred to as the Clopper-Pearson (1934) method, and this was the method used to obtain the fixed sample intervals in Tables 12.2 and 12.3. For the fixed sample problem, Sterne (1954) proposed an alternative method based on inverting a family of tests of $p = p_0$ versus $p \neq p_0$ whose acceptance regions $\mathcal{A}(p_0)$ have probability content under p_0 of at least $1 - \alpha$ and consist of the most probable outcomes under $p = p_0$. Duffy & Santner (1987) have extended Sterne's method to multi-stage designs and their Tables 2a to 2d enumerate intervals for the three-stage designs of Table 12.1. Duffy & Santner (1987, p. 89) note that their generalization suffers from several awkward features: interval endpoints are not necessarily non-decreasing with S_T, intervals may consist of just a single point, and computation of the intervals is not completely automated. Crow (1956) and Blyth & Still (1983) proposed a modification to Sterne's procedure which ensures interval confidence sets for p, and Duffy & Santner (1987, Section 4) have extended this method to multi-stage designs, producing confidence intervals without the awkward features noted above. Duffy & Santner do not provide tables, but Coe & Tamhane (1993, Table 2) list 90% intervals for the three-stage plan number 6 in our Table 12.1. In comparing different types of confidence interval, Coe & Tamhane note that those of Jennison & Turnbull (1983) tend to be wider and more conservative than the intervals obtained by Duffy & Santner's extension of the Crow-Blyth-Still method, although Jennison & Turnbull's intervals are perhaps easier to compute. It should also be noted that it may be inappropriate from a practical standpoint to exchange error probability freely between tails of a two-sided test or confidence interval when the errors associated with the two tails have quite different consequences. Although different in nature to confidence intervals upon termination, Coe & Tamhane also draw comparisons with repeated confidence intervals, the topic of our next section.

12.1.4 Repeated Confidence Intervals for a Bernoulli Probability p

Recall from Chapter 9 that a $(1-\alpha)$-level sequence of RCIs for the parameter p is a sequence of K intervals, $I_1, \ldots, I_K$, with the property that, for all p,

$$Pr_p\{p \in I_k \text{ for all } k = 1, \ldots, K)\} = 1 - \alpha. \tag{12.12}$$

Although RCIs can be used to define a group sequential stopping rule, their definition does not rely on any specific stopping rule being implemented. It is straightforward to use the normal approximation to construct such a sequence; see Jennison & Turnbull (1989, Section 5.1). At stage k the standardized statistic for testing a hypothesized success probability p is

$$Z_k(p) = \frac{S_k - n_k p}{\sqrt{\{n_k p(1-p)\}}}$$

and RCIs are given by

$$I_k = (p_{Lk}, p_{Uk}) = \{p\colon |Z_k(p)| \le c_k\}, \quad k = 1, \ldots, K, \tag{12.13}$$

where $c_1, \ldots, c_K$ are critical values of a group sequential test with two-sided error probability α, termed the *parent* test in Chapter 9. With equal group sizes, we could use the Pocock or O'Brien & Fleming tests defined by constants in Tables 2.1 and 2.3, or we could use any of the other tests described in Chapter 2. If group sizes are unequal, the same critical values $c_1, \ldots, c_K$ can be used to give an approximate method, as described in Section 3.3, or the more accurate treatment based on the error spending approach of Chapter 7 may be preferred. In general, the choice of parent test should reflect the use anticipated for the RCIs in deciding when a group sequential study should terminate. Note that even though the information $\mathcal{I}_k = n_k/\{p(1-p)\}$ depends on p (see Section 3.6.1), the correlations $Corr(Z_{k_1}(p), Z_{k_2}(p)) = \sqrt{(n_{k_1}/n_{k_2})}$, $1 \le k_1 \le k_2 \le K$, do not and hence the same sequence of constants $\{c_1, \ldots, c_K\}$ is applicable for all values of p.

Use of the normal approximation in constructing RCIs for p gives rise to the same difficulties noted in Section 12.1.1. Computation of exact RCIs for p is therefore desirable, and we shall adopt an error spending approach (see Section 7.2.1) in doing this. We start by specifying positive constants $\pi_1, \ldots, \pi_K$ summing to α, which represent the probability that a parent test should reject a hypothesized value of p at analyses $1, \ldots, K$. Then, for each value of p_0 we create a two-sided test of H_0: $p = p_0$ of the form (12.2) with critical values $a_k = a_k(p_0)$

and $b_k = b_k(p_0)$, $k = 1, \ldots, K$, defined for this particular p_0. Specifically, we choose the $a_k(p_0)$ to be the largest integers such that $r_k^L(p_0) \le \pi_k/2$ and the $b_k(p_0)$ the smallest integers such that $r_k^U(p_0) \le \pi_k/2$, where $r_k^L(p)$ and $r_k^U(p)$ are defined by (12.6). This family of tests, indexed by p_0, is then inverted to obtain the sequence of RCIs, as in Chapter 9. Since the π_k sum to α, each test in this family has two-sided Type I error probability of at most α; i.e., for each p_0,

$$Pr_{p=p_0}\{a_k(p_0) < S_k < b_k(p_0) \text{ for } k = 1, \ldots, K\}$$

$$\ge 1 - (\pi_1 + \ldots + \pi_K) = 1 - \alpha.$$

As the event $\{a_k(p) < S_k < b_k(p)\}$ corresponds exactly to the event that p_0 is contained in the kth RCI, it follows that the RCIs attain the confidence level $1-\alpha$ conservatively.

Coe & Tamhane (1993) note that if interval endpoints are required to be accurate to three decimal places, it suffices to determine whether each of the values $p_0 = 0.0005, 0.0015, 0.0025, \ldots, 0.9995$ is in each RCI and symmetry can be used to limit computations further to one half of these values with, say, $p_0 < 0.5$. The recursive method of calculation described in Section 12.1.2 may be used here to compute the values $a_k(p_0)$ and $b_k(p_0)$, $k = 1, \ldots, K$, for each p_0. We have followed this approach in calculating RCIs for outcomes arising in the three-stage plan number 6 of Table 12.1. The resulting 90% RCIs with error probability divided between the three stages as $\pi_1 = 0.0333$, $\pi_2 = 0.0334$ and $\pi_3 = 0.0333$ are listed in Tables 12.2 and 12.3 in the column headed "RCI". Since RCIs are valid and can be computed whether or not any particular stopping rule is adhered to, entries for RCIs appear in rows marked with a ‡ corresponding to outcomes that cannot occur under the original stopping rule. In contrast, the fixed sample intervals are not valid in the frequentist sense under any sequential stopping rule.

Construction of RCIs for a Bernoulli probability p using exact binomial calculations was first proposed by Coe & Tamhane (1993). The procedure described above produces equal-tailed intervals, analogous to the Clopper-Pearson method for a fixed sample experiment, whereas Coe & Tamhane used a group sequential adaptation of the Blyth & Still modification to Sterne's fixed sample construction, resulting in intervals with unequal tail probabilities but of shorter width. Comparison of the RCIs in Tables 12.2 and 12.3 with those in Table 1 of Coe & Tamhane (1993) shows that the two types of RCI do differ, but not to an extent that is likely to be of great practical significance .

12.2 Two Bernoulli Probabilities

12.2.1 Exact Calculations of Operating Characteristics

We turn now to the problem of comparing two treatment arms, A and B, with respect to a binary outcome. We assume responses $X_{A1}, X_{A2}, \ldots$ from subjects receiving treatment A are independent and distributed as Bernoulli $B(p_A)$ and, similarly, responses $X_{B1}, X_{B2}, \ldots$ on arm B are independent, Bernoulli $B(p_B)$.

We shall consider tests of the null hypothesis H_0: $p_A = p_B$ against either a two-sided alternative H_A: $p_A \neq p_B$ or a one-sided alternative such as H_A: $p_A > p_B$.

We suppose the data are collected group sequentially with a maximum of K stages. For treatment arm A, the kth group size is m_{Ak} and the cumulative sample size $n_{Ak} = m_{A1} + \ldots + m_{Ak}$, and we denote the cumulative number of successes by $S_{Ak} = X_{A1} + \ldots + X_{Ak}$. The quantities m_{Bk}, n_{Bk}, and S_{Bk}, $k = 1, \ldots, K$, are defined analogously for treatment B.

For a given sequence of sample sizes n_{Ak} and n_{Bk}, we can define a group sequential test based on successive pairs (S_{Ak}, S_{Bk}) in terms of decision regions and a continuation region at each stage. For each $k = 1, \ldots, K$, we let $\Omega_k = \{0, 1, \ldots, n_{Ak}\} \times \{0, 1, \ldots, n_{Bk}\}$ denote the set of possible values for (S_{Ak}, S_{Bk}) and we partition Ω_k into three mutually exclusive and exhaustive sets, $\mathcal{C}_k$, $\mathcal{A}_{0k}$ and $\mathcal{A}_{Ak}$. The group sequential test of H_0: $p_a = p_B$ is then:

$$
\begin{array}{lll}
\text{After group } k = 1, \ldots, K & & \\
\quad \text{if } (S_{Ak}, S_{Bk}) \in \mathcal{A}_{0k} & \text{stop and decide } H_0, \\
\quad \text{if } (S_{Ak}, S_{Bk}) \in \mathcal{A}_{Ak} & \text{stop and decide } H_A, \\
\quad \text{if } (S_{Ak}, S_{Bk}) \in \mathcal{C}_k & \text{continue to stage } k+1,
\end{array}
$$

where $\mathcal{C}_K = \emptyset$, the empty set, to ensure stopping by stage K. This formulation includes one-sided tests and two-sided tests with and without inner wedges to permit early stopping to accept H_0. In a two-sided test with no inner wedge, $\mathcal{A}_{0k} = \emptyset$ for $k = 1, \ldots, K-1$.

Exact formulae for a procedure's operating characteristics can be written down in a fashion analogous to that for the one-sample problem of Section 12.1.2. Let $C_k(y_A, y_B; p_A, p_B)$ be the probability under p_A and p_B of reaching stage k with $S_{Ak} = y_A$ and $S_{Bk} = y_B$. Then $C_1(y_A, y_B; p_A, p_B) = B_{m_{A1}}(y_A, p_A) \times B_{m_{B1}}(y_B, p_B)$, for $y_A = 0, \ldots, n_{A1}$ and $y_B = 0, \ldots, n_{B1}$, where $B_{m_k}(y, p)$ is the binomial probability mass function as defined in (12.4). For $k = 2, \ldots, K$, the following recursive formulae are analogous to (8.6) in the normal case:

$$
C_k(y_A, y_B; p_A, p_B) =
$$

$$
\sum_{(i,j) \in \mathcal{C}_{k-1}} \sum C_{k-1}(i, j; p_A, p_B) \times B_{m_{Ak}}(y_A - i, p_A) \times B_{m_{Bk}}(y_B - j, p_B)
$$

$$
\text{for } y_A = 0, \ldots, n_{Ak}, \; y_B = 0, \ldots, n_{Bk}. \tag{12.14}
$$

Recall that $B_m(y, p) = 0$ unless $y = 0, \ldots, m$, so there is no problem in having $y_A - i$ or $y_B - i$ negative or greater than m_{Ak} or m_{Bk}, respectively, in the above formula.

The expected total sample size is given by

$$
\sum_{k=1}^{K} \left\{ (n_{Ak} + n_{Bk}) \sum_{(i,j) \notin \mathcal{C}_k} \sum C_k(i, j; p_A, p_B) \right\} \tag{12.15}
$$

and the power function $\pi(p_A, p_B)$, the probability of rejecting H_0 as a function of p_A and p_B, by

$$\pi(p_A, p_B) = \sum_{k=1}^{K} \sum\sum_{(i,j) \in \mathcal{A}_{Ak}} C_k(i, j; p_A, p_B). \tag{12.16}$$

We define the size of the test to be its maximum Type I error probability over values of p_A and p_B satisfying H_0: $p_A = p_B$, i.e.,

$$\sup_{p_A = p_B} \pi(p_A, p_B). \tag{12.17}$$

The quantities (12.15), (12.16) and (12.17) can be evaluated for any group sequential design. As an example, consider the test discussed by O'Brien & Fleming (1979, Section 5) which has three stages and group sizes $m_{A1} = m_{A2} = m_{A3} = 7$ on treatment A and $m_{B1} = m_{B2} = m_{B3} = 14$ on treatment B. As explained in Section 3.6.2, the standardized statistics for testing H_0: $p_A = p_B$ at analyses $k = 1, 2$ and 3 are

$$\begin{aligned} Z_k &= (\hat{p}_A^{(k)} - \hat{p}_B^{(k)})\sqrt{\widehat{\mathcal{I}}_k} \\ &= \left(\frac{S_{Ak}}{n_{AK}} - \frac{S_{Bk}}{n_{BK}} \right) \left\{ (n_{Ak}^{-1} + n_{Bk}^{-1})\, \tilde{p}_k\, (1 - \tilde{p}_k) \right\}^{-1/2}, \end{aligned} \tag{12.18}$$

where $\tilde{p}_k = (S_{Ak} + S_{Bk})/(n_{Ak} + n_{Bk})$. A two-sided O'Brien & Fleming test (with no early stopping to accept H_0) rejects H_0 at stage k if

$$|Z_k| \geq C_B(3, 0.05)\sqrt{(3/k)} = 2.004\sqrt{(3/k)}.$$

Thus the test has continuation regions

$$\mathcal{C}_k = \{(S_{Ak}, S_{Bk}) \colon |Z_k| < 2.004\sqrt{(3/k)}\}$$

at analyses $k = 1$ and 2 and acceptance region of H_0

$$\mathcal{A}_{03} = \{(S_{A3}, S_{B3}) \colon |Z_3| < 2.004\}$$

at the third and final analysis.

The sets $\mathcal{C}_k$, $\mathcal{A}_{0k}$ and $\mathcal{A}_{Ak}$ can be evaluated in terms of the pairs (S_{Ak}, S_{Bk}) that each contains. As an example, at stage 1, the continuation region contains outcomes satisfying $|Z_1| < 3.471$, and if $S_{A1} = 0$ this requires $S_{B1} \leq 11$; if $S_{A1} = 1$ this requires $S_{B1} \leq 12$, etc. The continuation regions, $\mathcal{C}_1$ and $\mathcal{C}_2$, of this test and the final acceptance region $\mathcal{A}_{03}$ are shown in Table 12.4.

Using the recursion (12.14) to evaluate (12.16) with $p_A = p_B = p$ over a fine grid of values p we find the exact size of this test, as defined by (12.17), to be 0.0536 rather than the value 0.05, suggested by the normal approximation of Section 3.6.2. The same recursion can be used to evaluate the test at other values of p_A and p_B; for example, if $p_A = 0.4$ and $p_B = 0.1$, the test has power 0.797 and expected total sample size 53.30, and if $p_A = 0.1$ and $p_B = 0.4$, power is 0.743 and expected total sample size 56.86, showing some reduction in both cases below the maximum sample size of 63.

If it is desired to ensure that the test's maximum Type I error probability does not exceed 0.05, one could enlarge the acceptance region $\mathcal{A}_{03}$ at the final stage.

Table 12.4 *Continuation regions at analyses* 1 *and* 2 *and acceptance region at analysis* 3 *of a three-stage test of* H_0: $p_A = p_B$

Analysis 1	S_{A1}	S_{B1}	S_{A1}	S_{B1}
$\mathcal{C}_1 = \{(S_{A1}, S_{B1}): \lvert Z_1\rvert < 3.471\}$	0	0–11	4	0–14
	1	0–12	5	1–14
	2	0–13	6	2–14
	3	0–14	7	3–14
Analysis 2	S_{A2}	S_{B2}	S_{A2}	S_{B2}
$\mathcal{C}_2 = \{(S_{A2}, S_{B2}): \lvert Z_2\rvert < 2.454\}$	0	0–9	8	6–25
	1	0–12	9	8–26
	2	0–15	10	9–27
	3	1–17	11	11–27
	4	1–19	12	13–28
	5	2–20	13	16–28
	6	3–22	14	19–28
	7	5–23		
Analysis 3	S_{A3}	S_{B3}	S_{A3}	S_{B3}
$\mathcal{A}_{03} = \{(S_{A3}, S_{B3}): \lvert Z_3\rvert < 2.004\}$	0	0–7	11	12–32
	1	0–10	12	13–33
	2	1–13	13	15–35
	3	1–16	14	17–36
	4	2–18	15	19–38
	5	3–21	16	21–39
	6	4–23	17	24–40
	7	6–25	18	26–41
	8	7–27	19	29–41
	9	9–29	20	32–42
	10	10–30	21	35–42

Increasing the critical value for Z_3 from 2.004 to 2.036 accomplishes this, yielding an exact size of 0.0499 but reducing power to 0.792 at $(p_A, p_B) = (0.4, 0.1)$ and 0.734 at $(p_A, p_B) = (0.1, 0.4)$. The new acceptance region at stage 3 differs in just six entries from the previous one and is shown in Table 12.5.

As for the one-sample problem, we recommend a general strategy for designing a group sequential test whereby an initial design is chosen based on the normal approximation to the distribution of the standardized statistics Z_k and employing one of the testing boundaries described in Chapters 2 to 6. This test's exact operating characteristics can be computed from (12.15), (12.16) and 12.17) using the recursion (12.14). These properties are likely to be satisfactory for moderate or large group sizes, but if they are not, the initial design can be modified by trial and error until a satisfactory procedure is found. Lin, Wei & DeMets (1991) describe an alternative approach in which statistics Z_k, as defined in (12.18), are compared against critical values of the form used in Pocock or O'Brien & Fleming tests but

Table 12.5 *Acceptance region at analysis 3 of a modified three-stage test of* H_0: $p_A = p_B$

Analysis 3	S_{A3}	S_{B3}	S_{A3}	S_{B3}
$\mathcal{A}_{03} = \{(S_{A3}, S_{B3}): \lvert Z_3 \rvert < 2.036\}$	0	0–7	11	12–32
	1	0–10	12	13–34
	2	0–13	13	15–35
	3	1–16	14	17–36
	4	2–19	15	19–38
	5	3–21	16	21–39
	6	4–23	17	23–40
	7	6–25	18	26–41
	8	7–27	19	29–42
	9	8–29	20	32–42
	10	10–30	21	35–42

with new values of the constants C_P and C_B, chosen to ensure the tests have exact size no greater than α.

12.2.2 Exact Methods for Inference upon Termination

The methods of Section 12.1.3 are readily extended to the two-treatment problem. Suppose we are using a one-sided test or two-sided test with no inner wedge and we adopt the stage-wise ordering of the sample space as given by (A) in Section 8.4. Since the sufficient statistic (S_{Ak}, S_{Bk}) is two-dimensional, we still need to specify a criterion for ordering the sample space within each stage, and we shall order outcomes by the value of the standardized statistic Z_k given by (12.18).

We denote the upper part of the stopping region at stage k by $\mathcal{A}_k^+$ and the lower part by $\mathcal{A}_k^-$, for $k = 1, \ldots, K-1$. For a two-sided test of H_0: $p_A = p_B$ these regions are $\mathcal{A}_k^+ = \mathcal{A}_{Ak} \cap \{(S_{Ak}, S_{Bk}): Z_k > 0\}$ and $\mathcal{A}_k^- = \mathcal{A}_{Ak} \cap \{(S_{Ak}, S_{Bk}): Z_k < 0\}$; in the case of a one-sided test against $p_A > p_B$ they are $\mathcal{A}_k^+ = \mathcal{A}_{Ak}$ and $\mathcal{A}_k^- = \mathcal{A}_{0k}$, and these definitions are reversed when the alternative is $p_A < p_B$.

Let (k^*, z^*) denote the observed value of (T, Z_T). If (k^*, z^*) falls in the upper region, $\mathcal{A}_k^+$, or if $k^* = K$, we define

$$
\begin{aligned}
p_U(p_A, p_B) &= Pr_{(p_A, p_B)}\{(T, Z_T) \succeq (k^*, z^*)\} \\
&= \sum_{k=1}^{k^*} \sum_{(i,j) \in \mathcal{A}_k^+} \sum C_k(i, j; p_A, p_B) \\
&\quad + \sum_{\{(i,j) \in \Omega_{k^*}: Z_{k^*} \geq z^*\}} \sum C_{k^*}(i, j; p_A, p_B)
\end{aligned}
$$

and set $p_L(p_A, p_B) = 1 - p_U(p_A, p_B)$. If (k^*, z^*) falls in the lower region, $\mathcal{A}_k^-$, $p_L(p_A, p_B)$ is defined analogously to $p_U(p_A, p_B)$, but the two sums in the above expression are now over $\{(i, j) \in \mathcal{A}_k^-\}$ and $\{(i, j) \in \Omega_{k^*} : Z_{k^*} \leq z^*\}$. Again, $p_U(p_A, p_B) = 1 - p_L(p_A, p_B)$.

The above definitions imply that if the true success probabilities are $p_A = \tilde{p}_A$ and $p_B = \tilde{p}_B$ then, for any $0 < \epsilon < 1$,

$$Pr\{p_L(\tilde{p}_A, \tilde{p}_B) < \epsilon\} \leq \epsilon \quad \text{and} \quad Pr\{p_U(\tilde{p}_A, \tilde{p}_B) < \epsilon\} \leq \epsilon,$$

so $p_L(\tilde{p}_A, \tilde{p}_B)$ and $p_U(\tilde{p}_A, \tilde{p}_B)$ have the appropriate distribution to be P-values for testing H_0: $p_A = p_B$, with some conservatism due to the discreteness of the distribution of (T, Z_T). We shall use these two quantities as the basis for defining general P-values and confidence intervals.

Since the common success probability under H_0: $p_A = p_B$ is unknown, we allow for all possibilities in defining the one-sided upper and lower P-values for testing H_0 as

$$P_U = \sup_{p_A = p_B} p_U(p_A, p_B) \quad \text{and} \quad P_L = \sup_{p_A = p_B} p_L(p_A, p_B).$$

The two-sided P-value is twice the smaller of these two quantities.

Similar arguments show that a $(1 - \alpha)$-level confidence interval for the difference $\delta = p_A - p_B$ is (δ_L, δ_U) where

$$\sup_{p_A} p_U(p_A, p_A - \delta_L) = \alpha/2 \quad \text{and} \quad \sup_{p_A} p_L(p_A, p_A - \delta_U) = \alpha/2.$$

The suprema in these two equations are taken over $p_A \in [0, 1]$ such that $p_A - \delta_L \in [0, 1]$ and $p_A - \delta_U \in [0, 1]$, respectively. The roots δ_L and δ_U can be found by evaluating p_U and p_L over a grid of p_A and δ values.

The same approach can be taken to obtain a confidence interval for the ratio of two success probabilities or for their odds ratio. A $(1 - \alpha)$-level confidence interval for the ratio $\rho = p_A/p_B$ is (ρ_L, ρ_U) where

$$\sup_{p_A} p_U(p_A, p_A/\rho_L) = \alpha/2 \quad \text{and} \quad \sup_{p_A} p_L(p_A, p_A/\rho_U) = \alpha/2,$$

the suprema being taken over p_A values in the intervals $[0, \min(1, \rho_L)]$ and $[0, \min(1, \rho_U)]$, respectively. End points of a $(1 - \alpha)$-level confidence interval for the odds ratio $\phi = p_A(1 - p_B)/\{p_B(1 - p_A)\}$ are the solutions of

$$\sup_{p_A \in [0,1]} p_U\,(p_A, p_A/\{\phi_L(1 - p_A) + p_A\}) = \alpha/2$$

and

$$\sup_{p_A \in [0,1]} p_L\,(p_A, p_A/\{\phi_U(1 - p_A) + p_A\}) = \alpha/2.$$

12.2.3 Repeated Confidence Intervals

A $(1 - \alpha)$-level sequence of RCIs, $I_1, \ldots, I_K$, for the difference in success probabilities $\delta = p_A - p_B$ is required to have the property

$$Pr_{(p_A, p_B)}\{\delta \in I_k \text{ for all } k = 1, \ldots, K\} \geq 1 - \alpha \qquad (12.19)$$

for all p_A and p_B such that $p_A - p_B = \delta$. An approximate sequence obtained using a normal approximation is

$$I_k = (\hat{p}_A^{(k)} - \hat{p}_B^{(k)} \pm c_k \sqrt{\{\hat{p}_A^{(k)}(1 - \hat{p}_A^{(k)})/n_{Ak} + \hat{p}_B^{(k)}(1 - \hat{p}_B^{(k)})/n_{Bk}\}}),$$

where $\hat{p}_A^{(k)} = S_{Ak}/n_{Ak}$, $\hat{p}_B^{(k)} = S_{Bk}/n_{Bk}$ and $c_1, \ldots, c_K$ are the critical values of a group sequential test for normally distributed statistics with two-sided Type I error probability α. This "parent" test could be one of those described in Chapter 2, for example, that of Pocock or O'Brien & Fleming, but if increments in information are unequal and unpredictable, it is more accurate to define a test by the error spending approach of Chapter 7 with information levels estimated by

$$\mathcal{I}_k = \left\{ \frac{\hat{p}_A^{(k)}(1 - \hat{p}_A^{(k)})}{n_{Ak}} + \frac{\hat{p}_B^{(k)}(1 - \hat{p}_B^{(k)})}{n_{Bk}} \right\}^{-1}, \quad k = 1, \ldots, K.$$

We now turn to the construction of exact RCIs for $\delta = p_A - p_B$. We first specify positive constants $\pi_1, \ldots, \pi_K$, summing to α, to comprise the Type I error probabilities allocated at each analysis by the parent two-sided test. For each pair of probabilities (p_A^*, p_B^*), we form a group sequential test of H^*: $(p_A, p_B) = (p_A^*, p_B^*)$ which stops to reject H^* at stage $k = 1, \ldots, K$ if $Z_k \notin (a_k(p_A^*, p_B^*), b_k(p_A^*, p_B^*))$ and accepts H^* if stage K is reached without this hypothesis being rejected. Here the Z_k are the standardized statistics defined in (12.18), although these could be replaced by another choice of statistic such as $\hat{p}_A^{(k)} - \hat{p}_B^{(k)}$. For a fixed sequence of group sizes, the probabilities $C_k(y_A, y_B; p_A^*, p_B^*)$ defined in Section 12.2.1 can be used to construct critical values for the test of H^*. For each $k = 1, \ldots, K$, we take $a_k(p_A^*, p_B^*)$ to be the largest value of a_k such that

$$Pr_{(p_A^*, p_B^*)}\{a_j(p_A^*, p_B^*) < Z_j < b_j(p_A^*, p_B^*) \text{ for all } j = 1, \ldots, k-1 \text{ and } Z_k \le a_k\} \le \pi_k/2$$

and $b_k(p_A^*, p_B^*)$ is the smallest value of b_k satisfying

$$Pr_{(p_A^*, p_B^*)}\{a_j(p_A^*, p_B^*) < Z_j < b_j(p_A^*, p_B^*) \text{ for all } j = 1, \ldots, k-1 \text{ and } Z_k \ge b_k\} \le \pi_k/2.$$

By construction, the Type I error probability of this test of H^* does not exceed α. Let

$$a_k(\delta) = \inf_{p_A - p_B = \delta} a_k(p_A, p_B) \quad \text{and} \quad b_k(\delta) = \sup_{p_A - p_B = \delta} b_k(p_A, p_B)$$

for $k = 1, \ldots, K$; then, for any fixed δ between 0 and 1,

$$Pr_{(p_A, p_B)}\{a_k(\delta) < Z_k < b_k(\delta) \text{ for all } k = 1, \ldots, K\} \ge 1 - \alpha$$

whenever $p_A - p_B = \delta$. Thus, we have an acceptance region for testing a hypothesized value of δ at each stage $k = 1, \ldots, K$ with overall probability of wrong rejection of at most α. Inverting this family of group sequential tests of all possible values of δ, we obtain the RCI sequence

$$I_k = \{\delta : a_k(\delta) < Z_k < b_k(\delta)\}, \quad k = 1, \ldots, K.$$

Lin, Wei & DeMets (1991) present a similar construction, inverting a family of tests of $p_A - p_B = \delta$ of the same general form as their tests of $p_A - p_B = 0$.

In calculating these RCIs, consideration of any one δ requires the construction of group sequential boundaries at each of a grid of values for p_A. This requires a large amount of computation and there is a danger of numerical imprecision arising from the addition of a great many small probabilities; hence, this approach is only practicable for a small number of groups of fairly moderate size. Just as for confidence intervals upon termination, the above method can be adapted to give RCIs for the ratio or odds ratio between the success probabilities p_A and p_B .

The method we have described divides the error probability α equally between the two tails of each test of H^*: $(p_A, p_B) = (p_A^*, p_B^*)$ and, hence, between the two tails of the RCIs. Coe & Tamhane (1993) propose a construction based on a generalization of Blyth & Still's (1983) which is not equal tailed but which should result in somewhat narrower intervals. Computer programs implementing their procedure are available from Coe & Tamhane.

12.2.4 Conservatism Caused by Nuisance Parameters

The procedures we have described for comparing two Bernoulli distributions have an element of conservatism due to the need to guarantee appropriate properties under all values of a nuisance parameter. As an example, the size of an exact test of H_0: $p_A = p_B$, as defined in (12.17), may occur at a common value of p_A and p_B that is unlikely to be true.

One way to produce less conservative tests is to restrict the range of values of the nuisance parameter over which the various suprema are taken. An alternative approach is to operate adaptively, treating an estimate of the nuisance parameter at each stage as if it were exactly correct. We shall apply such adaptive methods in Chapter 14 to problems where the necessary sample size depends on unknown nuisance parameters. In Section 14.3.1 of that chapter we use the comparison of two Bernoulli probabilities to illustrate sample size re-estimation in error spending tests. It may sometimes be feasible to use exact calculation to check whether adaptive procedures attain their nominal properties accurately, but it is often simpler to use simulation to assess complex procedures.

12.3 The Odds Ratio and Multiple 2 × 2 Tables

A useful measure of the difference between two response probabilities p_A and p_B is the "odds ratio":

$$\psi = \frac{p_A(1 - p_B)}{p_B(1 - p_A)}.$$

This measure is used in the analysis of stratified two-by-two tables when it can be assumed that a common odds ratio occurs within each stratum. Of course, in the special case when there is only one stratum, this reduces to the problem of comparing two Bernoulli probabilities addressed in Section 12.2. We index the strata by $j = 1, \ldots, J$ and suppose that at the kth analysis n_{Ajk} and n_{Bjk} observations have accumulated in stratum j on treatments A and B, respectively, making $N_{jk} = n_{Ajk} + n_{Bjk}$ in total. All observations are assumed to be independent, with those on treatment A in stratum j distributed as $B(p_{Aj})$ and those on treatment B as $B(p_{Bj})$. For each analysis $k = 1, \ldots, K$ and stratum $j = 1, \ldots, J$, we define S_{Ajk} to be the sum of the n_{Ajk} responses on treatment A and S_{Bjk} the sum of the n_{Bjk} responses on treatment B.

In the constant odds ratio model, it is assumed that

$$\frac{p_{Aj}(1 - p_{Bj})}{p_{Bj}(1 - p_{Aj})} = \psi, \quad j = 1, \ldots, J.$$

Let $\theta = \log(\psi)$, the natural logarithm of ψ, and suppose we wish to test the null hypothesis H_0: $\theta = 0$, i.e., $p_{Aj} = p_{Bj}$ for each $j = 1, \ldots, J$. We use the well-known estimator of Mantel & Haenszel (1959). At each analysis $k = 1, \ldots, K$, the Mantel-Haenszel estimate of ψ is

$$\hat{\psi}^{(k)} = \sum_{j=1}^{J} \frac{S_{Ajk}(n_{Bjk} - S_{Bjk})}{N_{jk}} \Bigg/ \sum_{j=1}^{J} \frac{S_{Bjk}(n_{Ajk} - S_{Ajk})}{N_{jk}}$$

and we estimate θ by $\hat{\theta}^{(k)} = \log \hat{\psi}^{(k)}$. If $N_{jk} = 0$, a term $0/0$ occurs in the above formula; such terms should be interpreted as zero here and in subsequent formulae. Robins, Breslow & Greenland (1986) propose an estimator of the asymptotic variance of $\hat{\psi}^{(k)}$, denoted V_{US} in their paper, which is consistent as cell sizes increase in a fixed number of strata or when cell sizes are bounded and the number of strata increases. Let

$$P_{j,k} = \frac{S_{Ajk} + n_{Bjk} - S_{Bjk}}{N_{jk}}, \quad Q_{j,k} = \frac{S_{Bjk} + n_{Ajk} - S_{Ajk}}{N_{jk}},$$

$$R_{j,k} = \frac{S_{Ajk}(n_{Bjk} - S_{Bjk})}{N_{jk}}, \quad U_{j,k} = \frac{S_{Bjk}(n_{Ajk} - S_{Ajk})}{N_{jk}},$$

$$R_{+,k} = \sum_{j=1}^{J} R_{j,k} \text{ and } U_{+,k} = \sum_{j=1}^{J} U_{j,k}.$$

Then, the estimator of $Var(\hat{\theta}^{(k)})$ is

$$V_k = \frac{\sum_j P_{j,k}R_{j,k}}{2R_{+,k}^2} + \frac{\sum_j (P_{j,k}U_{j,k} + Q_{j,k}R_{j,k})}{2R_{+,k}U_{+,k}} + \frac{\sum_j Q_{j,k}U_{j,k}}{2U_{+,k}^2}$$

and we define

$$\mathcal{I}_k = V_k^{-1}, \quad k = 1, \ldots, K.$$

Here, $\mathcal{I}_k$ is not precisely the Fisher information for θ contained in the data at analysis k since the Mantel-Haenszel estimate is not 100% efficient for estimating θ. However, this estimate is still highly efficient in many situations and has other attractive features and $\mathcal{I}_k$ represents the effective information when θ is estimated in this way. The standardized statistics for testing H_0 are

$$Z_k = \hat{\theta}^{(k)} \sqrt{\mathcal{I}_k}, \quad k = 1, \ldots, K.$$

Jennison & Turnbull (1991c) have shown that $\{Z_1, \ldots, Z_K\}$ follows, approximately, the canonical joint distribution (3.1) with information levels

Table 12.6 *Hypothetical interim data for the Ille-et-Vilaine study (Breslow & Day, 1980, p. 137)*

Analysis	*Stratum*	*Cumulative frequencies* *			
		Cases		*Controls*	
		Exposed	*Unexposed*	*Exposed*	*Unexposed*
k	j	S_{Ajk}	$n_{Ajk}-S_{Ajk}$	S_{Bjk}	$n_{Bjk}-S_{Bjk}$
1	1	0	0	4	31
	2	2	2	8	60
	3	6	5	9	40
	4	20	19	5	30
	5	8	14	7	31
	6	2	3	0	9
2	1	1	0	6	66
	2	2	4	18	111
	3	18	14	19	89
	4	30	27	20	100
	5	11	22	12	57
	6	3	7	0	21
3	1	1	0	9	106
	2	4	5	26	164
	3	25	21	29	138
	4	42	34	27	139
	5	19	36	18	88
	6	5	8	0	31

* Entries are cumulative counts of exposed and unexposed cases and controls in each stratum at three interim analyses.

$\{\mathcal{I}_1, \ldots, \mathcal{I}_K\}$ for $\theta = \log(\psi)$ if (a) there is just one stratum, (b) sample sizes for each treatment within each stratum grow at the same rate, or (c) new strata are observed at each analysis but no new subjects are added to previous strata and the different strata form a random sample from some "super-population" of possible strata. Jennison & Turnbull (1989, Table 6) have used simulation to study the adequacy of the multivariate normal approximation to the distribution of $\{Z_1, \ldots, Z_K\}$ in the context of coverage probabilities of repeated confidence intervals. Their results illustrate its accuracy both for a fixed number of strata of increasing size and in matched pair comparisons which produce increasing numbers of strata of fixed size.

Given this standard distribution for $\{Z_1, \ldots, Z_K\}$, the group sequential tests of Chapters 2 to 10 can be used in the usual way. Either good initial estimates of p_{Aj} and p_{Bj} are needed at the design stage to determine the sample sizes needed to satisfy a given power condition, or otherwise, an adaptive strategy, as described in Chapter 14, could be used to achieve these information levels accurately.

The data in Table 12.6 were presented by Jennison & Turnbull (1989, Table 7)

Table 12.7 *Interim results for the data of Table 12.6 assuming the odds ratio ψ to be constant across the six strata*

Analysis k	$\hat{\theta} = \log \hat{\psi}$	$\sqrt{V_k}$	$\hat{\psi}$	*Pocock test-based 90% RCIs for* ψ	*O'Brien & Fleming 90% RCIs for* ψ
1	1.60	0.336	4.93	(2.5, 9.6)	(1.8, 13.4)
2	1.58	0.227	4.85	(3.1, 7.6)	(3.0, 7.8)
3	1.64	0.189	5.16	(3.5, 7.5)	(3.7, 7.1)

as an illustrative example with a fixed number of strata of increasing size. These are cumulative frequencies representing case-control data with six strata, collected in three stages. The frequencies at the third analysis are the Ille-et-Vilaine data set of Breslow & Day (1980, p. 137). The cumulative frequencies at the first and second analyses are hypothetical values which might have been observed had the study been conducted group sequentially. Table 12.7 shows the resulting sequences of 90% RCIs for the odds ratio ψ based on both a Pocock and an O'Brien & Fleming parent test with three analyses. The RCIs for θ are $\hat{\theta}_k \pm c_k \sqrt{V_k}$, $k = 1, \ldots, 3$, with constants $c_k = C_P(3, 0.1) = 1.992$ (from Table 2.1) and $c_k = C_B(3, 0.1)\sqrt{(3/k)} = 1.710\sqrt{(3/k)}$ (from Table 2.3), respectively, for the two types of RCI. The increments in information are approximately equal and so it is appropriate to follow the significance level approach of Section 3.3 in defining the parent test. The RCIs for ψ are obtained by exponentiating the endpoints of the corresponding intervals for θ. For both types of RCI, the first interval fails to include unity, indicating that an exposure effect might have been concluded at this point.

As an example with an increasing number of strata of fixed sizes, consider the data of Table 12.8, presented by Jennison & Turnbull (1989, Table 9). Each stratum is comprised of a case and four matched controls, and the exposure or non-exposure of each individual is recorded. The frequencies at the third analysis form the Leisure World data set of Breslow & Day (1980, p. 174), while data at analyses 1 and 2 are hypothetical counts that might have been observed under a group sequential design. Table 12.9 shows sequences of 90% RCIs for the odds ratio ψ based on both a Pocock and an O'Brien & Fleming parent test with $K = 3$ looks. By the second analysis, both types of RCI fail to include unity, and so an early decision in favor of an exposure effect might have been made.

12.4 Case-Control and Matched Pair Analyses

An important special case of the stratified designs discussed in Section 12.3 is the matched pair case-control or cohort study. The use of sequential methods in retrospective case-control studies has been described by O'Neill & Anello (1978) and by Pasternack & Shore (1982). Each stratum j now consists of two samples of

Table 12.8 *Hypothetical interim data for the Leisure World study (Breslow & Day, 1980, p. 174)*

Analysis k	*Case*	*Cumulative frequencies* * *Number of controls exposed* 0	1	2	3	4
1	*Exposed*	0	8	5	5	1
	Unexposed	0	1	0	1	0
2	*Exposed*	2	14	10	9	2
	Unexposed	0	3	0	1	1
3	*Exposed*	3	17	16	15	5
	Unexposed	0	4	1	1	1

* Entries are cumulative counts of each type of matched set, as specified by the exposure or non-exposure of the case and the number of exposed controls, at three interim analyses.

Table 12.9 *Interim results for the data of Table 12.8 assuming the odds ratio ψ to be constant across the six strata*

Analysis k	$\hat{\theta} = \log \hat{\psi}$	$\sqrt{V_k}$	$\hat{\psi}$	*Pocock test-based 90% RCIs for* ψ	*O'Brien & Fleming 90% RCIs for* ψ
1	2.28	0.831	9.74	(1.9, 51.1)	(0.8, 114.3)
2	2.07	0.538	7.90	(2.7, 23.1)	(2.6, 24.4)
3	2.14	0.463	8.46	(3.4, 21.3)	(3.8, 18.7)

size 1, i.e., $n_{Ajk} = n_{Bjk} = 1$, if the jth pair has been observed by the kth analysis and is empty otherwise.

Again assuming a common odds ratio ψ, the Mantel-Haenszel estimate $\hat{\psi}_k$ reduces to the McNemar estimate $\hat{\psi}_k = d_1(k)/d_2(k)$, where $d_1(k)$ and $d_2(k)$ are the number of discordant pairs of the first and second type, respectively, observed by the time of the kth analysis. Although the methods of Section 12.3 could be applied, it is easier to proceed directly. Let $d(k) = d_1(k) + d_2(k)$ be the total number of discordant pairs observed by the kth analysis. Then, conditional on $d(k)$, the variable $d_1(k)$ is binomial with success probability $p = (1+\psi)^{-1}$. Hence group sequential procedures can be constructed using the methods of Section 12.1 with $S_k = d_1(k)$ and $n_k = d(k)$. In particular, RCIs for ψ can be obtained by transforming intervals for p obtained using the methods of Section 12.1.4 .

12.5 Logistic Regression: Adjusting for Covariates

Consider the situation where binary observations $X_1, X_2, \ldots$ follow independent Bernoulli distributions with success probabilities given by a logit linear function of a parameter vector $\boldsymbol{\beta} = (\beta_1, \ldots, \beta_r)$. Thus, for $i = 1, 2, \ldots$, the observation X_i is distributed as $B(p_i)$, where

$$\log\{p_i/(1-p_i)\} = \sum_{j=1}^{r} d_{ij}\beta_j$$

and $(d_{i1}, \ldots, d_{ir})$ represents an r-vector of covariates associated with the ith subject. Typically, $d_{i1} = 1$ for all i and β_1 represents an intercept term. We suppose that the data are collected group sequentially and denote by $\widehat{\boldsymbol{\beta}}^{(k)}$ the maximum likelihood estimates of $\boldsymbol{\beta}$ based on data accumulated by each stage $k = 1, \ldots, K$. This is an example of a generalized linear model and, by the results of Section 11.6, estimates and related test statistics have, approximately, the standard group sequential distributions. In particular, proceeding as in Section 3.5.2, let $\boldsymbol{c}$ be a given vector of length r and $\mathcal{I}_k^{-1}$ a consistent estimate of the variance of $\boldsymbol{c}^T\widehat{\boldsymbol{\beta}}^{(k)}$. Then, if γ is a specified scalar, the standardized statistics

$$Z_k = (\boldsymbol{c}^T\widehat{\boldsymbol{\beta}}^{(k)} - \gamma)\sqrt{\mathcal{I}_k}, \quad k = 1, \ldots, K,$$

have approximately the canonical joint distribution (3.1) with $\theta = (\boldsymbol{c}^T\boldsymbol{\beta} - \gamma)$. Thus, we may construct group sequential tests of the hypothesis H_0: $\boldsymbol{c}^T\boldsymbol{\beta} = \gamma$ or repeated confidence intervals for $\boldsymbol{c}^T\boldsymbol{\beta}$.

An early example application of logistic regression modeling in a group sequential experiment described by Whitehead (1989) concerns a series of germination tests performed at periodic intervals to assess viability of seed samples. Other binary response regression models can also be employed in the group sequential framework. Jennison & Turnbull (1989, Section 5.5) propose a group sequential analysis of an odds ratio regression model in which the log odds ratio between a treatment and control group for an event of interest increases linearly in time, a reasonable model when the effect of treatment on a population is postulated to be gradual rather than immediate.

Returning to the Ille-et-Vilaine data of Table 12.6, we can analyze this data set with a logistic regression model in which the response variable is the indicator of an exposed/unexposed subject, a $0-1$ covariate indicates case or control and five $0-1$ dummy variables denote the stratum. The absence of any interaction terms in the model implies a constant odds ratio across strata, and so we have the same model as used in the analysis of this example in Section 12.3. However, we now use maximum likelihood estimation rather than the Mantel-Haenszel estimator. We are interested in the regression coefficient for the case/control indicator variable which is equal to the logarithm of the odds ratio. We therefore specify the vector $\boldsymbol{c}$ to have a 1 in the position for the case/control indicator and 0 in the other positions for the strata covariates. The logistic regressions can be readily performed using standard statistical software such as GLIM 3.77. Successive estimates for the log odds ratio based on cumulative data at stages 1,

2 and 3 are 1.617, 1.597 and 1.671 with standard errors 0.335, 0.228 and 0.190, respectively. These estimates and standard errors are almost identical to those in Table 12.7 obtained using the Mantel-Haenszel estimates and, hence, so will be related RCIs for the odds ratio .

12.6 Connection with Survival Analysis

A common situation where it is desired to compare two probabilities, as in Section 12.2, occurs in reliability tests or follow-up studies where two treatments are to be compared according to the proportions of subjects that have failed (or responded) within a fixed time horizon. If the actual times to failure or response are available, it is usually more appropriate to consider this as a problem with censored survival data. Group sequential procedures should then be based on the Kaplan-Meier (1958) estimates of the failure or response probabilities. This issue will be considered in Section 13.7 of the next chapter.

CHAPTER 13

Survival Data

13.1 Introduction

In many follow-up trials, the primary response variable is a subject's survival time or the time to occurrence of a particular event such as relapse or remission of symptoms. These are elapsed times measured from an origin pertinent to each subject, often the date of entry into the study. Although time is typically measured on a chronological scale of days, weeks or months, this need not always be so. In some epidemiological studies cumulative exposure plays the role of survival time, in a veterinary study of dairy cattle the equivalent measure might be cumulative milk production, or in a reliability strength test it could be the cumulative stress or load applied. We shall phrase the methods of this chapter in terms of "survival" or "failure" time measured from entry to a study. However, the same methods can be applied quite generally for any time to event response.

An individual's survival time may be censored if failure has not occurred when that individual is last seen or when the data are analyzed. In Section 3.7, we introduced the basic concepts of survival models, including the survival function $S(t)$ and hazard rate $h(t)$ of a response time distribution. We also described the two-sided, group sequential log-rank test for testing equality of two survival distributions. Suppose two sets of subjects, A and B, have respective hazard rates $h_A(t)$ and $h_B(t)$, then the log-rank test is used to test the null hypothesis H_0: $h_A(t) = h_B(t)$ for all $t > 0$, or equivalently $S_A(t) \equiv S_B(t)$, and is particularly powerful against "proportional hazards" alternatives where $h_B(t) \equiv \lambda h_A(t)$ for some constant λ. In Section 3.7 we followed the significance level approach which requires equal increments in information between successive analyses if the Type I error rate α is to be attained accurately. In a survival study, information is roughly proportional to the total number of observed failures and increments are usually unequal and unpredictable. The error spending approach of Chapter 7 is thus an attractive alternative, as illustrated in the example of Section 7.2.3.

In Section 13.2, we shall review the group sequential log-rank test described in Section 3.7, adding a modification to accommodate tied survival times. This test is further generalized in Section 13.3 to permit the inclusion of strata. In Section 13.4, we describe how to adjust the comparison of survival distributions for the effects of covariates through use of the proportional hazards regression model of Cox (1972) and we explain how to construct RCIs for a hazard ratio, λ, in Section 13.5. These methods are illustrated by a case study in Section 13.6. In Section 13.7, we show how successive Kaplan-Meier (1958) estimates of the survival function can be used as a basis for group sequential tests and repeated confidence intervals concerning survival probabilities and quantiles.

13.2 The Log-Rank Test

Consider the problem of testing the equality of survival distributions $S_A(t)$ and $S_B(t)$ for two treatment arms, A and B, based on accumulating survival data. At each analysis we observe a failure or censoring time for each subject, measured from that subject's date of entry or randomization as defined in the study protocol. Let d_k, $k = 1, \ldots, K$, denote the total number of uncensored failures observed across both treatment arms when analysis k is conducted. Some of these times may be tied and we suppose that d'_k of the d_k failure times are distinct, where $1 \leq d'_k \leq d_k$. We denote these distinct failure times by $\tau_{1,k} < \tau_{2,k} < \ldots < \tau_{d'_k,k}$ and let $r_{iA,k}$ and $r_{iB,k}$ denote the numbers at risk on treatment arms A and B, respectively, just before time $\tau_{i,k}$. Finally, let $\delta_{iA,k}$ and $\delta_{iB,k}$ denote the numbers on treatment arms A and B, respectively, that fail at time $\tau_{i,k}$ and define $\delta_{i,k} = \delta_{iA,k} + \delta_{iB,k}$ for $i = 1, \ldots, d'_{\ell k}$. If there are no ties, as assumed in Section 3.7, then $\delta_{i,k} = 1$ and either $\delta_{iA,k} = 1$ and $\delta_{iB,k} = 0$ or $\delta_{iA,k} = 0$ and $\delta_{iB,k} = 1$ for each pair i and k.

If the survival distributions $S_A(t)$ and $S_B(t)$ are equal, the conditional distribution of $\delta_{iB,k}$ given $r_{iA,k}$, $r_{iB,k}$ and $\delta_{i,k}$ is hypergeometric with expectation

$$e_{i,k} = \frac{r_{iB,k}\, \delta_{i,k}}{r_{iA,k} + r_{iB,k}}$$

and variance

$$v_{i,k} = \frac{r_{iA,k}\, r_{iB,k}\, \delta_{i,k}\, (r_{iA,k} + r_{iB,k} - \delta_{i,k})}{(r_{iA,k} + r_{iB,k} - 1)\, (r_{iA,k} + r_{iB,k})^2}.$$

The standardized log-rank statistic at analysis k is given by

$$Z_k = \frac{\sum_{i=1}^{d'_k} (\delta_{iB,k} - e_{i,k})}{\left(\sum_{i=1}^{d'_k} v_{i,k}\right)^{1/2}} \tag{13.1}$$

and the information $\mathcal{I}_k$ for the log hazard ratio is

$$\mathcal{I}_k = \sum_{i=1}^{d'_k} v_{i,k}. \tag{13.2}$$

In the absence of ties, the numerator of (13.1) reduces to the log-rank score statistic (3.17) and the information given by (13.2) is the same as (3.18).

The log-rank test has optimum power to detect alternatives when hazard rates in the two treatment arms are proportional, as described in Section 13.1. The sequence of log-rank statistics defined by (13.1) then has, approximately, the canonical joint distribution (3.1), given $\mathcal{I}_1, \ldots, \mathcal{I}_K$, with $\theta = \log(\lambda)$, the log hazard ratio; references to the derivation of this result were given in Section 3.7 and further references appear in Section 13.8.

Since the canonical joint distribution holds, the methods described in Chapter 7 can be used to construct group sequential error spending tests from the sequence of statistics Z_k and information levels $\mathcal{I}_k$. In designing a maximum information trial to meet a given power requirement, it is necessary to predict the information levels that will arise, especially that at the final possible analysis. Here, it is helpful to note that each $v_{i,k}$ is approximately $\delta_{i,k}/4$ if $r_{iA,k} \approx r_{iB,k}$ and either $\delta_{i,k} = 1$ or

$\delta_{i,k}$ is small relative to $r_{iA,k}+r_{iB,k}$. Hence, $\mathcal{I}_k$ will be approximately equal to $d_k/4$ and the final information level will be close to one quarter of the total number of observed failures. In Section 7.2.3, we applied a two-sided group sequential log-rank test to the BHAT data in the setting of a maximum duration trial. A further application, illustrating a one-sided test in a maximum information trial, will be described in Section 13.6.

13.3 The Stratified Log-Rank Test

We now suppose that each subject entering the trial can be classified as belonging to precisely one of L distinct categories or strata and it is desired to test the null hypothesis that survival distributions under treatments A and B are equal *within each stratum.* Specifically, if $h_{A\ell}(t)$ and $h_{B\ell}(t)$ denote the hazard rates for subjects in strata $\ell = 1, \ldots, L$ under treatments A and B respectively, then the null hypothesis is

$$H_0\colon\ h_{A\ell}(t) = h_{B\ell}(t) \quad \text{for all } t > 0 \text{ and } \ell = 1, \ldots, L.$$

The stratified log-rank test can be used in this situation and is particularly powerful against alternatives in which the hazard rates in the two treatment arms are proportional within each stratum with a common hazard ratio λ in each case, i.e., $h_{B\ell}(t) = \lambda h_{A\ell}(t)$ for all $t > 0$ and $\ell = 1, \ldots, L$. The test is described in the non-sequential setting in a number of textbooks on survival analysis, for example, Klein & Moeschberger (1997, Section 7.5).

Generalizing the notation of Sections 3.7 and 13.2, we let $d_{\ell k}$, $k = 1, \ldots, K$ and $\ell = 1, \ldots, L$, denote the number of uncensored failures in stratum ℓ observed when analysis k is conducted. Considering only those subjects in stratum ℓ, we suppose $d'_{\ell k}$ of the $d_{\ell k}$ failure times observed at analysis k are distinct and denote these times by $\tau_{1,\ell k} < \tau_{2,\ell k} < \ldots < \tau_{d'_{\ell k},\ell k}$. We also define $r_{iA,\ell k}$ and $r_{iB,\ell k}$, for $i = 1, \ldots, d'_{\ell k}$, to be the numbers at risk on each treatment arm, A and B, in stratum ℓ just before time $\tau_{i,\ell k}$. Finally, we let $\delta_{iA,\ell k}$ and $\delta_{iB,\ell k}$ denote the numbers that fail on treatments A and B at time $\tau_{i,\ell k}$ and define $\delta_{i,\ell k} = \delta_{iA,\ell k} + \delta_{iB,\ell k}$. In the absence of ties, $\delta_{i,\ell k} = 1$ and we must have either $\delta_{iA,\ell k} = 1$ and $\delta_{iB,\ell k} = 0$ or $\delta_{iA,\ell k} = 0$ and $\delta_{iB,\ell k} = 1$ for each triple i, ℓ and k.

Under H_0, the conditional distribution of $\delta_{iB,\ell k}$ given $r_{iA,\ell k}$, $r_{iB,\ell k}$ and $\delta_{i,\ell k}$ is hypergeometric with expectation

$$e_{i,\ell k} = \frac{r_{iB,\ell k}\,\delta_{i,\ell k}}{r_{iA,\ell k} + r_{iB,\ell k}}$$

and variance

$$v_{i,\ell k} = \frac{r_{iA,\ell k}\, r_{iB,\ell k}\, \delta_{i,\ell k}\, (r_{iA,\ell k} + r_{iB,\ell k} - \delta_{i,\ell k})}{(r_{iA,\ell k} + r_{iB,\ell k} - 1)\,(r_{iA,\ell k} + r_{iB,\ell k})^2}.$$

The stratified log-rank statistic at analysis k is defined as

$$Z_k = \frac{\sum_{\ell=1}^{L} \sum_{i=1}^{d'_{\ell k}} (\delta_{iB,\ell k} - e_{i,\ell k})}{\left(\sum_{\ell=1}^{L} \sum_{i=1}^{d'_{\ell k}} v_{i,\ell k}\right)^{1/2}} \tag{13.3}$$

and the information for the log hazard ratio is

$$\mathcal{I}_k = \sum_{\ell=1}^{L} \sum_{i=1}^{d'_{\ell k}} v_{i,\ell k}. \tag{13.4}$$

When $L = 1$ and there is only a single stratum, (13.3) reduces to (13.1) and (13.4) to (13.2). If, in addition, there are no ties the numerator in (13.3) is equal to the log-rank score statistic given by (3.17) and the information given by (13.4) reduces to (3.18). Large sample results for the non-stratified case can be extended to show that, if the numbers of failures in each stratum are large, the sequence of stratified log-rank statistics $Z_1, \ldots, Z_K$ also has, approximately, the canonical joint distribution (3.1), given $\mathcal{I}_1, \ldots, \mathcal{I}_K$, with $\theta = \log(\lambda)$. Group sequential tests can, therefore, be based on the statistics Z_k and information levels $\mathcal{I}_k$ in the usual way. As for the log-rank statistic, the information level $\mathcal{I}_k$ can be expected to equal roughly a quarter of the total number of deaths observed by analysis k, although slightly lower values will occur if the numbers at risk on the two treatment arms become uneven in any one stratum. An application of the group sequential stratified log-rank test will be presented in Section 13.6.

13.4 Group Sequential Methods for Survival Data with Covariates

13.4.1 The Cox Regression Model

Suppose independent subjects $i = 1, 2, \ldots$ are observed, each having a column vector of covariates $\boldsymbol{x}_i = (x_{i1}, \ldots, x_{ip})^T$. In the proportional hazards regression model (Cox, 1972), the survival distribution for subject i is continuous with hazard rate

$$h_i(t) = h_0(t)\, e^{\boldsymbol{\beta}^T \boldsymbol{x}_i}, \quad t > 0, \tag{13.5}$$

where $h_0(t)$ represents an unknown baseline hazard function and $\boldsymbol{\beta} = (\beta_1, \ldots, \beta_p)^T$ is a column vector of parameters to be estimated. The log-linear link function between covariate values x_{ij} and the hazard rate $h_i(t)$ is not as restrictive as might seem at first, since interactions and transformed covariates may be included in the vector $\boldsymbol{x}$. Entry of individuals to a study will usually be staggered and survival, measured as elapsed time from entry to the study, can be subject to competing risk censoring, which we shall assume to be non-informative (see Klein & Moeschberger, 1997, p. 91) as well as "end-of-study" censoring at interim and final analyses.

We use the same notation as in previous sections. For $k = 1, \ldots, K$, let d_k denote the total number of failures observed by the time the kth analysis is conducted. Supposing for now that there are no ties, we denote the survival times of the subjects observed to have failed at analysis k by $\tau_{1,k} < \tau_{2,k} < \ldots < \tau_{d_k,k}$. Let $\boldsymbol{x}^k_{(i)}$, $i = 1, \ldots, d_k$, denote the covariate vector associated with the individual who fails at time $\tau_{i,k}$ and define $\mathcal{R}_{i,k}$ to be the set of indices of individuals known at analysis k to have survived at least up to just before time $\tau_{i,k}$.

Following Cox (1972), we estimate the vector $\boldsymbol{\beta}$ at the kth analysis by the value maximizing the log partial likelihood

$$\mathcal{L}_k(\boldsymbol{\beta}) = \sum_{i=1}^{d_k} \left\{ \boldsymbol{\beta}^T \boldsymbol{x}_{(i)}^k - \log\left(\sum_{j \in \mathcal{R}_{i,k}} e^{\boldsymbol{\beta}^T \boldsymbol{x}_j} \right) \right\}. \qquad (13.6)$$

This estimate, denoted $\widehat{\boldsymbol{\beta}}^{(k)}$, satisfies the score equations

$$S(k, \boldsymbol{\beta}) = \frac{\partial\, \mathcal{L}_k(\boldsymbol{\beta})}{\partial \boldsymbol{\beta}} = \sum_{i=1}^{d_k} \left(\boldsymbol{x}_{(i)}^k - \frac{\sum_{j \in \mathcal{R}_{i,k}} \boldsymbol{x}_j\, e^{\boldsymbol{\beta}^T \boldsymbol{x}_j}}{\sum_{j \in \mathcal{R}_{i,k}} e^{\boldsymbol{\beta}^T \boldsymbol{x}_j}} \right) = 0. \qquad (13.7)$$

The expressions (13.6) and (13.7) can be adapted to accommodate ties; see, for example, Klein & Moeschberger (1997, Section 8.3).

The model (13.5) can also be modified to include strata with different baseline hazard rates, as in the stratified proportional hazards model of Section 13.3. In the stratified Cox regression model, the hazard rate for subject i in stratum ℓ, with covariate vector $\boldsymbol{x}_i$, is

$$h_{i\ell}(t) = h_{0\ell}(t)\, e^{\boldsymbol{\beta}^T \boldsymbol{x}_i}, \quad t > 0, \qquad (13.8)$$

the baseline hazard rate, $h_{0\ell}$, depending on the stratum ℓ but the vector of regression coefficients, $\boldsymbol{\beta}$, remaining constant across strata. If there are L strata, the log partial likelihood is a sum of L terms of the form (13.6) computed separately within each stratum. Differentiating this with respect to $\boldsymbol{\beta}$ produces a sum of L terms in the score equations corresponding to (13.7). For further details, see Klein & Moeschberger (1997, Section 9.3).

The score equations (13.7) must be solved numerically and many statistical computer software packages now include procedures to do this. The information matrix associated with $\widehat{\boldsymbol{\beta}}^{(k)}$ is $\mathcal{I}_k(\widehat{\boldsymbol{\beta}}^{(k)})$, where

$$\mathcal{I}_k(\boldsymbol{\beta}) = \frac{-\,\partial^2}{\partial \boldsymbol{\beta}^2} \mathcal{L}_k(\boldsymbol{\beta}).$$

This matrix and its inverse are routinely provided along with $\widehat{\boldsymbol{\beta}}^{(k)}$ in the output of statistical software packages.

It can be shown (see the references in Section 13.8) that the sequence of estimates $\widehat{\boldsymbol{\beta}}^{(1)}, \ldots, \widehat{\boldsymbol{\beta}}^{(K)}$ has, asymptotically, the standard multivariate normal joint distribution given by (11.1). Hence, the sequence of standardized vector statistics

$$\mathcal{I}_1(\widehat{\boldsymbol{\beta}}^{(1)})^{1/2}\, \widehat{\boldsymbol{\beta}}^{(1)}, \ldots, \mathcal{I}_K(\widehat{\boldsymbol{\beta}}^{(K)})^{1/2}\, \widehat{\boldsymbol{\beta}}^{(K)}$$

has an asymptotic joint distribution that is the multivariate analogue to the canonical joint distribution of (3.1). The remainder of this section describes important applications of this result.

13.4.2 A Two-Sample Test for Equality of Survival Distributions with Adjustment for Covariates.

We can now derive a generalization of the group sequential log-rank test incorporating adjustment for covariates. Suppose survival distributions are modeled by the Cox regression model (13.5) or its stratified version (13.8) and x_{i1} is a binary treatment indicator, so that the scalar coefficient β_1 represents the treatment effect. Our goal is to construct a group sequential test of H_0: $\beta_1 = 0$ in the presence of confounding variables $x_{i2}, \ldots, x_{ip}$ for each subject i. The maximum partial likelihood estimate of β_1 at stage k is $\hat{\beta}_1^{(k)}$ and the variance of this estimate is approximated by

$$v_k = [\{\mathcal{I}_k(\widehat{\boldsymbol{\beta}}^{(k)})\}^{-1}]_{11}, \tag{13.9}$$

the $(1,\ 1)$ element of the inverse of the information matrix $\mathcal{I}_k(\widehat{\boldsymbol{\beta}}^{(k)})$; see Jennison & Turnbull (1997a, Section 5.2). An alternative variance estimator, which is also consistent under H_0 and can be more accurate in small samples is obtained by replacing $\widehat{\boldsymbol{\beta}}^{(k)}$ in (13.9) with the value of $\boldsymbol{\beta}$ that maximizes (13.6) when β_1 is constrained to be zero. Defining the standardized statistics

$$Z_k = \hat{\beta}_1^{(k)} / \sqrt{v_k}, \quad k = 1, \ldots, K, \tag{13.10}$$

the results stated at the end of Section 13.4.1 imply that $Z_1, \ldots, Z_K$ have, approximately, the canonical joint distribution (3.1) when we equate θ with β_1 and $\mathcal{I}_k$ with v_k^{-1}.

Note that if $p = 1$, so the only regression term is for the treatment effect, the assumed model is identical to the proportional hazards model of Section 13.2, or the stratified proportional hazards model of Section 13.3 in the case of a stratified Cox regression model. The statistics (13.10) are then asymptotically equivalent to the standardized log-rank statistics and either statistic may be used to define a group sequential test.

The effects of covariates on the observed information add to the difficulty of organizing interim analyses to occur at pre-specified information levels, and the error spending method of Chapter 7 is the obvious choice for constructing testing boundaries. If randomization and similar patterns of survival on the two treatment arms lead to balance in covariate values between treatments throughout a study, information for β_1 will be roughly one quarter of the number of observed failures, as in the log-rank test. Thus, in designing a study to reach a target information level $\mathcal{I}_{max}$, it might be decided to enroll a total of $4\,\mathcal{I}_{max}/\gamma$ subjects, where γ is the estimated probability that any one subject will be observed to fail by the time of the last scheduled analysis. Alternatively, a somewhat higher sample size could be chosen to protect against errors in estimating the baseline failure rate, the level of competing risk censoring or the relation between number of failures and information.

13.4.3 Factorial Designs

Another application of the results of Section 13.4.1 is in making inferences about a linear combination of parameters of the form $\boldsymbol{d}^T\boldsymbol{\beta} = d_1\beta_1 + \ldots + d_p\beta_p$. This could be desirable if the x-variables represent factors in a factorial design with multiple treatments, an increasingly common feature of clinical trials (Natarajan et al. 1996). The vector $\boldsymbol{d} = (d_1, \ldots, d_p)^T$ might then be chosen so that $\boldsymbol{d}^T\boldsymbol{\beta}$ represents a main effect, a linear trend, or possibly an interaction. We can test the hypothesis H_0: $\boldsymbol{d}^T\boldsymbol{\beta} = 0$ by defining the sequence of test statistics

$$Z_k = \boldsymbol{d}^T \widehat{\boldsymbol{\beta}}^{(k)} \sqrt{\mathcal{I}_k}, \quad k = 1, \ldots, K,$$

where $\mathcal{I}_k = \{\boldsymbol{d}^T \mathcal{I}^{-1}(k, \widehat{\boldsymbol{\beta}}^{(k)})\boldsymbol{d}\}^{-1}$. This sequence has, approximately, the canonical joint distribution (3.1), given $\mathcal{I}_1, \ldots, \mathcal{I}_K$, and group sequential tests can be constructed in the usual way. Note, however, that in a factorial trial involving multiple treatments, more than one main effect may be designated a primary endpoint to be monitored. We discuss group sequential tests for multivariate endpoints in Chapter 15.

13.5 Repeated Confidence Intervals for a Hazard Ratio

Consider again the problem of comparing the survival distributions for two treatment groups with adjustment for covariates, as described in Section 13.4.2. We can use the arguments of Section 9.1 to construct RCIs for β_1, the log hazard ratio between treatments. These RCIs are obtained by inverting a family of group sequential tests of hypotheses H_0: $\beta_1 = \widetilde{\beta}_1$, where $\widetilde{\beta}_1$ ranges over the real line. The RCI for β_1 is the set of values of $\widetilde{\beta}_1$ for which H_0 is currently accepted.

A group sequential test of H_0: $\beta_1 = \widetilde{\beta}_1$ can be based on the standardized statistics

$$Z_k(\widetilde{\beta}_1) = (\hat{\beta}_1^{(k)} - \widetilde{\beta}_1)/\sqrt{v_k}, \quad k = 1, \ldots, K,$$

where $\hat{\beta}_1^{(k)}$ and v_k are as defined in Section 13.4.2. A sequence of RCIs for β_1 with overall confidence level $1 - \alpha$ is then given by

$$(\hat{\beta}_1^{(k)} \pm c_k(\alpha)\sqrt{v_k}), \quad k = 1, \ldots, K, \tag{13.11}$$

where $\pm c_k(\alpha)$, $k = 1, \ldots, K$, are critical values for a group sequential two-sided test with Type I error probability α based on standardized statistics $Z_1, \ldots, Z_K$ with the canonical joint distribution (3.1) for information levels $\mathcal{I}_k = v_k^{-1}$. If an error spending approach is used, each $c_k(\alpha)$ is obtained as the solution of (7.1) with π_k equal to the Type I error probability allocated to analysis k. RCIs for the hazard ratio e^{β_1} are found by exponentiating the limits in (13.11). RCIs can be constructed in a similar fashion for linear combinations of regression parameters, as described in Section 13.4.3.

Small sample accuracy may be improved by tailoring the estimate of the variance of $\hat{\beta}_1^{(k)}$ to each hypothesized value $\widetilde{\beta}_1$. This is done by replacing $\widehat{\boldsymbol{\beta}}^{(k)}$ in (13.9) with the maximum partial likelihood estimate of $\boldsymbol{\beta}$ subject to the constraint $\beta_1 = \widetilde{\beta}_1$, thereby defining a new variance estimate, $v_k(\widetilde{\beta}_1)$ say. The

kth RCI is then

$$\{\widetilde{\beta}_1 : \hat{\beta}_1^{(k)} \in \widetilde{\beta}_1 \pm c_k(\alpha)\sqrt{v_k(\widetilde{\beta}_1)}\,\}.$$

Computation of this RCI is less straightforward since a separate v_k must be found for each value of $\widetilde{\beta}_1$ considered, and the constrained estimation of variance is not so readily available in standard software packages. In principle, the critical values $c_1(\alpha), \ldots, c_K(\alpha)$ also depend on $\widetilde{\beta}_1$, since they are defined for the particular information sequence $\mathcal{I}_k = \{v_k(\widetilde{\beta}_1)\}^{-1}$, $k = 1, \ldots, K$; however, it should usually suffice to calculate the $c_k(\alpha)$ using the single sequence of information levels $\mathcal{I}_k = v_k^{-1}$ with v_k taken from (13.9) for $k = 1, \ldots, K$.

It is instructive to examine more closely the case $p = 1$ when the only regression term, x_1, is a binary treatment variable taking the value 0 for treatment A and 1 for treatment B (or equivalently 1 for A and 2 for B). We then have a two-sample comparison under the proportional hazards model of Section 13.2 or under a stratified proportional hazards model, as in Section 13.3. For simplicity, we consider the non-stratified proportional hazards model and suppose there are no ties; the stratified case is similar but with sums over strata in the formulae. We write $\theta = \beta_1$ so $\theta = \log(\lambda)$ if, as in Section 13.2, λ denotes the hazard ratio of treatment B to treatment A. Using the notation of Section 13.2, the partial likelihood for the data observed at analysis k is

$$\prod_{i=1}^{d_k} \left(\frac{r_{iA,k}}{r_{iA,k} + e^{\theta}\, r_{iB,k}} \right)^{\delta_{iA,k}} \left(\frac{e^{\theta}\, r_{iB,k}}{r_{iA,k} + e^{\theta}\, r_{iB,k}} \right)^{\delta_{iB,k}} . \tag{13.12}$$

The value $\hat{\theta}^{(k)}$ maximizing this expression is the maximum partial likelihood estimate, $\hat{\beta}_1^{(k)}$ in our previous notation for the Cox model. We can calculate $\hat{\theta}^{(k)}$ as the root of the score equation $S_k(\theta_0) = 0$, where

$$S_k(\theta_0) = \sum_{i=1}^{d_k} \left\{ \delta_{iB,k} - \frac{e^{\theta_0}\, r_{iB,k}}{r_{iA,k} + e^{\theta_0}\, r_{iB,k}} \right\} \tag{13.13}$$

is the score statistic for testing H_0: $\theta = \theta_0$ at analysis k, obtained as the derivative with respect to θ of the logarithm of (13.12) at $\theta = \theta_0$. The information for θ when $\theta = \theta_0$ is the second derivative of the log partial likelihood,

$$\mathcal{I}_k(\theta_0) = \sum_{i=1}^{d_k} \frac{e^{\theta_0}\, r_{iA,k}\, r_{iB,k}}{(r_{iA,k} + e^{\theta_0}\, r_{iB,k})^2} .$$

By definition, $\mathcal{I}_k(\hat{\theta}^{(k)})^{-1} = v_k$ and, hence, the RCI sequence (13.11) can also be written as

$$(\hat{\theta}^{(k)} \pm c_k(\alpha)\{\mathcal{I}_k(\hat{\theta}^{(k)})\}^{-1/2}), \quad k = 1, \ldots, K. \tag{13.14}$$

Tailoring the estimated variance of $\hat{\theta}^{(k)}$ to each hypothesized value of θ gives the alternative sequence

$$\{\theta_0 : \hat{\theta}^{(k)} \in \theta_0 \pm c_k(\alpha)\{\mathcal{I}_k(\theta_0)\}^{-1/2}\}, \quad k = 1, \ldots, K.$$

However, the sequence (13.14) is simpler to compute and Harrington (1989) notes that it is sufficient, in large samples, to base the RCI at analysis k on the single information estimate $\mathcal{I}_k(\hat{\theta}^{(k)})$.

If one wishes to avoid solving the score equations to find the maximum partial likelihood estimates $\hat{\theta}^{(k)}$, $k = 1, \ldots, K$, a sequence of RCIs can be constructed from the standardized log-rank statistics Z_k and associated information levels $\mathcal{I}_k$ given by (13.1) and (13.2) for the unstratified proportional hazards model or by (13.3) and (13.4) for the stratified model. These $\mathcal{I}_k$ are the same as $\mathcal{I}_k(0)$, $k = 1, \ldots, K$, in our current notation. Also, $Z_k = S_k(0)/\sqrt{\mathcal{I}_k(0)}$ where $S_k(0)$ is the log-rank score statistic for testing H_0: $\theta = 0$, referred to as S_k in Section 3.7. Under the assumption that the Z_k follow the canonical joint distribution (3.1) given information levels $\mathcal{I}_k$, we obtain the RCIs for θ:

$$(Z_k/\sqrt{\mathcal{I}_k} \pm c_k(\alpha)/\sqrt{\mathcal{I}_k}), \quad k = 1, \ldots, K, \tag{13.15}$$

where the constants $c_k(\alpha)$ are calculated using the observed values of $\mathcal{I}_1, \ldots, \mathcal{I}_K$. These RCIs are reliable if θ is close to zero but, when the true value of θ is away from zero, one should expect the intervals (13.14) to attain their nominal coverage probabilities more accurately.

Substituting $Z_k = S_k(0)/\sqrt{\mathcal{I}_k(0)}$ into (13.15) along with the approximation $\mathcal{I}_k(0) \approx d_k/4$, which is appropriate if the numbers at risk on the two treatment arms remain roughly equal and θ is close to zero, we obtain the RCIs for θ:

$$\left(\frac{4\, S_k(0)}{d_k} \pm \frac{2\, c_k(\alpha)}{\sqrt{d_k}} \right), \quad k = 1, \ldots, K. \tag{13.16}$$

This formula, first given in Jennison & Turnbull (1984, Eqs. 1, 2, and 1989, Eq. 4.4), is attractive for its computational simplicity. However, simulation studies such as those reported in Jennison & Turnbull (1984, 1989) suggest that the intervals given by (13.16) may fail to maintain a coverage probability adequately close to $1 - \alpha$ when θ is not close to zero or censoring patterns differ in the two treatment groups. The approximation $\mathcal{I}_k \approx d_k/4$ is useful in its own right and can help when designing a group sequential study to reach a target information level.

13.6 Example: A Clinical Trial for Carcinoma of the Oropharynx

13.6.1 Description of the Study

We shall illustrate the methods just described by applying them to a clinical trial conducted by the Radiation Therapy Oncology Group in the U.S. to investigate treatments of carcinoma of the oropharynx. We use the data from six of the larger institutions participating in this trial as recorded by Kalbfleisch & Prentice (1980, Appendix II). Subjects were recruited to the study between 1968 and 1972 and randomized to either a standard radiotherapy treatment or an experimental treatment in which the radiotherapy was supplemented by chemotherapy. The major endpoint was patient survival and patients were followed until around the end of 1973. Several baseline covariates, thought to have strong prognostic value, were also recorded.

The conduct of the study did not follow a group sequential plan but, for purposes of illustration, we have reconstructed patients' survival times and their status, dead or censored, at times 720, 1080, 1440, 1800 and 2160 days from the beginning of 1968. As the central survival records would not have been updated continuously, our constructed data sets most likely resemble the information that would have been available at interim analyses conducted a month or two after these times, and so they are an approximation to the data that could have been studied by a monitoring committee meeting at dates a little after 2, 3, 4, 5 and 6 years from the start of the study. The longer waiting period to the first interim analysis is intended to compensate for the slow initial accrual of survival information while only a few patients had been entered to the trial.

Since the experimental treatment involved chemotherapy as well as radiotherapy, the researchers would have been looking for a substantive improvement in survival on this treatment in return for the additional discomfort and short term health risks. A one-sided testing formulation is, therefore, appropriate and we shall conduct our retrospective interim analyses as a group sequential test of the null hypothesis of no treatment difference against the one-sided alternative that the new combination therapy is superior to the standard treatment of radiotherapy alone. For the sake of illustration, we suppose the experiment was designed to achieve a Type I error probability of $\alpha = 0.05$ and power $1 - \beta = 0.95$ when the log hazard ratio for the experimental treatment to the standard is equal to 0.6. By (4.1), our stated Type I error and power condition lead to a required information level

$$\mathcal{I}_{f,1} = \{2\,\Phi^{-1}(0.95)\}^2/0.6^2 = 30.06$$

for a single fixed sample test and we shall multiply this by the appropriate factor R to find the target maximum information level in a group sequential test.

13.6.2 A Group Sequential Stratified Log-Rank Test

We first consider group sequential monitoring using the log-rank test. The study protocol allowed patients to receive additional medical care "as deemed prudent" and with no restrictions, except a prohibition of the study treatment, after the initial 90 day treatment period. Kalbfleisch & Prentice (1980, p. 91) note that decisions on such medical care were liable to be made on an institutional basis and so it is reasonable to allow for a possible effect on baseline survival patterns by stratifying the log-rank test with respect to institution.

For $k = 1, \dots, 5$, let Z_k denote the standardized, stratified log-rank statistic (13.3) computed at analysis k and $\mathcal{I}_k$ the associated information (13.4). We have taken treatment A here to be the experimental treatment and B the standard, so that the Z_k have positive expectation under the alternative that the experimental treatment improves survival. The stratified log-rank test is particularly appropriate if survival times follow a stratified proportional hazards model in which the hazard rate at time t is $h_{0\ell}(t)$ or $\lambda h_{0\ell}(t)$ for a subject in stratum ℓ on the experimental or standard treatment, respectively. For this model, we denote the log hazard ratio between treatments by $\theta = \log(\lambda)$. The following analysis is based on the assumption that $Z_1, \dots, Z_5$ follow the standard joint distribution (3.1), given information levels $\mathcal{I}_1, \dots, \mathcal{I}_5$.

The observed information level at each analysis depends primarily on the total number of deaths at that time and, thus, is subject to considerable random variability. It is unlikely that observed information levels at interim analyses conducted on pre-specified dates will be equally spaced and we therefore adopt the error spending approach to control Type I and Type II error rates, following the description for one-sided tests in Section 7.3. We shall work in the maximum information paradigm of Section 7.2.2, using error spending functions $f(\tilde{t}) = \min\{\alpha\tilde{t}^2, \alpha\}$ and $g(\tilde{t}) = \min\{\beta\tilde{t}^2, \beta\}$ for Type I and II errors, respectively, where $\tilde{t}$ represents the ratio of the current information level to $\mathcal{I}_{max}$, the target maximum information level (we denote the information fraction by $\tilde{t}$ here to avoid confusion with t, an individual's survival time). This form of error spending function was considered in Section 7.3 and shown to provide good opportunity for early stopping with about a 10% increase in the maximum information level over that needed for a fixed sample test.

With $\alpha = \beta = 0.05$ and $K = 5$ analyses planned, we multiply $\mathcal{I}_{f,1}$, the information for θ required in a fixed sample test, by $R_{OS}(5, 0.05, 0.05, 2) = 1.101$, taken from Table 7.6, to obtain the maximum information level

$$\mathcal{I}_{max} = 1.101 \times 30.06 = 33.10.$$

If numbers at risk remain roughly equal on the two treatment arms, each observed death contributes about 0.25 to the information for the log hazard ratio, so an information level of 33.1 would need a total of around 132 deaths. We shall assume this maximum information level appeared plausible to the organizers of our hypothetical group sequential study. In principle, the target information level, $\mathcal{I}_{max}$, must be reached eventually but this is not easy to guarantee in a survival study as loss to follow-up or extended survival may staunch the flow of deaths after patient accrual is complete. As explained in Section 7.2.2, this problem of "under-running" can be handled by spending all the remaining Type I error probability at a pre-planned final analysis, whether or not $\mathcal{I}_{max}$ has been achieved.

We conduct our group sequential test according to a rule of the form (4.2), stopping at analysis k with a recommendation for the experimental combination treatment if $Z_k \geq b_k$ and stopping to accept H_0: "No treatment difference" if $Z_k \leq a_k$. The critical values a_k and b_k are found as the solutions to (7.11) and (7.12) and only become known as analysis k is reached. Observed information levels $\mathcal{I}_k$ and the resulting boundary values, a_k and b_k, are displayed in Table13.1. We have included information levels and boundary values for all 5 analyses for completeness although, with early stopping, the later values might not in fact have become known. The $\mathcal{I}_k$s are unequally spaced and the final information level is a little greater than the target of 33.10. Conditional on these information levels, numerical calculations under the approximation (3.1) to the distribution of $Z_1, \ldots, Z_5$ show the test attains a power of 0.952 when θ is 0.6, still very close to the design value of 0.95. By construction, the Type I error probability is exactly 0.05 under this normal approximation.

Inspection of the observed statistics Z_k shows that the lower boundary is crossed at the second analysis and the test would have stopped to accept H_0 at that point. This decision is very much a consequence of the one-sided testing formulation. The negative value of Z_2 indicates that *observed* survival is worse on the experimental treatment than on the standard but the question of whether the

Table 13.1 *Summary data and critical values for a group sequential stratified log-rank test in the clinical trial for carcinoma of the oropharynx. Critical values* a_k *and* b_k *are for a test of* H_0*: "No treatment difference" against the one-sided alternative that the experimental treatment is superior.*
The test uses stratified log-rank statistics (13.3) *and the associated information levels given by* (13.4). *It is constructed using error spending functions* $f(\tilde{t}) = \min\{\alpha\tilde{t}^2, \alpha\}$ *and* $g(\tilde{t}) = \min\{\beta\tilde{t}^2, \beta\}$, *and is designed to attain Type I and Type II error probabilites* $\alpha = \beta = 0.05$ *under five equally spaced information levels concluding with* $\mathcal{I}_5 = 33.10$.

k	*Number entered*	*Number of deaths*	*Stratified log-rank score*	$\mathcal{I}_k$	a_k	b_k	Z_k
1	83	27	−2.41	5.43	−1.60	3.00	−1.04
2	126	58	−3.55	12.58	−0.37	2.49	−1.00
3	174	91	−5.56	21.11	0.63	2.13	−1.21
4	195	129	−4.05	30.55	1.51	1.81	−0.73
5	195	142	−5.03	33.28	1.73	1.73	−0.87

log hazard ratio, θ, is greater or less than zero is not resolved conclusively at this point. However, the results are not consistent with a value of θ as high as 0.6 and so the one-sided test is able to stop in favor of H_0.

Instead of applying a formal stopping rule, the study could have been monitored by repeated confidence intervals. Since a Type I error arises from an error in one tail of an RCI and a Type II error from an error in the other tail, it is appropriate to base decisions on a sequence of 90% RCIs for θ to achieve Type I and II error probabilities each of 0.05 (see the discussion of one-sided derived tests in Section 9.3.2). Table 13.2 shows the sequence of 90% RCIs for the log hazard ratio, θ, in an assumed stratified proportional hazards model. The RCIs are computed from formula (13.15), in keeping with the assumption that $Z_1, \ldots, Z_5$ have the canonical joint distribution (3.1). The critical values $c_k(\alpha)$ are based on the two-sided error spending function $f(\tilde{t}) = \min(0.1\,\tilde{t}^2, 0.1)$, which allocates the same error probabilities in either tail as the two error spending functions in the earlier one-sided test allocate separately to Type I and Type II errors.

If $\theta = 0.6$ had been specified as the treatment effect researchers hoped to detect with power 0.95, the study could have been terminated at the second analysis as the RCI at that point, $(-0.98, 0.42)$, is well below 0.6. Formalizing such decisions into a rule in which the study is stopped the first time an RCI fails to contain either 0 or 0.6 gives a "derived test", as described in Section 9.3, and as long as the final RCI for θ has width at most 0.6 this derived test will have Type I and II error rates of less than 0.05, the overall error probability in either tail of the RCI sequence. In fact, for the observed sequence of information levels, the Type I error of the one-sided derived test, calculated under the normal approximation to the distribution of $\{Z_1, \ldots, Z_5\}$, is 0.047 and, since the width of the final RCI is a little greater than 0.6, its Type II error rate at $\theta = 0.6$ is slightly higher than 0.05 at 0.053.

Table 13.2 *Repeated confidence intervals for* θ*, the log hazard ratio, using the stratified log-rank statistics* (13.3) *and associated information levels* (13.4) *in formula* (13.15) *for the oropharynx trial data.*

Analysis, k	$\mathcal{I}_k$	$Z_k/\sqrt{\mathcal{I}_k}$	*90% RCI,* $(\underline{\theta}_k, \overline{\theta}_k)$
1	5.43	−0.45	(−1.73, 0.84)
2	12.58	−0.28	(−0.98, 0.42)
3	21.11	−0.26	(−0.73, 0.20)
4	30.55	−0.13	(−0.46, 0.20)
5	33.28	−0.15	(−0.47, 0.17)

The RCI approach has the advantage of flexibility and RCIs remain valid whether or not a formal stopping rule is obeyed. Thus, if researchers had decided to continue past the second analysis, despite the low upper limit of the RCI, it would still have been permissible to quote the RCIs at later analyses with an overall confidence level of 90%: in this case, it is likely that the study would have been terminated at the third analysis in favor of the null hypothesis.

We have also calculated RCIs from formula (13.14), finding the maximum partial likelihood estimates $\hat{\theta}^{(k)}$ by fitting a Cox regression model, stratified by institution and with a single x-variable for treatment. Each of these estimates was within 0.01 of the corresponding estimate $Z_k/\sqrt{\mathcal{I}_k}$ in Table 13.2 and the information levels $\mathcal{I}_k(\hat{\theta}^{(k)}) = v_k^{-1}$ were one or two percent higher than the values of $\mathcal{I}_k$ in that table. Endpoints of the resulting intervals differed by at most 0.02 from the values shown in Table 13.2. On the other hand, there are substantial differences between the values $\mathcal{I}_k$ in Table 13.2 and the simple estimates of information, $d_k/4$, where d_k is the number of observed deaths at analysis k listed in Table 13.1, and thus the simplest expression for RCIs (13.16) would not be reliable in this instance.

13.6.3 A Group Sequential Test using the Cox Regression Model

Kalbfleisch & Prentice (1980, p. 3) remark on the importance of adjusting for possible imbalance with regard to baseline covariates in assessing the effect of treatment on survival. The stratified log-rank test does not make such adjustments, relying instead on randomization to balance subjects with respect to important prognostic variables. Use of this test can lead to an awkward situation if randomization happens to produce imbalance with respect to a variable which is known or suspected to have a substantial affect on survival.

As explained in Section 13.4.1, the proportional hazards regression model (Cox, 1972) allows covariates to be modeled either as variables in the regression term for the log hazard ratio or as stratification variables defining separate baseline hazard rates for each stratum. We have conducted a retrospective group sequential

Table 13.3 *Group sequential estimates of Cox model parameters $\beta_1, \ldots, \beta_7$ and their standard errors for the oropharynx trial data. The table shows estimates $\hat{\beta}_j^{(k)}$ at analyses $k = 1, \ldots, 5$, with the standard error of each estimate in parentheses.*

k	*Treatment,* β_1	*Gender,* β_2	*Condition,* β_3	*T-staging,* β_4
1	−0.79 (0.49)	−0.95 (0.82)	1.24 (0.39)	0.31 (0.38)
2	−0.14 (0.30)	−0.76 (0.42)	1.30 (0.26)	0.32 (0.22)
3	−0.08 (0.23)	−0.50 (0.30)	1.19 (0.21)	0.32 (0.17)
4	0.04 (0.19)	−0.59 (0.24)	1.08 (0.17)	0.32 (0.14)
5	0.01 (0.18)	−0.40 (0.22)	1.04 (0.17)	0.25 (0.13)

k	*N-staging,* β_5	*Site* 1, β_6	*Site* 2, β_7
1	0.73 (0.28)	−0.18 (0.30)	0.10 (0.20)
2	0.35 (0.15)	−0.32 (0.18)	−0.08 (0.11)
3	0.17 (0.10)	−0.10 (0.15)	−0.03 (0.08)
4	0.16 (0.09)	−0.11 (0.12)	−0.04 (0.07)
5	0.17 (0.08)	−0.13 (0.11)	−0.03 (0.06)

analysis assuming a model of the form

$$h_{i\ell}(t) = h_{0\ell}(t)\, e^{\boldsymbol{\beta}^T \boldsymbol{x}_i}, \quad t > 0,$$

for the hazard rate of subject i in stratum ℓ. We have taken six strata, corresponding to the six participating institutions, and the following x variables which were identified as important prognostic indicators prior to the study's commencement:

x_{i1}	Treatment	1 = experimental, 2 = standard
x_{i2}	Gender	1 = male, 2 = female
x_{i3}	Condition	1 = no disability, 2 = restricted work 3 = assistance with self care, 4 = bed confined
x_{i4}	T-staging	1, 2, 3, 4 with increasing size of primary tumor
x_{i5}	N-staging	0, 1, 2, 3 with increasing incidence of metastases
x_{i6}	Site 1	1 for faucial arch, 0 for other two sites
x_{i7}	Site 2	1 for tonsillar fossa, 0 for other two sites.

The first variable shows the treatment received and its coefficient, β_1, is the log hazard ratio between the standard and experimental treatment, a positive value indicating an improvement in survival for the experimental treatment. Tumors were classified as occurring at one of three different sites, and the coefficients β_6 and β_7 represent differences in log hazard rates at each of the two named sites relative to the third, the pharyngeal tongue. Table 13.3 shows the estimates of each element of β and their associated standard errors at the five analyses, based on survival data up to times 720, 1080, 1440, 1800 and 2160 days from the beginning of 1968. The models were fitted in S-PLUS (MathSoft Inc., 1998)

Table 13.4 *Test statistics and critical values for a group sequential test based on a Cox regression model for the oropharynx trial data.*
Critical values a_k and b_k are for a test of H_0: $\beta_1 = 0$ against the one-sided alternative $\beta > 0$ under which the experimental treatment is superior. The test is constructed using error spending functions $f(\tilde{t}) = \min\{\alpha\tilde{t}^2, \alpha\}$ and $g(\tilde{t}) = \min\{\beta\tilde{t}^2, \beta\}$, and is designed to attain Type I and Type II error probabilites $\alpha = \beta = 0.05$ under five equally spaced information levels concluding with $\mathcal{I}_5 = 33.10$.
The sequence of RCIs is based on the same form of error spending function and has overall coverage probability 0.9 under the usual normal approximation.

k	$\mathcal{I}_k$	a_k	b_k	$\hat{\beta}_1^{(k)}$	Z_k	90% RCI, $(\underline{\beta}_{1k}, \overline{\beta}_{1k})$
1	4.11	−1.95	3.17	−0.79	−1.60	(−2.35, 0.77)
2	10.89	−0.61	2.59	−0.14	−0.45	(−0.92, 0.65)
3	19.23	0.43	2.20	−0.08	−0.33	(−0.58, 0.43)
4	28.10	1.28	1.90	0.04	0.20	(−0.32, 0.40)
5	30.96	1.86	1.86	0.01	0.04	(−0.33, 0.35)

using the routine “coxph”. The stratified Cox model can also be fitted by the SAS procedure PROC PHREG (SAS Institute Inc., 1996) or the STATA command “stcox” (Stata Corporation, 1997).

A group sequential test can be based on the sequence of estimates of the treatment effect, $\hat{\beta}_1^{(k)}$, $k = 1, \ldots, 5$, and information levels $\mathcal{I}_k$, which are simply the reciprocals of the squares of the standard errors of the $\hat{\beta}_1^{(k)}$. These estimates and information levels are shown in Table 13.4, as are the standardized test statistics $Z_k = \beta_1^{(k)} \sqrt{\mathcal{I}_k}$, $k = 1, \ldots, 5$.

In deriving a group sequential test, we make the approximation that the sequence $Z_1, \ldots, Z_5$ follows the canonical joint distribution (3.1) with $\theta = \beta_1$, given the observed information levels $\mathcal{I}_1, \ldots, \mathcal{I}_5$. Table 13.4 shows the critical values a_k and b_k for a test of the null hypothesis of no treatment difference, H_0: $\beta_1 = 0$ against the one-sided alternative $\beta_1 > 0$. As for the earlier stratified log-rank test, this test is designed to achieve a Type I error probability of $\alpha = 0.05$ and power $1 - \beta = 0.95$ if $\beta_1 = 0.6$ and uses error spending functions $f(\tilde{t}) = \min\{\alpha\tilde{t}^2, \alpha\}$ and $g(\tilde{t}) = \min\{\beta\tilde{t}^2, \beta\}$ for Type I and II errors, respectively. The table also shows a 90%-level RCI sequence, given by (13.11) with critical values $c_k(\alpha)$ based on the two-sided error spending function $f(\tilde{t}) = \min(0.1\,\tilde{t}^2, 0.1)$ and relying on the same distributional assumptions for $Z_1, \ldots, Z_5$.

It is evident that the covariate adjustment has affected the standardized statistics, Z_k, the observed information levels, $\mathcal{I}_k$, and the RCI sequence. This time the test would have stopped at the third analysis, again in favor of H_0. Similarly, a “derived test” based on a sequence of 90% RCIs for β_1 would have stopped at the third analysis since the RCI is completely below 0.6 for the first time on this occasion.

13.7 Survival Probabilities and Quantiles

A time to response variable is more informative than a binary outcome indicating whether or not failure has occurred within a fixed time period of, say, τ years. However, it is sometimes useful to consider a "two-year recurrence rate" or a "five-year survival rate" as a primary outcome. A simple proportion of those surviving the time period will be a biased estimate of the survival rate if not all subjects are followed for the full period, and omitting those subjects with potential censoring times less than τ is inefficient. These difficulties are overcome by use of the Kaplan-Meier estimate (Kaplan & Meier, 1958) of the survival function $S(t)$.

As an example, consider a study of the effect of short-course zidovudine (ZDV) on the mother-to-infant HIV transmission rate among HIV infected mothers in a developing country. The primary response here is time from birth to the first positive PCR test in the infant, indicating the presence of the HIV virus. For a non-breast feeding population, the proportion of infants with a positive PCR within $\tau = 3$ months of birth is a reasonable outcome measure since any perinatal HIV infection will generally lead to a positive PCR test within three months. For a breast feeding population, a horizon of $\tau = 24$ months would be a more suitable choice as infants have continued high exposure to infection. It is likely, because of ethical considerations, that such a trial would be uncontrolled, in which case we have a one-sample problem and must compare the infection rate by time τ with the historical rate.

For $k = 1, \ldots, K$, let d_k denote the total number of failures observed to have occurred by the time of the kth analysis. Let d'_k be the number of distinct failure times and denote these times $\tau_{1,k} < \tau_{2,k} < \ldots < \tau_{d'_k,k}$. Here, $d'_k \leq d_k$ with $d'_k = d_k$ if there are no ties. For the data available at the kth analysis, let $r_{i,k}$ denote the number at risk just before time $\tau_{i,k}$ and $\Delta_{i,k}$ the number of failures at $\tau_{i,k}$, for $i = 1, \ldots, d'_k$. If there are no ties, then each $\Delta_{i,k}$ is equal to one.

The Kaplan-Meier estimate of the survival probability $S_k(t)$ at time t based on data available at analysis k is

$$\widehat{S}_k(t) = \prod_{i:\, \tau_{i,k} \leq t} \left(1 - \frac{\Delta_{i,k}}{r_{i,k}}\right).$$

For a given value of τ, assuming that $0 < S(\tau) < 1$ and there is a positive probability of having an uncensored observation greater than τ, Jennison & Turnbull (1985) show that the sequence

$$Z_k = \{\widehat{S}_k(\tau) - S(\tau)\}/\sqrt{Var\{\widehat{S}_k(\tau)\}}, \quad k = 1, \ldots, K, \tag{13.17}$$

has, asymptotically, the canonical joint distribution (3.1) with $\theta = S(\tau)$ and information levels $\mathcal{I}_k = [Var\{\widehat{S}_k(\tau)\}]^{-1}$.

Greenwood's formula provides a consistent estimate of the variance of $\widehat{S}_k(\tau)$,

$$\widehat{V}_k(\tau) = \widehat{S}_k^2(\tau) \sum_{i:\, \tau_{i,k} \leq \tau} \frac{\Delta_{i,k}}{r_{i,k}(r_{i,k} - \Delta_{i,k})}. \tag{13.18}$$

Hence, a group sequential test of the hypothesis H_0: $S(\tau) = p_0$, where τ and p_0

are specified, can be based on the standardized statistics

$$Z_k = \{\widehat{S}_k(\tau) - p_0\}/\sqrt{\{\widehat{V}_k(\tau)\}}, \quad k = 1, \ldots, K, \tag{13.19}$$

and associated information levels $\mathcal{I}_k = \{\widehat{V}_k(\tau)\}^{-1}$. Since information depends on the number and times of observed failures, the error spending approach of Chapter 7 is to be recommended for constructing such tests.

Repeated confidence intervals for a survival probability can be obtained by inverting a family of two-sided tests, as described in Chapter 9. A sequence of $(1-\alpha)$-level RCIs for $S(\tau)$ has the form

$$(\widehat{S}_k(\tau) \pm c_k(\alpha)\sqrt{\{\widehat{V}_k(\tau)\}}), \quad k = 1, \ldots, K, \tag{13.20}$$

where $\pm c_k(\alpha)$, $k = 1, \ldots, K$, are the critical values of a group sequential two-sided test with Type I error probability α based on standardized statistics with the joint distribution (3.1) for information levels $\mathcal{I}_k = \{\widehat{V}_k(\tau)\}^{-1}$.

Thomas & Grunkemeier (1975, Section 4) propose an alternative estimate of the variance of $\widehat{S}_k(\tau)$ under H_0: $S(\tau) = p_0$, derived in a similar manner to Greenwood's formula but with estimation of $S(t)$, $0 < t \leq \tau$, constrained to agree with the hypothesis H_0. At analysis k, the generalized nonparametric estimate of $S(t)$, $0 < t \leq \tau$, satisfying $S(\tau) = p_0$ is

$$\widetilde{S}_k(t) = \prod_{i:\, \tau_{i,k} \leq t} \left(1 - \frac{\Delta_{i,k}}{r_{i,k} + \eta_k}\right),$$

where η_k is the value for which this expression gives $\widetilde{S}_k(\tau) = p_0$. The "constrained variance" estimate of Thomas & Grunkemeier (1975, Eq. 4.5) is

$$\widetilde{V}_k(\tau) = \hat{p}_0^2 \sum_{i:\, \tau_{i,k} \leq \tau} \frac{\Delta_{i,k}}{r_{i,k}\,(r_{i,k} + \eta_k - \Delta_{i,k})} \frac{\widehat{S}_k(\tau_{i,k}-)}{\widetilde{S}_k(\tau_{i,k}-)}, \tag{13.21}$$

where $\widehat{S}_k(t-)$ and $\widetilde{S}_k(t-)$ denote values of the functions $\widehat{S}_k$ and $\widetilde{S}_k$ just before time t. In the absence of censoring, $\widetilde{V}_k(\tau)$ simplifies to the correct binomial variance under H_0, namely $p_0(1 - p_0)/r_{1,k}$, whereas the Greenwood estimate $\widehat{V}_k(\tau)$ is equal to $\widehat{S}_k(\tau)\{1 - \widehat{S}_k(\tau)\}/r_{1,k}$. Simulations for fixed sample tests reported by Thomas & Grunkemeier (1975) and Barber & Jennison (1999) suggest that use of $\widetilde{V}_k(\tau)$ rather than $\widehat{V}_k(\tau)$ in test statistics (13.19) or RCIs (13.20) should lead to more accurate attainment of error rates and coverage probabilities, respectively. The constrained variance estimate, $\widetilde{V}_k(\tau)$, is not typically provided by statistical software packages, but the calculation is straightforward to program. The Greenwood estimate, $\widehat{V}_k(\tau)$, is a little easier to calculate and is usually available in the output of standard statistical computer software for estimating survival curves.

Sometimes, interest is in a certain *quantile* of the survival distribution. As an example, in a trial of a vaccine for Stage IV melanoma patients it was desired to estimate the median survival time and to compare it with the figure of six months suggested by historical data. For $0 < p < 1$, we define the pth quantile of the survival distribution $S(t)$ to be $t_p = \inf\{t : S(t) \geq p\}$. Assuming $S(t)$ to be strictly decreasing in t, a group sequential test of H_0: $t_p = t^*$ for specified t^*

and p is equivalent to a test of H_0: $S(t^*) = p$ and the test statistics (13.19) can be used with $\tau = t^*$ and $p_0 = p$.

We can also invert a family of group sequential tests with fixed p and varying t to obtain a sequence of RCIs for a quantile t_p. A $(1-\alpha)$-level sequence of RCIs for t_p has the form

$$\{t\colon |\widehat{S}_k(t) - p| \le c_k(\alpha)\sqrt{V_k(t)}\}, \quad k = 1, \ldots, K, \tag{13.22}$$

where $\pm c_k(\alpha)$, $k = 1, \ldots, K$, are critical values for standardized statistics in a group sequential, two-sided test with Type I error probability α. For $V_k(t)$, we can use either the Greenwood estimate $\widehat{V}_k(t)$ given by (13.18) with $\tau = t$, which produces the interval proposed by Brookmeyer & Crowley (1982) in the fixed sample case, or the constrained variance estimate $\widetilde{V}_k(t)$ with $p_0 = p$ and the appropriate $\widetilde{S}_k$ in (13.21). The critical values $c_k(\alpha)$ should be derived for the observed information sequence $\mathcal{I}_k = \{V_k(t)\}^{-1}$, $k = 1, \ldots, K$. They will therefore vary with t, whichever variance estimate is used, but in practice it should suffice to calculate their values using a single, representative value of t at each analysis. Jennison & Turnbull (1985, Tables 1, 2) present simulation results for the coverage probabilities of a single confidence interval or sequences of 5 or 10 RCIs for the median survival time. They find the intervals based on the constrained variance estimate to have error rates in each tail closer to the nominal value $\alpha/2$ than those based on the Greenwood estimate, which tend to be anti-conservative as estimated variances are often too small.

Lin, Shen, Ying & Breslow (1996) have further developed group sequential procedures for monitoring the survival probability up to a fixed time, using Kaplan-Meier estimates. They give a detailed example of designing a trial for treatments of Wilms tumor where it is desired to base decisions on the two-year relapse free survival rate.

Analogous methods can also be used in a two-sample comparison. If $S_A(t)$ and $S_B(t)$ denote survival functions on treatments A and B in a randomized trial, a test of H_0: $S_A(\tau) = S_B(\tau)$, for a given choice of τ, can be based on successive statistics

$$Z_k = \{\widehat{S}_{Ak}(\tau) - \widehat{S}_{Bk}(\tau)\}/\sqrt{\{\widetilde{V}_{Ak}(\tau) + \widetilde{V}_{Bk}(\tau)\}}, \quad k = 1, \ldots, K,$$

where $\widehat{S}_{Ak}(\tau)$ and $\widehat{S}_{Bk}(\tau)$ are Kaplan-Meier estimates of $S_A(\tau)$ and $S_B(\tau)$, respectively, at analysis k and $\widetilde{V}_{Ak}(\tau)$ and $\widetilde{V}_{Bk}(\tau)$ their estimated variances. The problem of comparing the pth quantiles of two survival distributions has been addressed by Keaney & Wei (1994).

13.8 Bibliography and Notes

The asymptotic joint distributions of successively computed log-rank statistics and Cox partial likelihood estimates have been proved under differing degrees of generality by Tsiatis (1981); Sellke & Siegmund (1983); Slud (1984); Tsiatis, Rosner & Tritchler (1985); Gu & Ying (1995); Jennison & Turnbull (1997a); Scharfstein, Tsiatis & Robins (1997); and Bilias, Gu & Ying (1997).

The weighted log-rank statistic generalizes (13.1) to

$$Z_k = \frac{\sum_{i=1}^{d'_k} w_{i,k} \, (\delta_{iA,k} - e_{i,k})}{\left(\sum_{i=1}^{d'_k} w_{i,k}^2 \, v_{i,k}\right)^{1/2}},$$

incorporating weights $w_{1,k}, \ldots, w_{d'_k,k}$. Setting unit weights, $w_{i,k} = 1$ for all i and k, recovers the log-rank test. Weights $w_{i,k} = r_{iA,k} + r_{iB,k}$ yield Gehan's (1965) modification of the Wilcoxon test for censored data. This choice places greater emphasis on differences between observed and expected numbers of failures at earlier follow-up times, yielding a test that is sensitive to early differences between the two survival curves. However, Slud and Wei (1982) show that use of such weights leads to test statistics $Z_1, Z_2, \ldots$ which do *not* necessarily follow the canonical joint distribution (3.1) when there is staggered entry; see also the discussion in Section 11.7. Bilias, Gu & Ying (1997, Corollary 5.1) give the asymptotic distribution of successive weighted log-rank statistics and conditions on the weights for (3.1) to hold.

An example of the use of a group sequential Cox regression analysis is provided by Gu & Ying (1995) in an application to the prostate cancer survival data of Byar (1985). Lin, Yao & Ying (1999) present a thorough investigation into the use of methods for censored survival data in the context of the conditional power approach to stochastic curtailment and include an illustration with data from a colon cancer trial.

Li (1999) describes an alternative to the group sequential log-rank test for testing equality of two survival distributions appropriate when the proportional hazards assumption may not hold under the alternative hypothesis. This procedure is based on monitoring the Pepe-Fleming (1989) statistic, which is a weighted difference between the two Kaplan-Meier curves.

The accelerated life model appears to be an attractive alternative to the proportional hazards model for censored survival data with covariates. However, it has proved cumbersome to deal with, both analytically and computationally. Lin (1992) has considered sequential procedures using this model

Tsiatis, Boucher & Kim (1995) prove results for a parametric survival model under quite general conditions, obtaining analogues to the nonparametric and semi-parametric results of this chapter. Lee & Sather (1995) consider group sequential methods for testing equality of cure rates in survival models where a fraction of each population is not susceptible to failure. They present both parametric and nonparametric procedures and illustrate these with data from a childhood leukemia trial.

Jennison & Turnbull (1984) provide a numerical example of the computation of RCIs for a hazard ratio based on a group sequential log-rank test. Jennison & Turnbull (1985) use the same set of data analyzed in Section 13.6 to illustrate construction of RCIs for a median survival time. Keaney & Wei (1994) illustrate their method of finding a sequence of RCIs for the difference in medians of two survival distributions with an application to AIDS data.

CHAPTER 14

Internal Pilot Studies: Sample Size Re-estimation

14.1 The Role of an Internal Pilot Phase

In setting the sample size for a study, one may find the power calculation requires knowledge of an unknown parameter, such as a response variance or an event rate, which can only be estimated from the data to be collected in the study. One solution to this problem is to carry out a preliminary pilot study before commencing the main trial. There may be other uses for such a pilot study: checking whether a treatment process is feasible, refining the definition of a treatment, learning how to identify suitable participants, or ensuring that randomization and data collection run smoothly. However, if organizers are confident that their treatments and experimental procedures are already well defined, they may wish to launch into the main study without delay. Wittes & Brittain (1990) quote W. G. Cochran's warning that over-interpretation of results from a small pilot study, either positive or negative, may undermine support for the major investigation. Their solution is to forego an "external" pilot study but treat the first part of the main study as an "internal pilot" and re-calculate the overall sample size using estimates of the relevant parameters obtained from the internal pilot data.

Wittes & Brittain emphasize the need to estimate parameters governing sample size from the actual study population, and they cite examples of clinical trials where initial estimates of response variance, recruitment rate or mortality rate were wildly inaccurate. They note the efficiency gained by using data obtained during an internal pilot phase in the end of study analysis, whereas data from an external pilot study would normally be discarded from the main analysis.

Re-estimation of sample size from internal pilot data is simplest when the study will have a single analysis of the major outcome measure once sampling is complete. Thus, the experimental design is sequential only in that interim data are used to modify a fixed sample design. In this case, the mathematical details are quite straightforward. Suppose hypotheses and Type I and II error rates have been specified and the sample size needed for a fixed sample study can be expressed as a function $n(\phi)$ of the unknown parameter ϕ. Based on a pre-study estimate $\hat{\phi}_0$, the study commences with target sample size $n(\hat{\phi}_0)$. After a certain fraction of this sample has been obtained, a new estimate, $\hat{\phi}_1$, is found from the data available. The study then continues with $n(\hat{\phi}_1)$ as the target for its overall sample size, and all data are analyzed at the end as if they had been collected in a fixed sample study. Variations on this scheme are possible. Wittes & Brittain (1990) treat $n(\hat{\phi}_0)$

as a minimum sample size and continue to take at least $n(\hat{\phi}_0)$ observations even if $n(\hat{\phi}_1) < n(\hat{\phi}_0)$. Gould (1992) proposes retaining the initial choice of sample size unless $n(\hat{\phi}_1) > \gamma\, n(\hat{\phi}_0)$, where $\gamma > 1$, and restricting sample size to a maximum of $\omega\, n(\hat{\phi}_0)$, where $\omega > 1$, suggesting possible values $\gamma = 1.33$ and $\omega = 2$ for the two constants. If $n(\hat{\phi}_1)$ is particularly high, organizers may decide to abandon a study on the grounds that it is not feasible to recruit sufficient subjects to achieve acceptable power: this is exactly what happened in the clinical trial of treatments for rheumatoid arthritis reported by Pedersen & Starbuck (1992) when the required sample size was re-estimated three years after the start of patient enrollment.

There is one important proviso when data from a study's internal pilot phase are used to re-calculate the overall sample size. If sample size is allowed to depend on observed responses, it is possible to construct sampling rules which inflate the Type I error rate significantly (adapting the first type of example in Section 7 of Proschan, Follmann & Waclawiw (1992) to this setting gives a rule which can more than double the Type I error probability). Thus, it is crucial that the new sample size be based *only* on estimates of parameters controlling the variance of the major response variable and *not* on any comparison of observed responses between treatment groups. Gould (1992, 1995a), Gould & Shih (1992, 1998) and Shih (1992) advocate maintaining the blinding of treatment codes when analyzing the internal pilot data in order to guard against any possibility of inappropriate practices. Sample size must then be re-estimated from the set of response values pooled across treatment groups. Other authors, for example Herson & Wittes (1993), propose schemes in which a data analyst is allowed access to response variables and treatment codes, but only those data summaries relevant to the sample size calculation are revealed to the Data Monitoring Board, and even this information is not passed on to investigators administering the treatments to patients. Since these analyses of internal pilot data do not allow early termination on the grounds of an observed treatment difference, they may be regarded as "administrative analyses" in the nomenclature of Enas et al. (1989); indeed, study monitors might take the opportunity to make the checks on patient compliance, safety variables, etc., usually associated with an administrative analysis, when meeting to decide on a revised sample size.

Wittes & Brittain (1990) note that adjusting sample size on the basis of an estimated variance may affect the Type I error probability. Typically, the additional sample size is larger when the estimated variance is high; thus over-estimates of variance will be diluted by more additional data than under-estimates, and the final estimate of variance will be biased downward. If this bias is large, one would expect the Type I error to rise. In fact, effects on Type I error rate are usually slight, as we shall see in applications of sample size re-estimation to binary data in Section 14.2.1 and normal data in Section 14.2.2. The most serious difficulties arise when the variance of a normal response is estimated with fewer than 10 degrees of freedom, and we shall describe adjustments to the simple sample size calculations which protect the Type I error in such situations.

The approach outlined above has been used successfully to produce tests with a specified power, often achieving this with an expected sample size close to that of the fixed sample test. Not surprisingly, the expected sample size increases and additional power is achieved as the number of observations in the pilot phase approaches or exceeds the fixed sample size. The general method can be used to update the target sample size or information level for many forms of response distribution. There are however practical limitations; for example, in a survival study the decision on when to terminate patient accrual may have to be taken before information on long-term survival is available. If there are doubts about the practicality of sample size re-estimation or its effects on Type I error or power in a particular application, it is advisable to investigate achieved error probabilities by simulations of the type we report later in this chapter.

Sample size re-estimation can also be combined with group sequential testing. Indeed, in the maximum information paradigm for error spending tests sample size is automatically adjusted, in order to reach the target set for the final information level. Problems may arise in implementing a group sequential test when observed information levels must be estimated and estimates at early analyses have significant variance. There is then a danger that error rates will stray from their intended values and care must be taken to avoid this. We shall address these issues in Section 14.3, where we discuss sample size re-estimation in group sequential tests.

14.2 Sample Size Re-estimation for a Fixed Sample Test

14.2.1 Binary Data

In this section we consider the comparison of binary responses from subjects randomized between two treatment arms. Suppose observations $X_{A1}, X_{A2}, \ldots$ and $X_{B1}, X_{B2}, \ldots$ are independent and take values 0 or 1 with $Pr\{X_{Ai} = 1\} = p_A$ and $Pr\{X_{Bi} = 1\} = p_B$ for $i = 1, 2, \ldots$. If n observations from each distribution are used to test H_0: $p_A = p_B$, we have, approximately,

$$\bar{X}_A - \bar{X}_B \sim N(0, \frac{2}{n} p(1-p))$$

under H_0, where $\bar{X}_A = (X_{A1} + \ldots + X_{An})/n$, $\bar{X}_B = (X_{B1} + \ldots + X_{Bn})/n$ and p denotes the common value of p_A and p_B. Estimating p by

$$\hat{p} = \frac{1}{2n}\left(\sum_{i=1}^{n} X_{Ai} + \sum_{i=1}^{n} X_{Bi}\right), \tag{14.1}$$

we obtain the two-sided test with Type I error probability α which rejects H_0 if

$$|\bar{X}_A - \bar{X}_B| > z_{\alpha/2}\sqrt{\{2\hat{p}(1-\hat{p})/n\}}. \tag{14.2}$$

Here $z_{\alpha/2}$ denotes the upper $\alpha/2$ tail point of a standard normal distribution.

For general p_A and p_B, the distribution of $\bar{X}_A - \bar{X}_B$ is approximately

$$\bar{X}_A - \bar{X}_B \sim N(p_A - p_B, \{p_A(1-p_A) + p_B(1-p_B)\}/n).$$

Suppose $|p_A - p_B|$ is sufficiently large that we can neglect the probability of rejecting H_0 with the sign of $\bar{X}_A - \bar{X}_B$ opposite to that of $p_A - p_B$. The expectation of $\hat{p}$ defined by (14.1) is $(p_A + p_B)/2$, which we denote by $\bar{p}$. Substituting $\bar{p}$ for $\hat{p}$ in (14.2), we find the power of the above test is approximately

$$\Phi^{-1}\left\{\frac{|p_A - p_B|\sqrt{n}}{\sqrt{\{p_A(1-p_A) + p_B(1-p_B)\}}} - \frac{z_{\alpha/2}\sqrt{\{2\,\bar{p}(1-\bar{p})\}}}{\sqrt{\{p_A(1-p_A) + p_B(1-p_B)\}}}\right\}.$$

Using the further approximation

$$\frac{2\,\bar{p}(1-\bar{p})}{p_A(1-p_A) + p_B(1-p_B)} \approx 1, \tag{14.3}$$

we see that power $1 - \beta$ is achieved at a specific pair of values (p_A, p_B) by a sample size

$$n = \frac{(z_{\alpha/2} + z_\beta)^2\{p_A(1-p_A) + p_B(1-p_B)\}}{(p_A - p_B)^2} \tag{14.4}$$

from each treatment arm. Replacing $p_A(1 - p_A) + p_B(1 - p_B)\}$ in (14.4) by $2\,\bar{p}(1 - \bar{p})$ gives the alternative approximation:

$$n = \frac{(z_{\alpha/2} + z_\beta)^2\, 2\,\bar{p}(1-\bar{p})}{(p_A - p_B)^2}, \tag{14.5}$$

which agrees with that given by Gould (1992) for a test of H_0: $p_A = p_B$ based on the χ^2 statistic for the 2×2 table of responses on the two treatments.

Suppose one wishes to achieve power $1 - \beta$ if $p_B = p_A + \Delta$, where Δ is specified but not p_A. We can substitute Δ for $p_A - p_B$ in the denominator of (14.4) or (14.5), but estimates of p_A and p_B are needed to evaluate the numerator of either function. In the internal pilot approach, we use initial estimates of response rates p_A and p_B that satisfy the alternative hypothesis $p_B = p_A + \Delta$ to calculate a first approximation to the required sample size. We then sample a fraction of these observations, n_0 say, from each treatment arm in the study's internal pilot phase. Estimates of p_A and p_B from pilot phase data are used to re-calculate the total sample size. If the new value for the sample size is n_1 per treatment, we sample a further $n_1 - n_0$ observations from each arm. Exceptions to this rule arise if n_0 already exceeds n_1, in which case no further observations are necessary, or if other constraints are set on the second stage sample size. When sampling is completed, the test of H_0 is applied as defined by (14.1) and (14.2) with n equal to the total sample size actually observed from each arm, or with the appropriate correction if sample sizes on the two arms are not exactly equal.

In analyzing the pilot phase data, Gould (1992) recommends use of (14.5) with $\bar{p}$ estimated by

$$\frac{1}{2n_0}\left(\sum_{i=1}^{n_0} X_{Ai} + \sum_{i=1}^{n_0} X_{Bi}\right).$$

An advantage of this method is that $\bar{p}$ depends only on the pooled response data, and it is not necessary to unblind treatment allocations to find $\bar{p}$.

Herson & Wittes (1993) adopt a different approach in a problem where the X_{Ai}s and X_{Bi}s are responses on standard and experimental treatments, respectively. They use the pilot phase data just to obtain an estimate, $\hat{p}_A$, of the response rate on the standard treatment and calculate the required sample size by pairing this with the value of p_B that satisfies the alternative hypothesis. Thus, a test with approximate power $1 - \beta$ at $p_B = p_A + \Delta$ is obtained by substituting $p_A = \hat{p}_A$ and $p_B = \hat{p}_A + \Delta$ in (14.4). This approach requires unblinding of treatment allocations, at least for the data analyst.

The power requirement can be specified in other ways, for example, in terms of the ratio p_A/p_B. If power $1 - \beta$ is required when $p_B = p_A/\rho$, formula (14.5) becomes

$$n = \frac{(z_{\alpha/2} + z_\beta)^2 \, (1 - \bar{p}) \, (\rho + 1)^2}{2 \, \bar{p} \, (\rho - 1)^2} \tag{14.6}$$

and Gould's method of substituting an estimate of $\bar{p}$ from the pooled response data, without unblinding, can still be employed. Alternatively, one can follow Herson & Wittes' approach, writing (14.4) under $p_B = p_A/\rho$ as

$$n = \frac{(z_{\alpha/2} + z_\beta)^2 \{p_A(1 - p_A) + (p_A/\rho)(1 - p_A/\rho)\}}{(p_A - p_A/\rho)^2} \tag{14.7}$$

and substituting the estimate $\hat{p}_A$ obtained from pilot phase observations on the first treatment arm. Gould (1992) also gives a formula for the sample size necessary to achieve a specific power under a given odds ratio $p_A(1 - p_B)/\{p_B(1 - p_A)\}$.

Tables 14.1 and 14.2 show the results of applying the two approaches described above to construct tests with power $1 - \beta = 0.9$ when $p_B = p_A + \Delta$. The tests reported in Table 14.1 use Herson & Wittes' method, taking an estimate $\hat{p}_A$ from pilot phase data on the first treatment and calculating the overall sample size per treatment arm from (14.4) with $p_A = \hat{p}_A$ and $p_B = \hat{p}_A + \Delta$. Since p_B can be at most 1, $\hat{p}_A$ is truncated to $1 - \Delta$ if it exceeds this value. Note that the sample size formula involves $\hat{p}_A$ and Δ but does not depend on the responses from treatment arm B. This explains why the same means and standard deviations of the sample size distribution are seen in the top and bottom halves of Table 14.1. Table 14.2 concerns tests using Gould's method in which an estimate of $\bar{p}$ from the pooled pilot phase data is substituted into (14.5). As this calculation implicitly assumes the values $p_A = \bar{p} - \Delta/2$ and $p_B = \bar{p} + \Delta/2$, values of $\bar{p}$ are restricted to the interval $(\Delta/2, 1 - \Delta/2)$, and if response rates outside this range are observed, the estimate of $\bar{p}$ is shifted upward to $\Delta/2$ or downward to $1 - \Delta/2$ as necessary.

It is evident from the tables that Type I error rates are only slightly perturbed from their nominal value of 0.05, rising to around 0.06 in a few examples with low n_0 and low total sample size. Power is close to its nominal value of 0.9, lying between 0.86 and 0.93 for the Herson & Wittes approach and in the range 0.89 to 0.91 for Gould's method. These results are in general agreement with those reported by other authors and support Gould's (1992) claim that re-estimation of sample size "does not materially affect the Type I error rates".

Sample sizes under H_0: $p_A = p_B$ differ between the two methods since different alternatives satisfying $p_B = p_A + \Delta$ are considered in each case. In Herson & Wittes' approach p_A is set first and Δ added to give the value for p_B; we have followed this procedure, using the true value of p_A, in calculating the fixed sample sizes in Table 14.1. Gould's approach starts with a value for the mean response rate $\bar{p}$ and then sets the individual probabilities at $p_A = \bar{p} - \Delta/2$ and $p_B = \bar{p} + \Delta/2$; the fixed sample sizes in Table 14.2 are calculated by this

Table 14.1 *Properties of "internal pilot" tests of two binary responses with power at* $p_B = p_A + \Delta$ *constructed using Herson & Wittes' (1993) approach.*
An initial sample of n_0 *is observed on each arm and the overall sample size calculated from* (14.4) *with* $\alpha = 0.05$, $\beta = 0.1$, $p_A = \hat{p}_A$ *and* $p_B = \hat{p}_A + \Delta$. *The tabulated fixed sample size gives power* $1 - \beta$ *under the true value of* p_A *and* $p_B = p_A + \Delta$.
Results are based on simulations with one million replicates; standard errors are 0.0002 *for Type I errors,* 0.0003 *for power, and well below* 0.1 *for the mean and standard deviation of the total sample size.*

Δ	p_A	p_B	*Pilot size* n_0	*Fixed sample*	*Total sample size* *Mean*	*St. dev.*	*Type I error probability*
0.3	0.1	0.1	10	39	36.8	9.6	0.059
	0.1	0.1	20	39	38.0	7.2	0.061
	0.2	0.2	20	48	46.3	6.1	0.056
	0.2	0.2	30	48	47.1	5.0	0.055
	0.3	0.3	30	53	51.4	2.9	0.053
	0.3	0.3	40	53	51.6	2.3	0.053
	0.4	0.4	30	53	51.2	3.5	0.054
0.2	0.1	0.1	30	79	77.6	16.6	0.056
	0.1	0.1	50	79	78.3	12.8	0.053
	0.2	0.2	50	106	103.9	11.8	0.053
	0.2	0.2	70	106	104.4	9.9	0.052
	0.3	0.3	60	121	119.4	6.4	0.052
	0.3	0.3	90	121	120.1	5.2	0.051
	0.4	0.4	60	127	124.3	3.0	0.050
							Power
0.3	0.1	0.4	10	39	36.8	9.6	0.897
	0.1	0.4	20	39	38.0	7.2	0.919
	0.2	0.5	20	48	46.4	6.1	0.898
	0.2	0.5	30	48	47.1	5.0	0.903
	0.3	0.6	30	53	51.4	2.9	0.879
	0.3	0.6	40	53	51.6	2.3	0.880
	0.4	0.7	30	53	51.2	3.5	0.859
0.2	0.1	0.3	30	79	77.6	16.6	0.921
	0.1	0.3	50	79	78.4	12.8	0.931
	0.2	0.4	50	106	103.9	11.8	0.910
	0.2	0.4	70	106	104.4	9.9	0.914
	0.3	0.5	60	121	119.4	6.4	0.898
	0.3	0.5	90	121	120.0	5.2	0.900
	0.4	0.6	60	127	124.3	3.0	0.886

Table 14.2 *Properties of "internal pilot" tests of two binary responses with power at* $p_B = p_A + \Delta$ *constructed using Gould's (1992) approach.*
An initial sample of n_0 *is observed on each arm and the overall sample size calculated from* (14.5) *with* $\alpha = 0.05$, $\beta = 0.1$ *and* $\bar{p}$ *estimated from the pooled pilot phase data. The tabulated fixed sample size gives power* $1 - \beta$ *under* $p_A = \bar{p} - \Delta/2$ *and* $p_B = \bar{p} - \Delta/2$, *where* $\bar{p}$ *is the mean of the true* p_A *and* p_B.
Results are based on simulations with one million replicates; standard errors are 0.0002 *for Type I errors,* 0.0003 *for power, and well below* 0.1 *for the mean and standard deviation of the total sample size.*

Δ	p_A	p_B	*Pilot size* n_0	*Fixed sample*	*Total sample size* *Mean*	*St. dev.*	*Type I error probability*
0.3	0.1	0.1	10	22	31.4	3.9	0.057
	0.1	0.1	20	22	30.6	2.2	0.056
	0.2	0.2	20	38	38.0	7.0	0.051
	0.2	0.2	30	38	37.8	6.0	0.049
	0.3	0.3	30	50	48.8	5.6	0.051
	0.3	0.3	40	50	49.2	4.6	0.051
	0.4	0.4	30	57	55.7	3.2	0.050
0.2	0.1	0.1	30	48	53.9	9.1	0.057
	0.1	0.1	50	48	53.8	6.4	0.049
	0.2	0.2	50	85	83.8	12.5	0.051
	0.2	0.2	70	85	84.6	9.5	0.050
	0.3	0.3	60	111	109.9	8.9	0.050
	0.3	0.3	90	111	110.2	7.1	0.051
	0.4	0.4	60	127	125.7	4.9	0.050
							Power
0.3	0.1	0.4	10	44	43.3	9.0	0.893
	0.1	0.4	20	44	43.5	7.1	0.901
	0.2	0.5	20	54	52.6	5.3	0.903
	0.2	0.5	30	54	52.9	4.3	0.907
	0.3	0.6	30	58	57.5	1.9	0.908
	0.3	0.6	40	58	57.8	1.6	0.910
	0.4	0.7	30	58	57.5	1.9	0.908
0.2	0.1	0.3	30	85	83.3	15.4	0.889
	0.1	0.3	50	85	83.9	12.1	0.897
	0.2	0.4	50	111	109.9	9.4	0.901
	0.2	0.4	70	111	110.1	8.0	0.903
	0.3	0.5	60	127	125.7	4.8	0.903
	0.3	0.5	90	127	126.0	3.9	0.904
	0.4	0.6	60	132	131.0	1.5	0.911

method using the true value of $\bar{p}$. Note that although sample sizes under H_0 are consistently smaller in Table 14.2 than in Table 14.1, the position can be reversed in other situations not presented here. Minor differences between the fixed sample sizes in the two tables when $p_B = p_A + \Delta$ arise because of the different variance estimates in formulae (14.4) and (14.5), and evaluating the numerators of these formulae using estimates of p_A and $\bar{p}$, respectively, leads to further variation between the two methods.

Table 14.3 shows properties of tests constructed to satisfy a power requirement when $p_B = p_A/\rho$ for a specified constant ρ; the cases shown here were selected as representative examples from a more extensive study. In Herson & Wittes' tests, the pilot phase data are used to estimate p_A and the overall sample size per arm is found by substituting $\hat{p}_A$ for p_A in (14.7). If $\rho < 1$ and $\hat{p}_A > \rho$, $\hat{p}_A$ is truncated to ρ so that $\hat{p}_A/\rho$ does not exceed 1. If all observations on arm 1 in the pilot phase were zero, we set $\hat{p}_A = 0.5/n_0$ to ensure that (14.7) could still be used. Herson & Wittes' sample size formula involves $\hat{p}_A$ and ρ but not the responses from treatment arm B. Hence, the pattern of means and standard deviations for the sample size distribution is repeated in the second group of four Herson & Wittes tests when p_A and ρ take the same values as in the first four tests but p_B is different. Gould's tests are carried out using sample size formula (14.6) with $\bar{p}$ estimated from the pooled pilot phase data. For $\rho > 1$, any estimate of $\bar{p}$ greater than $(1+\rho)/(2\rho)$ is reduced to this value so that the value of p_A implicit in (14.6) does not exceed 1; similarly, for $\rho < 1$, high estimates of $\bar{p}$ are reduced to $(1+\rho)/2$ so that $p_B = 2\bar{p}/(1+\rho)$ is not greater than 1. If all pilot phase observations on both treatment arms were zero, we set $\hat{p}_A = 0.5/(2n_0)$. In all these simulations the second stage sample size was restricted to 1000 observations per treatment arm.

Once again, Type I error rates are in close agreement with their nominal value, $\alpha = 0.05$. However, for this problem the power shows greater variation above and below its target of 0.9. It is notable that the standard deviation of the total sample size is very high both under H_0 and when $p_B = p_A/\rho$. This variability in sample size can be attributed to the sensitivity of the formulae (14.7) and (14.6) to changes in p_A and $\bar{p}$, respectively, and the fact that both these quantities may be estimated quite poorly from the pilot phase data. The fact that Type I error rates are not affected in this situation lends further support to claims of robustness of the Type I error probability to sample size re-estimation.

The testing problem considered in this section has the special feature that variances of thc estimates of response probability differ on the two treatment arms when $p_A \neq p_B$. Consequently, the variance of the final estimate of $p_A - p_B$ could be reduced by allocating observations unequally between the two treatment arms. This possibility has not been exploited in the methods reported here, but it might prove a useful addition to two-stage experimental designs .

14.2.2 Normal Data with Unknown Variance

One of the most common difficulties in carrying out sample size calculations arises from the lack of an accurate estimate of the variance of normally distributed

Table 14.3 *Properties of "internal pilot" tests of two binary responses with power at* $p_B = p_A/\rho$.
An initial sample of n_0 *is observed on each arm. For Herson & Wittes' (1993) tests, the overall sample size is found from* (14.7) *with* $\alpha = 0.05$, $\beta = 0.1$, *and* p_A *estimated from the pilot phase data. In Gould's (1992) approach, formula* (14.6) *is used with an estimate of* $\bar{p}$ *from the pooled pilot phase data.*
The tabulated fixed sample size gives power $1 - \beta$ *under the true value of* p_A *and* $p_B = p_A/\rho$ *for Herson & Wittes' tests, and under values* p_A *and* p_B *with mean equal to the true* $\bar{p}$ *and satisfying* $p_B = p_A/\rho$ *for Gould's tests.*
Results are based on simulations with one million replicates; standard errors are 0.0002 *for Type I errors,* 0.0003 *for power and at most* 0.3*, but usually much less, for the mean and standard deviation of the total sample size.*

Herson & Wittes' tests

ρ	p_A	p_B	*Pilot size* n_0	*Fixed sample*	*Total sample size* *Mean*	*St. dev.*	*Type I error probability*
1.5	0.75	0.75	20	74	77.8	30.3	0.054
1.25	0.75	0.75	80	200	202.8	41.6	0.052
0.5	0.2	0.2	80	106	116.9	40.2	0.048
0.25	0.1	0.1	30	39	71.4	68.8	0.051
							Power
1.5	0.75	0.5	20	74	77.8	30.3	0.917
1.25	0.75	0.6	80	200	202.8	41.6	0.927
0.5	0.2	0.8	80	106	116.9	40.4	0.834
0.25	0.1	0.4	30	39	71.3	68.7	0.832

Gould's tests

ρ	p_A	p_B	*Pilot size* n_0	*Fixed sample*	*Total sample size* *Mean*	*St. dev.*	*Type I error probability*
1.5	0.75	0.75	20	44	46.3	16.1	0.052
1.25	0.75	0.75	80	142	143.6	26.1	0.050
0.5	0.2	0.2	80	190	195.7	40.8	0.050
0.25	0.1	0.1	30	132	165.6	115.5	0.051
							Power
1.5	0.75	0.5	20	79	82.4	26.7	0.882
1.25	0.75	0.6	80	205	207.1	34.6	0.894
0.5	0.2	0.8	80	111	113.2	19.3	0.909
0.25	0.1	0.4	30	44	47.3	14.4	0.936

responses. Suppose X_{Ai} and X_{Bi}, $i = 1, 2, \ldots$, are responses of subjects allocated to treatments A and B, respectively, and these are independently distributed as $X_{Ai} \sim N(\mu_A, \sigma^2)$ and $X_{Bi} \sim N(\mu_B, \sigma^2)$, $i = 1, 2, \ldots$. We shall consider the problem of testing H_0: $\mu_A = \mu_B$ against the two-sided alternative $\mu_A \neq \mu_B$ with Type I error probability α and power $1 - \beta$ at $\mu_A - \mu_B = \pm\delta$.

If n responses have been observed on each treatment, the t-test with two-sided Type I error probability α rejects H_0 if

$$\frac{|\bar{X}_A - \bar{X}_B|}{\sqrt{(2s^2/n)}} > t_{2n-2,\alpha/2} \, ,$$

where $t_{\nu,q}$ denotes the upper q tail-point of a t-distribution on ν degrees of freedom. Here, $\bar{X}_A$ is the mean of $X_{A1}, \ldots, X_{An}$, $\bar{X}_B$ the mean of $X_{B1}, \ldots, X_{Bn}$ and s^2 the standard unbiased estimate of σ^2. When $\mu_A - \mu_B = \delta$, the statistic $(\bar{X}_A - \bar{X}_B)/\sqrt{(2s^2/n)}$ has a non-central t-distribution on $2n - 2$ degrees of freedom with non-centrality parameter $\delta\sqrt{\{n/(2s^2)\}}$, which we shall write as $T(2n - 2; \delta\sqrt{\{n/(2s^2)\}})$. Thus, in order to meet the power condition, n must be large enough that

$$Pr\{T(2n-2; \delta\sqrt{\{n/(2s^2)\}}) > t_{2n-2,\alpha/2}\} \geq 1 - \beta. \qquad (14.8)$$

Taking α, β and δ as fixed, we denote the smallest value of n satisfying (14.8) as $N_f(\sigma^2)$, representing the required number of observations per treatment arm to provide the stated error probabilities for a given true value of σ^2.

Wittes & Brittain (1990) propose the following general strategy for using an internal pilot study to re-estimate sample size. One first calculates the sample size, $N_f(\sigma_0^2)$, required if σ^2 were equal to an initial estimate of its value, σ_0^2. In the internal pilot phase, a fraction of this sample, $\pi N_f(\sigma_0^2)$ per treatment arm, is observed and s_0^2, the usual unbiased estimate of σ^2, is calculated from these data. The overall sample size is then re-estimated as $N_f(s_0^2)$ per treatment. At this point, various options are available. Wittes & Brittain recommend taking the maximum of $N_f(s_0^2)$ and the original figure $N_f(\sigma_0^2)$ as the new total sample size per treatment, partly out of concern that reducing the sample size below $N_f(\sigma_0^2)$ may lead to an increase in the Type I error probability. Gould & Shih (1992) suggest retaining the initial target of $N_f(\sigma_0^2)$ unless $N_f(s_0^2)$ is substantially higher, say by more than 25%, and they also propose truncating excessive values of $N_f(s_0^2)$ to a practical level such as $2N_f(\sigma_0^2)$. In assessing this method of sample size re-estimation, we have followed Birkett & Day's (1994) example and simply set the new total sample size per treatment as the maximum of n_0 and $N_f(s_0^2)$, where n_0 is the sample size already observed in the pilot phase. In any event, if a total of n_1 observations per treatment is deemed appropriate after examining the pilot phase data, one continues to observe a further $n_1 - n_0$ responses on each arm and then conducts a test of H_0 using the full set of data. In this test, H_0 is rejected if

$$\frac{|\bar{X}_A - \bar{X}_B|}{\sqrt{(2s_1^2/n_1)}} > t_{2n_1-2,\alpha/2} \, ,$$

where now $\bar{X}_A$ and $\bar{X}_B$ are the means of $X_{A,1}, \ldots, X_{A,n_1}$ and $X_{B,1}, \ldots, X_{B,n_1}$,

Table 14.4 *Properties of Wittes & Brittain (1990) and Birkett & Day (1994) "internal pilot" tests for two normal distributions of unknown variance.*
An initial sample of n_0 is observed on each arm and the overall sample size, n_1, set as the minimum of n_0 and $N_f(s_0^2)$, as defined by (14.8) *with Type I error probability $\alpha = 0.05$ and power $1 - \beta = 0.9$ at $\mu_A - \mu_B = \pm\delta = \pm 1$.*
Results are based on simulations with one million replicates; standard errors are at most 0.0001 *for Type I errors,* 0.0002 *for power and* 0.1 *for the mean and standard deviation of the total sample size, n_1.*

σ^2	*Fixed size per arm* $N_f(\sigma^2)$	*Pilot size per arm* n_0	*Total sample size per arm, n_1* Mean	St. dev.	*Type I error rate*	*Power at* $\mu_A - \mu_B = \pm 1$
0.3	8	2	8.0	6.2	0.090	0.829
	8	3	8.0	4.4	0.076	0.893
	8	5	8.1	2.9	0.062	0.931
	8	10	10.2	0.7	0.050	0.977
0.5	12	2	12.2	10.4	0.085	0.781
	12	3	12.1	7.4	0.074	0.851
	12	5	12.1	5.2	0.065	0.897
	12	10	12.6	2.9	0.055	0.931
1.0	23	3	22.6	14.8	0.065	0.810
	23	5	22.6	10.5	0.060	0.862
	23	10	22.5	7.0	0.057	0.898
	23	20	23.4	3.8	0.053	0.921
2.0	44	3	43.5	29.7	0.058	0.786
	44	5	43.5	21.0	0.055	0.842
	44	10	43.5	14.0	0.054	0.880
	44	20	43.5	9.6	0.053	0.898
4.0	86	5	85.5	42.1	0.052	0.832
	86	10	85.5	28.0	0.052	0.871
	86	20	85.5	19.3	0.052	0.890
	86	40	85.6	13.5	0.051	0.899

respectively, and s_1^2 is the usual estimate of σ^2 calculated from all $2n_1$ observations.

Table 14.4 shows properties of tests of the above form when n_1 is set equal to the maximum of n_0 and $N_f(s_0^2)$. Values of s_0^2 and, hence, n_1 and s_1^2 were generated by simulation, and the conditional probability of rejecting H_0 was then found exactly as a tail point of the standard normal distribution. In the examples considered here, $\alpha = 0.05$ and tests are intended to achieve power $1 - \beta = 0.9$ at $\mu_A - \mu_B = \pm 1$. The true values of σ^2 are such that the necessary fixed sample size ranges from 8 to 86 per treatment arm. The problem depends on σ^2 and δ only through σ^2/δ^2, so the reported results also apply to other situations with the same value of this ratio.

Examples with low values for n_0 and $N_f(\sigma^2)$ are included to demonstrate just where the method starts to break down. In Section 14.1 we noted Wittes &

Brittain's concern that the negative bias in s_1^2, the final variance estimate, might inflate the Type I error rate. The tabulated results show that this problem does indeed occur, but only at extremely low sample sizes. For practical purposes, the attained Type I error rates may be regarded as sufficiently close to the target of 0.05 as long as the initial sample contains at least 10 observations on each treatment. Errors in estimating σ^2 from a small pilot phase have a noticeable effect on the attained power, and an initial sample of at least 10 observations per treatment also appears necessary for adequate power to be reliably achieved. Of course, an initial sample greater than or equal to $N_f(\sigma^2)$ leads to attained power in excess of the specified $1 - \beta$.

We have obtained similar results in further simulation studies and have found the general pattern of results to be only slightly affected by variations to the sampling rule. We found that Wittes & Brittain's proposal of setting a lower limit on n_1 does indeed reduce inflation in the Type I error probability when n_0 and $N_f(\sigma^2)$ are very low. If sample sizes are high, the method can be simplified by replacing $N_f(\sigma^2)$ with the sample size formula for a known variance problem:

$$(z_{\alpha/2} + z_\beta)^2 \, \frac{2\sigma^2}{\delta^2}.$$

However, if either n_0 or $N_f(\sigma^2)$ is small, this can lead to slightly higher Type I error rates and, since the resulting sample size is uniformly lower, some loss of power.

Gould & Shih (1992) propose a method for re-estimating sample size without the need to unblind treatment allocations. At the end of the study's pilot phase, they model the pooled responses from both treatment arms as a mixture of two normal distributions of unknown means and common variance σ^2, using the EM algorithm to find the maximum likelihood estimate of σ^2. This variance estimate is used to calculate the overall sample size and, after the necessary additional data have been collected, treatment allocations are unblinded and a standard t-test performed. Simulation results presented by Gould & Shih demonstrate the effectiveness of their procedure in estimating σ^2 from pooled observations and show that the resulting two-stage test attains its nominal Type I error rate accurately in a range of examples. Given that this method has to make do with less information about σ^2, we would expect it to experience problems for small n_0 and $N_f(\sigma^2)$ on at least the same scale as methods using the standard variance estimate based on knowledge of treatment allocations.

Gould & Shih (1992) recommend a straightforward approach to study design, allowing reconsideration of the overall sample size at just one interim inspection of the data and only modifying the initial choice of sample size if this is clearly inadequate, for example, less that 80% of the new estimate. They suggest conducting this sample size analysis as soon as sufficient data are available to give a reliable estimate of σ^2 since, from an administrative perspective, changes in design are easier to implement early on in a study. In contrast, Sandvik et al. (1996) conclude that re-analysis of sample size should occur rather later if the major objective is to estimate σ^2 as accurately as possible, subject to a limit on the probability that the internal pilot sample exceeds the sample size needed for the entire study. Most of the standard deviations of n_1 shown in Table 14.4 are quite substantial, reflecting the high variability of estimates of σ^2 based on pilot phase data. Hall (1981) has suggested the addition of a small third study phase to bring the total sample size up to a value calculated using information on σ^2 from the pilot phase and the main body of observations. While this modification can assist in stabilizing the final choice of sample size, there may sometimes be practical difficulties in adjusting targets for patient accrual so late in the course of a study.

The methods discussed so far make no allowance for the fact that an estimate of variance is used in setting the overall sample size. It should not, therefore, be surprising that values for power at $\mu_A - \mu_B = \pm 1$ reported in Table 14.4 can be well below the target of 0.9 when σ^2 is estimated from a small pilot sample. One may try to compensate for the possibility that an under-estimate of σ^2 has been observed (see, for example, Browne, 1995, and Betensky & Tierney, 1997). However, an elegant and precise way of dealing with the sampling distribution of s_0^2 is provided in Stein's (1945) two-stage test, which has Type I error rate exactly equal to its nominal level α and guarantees the specified power conservatively. In Stein's test, an estimate s_0^2 on $2n_0 - 2$ degrees of freedom is obtained from pilot phase data and the total sample size per treatment, n_1, is taken to be the maximum of n_0 and

$$(t_{2n_0-2,1-\alpha/2} + t_{2n_0-2,1-\beta})^2 \, \frac{2s_0^2}{\delta^2} \, . \tag{14.9}$$

On termination, H_0: $\mu_A - \mu_B = 0$ is rejected if

$$\frac{|\bar{X}_A - \bar{X}_B|}{\sqrt{(2s_0^2/n_1)}} > t_{2n_0-2,\alpha/2} .$$

Use of the initial variance estimate, s_0^2, in this rule ensures that the test has the stated error probabilities but detracts from its appeal as a practical method. If the estimate s_1^2 calculated from the final data set differs substantially from s_0^2, it is difficult to justify a decision which relies on use of s_0^2, rather than s_1^2, in the final t-test.

Denne & Jennison (1999a) present a two-stage test using Stein's sample size formula (14.9), but with the natural choice of variance estimate, s_1^2, in the final test statistic. This test rejects H_0 if

$$\frac{|\bar{X}_A - \bar{X}_B|}{\sqrt{(2s_1^2/n_1)}} > t_{2n_0-2+2\epsilon(n_1-n_0),\alpha/2} \, , \tag{14.10}$$

where the constant ϵ can be varied between 0 and 1 to fine-tune the test and a value $\epsilon = 1/8$ is recommended for accurate attainment of both Type I error and Type II error probabilities. Properties of this test are shown in Table 14.5. It is evident that Stein's sampling rule increases the expected sample size over the corresponding values in Table 14.4, especially under low values of n_0, and this helps increase power toward the target of 0.9.

It is surprising that some tests in Table 14.5 should have Type I error rate greater than $\alpha = 0.05$ and power less than $1-\beta = 0.9$ when $\mu_A - \mu_B = \pm 1$, since Stein's original procedure uses the same samples to produce a test with Type I error rate

Table 14.5 *Properties of Denne & Jennison's (1999a) "internal pilot" tests for two normal distributions of unknown variance.*
An initial sample of n_0 is observed on each arm and the overall sample size, n_1, set as the minimum of n_0 and the expression (14.9). *On termination the test is conducted using rule* (14.10).
Results are based on simulations with one million replicates; standard errors are at most 0.0001 *for Type I errors,* 0.0002 *for power and* 0.1 *for the mean and standard deviation of the total sample size, n_1.*

σ^2	*Fixed size per arm* $N_f(\sigma^2)$	*Pilot size per arm* n_0	*Total sample size per arm, n_1* *Mean*	*St. dev.*	*Type I error rate*	*Power at* $\mu_A - \mu_B = \pm 1$
0.3	8	2	23.5	22.9	0.055	0.861
	8	3	11.7	7.8	0.053	0.900
	8	5	8.9	3.9	0.056	0.933
	8	10	10.2	0.8	0.050	0.977
0.5	12	2	38.8	38.2	0.053	0.855
	12	3	19.1	13.1	0.047	0.875
	12	5	14.2	6.8	0.052	0.905
	12	10	12.9	3.3	0.053	0.933
1.0	23	3	37.6	26.2	0.041	0.862
	23	5	27.9	13.7	0.044	0.882
	23	10	24.1	7.8	0.051	0.903
	23	20	23.5	4.1	0.052	0.922
2.0	44	3	74.8	52.5	0.041	0.863
	44	5	55.3	27.4	0.042	0.875
	44	10	47.6	15.7	0.046	0.891
	44	20	44.8	10.2	0.050	0.901
4.0	86	5	110.1	54.9	0.044	0.877
	86	10	94.7	31.4	0.046	0.888
	86	20	89.1	20.3	0.048	0.895
	86	40	86.8	13.8	0.050	0.901

exactly equal to α and power at least $1 - \beta$. Denne & Jennison (1999b) attribute this efficiency to the way in which Stein's test implicitly allocates Type I error conditionally on the value of s_0^2 and, hence, n_1. This distribution of conditional Type I error over values of n_1 happens to produce high overall power in this instance. In contrast, by using s_1^2 in the final t-test, the modified test evens out the conditional Type I error over values of n_1 and this reduces overall power. Denne & Jennison (1999b) provide further discussion of the conditional properties of Stein's test. Although a simple comparison of Type I error and power may suggest advantages to Stein's original procedure, there is little practical value in having a significance test reject the null hypothesis using one estimate of variance when further information, not used in the test, indicates that this estimate is too low.

We would therefore recommend using the standard variance estimate from all available data on conclusion of a study incorporating sample size re-estimation.

14.3 Sample Size Re-estimation in Group Sequential Tests

14.3.1 The Error Spending Approach

The maximum information formulation of the error spending method, described in Section 7.2.2, accommodates sample size re-estimation very naturally. In the simplest types of application, the information accruing by a given analysis is affected by unknown parameters, but this information level can be accurately assessed at the time the analysis is conducted. If, instead, information levels are functions of an unknown parameter and so have to be estimated along with that parameter, some modifications to the basic approach become necessary.

As an example where information levels are readily available, consider a comparison of two survival distributions using a group sequential log-rank test. The observed information $\mathcal{I}_k$ at analysis k can be calculated from equation (13.2) and is roughly proportional to the total number of observed deaths. Thus, the level of information is affected by the accrual rate, the average survival curve and the amount of competing risk censoring. The error spending methods of Chapter 7 can be used to conduct a group sequential test conditionally on observed information levels $\{\mathcal{I}_1, \mathcal{I}_2, \ldots\}$, the one requirement in the maximum information paradigm being that information should eventually reach a pre-specified target, $\mathcal{I}_{max}$. In this instance, the maximum information that can become available is determined by the number of patients accrued and the total length of follow-up and changing these features of the experimental design forms the analogue of sample size re-estimation in other contexts. The papers by Scharfstein, Tsiatis & Robins (1997) and Scharfstein & Tsiatis (1998) illustrate how such design changes can be planned so that a target information level will ultimately be reached.

Now consider a comparison of the success probabilities p_A and p_B in two binary outcomes, to be conducted to achieve a certain power when $|p_A - p_B| = \Delta$. Suppose a group sequential test is being performed and n_k observations of each type are available at analysis k. The variance of the usual estimate $\hat{p}_A - \hat{p}_B$ is approximately $\bar{p}(1-\bar{p})/n_k$, where $\bar{p}$ is the mean of the true p_A and p_B. Thus, the information for $p_A - p_B$ depends on the unknown $\bar{p}$ and is approximately $\mathcal{I}_k = n_k/\{\bar{p}(1-\bar{p})\}$. If $\tilde{p}_k$ denotes the estimate of $\bar{p}$ based on the data at analysis k, we can estimate $\mathcal{I}_k$ by

$$\hat{\mathcal{I}}_k = \frac{n_k}{\tilde{p}_k(1-\tilde{p}_k)}, \quad k = 1, 2, \ldots,$$

and construct an error spending test using these estimated information levels. In re-calculating suitable sizes for future groups of observations, the experimenter should aim for a final sample, if the test does not stop earlier, of n observations from each distribution, where n satisfies

$$\mathcal{I}_{max} = \frac{n}{\bar{p}(1-\bar{p})}. \tag{14.11}$$

Here, $\mathcal{I}_{max}$ is the target maximum information level appropriate to the form of group sequential test, the chosen error probabilities and Δ. Substituting the current estimate of $\bar{p}$ after the kth analysis into (14.11) gives a target of $n = \mathcal{I}_{max}/\{\tilde{p}_k(1-\tilde{p}_k)\}$ to aim for in the remainder of the study.

One complication in calculating the testing boundary at analysis k is that the current estimate of $\bar{p}$ is more reliable than earlier estimates used in constructing previous boundary points, and it may now be evident that error probabilities spent at previous analyses were not in fact equal to their desired values. It is not possible to go back and change the stopping rule at analyses $1, \ldots, k-1$. However, corrections to earlier inaccuracies can be made by using the current estimate, $\tilde{p}_k$, in approximating the joint distribution of the first k test statistics when the current boundary point is being chosen to give a specified cumulative error probability. Details of this calculation for tests on binary data are given by Jennison & Turnbull (1993a, Section 3.3) and Jennison & Turnbull (1993b, Section 3.3).

When sample size is re-estimated or other aspects of an experimental design modified in response to estimated information levels, the possible effects on a group sequential test's error rates should be considered. Suppose the variance of the parameter of interest is under-estimated at a particular analysis. Then, the observed information is over-estimated and the error spending rule will allocate an increased cumulative error probability; at the same time, the under-estimate of variance enhances the probability of observing a large standardized test statistic, increasing the chance of an error. The net effect is that error spending methods will allocate proportionately more error probability to analyses where the variance estimate is low, and this can be expected to increase the overall probability of error. If sample sizes are large, errors in estimated information levels will be small and problems should not arise: Jennison & Turnbull (1993a,b) report simulation results for tests of binary data involving several hundred observations per distribution, and these show no evidence of inflated error probabilities. However, we would urge a degree of caution when new methods are developed, and we recommend investigating group sequential tests' error rates by simulation to check that sample size re-estimation does not seriously inflate error probabilities.

14.3.2 Normal Data with Unknown Variance

In the group sequential t-tests comparing two normal distributions which we presented in Chapters 3 to 6, sample sizes are pre-specified and a given power is attained when the difference in means is a fixed multiple of σ. We now consider the problem of achieving power at a difference in means specified in absolute terms, rather than as a multiple of the unknown σ. The methods of Section 14.2.2 use sample size re-estimation to achieve this objective when a single test is applied at the end of a study: in this section we discuss extensions of these methods to the group sequential setting.

We consider the problem of Section 14.2.2 in which responses X_{Ai} and X_{Bi}, $i = 1, 2, \ldots$, of subjects allocated to treatments A and B, respectively, are independently distributed as $X_{Ai} \sim N(\mu_A, \sigma^2)$ and $X_{Bi} \sim N(\mu_B, \sigma^2)$. We shall consider group sequential two-sided tests of H_0: $\mu_A = \mu_B$ designed to have Type I error probability α and power $1 - \beta$ at $\mu_A - \mu_B = \pm\delta$.

Gould & Shih (1998) adapt their earlier proposals (Gould & Shih, 1992) to produce a group sequential test with two or possibly three analyses. An initial sample is taken from each treatment arm and σ^2 estimated from the pooled observations, as before, without unblinding treatment allocation. This estimate of σ^2 is then used to determine the course of the remainder of the experiment. Simulation results reported by Gould & Shih (1998) show that their tests achieve the nominal Type I error rate quite accurately, but power is variable, ranging from 0.8 to 0.95 in a variety of examples where the intended power is 0.9. In some instances expected sample size is reduced below that necessary for a fixed sample test. If the number of analyses in the group sequential test were increased, one might expect greater reductions in expected sample size, as seen in tests for the known variance problem.

Gould & Shih impose the restriction that all future sample sizes should be fixed and tests specified by the time treatment allocations are unblinded. Thus, any sample size re-estimation must occur before the first analysis in the group sequential test. Relaxing this restriction would provide the opportunity to use improved estimates of σ^2 to update the required sample size later in the study and, hence, attain specified power more closely. However, care is necessary as information on the observed sample means would then be available at times when sample size is re-estimated or the testing procedure revised. Since such amendments should not be allowed to depend on the sample means, it is essential that they follow a pre-specified formula: rules governing the overall experimental design, including adaptation to new variance estimates, should therefore be clearly stated in a study's protocol and adhered to as the study proceeds.

Adaptation of known variance group sequential tests to the unknown variance problem in a way which accurately attains nominal Type I error probability and power at a stipulated value of $\mu_A - \mu_B$ has proved problematic. Facey (1992) applies Whitehead's triangular test to normal responses with unknown variance using two different formulations of a one-sided testing problem. In the first parameterization the power condition is set at a value of $(\mu_A - \mu_B)/\sigma$ and Type I error rates and power are achieved quite accurately—however, this does not solve our current problem. In the second parameterization, where power is specified at a value of $\mu_A - \mu_B$, results are less satisfactory. In examples with intended one-sided Type I error 0.05 and power 0.9, actual Type I error rates range from 0.06 to 0.08 and the achieved power varies from 0.78 to 0.84.

Denne (1996) reports similar difficulties in applying two-sided error spending tests defined for the case of known variance to the unknown variance problem. Tests are adapted by substituting a current estimate of σ^2 at each analysis in formulae for the test statistic and the target maximum sample size. In order to allow for error in estimating σ^2, critical values for Z-statistics are converted to the corresponding points of the appropriate t-distributions, following the "significance level" approach of Section 3.8. The resulting tests have Type I error rates of the order of 0.06 and 0.07 when the nominal rate is 0.05 and their achieved power is often well below its target.

It is, perhaps, not surprising that error probabilities should be larger than desired when sample sizes are computed simply by substituting an estimate of σ^2 in a known variance formula. Variance estimates, even on moderately high degrees of freedom, are highly variable, and consequently so are estimates of required sample size. Once again, it helps to remember Stein's (1945) precise method of compensating for the variance of an initial estimate of σ^2, and the idea which underpins this method has been exploited in a variety of sequential tests; see Baker (1950), Hall (1962), Hochberg & Marcus (1983) and Arghami & Billard (1991, 1992).

More recently, Denne (1996) and Denne & Jennison (1999c) have used Stein's approach in creating group sequential t-tests. Full details of this work are presented by Denne (1996) in the context of testing the value of a single normal mean. We shall complete this chapter by presenting an outline of this method, modified to treat the problem of testing equality of two normal means.

As an initial step, Denne defines a test using the estimate s_0^2 from the pilot sample as its only estimate of σ^2 at any stage. Although the ultimate goal is to use the current variance estimate at each point, this initial test is of value in establishing formulae for sample size and boundary values in a tractable framework. The overall form of the test is determined by an error spending function, rising from zero to α in the usual manner, and a planned number of analyses $\tilde{K}$. After a pilot phase sample of n_0 observations on each treatment arm, s_0^2 is found on $\eta_0 = 2n_0 - 2$ degrees of freedom. The maximum sample size per treatment is then given as a multiple of s_0^2,

$$n_{max} = \tau s_0^2, \tag{14.12}$$

and, assuming equally spaced analyses are desired, these are set at cumulative sample sizes:

$$n_k = \frac{k}{\tilde{K}} \tau s_0^2, \quad k = 1, \ldots, \tilde{K}.$$

It is, of course, possible that n_0 will already exceed the first one or more of these sample sizes and the prescribed plan cannot be followed exactly, but this eventuality is ignored for the moment. The t-statistics used to test the null hypothesis H_0: $\mu_A - \mu_B = 0$ at analyses 1 to $\tilde{K}$ are

$$T_k = \frac{\bar{X}_A^{(k)} - \bar{X}_B^{(k)}}{\sqrt{(2s_0^2/n_k)}}, \quad k = 1, \ldots, \tilde{K},$$

where $\bar{X}_A^{(k)}$ and $\bar{X}_B^{(k)}$ are the sample means of the n_k observations on treatments A and B. Setting sample sizes proportional to s_0^2 ensures that under the idealized assumption that n_1 is never smaller than n_0, the joint distribution of $\{T_1, \ldots, T_{\tilde{K}}\}$ is independent of σ^2. This distribution is sufficiently tractable that an error spending boundary can be computed (the calculation involves an integral over the distribution of s_0^2 as well as the sequence of values of the $\bar{X}_A^{(k)} - \bar{X}_B^{(k)}$, but this is quite manageable). The value of τ in (14.12) needed to satisfy the power requirement also follows from this calculation. The error spending method can be formally applied to create boundaries for any sequence of group sizes, including instances where the plan has to be amended because n_0 exceeds one or more of the specified sample sizes, and although the underlying theory is no longer exactly correct, the consequences of any inaccuracies on achieved error rates are found to be minor.

Having constructed a test with the desired Type I error and power, it remains to modify this test to use updated variance estimates throughout the study. In doing this, Denne (1996) defines an effective number of degrees of freedom at analysis k,

$$\eta_k = 2n_0 - 2 + \epsilon(2n_k - 2n_0),$$

where $\epsilon \in (0, 1)$ is used as a fine-tuning parameter; a value of $\epsilon = 1/4$ is recommended as producing error probabilities close to their nominal values over a range of problems. The t-statistics at each analysis are now

$$T_k = \frac{\bar{X}_A^{(k)} - \bar{X}_B^{(k)}}{\sqrt{(2s_k^2/n_k)}}, \quad k = 1, \ldots, \tilde{K},$$

where s_k^2 is the standard estimate of σ^2 from the $2n_k$ observations at analysis k, and the critical value for each of these statistics is re-computed using η_k in place of η_0 in the earlier calculation of the error spending boundary. The target maximum sample size is also re-estimated at each analysis, with s_0^2 replaced in (14.12) by s_k^2 and τ re-computed using degrees of freedom η_k in place of η_0; subsequent group sizes are then modified accordingly. Although these adjustments to the initial form of test introduce a number of new approximations, they have only slight effects on the test's achieved error rates, and results reported by Denne (1996) and Denne & Jennison (1999c) show the final test has both Type I error and power close to their nominal values in a variety of examples. As hoped, increasing the number of groups helps reduce expected sample size on a scale comparable with that seen for group sequential tests for known σ^2.

CHAPTER 15

Multiple Endpoints

15.1 Introduction

Interim analyses in clinical trials often include the examination of a number of patient outcome measures. For example, Pocock, Geller & Tsiatis (1987) describe a crossover trial of chronic respiratory disease in which active drug and placebo were compared with respect to three lung function measurements: peak expiratory flow rate, forced expiratory volume and forced vital capacity. This is an example where the outcome variables might be regarded as *unordered* since one does not take priority over another. Another example occurred in the NINDS Stroke Trial (Tilley et al., 1996) in which treatment effect in patients with acute ischemic stroke was measured on four different ratings scales. In an extreme example, O'Brien (1984) described a study of diabetes patients in which improvements in nerve function were measured on 34 electromyographic variables.

In other trials there will be an ordering of importance of the outcome variables. Jennison & Turnbull (1993c) describe a clinical trial of an analgesic drug used to relieve arthritic pain. The primary endpoint was a measure of the amount of pain relief experienced by the patient, but a secondary endpoint concerned a possible effect on the arthritic condition of the joint. It was thought that the two outcome measures might be related, if for no other reason than that the drug's success in relieving pain may lead the patient to be less careful in protecting the joint. When the primary outcome measure is a rare event, consideration of additional intermediate endpoints can lead to lower sample sizes or higher power. For instance, in evaluating therapies for acute myocardial infarction (MI), mortality will be the most important endpoint but other clinically meaningful endpoints that are correlated with adverse long-term outcome, such as recurrent MI or ventricular dysfunction, may also be considered (Cannon, 1997).

Sometimes it is reasonable to adopt a strategy of assigning a composite score or summary scalar measure to each subject based on all of that individual's responses. The problem is then reduced to one of univariate response and the methods described in preceding chapters for monitoring a Z-statistic or a Student's t-statistic can be applied to the summary measure. This approach is suitable when the outcome variables all attempt to measure a common underlying response. In quality of life studies, several responses may be combined into a single index, based perhaps on a multivariate trait analysis. Another example is a study of efficacy of chemoprophylaxis for tuberculosis (TB) in HIV+ patients with two binary endpoints: suspected TB (a positive culture or smear) and confirmed TB. We could turn this into a single ordinal response with a score of 0 for no TB, 1 for suspected TB, or 2 for confirmed TB. In a more complicated example, the Hormone Replacement Trial of the Women's Health Initiative considered a "weighted combined index" involving five binary outcomes: incidence of coronary heat disease, hip fracture, breast cancer, endometrial cancer and death from other causes. These outcomes were assigned weights using data external to the trial of 0.5, 0.18, 0.35, 0.15 and 1.00, respectively; see Freedman et al. (1996, Table 1). When the multiple outcomes are survival times, time to the first occurring event can be used. Examples of such composite endpoints might include "total" or "all-cause" mortality, "total morbidity", "cancer mortality" or "cancer incidence". Cannon (1997) describes similar composite survival endpoints that have been used in large trials of acute MI. Gent (1997) discusses some of the issues in the construction of composite event outcomes.

The strategy of using a summary score or composite endpoint obviates the problem of multiple endpoints. However, using a group sequential rule based on several outcome measures rather than a rule based on a single primary outcome measure is sometimes desirable for two reasons. First, specific stopping guidelines are defined that recognize separately the presence of all important variables and, second, consideration of the multivariate structure of the observations can lead to more sensitive and powerful group sequential tests.

Setting aside essentially univariate methods based on a summary response for each subject, most multiple-endpoint procedures can be classified into two general categories. In the first, univariate procedures are applied to each outcome variable separately with allowance made for the multiplicity effect which would otherwise increase the *experiment-wise error rate*, defined as the probability of rejecting at least one true hypothesis. In the second category, stopping decisions are based on a single "global" univariate statistic, constructed from the accumulated results on all variables, then a step-down method is employed to make inferences about individual response variables or subsets of variables. In the next sections, we describe a variety of methods from both these categories.

15.2 The Bonferroni Procedure

A simple strategy when monitoring multiple outcomes is to run separate univariate group sequential tests on each variable, stopping the first time any one of the individual tests so indicates, but using a Bonferroni adjustment to account for the multiplicity of tests. For instance, with p response variables, each group sequential test would be conducted at level α/p to restrict the overall probability of a Type I error to at most α. We need to expand the tables of Chapter 2 to obtain critical values for these stopping rules. Tables 15.1 and 15.2 give the constants needed to construct two-sided Pocock or O'Brien & Fleming tests with Type I error probability α/p for $\alpha = 0.05$ and $p = 1, \ldots, 6$ and $p = 10$. These two tables can be considered as extensions of Tables 2.1 and 2.3, respectively.

Example

Suppose a trial has $K = 4$ planned analyses and $p = 3$ outcome variables and we choose to run an O'Brien & Fleming test on each endpoint with an experiment-wise Type I error probability of $\alpha = 0.05$. The critical values in each test are

Table 15.1 *Pocock tests: constants $C_P(K, 0.05/p)$ for two-sided tests with K groups of observations and Type I error probability $\alpha = 0.05/p$, for use with Bonferroni procedures with p endpoints*

	$C_P(K, 0.05/p)$						
K	$p = 1$	$p = 2$	$p = 3$	$p = 4$	$p = 5$	$p = 6$	$p = 10$
1	1.960	2.241	2.394	2.498	2.576	2.638	2.807
2	2.178	2.449	2.596	2.696	2.772	2.832	2.995
3	2.289	2.556	2.700	2.799	2.873	2.932	3.093
4	2.361	2.625	2.768	2.865	2.939	2.997	3.156
5	2.413	2.675	2.817	2.913	2.986	3.045	3.203
10	2.555	2.811	2.950	3.045	3.117	3.174	3.329

then

$$c_k = C_B(4, 0.05/3)\sqrt{(4/k)}, \quad k = 1, \ldots, 4,$$

where we find $C_B(4, 0.05/3) = 2.435$ from Table 15.2. The resulting values, $c_1 = 4.870$, $c_2 = 3.444$, $c_3 = 2.812$ and $c_4 = 2.435$, correspond to two-sided nominal significance levels of $\alpha'_1 = 0.000001$, $\alpha'_2 = 0.0006$, $\alpha'_3 = 0.0049$ and $\alpha'_4 = 0.0149$. At each stage $k = 1, \ldots, 4$, the marginal two-sided significance level for each of the p variables is obtained and compared with α'_k, and stopping occurs if any one value falls below α'_k. If no Bonferroni adjustment for the multiple endpoints were made and we used $C_B(4, 0.05) = 2.024$ in place of $C_B(4, 0.05/3)$, the nominal significance levels for each endpoint would be 0.0001, 0.0042, 0.0194 and 0.0430 at the four analyses and each test on an individual outcome would have a Type I error rate of 0.05, giving an experiment-wise Type I error probability considerably larger than this.

In the above example, we have assumed the sequence of standardized test statistics for each endpoint follows the standard joint distribution (3.1). This assumption is not crucial and methods for other types of distribution may be used, as long as the Type I error probability for each test is controlled at the specified level. It is not necessary that the total Type I error probability α be allocated equally among the p endpoints. When one endpoint is designated as being the primary outcome and the remaining $p - 1$ are all secondary outcomes, Davis (1997) and Prentice (1997) discuss the merits of allocating $\alpha/2$ to the test of the primary endpoint and $\alpha/(2p - 2)$ to tests for each secondary endpoint. In a similar spirit, the Data Safety Monitoring Board of the NPC trial described in Section 1.4.5 (Clark et al., 1996) proposed using Haybittle-Peto boundaries of Section 2.7.2 with interim boundary values for standardized statistics of 3.0 for the primary endpoint (incidence of squamous cell carcinoma of the skin), of 3.5 for secondary endpoints (incidence of other site-specific cancers, etc.) and of 2.0 for all-cause mortality. This type of approach had been suggested by Cox (1989).

Table 15.2 *O'Brien & Fleming tests: constants $C_B(K, 0.05/p)$ for two-sided tests with K groups of observations and Type I error probability $\alpha = 0.05/p$, for use with Bonferroni procedures with p endpoints*

	$C_B(K, 0.05/p)$						
K	$p=1$	$p=2$	$p=3$	$p=4$	$p=5$	$p=6$	$p=10$
1	1.960	2.241	2.394	2.498	2.576	2.638	2.807
2	1.977	2.250	2.400	2.502	2.580	2.641	2.809
3	2.004	2.272	2.419	2.519	2.595	2.656	2.820
4	2.024	2.289	2.435	2.534	2.609	2.669	2.833
5	2.040	2.303	2.448	2.547	2.621	2.681	2.843
10	2.087	2.346	2.489	2.586	2.660	2.719	2.879

The Bonferroni procedure is very simple to carry out. The endpoints can be of differing types, continuous, binary, time-to-event, etc., and information levels for each variable do not need to be the same at a given analysis. Indeed, different boundaries (Pocock, O'Brien & Fleming, etc.) could be used for different endpoints. This procedure does not take into account how many outcome variables appear discrepant from the null hypothesis as judged by their standardized test statistics or nominal P-values: stopping occurs if just one of the p tests on different variables yields a decision, or if many do. The Bonferroni approach can be inefficient because it does not take into account the correlation structure of the response variables. In particular, it will be very conservative if outcomes are highly positively correlated, as might be expected in the pulmonary trial example cited in Section 15.1. Such conservatism does not arise in the alternative methods considered in the following sections, which monitor a single summary statistic or monitor several outcomes in an integrated manner.

15.3 A Group Sequential Hotelling Test

Suppose a group sequential study with a maximum of K analyses yields a sequence of summary statistics $\boldsymbol{Y}_k$, $k = 1, \ldots, K$, where each $\boldsymbol{Y}_k$ is a column vector of length p. We shall consider tests of the null hypothesis H_0, that each element of $\boldsymbol{Y}_k$ has expectation zero, against a general alternative. We first assume that the covariance matrices of the $\boldsymbol{Y}_k$, denoted $\mathbf{Var}(\boldsymbol{Y}_k)$, $k = 1, \ldots, K$, are completely known so we can divide each element of $\boldsymbol{Y}_k$ by its standard deviation to create standardized statistics $\boldsymbol{Z}_k = (Z_{1k}, \ldots, Z_{pk})^T$, where each Z_{jk} has unit variance and mean zero under H_0. The relation between the $\boldsymbol{Z}_k$ and the original observations will depend on the underlying data structure. As an example, in a two-treatment parallel comparison $\boldsymbol{Z}_k$ is formed, component by component, as the vector analogue of the univariate Z_k defined in Section 3.1.1. Similarly, vector analogues of expressions for Z_k in Sections 3.1.2, 3.1.3 and 3.1.4 can be defined for the single sample problem, the two-treatment paired comparison and the simple two-period crossover design, respectively.

For $k = 1, \ldots, K$, let $\boldsymbol{\Sigma}_k$ denote the correlation matrix of $\boldsymbol{Y}_k$, and therefore of $\boldsymbol{Z}_k$. If the underlying data are multivariate normal, the quantity

$$\boldsymbol{Z}_k^T \boldsymbol{\Sigma}_k^{-1} \boldsymbol{Z}_k \tag{15.1}$$

has a χ^2_p distribution under H_0. Jennison & Turnbull (1991b, Section 2.2; 1997b, Section 5) show that the sequence $\{\boldsymbol{Z}_k^T \boldsymbol{\Sigma}_k^{-1} \boldsymbol{Z}_k;\ k = 1, \ldots, K\}$ is Markov and derive its joint distribution. The constants in Table 2 of Jennison & Turnbull (1991b) for group sequential chi-square tests can be used to construct boundary values for the statistics (15.1) which give tests with a stated Type I error probability α. The table gives values for $\alpha = 0.01, 0.05$ and 0.10, $p = 1$ to 5, and $K = 1$ to 10, 20 and 50.

We now suppose the covariance matrices of the summary statistics $\boldsymbol{Y}_k$ are not known. One possibility is that variances and covariances are partly known and each $\mathbf{Var}(\boldsymbol{Y}_k)$ can be written as the product of a known matrix and an unknown scale factor. In this case, a group sequential F-test can be used; see Jennison & Turnbull (1991b, Section 2.3; 1997b, Section 5).

When multiple endpoints arise in a clinical trial, it is likely that the matrices $\mathbf{Var}(\boldsymbol{Y}_k)$ are completely unknown. In this case, at analysis k, we create a Studentized statistic t_{jk} for each $j = 1, \ldots, p$ using an estimate of $Var(Y_{jk})$ calculated from the original observations. The form of this variance estimate will depend on the original data structure but, since only one endpoint is involved at a time, the variance estimation problem is the same as that for a single endpoint. As before, we denote by $\boldsymbol{\Sigma}_k$ the correlation matrix of $\boldsymbol{Y}_k$ but now the observed data are used to obtain an estimate of this matrix, $\widehat{\boldsymbol{\Sigma}}_k$. The quantity

$$\boldsymbol{t}_k^T \widehat{\boldsymbol{\Sigma}}_k^{-1} \boldsymbol{t}_k \tag{15.2}$$

then has, marginally, a Hotelling's $\mathcal{T}^2_p(\nu_k)$ distribution, where ν_k denotes the degrees of freedom for $\widehat{\boldsymbol{\Sigma}}_k$. (See, for example, Chatfield & Collins, 1980, Chapter 7.) In the one-sample problem, $\widehat{\boldsymbol{\Sigma}}_k$ is the usual sample correlation matrix based on all data accumulated so far and $\nu_k = n_k - 1$; for the paired treatment comparison, it is the within-pair sample correlation matrix and $\nu_k = n_k - 1$; for the two-treatment parallel design with common covariance matrices, $\widehat{\boldsymbol{\Sigma}}_k$ is the pooled within-treatment sample correlation matrix and $\nu_k = n_{Ak} + n_{Bk} - 2$; in the simple two-period crossover design, assuming the covariance matrix is the same for subjects on either treatment ordering, $\widehat{\boldsymbol{\Sigma}}_k$ is the sample correlation matrix pooled across both treatment orderings and again $\nu_k = n_{Ak} + n_{Bk} - 2$.

Jennison & Turnbull (1991b, Section 2.4) point out that an exact theory for the joint distribution of successive Hotelling's $\mathcal{T}^2$ statistics would be very complicated, involving joint distributions of repeated Wishart variables. As an alternative, we shall adopt the "significance level approach" of Section 3.3 and compare successive values of (15.2) with percentiles of the $\mathcal{T}^2_p(\nu)$ distribution corresponding to the significance levels of the normal theory tests of Chapter 2. Percentiles of Hotelling's $\mathcal{T}^2_p(\nu)$ distribution can be obtained from tables of the

F-distribution by using the well-known relation

$$\mathcal{T}_p^2(\nu) = \frac{p\,\nu}{\nu - p + 1} F_{p,\,\nu-p+1}, \tag{15.3}$$

where $F_{\nu_1,\,\nu_2}$ denotes an F-distribution on ν_1 and ν_2 degrees of freedom; see, for example, Chatfield & Collins (1980, Eq. 6.26).

An Example

Consider an example with $p = 3$ outcome variables and a maximum of $K = 4$ stages. Suppose the covariance matrices of summary statistics are unknown and we observe the following results. Here, $\boldsymbol{t}_k$ is the vector of Studentized statistics at stage k and $\widehat{\boldsymbol{\Sigma}}_k$ the estimated correlation matrix on ν_k degrees of freedom.

$$\textit{Stage } 1 \quad \nu_1 = 12 \quad \boldsymbol{t}_1 = \begin{pmatrix} 2.01 \\ 1.92 \\ 1.39 \end{pmatrix} \quad \widehat{\boldsymbol{\Sigma}}_1 = \begin{pmatrix} 1 & 0.20 & 0.02 \\ 0.20 & 1 & 0.03 \\ 0.02 & 0.03 & 1 \end{pmatrix}$$

$$\textit{Stage } 2 \quad \nu_2 = 25 \quad \boldsymbol{t}_2 = \begin{pmatrix} 1.86 \\ 2.00 \\ 1.55 \end{pmatrix} \quad \widehat{\boldsymbol{\Sigma}}_2 = \begin{pmatrix} 1 & 0.21 & 0.03 \\ 0.21 & 1 & 0.05 \\ 0.03 & 0.05 & 1 \end{pmatrix}$$

$$\textit{Stage } 3 \quad \nu_3 = 35 \quad \boldsymbol{t}_3 = \begin{pmatrix} 1.89 \\ 2.15 \\ 1.53 \end{pmatrix} \quad \widehat{\boldsymbol{\Sigma}}_3 = \begin{pmatrix} 1 & 0.17 & 0.02 \\ 0.17 & 1 & 0.04 \\ 0.02 & 0.04 & 1 \end{pmatrix}$$

$$\textit{Stage } 4 \quad \nu_4 = 48 \quad \boldsymbol{t}_4 = \begin{pmatrix} 1.92 \\ 1.93 \\ 1.74 \end{pmatrix} \quad \widehat{\boldsymbol{\Sigma}}_4 = \begin{pmatrix} 1 & 0.12 & 0.02 \\ 0.12 & 1 & 0.03 \\ 0.02 & 0.03 & 1 \end{pmatrix}$$

Calculation shows the successive $\mathcal{T}^2$ statistics (15.2) are 8.155, 8.193, 9.045 and 9.356. Suppose it was decided to base stopping criteria on significance levels from an O'Brien & Fleming test with Type I error probability $\alpha = 0.05$. From Table 2.3, we have $C_B(4, 0.05) = 2.024$ and the corresponding nominal significance levels are

$$\alpha_1' = 2\{1 - \Phi(4.048)\} = 0.0001,$$

where Φ is the standard normal cdf, and similarly $\alpha_2' = 0.0042$, $\alpha_3' = 0.0194$ and $\alpha_4' = 0.0430$. At stage 1, we compute the significance level

$$Pr\{\mathcal{T}_3^2(\nu_1) > 8.155\} = Pr\{F_{3,10} > 2.265\} = 0.1433$$

and since this exceeds α_1', the procedure continues to stage 2. We can draw up a worksheet as displayed in Table 15.3 to assist in applying the stopping rule. The value F in this worksheet is the $\mathcal{T}^2$ statistic multiplied by $(\nu_k - p + 1)/(p\,\nu_k)$, i.e., by $(\nu_k - 2)/(3\,\nu_k)$, to produce a statistic with null distribution $F_{p,\,\nu_k-p+1} = F_{3,\nu_k-2}$.

Table 15.3 *Worksheet for a group sequential test using Hotelling's $\mathcal{T}^2$ statistic*

k	ν_k	$\mathcal{T}^2$	F	$Pr\{F_{3,\nu_k-2} > F\}$	*Nominal significance level,* α'_k
1	12	8.155	2.265	0.1433	0.0001
2	25	8.193	2.512	0.0838	0.0042
3	35	9.045	2.843	0.0527	0.0194
4	48	9.356	2.989	0.0406	0.0430

The results show that the test continues to the last stage, $K = 4$, at which point it rejects the null hypothesis of zero means.

We may compare this test with the Bonferroni procedure of the previous section. For that test, since each t_{jk}, $j = 1, \ldots, 3$, is compared to the same critical value, the outcome of stage k is determined by the maximum of $|t_{1k}|$, $|t_{2k}|$ and $|t_{3k}|$, which takes values 2.01, 2.00, 2.15 and 1.93 at stages $k = 1, 2, 3$ and 4, respectively. These values have nominal significance levels 0.067, 0.056, 0.039 and 0.060 relative to the appropriate F-distributions and these significance levels do not come close to falling below the critical values $\alpha'_1 = 0.000001$, $\alpha'_2 = 0.0006$, $\alpha'_3 = 0.0049$ and $\alpha'_4 = 0.0149$ derived in Section 15.2. Thus the Bonferroni procedure is unable to reject the null hypothesis at any stage. In fact, even if we applied significance levels of an O'Brien & Fleming procedure test with a Type I error rate of 0.05 for each endpoint separately, without any adjustment for multiplicity, the null hypothesis would not be rejected at any stage. The $\mathcal{T}^2$ statistic combines the moderate evidence against H_0 from each of the three endpoints to produce a significant result, demonstrating the advantage of combining endpoints when each mean is a small distance from the value zero specified in H_0.

The Hotelling's $\mathcal{T}^2$ test is appropriate if any departure from H_0, in whatever direction, is of interest. It has found application in multivariate control charts in industrial quality control, where it is important to detect the departure of any output variable from its usual distribution. The test is not used much in clinical trials where such an "omnibus" test, designed to have power against all alternatives to H_0, is usually less suitable. Suppose the above example concerned a two-treatment comparison with each endpoint defined so that a positive value indicates the superiority of one treatment and a negative value superiority of the other. If the value of $\boldsymbol{t}_3$ had been equal to (1.89, −2.15, 1.53), we would have found $\mathcal{T}_3^2 = 12.239$, giving an F value of 3.891 and significance level $Pr\{F_{3,33} > 3.891\} = 0.017$, and the procedure would have stopped to reject H_0 at the third stage. (Because of the positive correlations, the negative component of $\boldsymbol{t}_3$ now provides stronger evidence against the null hypothesis, even though its magnitude is unchanged.) However, these data show that one treatment has a better response in two endpoints and a poorer response for the other endpoint — which is not particularly helpful as a recommendation for either treatment. The major interest in such a comparison is in alternatives where the treatment difference is in the same direction for all variables. By giving up power against alternatives where the null hypothesis fails because some endpoints respond well to the first treatment and others to the second, we can design procedures which are more sensitive to the most relevant alternatives: we consider such procedures in the next section.

15.4 A Group Sequential Version of O'Brien's Test

O'Brien (1984) proposed a test of the null hypothesis that a multivariate distribution has mean zero against alternatives under which means of all elements have the same sign. With suitably defined response variables, this is the appropriate formulation for detecting an improvement of one treatment over another across the range of outcome measures. O'Brien considered parametric and nonparametric test statistics but we shall pursue the parametric case here, and the multivariate normal response distribution in particular. Pocock et al. (1987) illustrate O'Brien's test in a number of examples and we follow their notation in this section. Adaptation of O'Brien's test to a group sequential setting has been described by Tang, Gnecco & Geller (1989a) and Tang, Geller & Pocock (1993).

We first consider the case where variances and correlations of the different endpoints are known so that at each stage k we can create a vector of p standardized statistics $\boldsymbol{Z}_k = (Z_{1k}, \ldots, Z_{pk})^T$, for which each Z_{jk} has unit variance and mean zero under the null hypothesis H_0. O'Brien's generalized least square (GLS) statistic is then

$$\mathcal{Z}_k = \frac{\boldsymbol{J}^T \boldsymbol{\Sigma}_k^{-1} \boldsymbol{Z}_k}{(\boldsymbol{J}^T \boldsymbol{\Sigma}_k^{-1} \boldsymbol{J})^{1/2}}, \tag{15.4}$$

where $\boldsymbol{\Sigma}_k$ is the correlation matrix of $\boldsymbol{Z}_k$. The components of the vector $\boldsymbol{J}$ are positive and, typically, represent the relative differences of interest in each of the p endpoints, measured on the standardized scale. The common choice $\boldsymbol{J} = (1, \ldots, 1)^T$ is optimal for testing alternatives in which the improvements of the treatment are the same, on the standardized scale, for each endpoint. In this case, $\mathcal{Z}_k$ is a linear combination of Z_{1k} to Z_{pk} in which those variables that are less highly correlated with others receive correspondingly larger weights.

Other choices for $\boldsymbol{J}$ can be made if sensitivity of the test to departures from the null hypothesis in other directions is preferred. However, Tang et al. (1993, p. 25) point out that for certain choices of $\boldsymbol{J}$, and even for $\boldsymbol{J} = (1, \ldots, 1)^T$, the vector $\boldsymbol{\Sigma}_k^{-1} \boldsymbol{J}$ can possibly have negative components, leading to negative weights in $\mathcal{Z}_k$ for some endpoints. In this case, if the mean of $\boldsymbol{Z}_k$ lies along certain directions in the positive or negative orthants, the GLS statistic (15.4) has expectation zero. Hence, tests have power of only α in parts of the alternative hypothesis where high power might be expected. To avoid this possibility, Tang et al. (1993) recommend a choice of $\boldsymbol{J}$ which guarantees that $\boldsymbol{\Sigma}_k^{-1} \boldsymbol{J}$ will have no negative components and is also optimal with regard to maximizing the minimum power over the positive or negative orthant. In the context of a non-sequential test, their choice is

$$\boldsymbol{J}^T = (\phi_1, \ldots, \phi_p)\, \boldsymbol{\Sigma} \tag{15.5}$$

where $\boldsymbol{\Sigma}$ is the correlation matrix of the vector of standardized statistics and ϕ_j^2

is the jth diagonal element of Σ^{-1}. In a group sequential test, this J can be used with $\Sigma = \Sigma_k$ when the correlation matrices Σ_k do not vary with k, a typical property which we shall see in the following examples; in other cases, a value of Σ could be chosen to capture the key features of all the Σ_ks.

In applications where each Z_{jk} is a multiple of a sample mean or of the difference in the means of two samples, it is straightforward to check that the sequence $\{\mathcal{Z}_1, \ldots, \mathcal{Z}_K\}$ has the canonical joint distribution (3.1) for suitably defined θ and $\mathcal{I}_1, \ldots, \mathcal{I}_K$, either exactly when observations are multivariate normal or approximately for other response distributions. In other problems where each $\Sigma_k^{-1} Z_k$ is a fixed linear function of an estimated parameter vector at analysis k, the same result can be deduced using the theory of Chapter 11. Hence, in order to apply the methods of earlier chapters to the GLS statistic (15.4), we need only identify the quantities θ and $\mathcal{I}_k$ and their interpretation in the particular problem being considered.

The One-Sample Problem

In the one-sample problem analogous to the one-sample univariate problem of Section 3.1.2, we observe independent, multivariate normal p-vectors $X_1, X_2, \ldots$ with common mean vector μ and covariance matrix $\widetilde{\Sigma}$, say. Suppose we wish to test H_0: $\mu = \mu_0$. If n_k observations have accumulated by analysis k, let $\bar{X}_k = (\bar{X}_{1k}, \ldots, \bar{X}_{pk})^T$ denote the mean of these n_k observation vectors. The jth component of Z_k is

$$Z_{jk} = \frac{\bar{X}_{jk} - \mu_{0j}}{\sqrt{(\sigma_j^2/n_k)}},$$

where σ_j^2 is the variance of the jth element of X, i.e., the jth diagonal element of $\widetilde{\Sigma}$. We can also write

$$Z_k = M(\bar{X}_k - \mu_0)\sqrt{n_k}$$

where M is a diagonal matrix with jth diagonal entry $1/\sigma_j$, $j = 1, \ldots, p$, and all other entries equal to zero. Since, marginally,

$$\bar{X}_k \sim N_p(\mu, \widetilde{\Sigma}/n_k),$$

where N_p denotes a p-dimensional multivariate normal distribution, it follows that

$$Z_k \sim N_p(M(\mu - \mu_0)\sqrt{n_k}, M\widetilde{\Sigma}M). \quad (15.6)$$

Thus, Σ_k in (15.4) does not depend on k and is equal to $M\widetilde{\Sigma}M$. Writing $J^T = (J_1, \ldots, J_p)$, define

$$\delta^T = J^T M^{-1} = (J_1\sigma_1, \ldots, J_p\sigma_p), \quad (15.7)$$

then it follows from (15.4) and (15.6) that, marginally, $\mathcal{Z}_k \sim N(\theta\sqrt{\mathcal{I}_k}, 1)$, where

$$\theta = \frac{\delta^T \widetilde{\Sigma}^{-1}(\mu - \mu_0)}{\delta^T \widetilde{\Sigma}^{-1} \delta} \quad \text{and} \quad \mathcal{I}_k = n_k\,(\delta^T \widetilde{\Sigma}^{-1} \delta).$$

If $\mu - \mu_0$ is assumed to be a multiple of δ, we have the model $\mu - \mu_0 = \lambda\,\delta$

and the GLS statistic can be written as

$$\mathcal{Z}_k = \hat{\lambda}_k / \sqrt{\{Var(\hat{\lambda}_k)\}},$$

where

$$\hat{\lambda}_k = \boldsymbol{\delta}^T \widetilde{\boldsymbol{\Sigma}}^{-1} \bar{\boldsymbol{X}}_k / (\boldsymbol{\delta}^T \widetilde{\boldsymbol{\Sigma}}^{-1} \boldsymbol{\delta})$$

is the GLS estimate of λ based on the data at stage k.

Two-Sample Problems

In the balanced two-treatment problem, suppose there are n_k multivariate normal p-vectors from each treatment at stage k, with observations $\boldsymbol{X}_{A1}, \ldots, \boldsymbol{X}_{An_k}$ from treatment A distributed as $N_p(\boldsymbol{\mu}_A, \widetilde{\boldsymbol{\Sigma}})$ and $\boldsymbol{X}_{B1}, \ldots, \boldsymbol{X}_{Bn_k}$ from treatment B distributed as $N_p(\boldsymbol{\mu}_B, \widetilde{\boldsymbol{\Sigma}})$. Suppose response variables have been defined so that high values are desirable and consider a test of H_0: $\boldsymbol{\mu}_A = \boldsymbol{\mu}_B$ against alternatives in which each element of $\boldsymbol{\mu}_A - \boldsymbol{\mu}_B$ has the same sign. Let σ_j^2 be the variance of the jth element of each $\boldsymbol{X}_{Ai}$ or $\boldsymbol{X}_{Bi}$, i.e., the jth diagonal element of $\widetilde{\boldsymbol{\Sigma}}$. Using obvious notation for the means on treatments A and B, the jth component of the standardized statistic $\boldsymbol{Z}_k$ is

$$Z_{jk} = \frac{\bar{X}_{Ajk} - \bar{X}_{Bjk}}{\sqrt{(2\sigma_j^2/n_k)}}$$

and $\mathcal{Z}_k$ is defined from $\boldsymbol{Z}_k = (Z_{1k}, \ldots, Z_{pk})^T$ by (15.4).

Defining $\boldsymbol{M}$ be the matrix with diagonal entries $1/\sigma_1, \ldots, 1/\sigma_p$, and all other entries equal to zero, we have

$$\boldsymbol{Z}_k = \boldsymbol{M}(\bar{\boldsymbol{X}}_{Ak} - \bar{\boldsymbol{X}}_{Bk})\sqrt{(n_k/2)}$$

and

$$\boldsymbol{Z}_k \sim N_p(\boldsymbol{M}(\boldsymbol{\mu}_A - \boldsymbol{\mu}_B)\sqrt{(n_k/2)},\ \boldsymbol{M}\widetilde{\boldsymbol{\Sigma}}\boldsymbol{M}),$$

so again $\boldsymbol{\Sigma}_k$ does not depend on k. As for the one-sample problem, define $\boldsymbol{\delta}$ by (15.7). Then $\mathcal{Z}_k$ again has an interpretation as the standardized value of a generalized least squares estimator, this time of λ in the model $\boldsymbol{\mu}_A - \boldsymbol{\mu}_B = \lambda\,\boldsymbol{\delta}$ for given $\boldsymbol{\delta}$.

Similar calculations to those for the one-sample problem show that, marginally,

$$\mathcal{Z}_k \sim N(\theta\sqrt{\mathcal{I}_k}, 1), \quad k = 1, \ldots, K,$$

where

$$\theta = \frac{\boldsymbol{\delta}^T \widetilde{\boldsymbol{\Sigma}}^{-1} (\boldsymbol{\mu}_A - \boldsymbol{\mu}_B)}{\boldsymbol{\delta}^T \widetilde{\boldsymbol{\Sigma}}^{-1} \boldsymbol{\delta}} \quad \text{and} \quad \mathcal{I}_k = n_k\,(\boldsymbol{\delta}^T \widetilde{\boldsymbol{\Sigma}}^{-1} \boldsymbol{\delta})/2,$$

and the sequence $\mathcal{Z}_1, \ldots, \mathcal{Z}_K$ has the canonical joint distribution (3.1).

If $\boldsymbol{\mu}_A - \boldsymbol{\mu}_B$ is in the direction $\boldsymbol{\delta}$ then θ is positive, and if $\boldsymbol{\mu}_A - \boldsymbol{\mu}_B$ is in the opposite direction θ is negative. More generally, since every component of $\boldsymbol{J}$ is positive, θ will usually be positive when treatment A is superior across all endpoints, and certainly so if (15.5) is used to define $\boldsymbol{J}$. Similarly, θ will usually be negative when treatment B is superior across all endpoints. Thus, one-sided or two-sided tests, as described in Chapters 2 to 6, can be constructed using the sequence of $\mathcal{Z}_k$ statistics. One-sided tests are appropriate when it is desired to show that *one specific* treatment is superior to the other on the basis of its combined performance over all endpoints. Two-sided tests should be used to detect an overall superiority of *either* treatment. In either case, a test will have high power when the superior treatment is equal to or better than the other in respect of all p endpoints. GLS statistics following the canonical joint distribution (3.1) can be derived in a similar fashion for multivariate data from paired sample, crossover or other designs, and used to construct group sequential tests in the usual way.

In practice, the covariance matrix of multivariate observations will often be unknown. As in the development of the procedure based on Hotelling's statistic, components of the standardized statistics $\boldsymbol{Z}_k$ can be replaced by t-statistics and an estimate $\widehat{\boldsymbol{\Sigma}}_k$ substituted for the correlation matrix. The GLS statistic (15.4) at stage k then becomes (Pocock et al. 1987)

$$\mathcal{Z}_k = \frac{\boldsymbol{J}^T \widehat{\boldsymbol{\Sigma}}_k^{-1} \boldsymbol{t}_k}{(\boldsymbol{J}^T \widehat{\boldsymbol{\Sigma}}_k^{-1} \boldsymbol{J})^{1/2}} . \tag{15.8}$$

For example, in the two-treatment problem above, the p components of $\boldsymbol{t}_k$ are the two-sample t-statistics corresponding to each variable by variable comparison, and $\widehat{\boldsymbol{\Sigma}}_k$ is the pooled within-treatment estimate of the correlation matrix.

The statistic (15.8) is a combination of t-statistics. It does not itself have a Student's t-distribution, but it is asymptotically normal. Simulations reported by Pocock et al. (1987) for the fixed sample problem suggest that the normal approximation for (15.8) is good for small dimensions of $p = 2$ or 3, even when the degrees of freedom ν_k associated with $\widehat{\boldsymbol{\Sigma}}_k$ are as low as 10. However, they report that the normal approximation is not nearly so accurate as the dimension p increases. More work needs to be done here to find critical values to achieve a specified Type I error probability.

The elements of $\boldsymbol{t}_k$ have greater variance than the standard normal variates Z_k. Compensation for this additional variability can be made by basing critical values for successive statistics (15.8) on percentiles of Student's t-distribution with ν_k degrees of freedom when using significance levels taken from tests for normal data of known variance, in keeping with the "significance level approach" of Section 3.3. We have applied this procedure to construct a group sequential two-sided test for the example discussed earlier in this chapter. We used $\boldsymbol{J} = (1, 1, 1)^T$ in defining the statistics $\mathcal{Z}_k$ and based boundaries on an O'Brien & Fleming test with two-sided Type I error probability 0.05, supposing there is particular interest in rejecting H_0 when the elements of $\boldsymbol{t}_k$ are all positive or all negative.

The results of our computations are shown in Table 15.4. The column headed $Pr\{|t_{\nu_k}| > |\mathcal{Z}_k|\}$ shows the two-sided significance level of the observed $\mathcal{Z}_k$. The test stops to reject H_0 if this significance level is less than the value α'_k in the final column. Using this procedure, the trial would stop to reject H_0 at the third stage, one stage earlier than the procedure based on Hotelling's $\mathcal{T}^2$. This is to be expected as the O'Brien GLS test is most sensitive to alternatives in which all the endpoints depart from H_0 in the same direction. On the other hand, if the sign of the second component of $\boldsymbol{t}_k$ is switched to create a negative value at every stage,

Table 15.4 *Worksheet for a group sequential test using O'Brien's GLS statistic*

k	ν_k	$\mathcal{Z}_k$	$Pr\{\lvert t_{\nu_k}\rvert > \lvert\mathcal{Z}_k\rvert\}$	*Nominal significance level,* α'_k
1	12	2.811	0.0049	0.0001
2	25	2.843	0.0045	0.0042
3	35	2.974	0.0029	0.0194
4	48	3.055	0.0023	0.0430

the GLS statistics become $\mathcal{Z}_1 = 0.889$, $\mathcal{Z}_2 = 0.872$, $\mathcal{Z}_3 = 0.795$ and $\mathcal{Z}_4 = 1.020$, and the procedure continues to the last stage and fails to reject H_0. In contrast, the Hotelling's $\mathcal{T}^2$ procedure stopped at stage $k = 3$ to reject H_0 for this set of data.

In designing a trial, one may need to choose between a group sequential test based on a single particular endpoint and one based on the GLS statistic using multiple endpoints. Tang et al. (1989a) show there can be substantial savings in sample size if the GLS statistic is used, rather than a single selected endpoint, when there are multiple correlated endpoints.

In planning a group sequential study based on the GLS statistic, the maximum sample size needed to assure Type I error and power requirements depends on the correlation matrix of the standardized variables $\boldsymbol{Z}_k$, and this is typically unknown at the design stage. However, Tang et al. (1989a) prove that the sample size needed is no greater than the smallest required for any of the corresponding univariate tests. Thus, if a good prior estimate of the correlation matrix is not available, a conservative strategy is to use that smallest maximum sample size. Significant efficiency gains will still result.

15.5 Tests Based on Other Global Statistics

As an alternative to tests based on (15.8), Tang et al. (1993) describe group sequential tests based on the approximate likelihood ratio (ALR) statistic of Tang, Gnecco & Geller (1989b). A computational problem with the latter approach is that the statistics have a chi-bar-squared distribution (Robertson, Wright & Dykstra, 1988) which is not easily handled by standard numerical methods. The statistics are not asymptotically normally distributed, so critical values tabulated in earlier chapters are not applicable. However, simulation methods can be used to generate appropriate boundaries. Tang et al. (1993) provide details and give tables of critical values for sequences of ALR statistics for use in group sequential tests with Type I error probability $\alpha = 0.05$ corresponding to two boundary shapes. The first is a repeated significance test with constant significance level (Pocock, 1977); the second is a Lan & DeMets (1983) error spending test that allocates a Type I error probability of 0.01 to each interim analysis and all remaining error probability to the final analysis. The tables are for tests with $K = 1, \ldots, 5$ stages and $p = 2, 3, 4$ and 5 outcome variables.

Nonparametric tests are of value when data depart substantially from normality.

O'Brien (1984) considers rank-sum statistics as well as the parametric models that lead to the GLS statistic (15.4). Similarly, Wei & Johnson (1985) define tests in terms of linear combinations of U-statistics to combine results on separate endpoints. Su & Lachin (1992) describe a group sequential test based on a summary rank statistic and Lin (1991) proposes use of a summary statistic based on ranks in a group sequential test for multivariate survival data.

15.6 Tests Based on Marginal Criteria

A problem with combining data from different endpoints is that the resulting summary measure may have little clinical meaning. If the endpoints are quite different in nature, it may not really be appropriate to combine them at all: this could be the case, for example, if one outcome is an efficacy variable and a second is a safety variable (e.g., toxicity). Then, it may be important to monitor each variable separately but still control the overall error rates of making any incorrect inferences. An alternative strategy whereby a group sequential test is used only for the efficacy variable has the defect of not providing any guidelines for monitoring the safety endpoint. Thus we are led to consider methods that retain the identity of the different endpoints but are more efficient than the simple Bonferroni procedure described previously. Most work to date on constructing stopping boundaries for monitoring multivariate test statistics has concentrated on the bivariate case, although with some computational effort methods can be extended in an obvious way to three or more endpoints.

We begin by stating the multivariate analogue of the unified formulation of Chapter 3 that enables us to handle a variety of problems, including the one-sample problem, paired and unpaired two-treatment comparisons, and the two-period crossover design. We suppose the covariance matrix of the response vector is known and, as before in this chapter, a standardized p-variate statistic $\boldsymbol{Z}_k = (Z_{1k}, \ldots, Z_{pk})^T$ is created at each analysis $k = 1, \ldots, K$. The distribution of $\boldsymbol{Z}_k$ is assumed to be multivariate normal with mean $(\theta_1\sqrt{\mathcal{I}_{1k}}, \ldots, \theta_p\sqrt{\mathcal{I}_{pk}})^T$ and correlation matrix $\boldsymbol{\Sigma}_k$. The information levels $\mathcal{I}_{jk}$ and the matrix $\boldsymbol{\Sigma}_k$ are taken to be known and we suppose the unknown parameter vector $\boldsymbol{\theta} = (\theta_1, \ldots, \theta_p)^T$ lies in a p-dimensional parameter space Ω, say.

Consider a two-decision problem where we must decide whether to accept a new treatment over a standard or control based on trial data. Acceptance might mean proceeding to submit a New Drug Application to a regulatory body. For each variable j, the range of possible values of the parameter θ_j is divided into three exhaustive and non-overlapping sets in which, with regard to this variable:

(i) the new treatment is clearly acceptable,

(ii) the new treatment is clearly unacceptable, and

(iii) the new treatment does not differ from the standard or control by a clinically significant amount.

This leads to a partition of the p-dimensional parameter space Ω into 3^p regions, which we need to collapse into just two regions corresponding to acceptance and rejection of the new treatment. This mapping will depend on the nature of the variables and on clinical assessment of the trade-offs between them.

In an equivalence trial, the new treatment may be deemed acceptable if θ is in a region of the form

$$\Omega_A = \{\boldsymbol{\theta}\colon \epsilon_j < \theta_j < \delta_j \text{ for all } j = 1, \ldots, p\},$$

for specified pairs $\epsilon_j < \delta_j$, $j = 1, \ldots, p$. If for certain endpoints, it is desired only to show that a test formulation is at least as good as a standard or not worse by more than a certain amount, a "one-sided" criterion (see Section 6.2), then the corresponding constants δ_j may be set at $+\infty$.

For efficacy trials, Jennison & Turnbull (1993c) argue that, after a suitable translation of the parameters θ_j, the set of values of $\boldsymbol{\theta}$ for which the new treatment is acceptable can often be represented in the form

$$\Omega_A = \{\boldsymbol{\theta}\colon \theta_j > 0 \text{ for all } j = 1, \ldots, p\}. \qquad (15.9)$$

Let Ω_R denote complement of Ω_A in Ω, i.e.,

$$\Omega_R = \Omega \setminus \Omega_A.$$

Then, if $\boldsymbol{\theta}$ is in Ω_R the new treatment should be rejected.

For a given testing procedure, fixed or sequential, let $\pi(\boldsymbol{\theta})$ denote the probability of deciding in favor of the new treatment for a given value of $\boldsymbol{\theta}$. We regard acceptance of the new treatment when $\boldsymbol{\theta} \in \Omega_R$ as a Type I error and impose the requirement that the size of the test, i.e., the maximum probability of accepting the new treatment over $\boldsymbol{\theta} \in \Omega_R$, should be at most α, that is,

$$\sup_{\boldsymbol{\theta} \in \Omega_R} \{\pi(\boldsymbol{\theta})\} \leq \alpha. \qquad (15.10)$$

For an efficacy trial, with Ω_A given by (15.9), Jennison & Turnbull (1993c) suggest a procedure which combines univariate, one-sided group sequential tests defined separately for each variable. Tests may be chosen from the families described in Chapter 4 with the null hypothesis taken to mean that the new treatment does not improve on the standard treatment for the endpoint in question. Thus, a decision to accept H_0 indicates rejection of the new treatment and a decision to reject H_0 shows the new treatment is acceptable for this endpoint.

Suppose the univariate test for each endpoint j is defined as in (4.2) with critical values a_{jk} and b_{jk}, $k = 1, \ldots, K$, for statistics Z_{j1} to Z_{jK}, respectively. In combining the p tests on different endpoints, the trial is stopped to accept the new treatment if *all* univariate tests stop to reject their H_0s at the same stage, and the trial stops to reject the new treatment if *any* one univariate test accepts its H_0.

Thus, the sequential decision rule has the form:

$$
\begin{array}{ll}
\text{After stage } k = 1, \ldots, K-1 & \\
\quad \text{if } \boldsymbol{Z}_k \in \mathcal{A}_k & \text{stop, accept the new treatment} \\
\quad \text{if } \boldsymbol{Z}_k \in \mathcal{R}_k & \text{stop, reject the new treatment} \\
\quad \text{if } \boldsymbol{Z}_k \in \mathcal{C}_k & \text{continue to group } k+1, \\
\text{after group } K & \\
\quad \text{if } \boldsymbol{Z}_K \in \mathcal{A}_K & \text{stop, accept the new treatment} \\
\quad \text{if } \boldsymbol{Z}_K \in \mathcal{R}_K & \text{stop, reject the new treatment,}
\end{array}
$$

where the acceptance, rejection and continuation regions at stage k are

$$
\begin{aligned}
\mathcal{A}_k &= \{\boldsymbol{Z}_k\colon\ Z_{jk} \geq b_{jk} \text{ for all } j = 1, \ldots, p\}, \\
\mathcal{R}_k &= \{\boldsymbol{Z}_k\colon\ Z_{jk} \leq a_{jk} \text{ for at least one } j = 1, \ldots, p\}
\end{aligned}
$$

and

$$
\begin{aligned}
\mathcal{C}_k = \{\boldsymbol{Z}_k\colon\ Z_{jk} > a_{jk} &\text{ for all } j = 1, \ldots, p \\
\text{and } Z_{jk} < b_{jk} &\text{ for at least one } j\}.
\end{aligned}
$$

Since the univariate tests have $a_{jK} = b_{jK}$ for each j, the test is sure to terminate with a decision at analysis K.

For $p = 2$, the continuation regions are "L-shaped"; see Jennison & Turnbull (1993c, Figure 3). It turns out that if each univariate test is defined to achieve Type I error probability α, the constraint (15.10) will be met, whatever the correlation matrix $\boldsymbol{\Sigma}_k$. This is because the supremum in (15.10) occurs when one component of $\boldsymbol{\theta}$ is zero, θ_j say, and all the others are infinite (Jennison & Turnbull 1993c, Section 4) so the overall conclusion is determined by the outcome of the jth univariate test. The power function $\pi(\boldsymbol{\theta})$ and expected sample size of the overall test do depend on $\boldsymbol{\Sigma}_k$ and multivariate calculations are required to evaluate such properties, even if endpoints are uncorrelated. Computation of $\pi(\boldsymbol{\theta})$ is needed to establish the group size which will satisfy a power requirement of the form

$$\pi(\boldsymbol{\theta}) \geq 1 - \beta \quad \text{whenever } \theta_j \geq \theta_j^* \text{ for all } j = 1, \ldots, p$$

for specified values θ_j^*. These calculations involve a multivariate analogue of the recursion formulae described in Chapter 19. Further details are given in the appendix of Jennison & Turnbull (1993c).

Cook & Farewell (1994) present a similar procedure for a bivariate outcome with one efficacy and one toxicity response. Their procedure is asymmetric in that a two-sided, rather than one-sided, group sequential test is proposed for monitoring the efficacy response. The Type I error probability is controlled at $\theta_1 = \theta_2 = 0$ and bivariate calculations involving the correlation matrices $\boldsymbol{\Sigma}_k$ are needed to construct the testing boundaries. An error spending approach (Chapter 7) is taken in designing the boundaries, with the error spent at each stage apportioned between the two endpoints. When correlations are unknown, an adaptive procedure is proposed whereby the correlation matrix is estimated from the data currently available at each stage. Results of a small simulation study reported by Cook & Farewell (1994) with $K = 2$ stages and $p = 2$ uncorrelated endpoints suggest the adaptive procedure gives close to nominal error rates.

Cook (1994) also considers the case of a bivariate outcome and defines a procedure similar to that of Cook & Farewell (1994), except that both univariate tests are two-sided. The resulting bivariate group sequential test can be inverted to obtain repeated confidence *regions* for (θ_1, θ_2) analogous to the repeated confidence intervals described in Chapter 9 for a one-dimensional parameter. Cook (1994) goes on to describe how a group sequential equivalence test for a bivariate response can be derived from the repeated confidence regions, just as "derived tests" for a univariate response were created from RCIs in Section 9.3. It should be noted that repeated confidence regions generated by bivariate group sequential tests of the form considered in this section lead to rectangular repeated confidence regions. Elliptical repeated confidence regions can be obtained by inverting the group sequential Hotelling's $\mathcal{T}^2$ test of Section 15.3. However, for the reasons expressed at the beginning of this section concerning disadvantages of the use of global statistics, rectangular regions are to be preferred; for more discussion, see Cook (1994, p. 190).

15.7 Bibliography and Notes

All the methods in this chapter are designed to control the overall experiment-wise Type I error rate. Cook & Farewell (1996) have argued that there are situations when this criterion may not be relevant and tests on the different endpoints should be designed with reference to marginal rather than experiment-wise Type I error rates; for example, if the marginal test results have separate implications on treatment evaluation and prescription. Cook (1996) describes a "coupled error spending" function approach similar to those presented at the end of Section 15.6 but in which separate marginal error spending functions are specified for the different outcome variables.

We have concentrated here on continuous outcomes that can be considered multivariate normally distributed, at least approximately. As in the univariate case, the ideas are readily adapted to other types of endpoint. Cook (1994) and Cook & Farewell (1994) have considered application of their procedures to bivariate failure time responses. Williams (1996) discusses several different methods for constructing repeated joint confidence regions for monitoring two hazard ratios with bivariate survival data. Group sequential designs for multinomial outcomes are considered by Cook (1994) and by Conaway & Petroni (1995). Bayesian monitoring procedures for multinomial data have been proposed by Thall, Simon and Estey (1995). Etzioni & Pepe (1994) also propose a Bayesian monitoring scheme for multinomial data, combined with frequentist inference upon termination using ideas similar to those described in Chapter 8.

In this section we have concentrated on multiple outcomes, all of which can be used to influence early stopping. Another situation occurs when a univariate group sequential procedure is used to monitor a single response variable Z_1 but, upon termination, it is desired to make inferences about a parameter θ_2 associated with a secondary response variable Z_2 which is correlated with Z_1. A confidence interval for θ_2 will depend on the joint distribution of $\{(Z_{1k}, Z_{2k}); k = 1, \ldots, K\}$ and the boundary used to monitor Z_{1k}. Whitehead (1986b) has proposed a method for constructing such a confidence interval; the same computational methods referred to in Section 15.6 allow exact numerical calculation of the coverage probabilities of such confidence intervals for θ_2 under specific values of θ_1; see the comments in Jennison & Turnbull (1993c, p. 750).

Pocock (1997) gives a very comprehensive account of some of the statistical and practical issues in handling multiple outcomes, with examples from several clinical trials. Multivariate responses can also arise in industrial acceptance sampling (see Jackson & Bradley, 1961; Baillie, 1987a,b; and Hamilton & Lesperance, 1991), and the methods of this chapter can be applied there also.

CHAPTER 16

Multi-Armed Trials

16.1 Introduction

It is becoming increasingly common to conduct trials with three or more treatment arms. The substantial overhead expense in setting up a large clinical trial means that there are economies of scale and time if several competing treatments can be compared in the same trial. Follmann, Proschan & Geller (1994, p. 331) describe an example of a hypertension prevention trial in which subjects were randomized either to a control group or to one of three interventions, weight loss, sodium restriction, or stress management, making a total of four treatment arms. The primary endpoint was change in diastolic blood pressure from a baseline measurement taken on entry to the study.

We illustrate the methods for multi-armed trials in the simplest case of a balanced one-way layout comparing the means of J univariate normal distributions, where $J \geq 3$. Extensions to other situations will be referred to later. Independent observations are available from each arm $j = 1, \dots, J$, and these are assumed to be normally distributed with unknown mean μ_j and common variance σ^2. Observations are taken in groups of g per treatment arm. For $j = 1, \dots, J$ and $k = 1, \dots, K$, let $\bar{X}_{jk}$ denote the sample mean of the $n_k = g\,k$ responses from treatment arm j available at stage k. Also, let s_k^2 denote the pooled within-arms estimate of σ^2 available at stage k.

16.2 Global Tests

16.2.1 Group Sequential Chi-Squared Tests

In some circumstances it may be appropriate to monitor a single global test statistic. For testing the hypothesis of homogeneity of J normal means, we can consider group sequential tests based on monitoring successive chi-squared and F-statistics. For known σ^2, the test of H_0: $\mu_1 = \dots = \mu_J$ is based on values of the standardized between-arms sum of squares statistic

$$S_k = \frac{n_k}{\sigma^2} \sum_{j=1}^{J} (\bar{X}_{jk} - \bar{X}_{\cdot k})^2, \quad k = 1, \dots, K. \tag{16.1}$$

Here $n_k = gk$, the cumulative sample size on each arm, and

$$\bar{X}_{\cdot k} = \frac{1}{J} \sum_{j=1}^{J} \bar{X}_{jk}$$

is the overall mean at analysis k.

We consider a group sequential chi-squared test which stops to reject H_0 the first time $S_k \geq c_k$ and accepts H_0 at the final stage, K, if $S_K < c_K$. Critical values $c_1, \ldots, c_K$ are to be constructed so that the test has a specified Type I error probability α. The marginal distribution of S_k is chi-squared with $p = J - 1$ degrees of freedom and noncentrality parameter

$$n_k \sum_{j=1}^{J} (\mu_j - \bar{\mu})^2 / \sigma^2,$$

where $\bar{\mu} = (\mu_1 + \ldots + \mu_J)/J$. The joint distribution of $S_1, \ldots, S_K$ does not have the canonical distribution (3.1). However, by using the Helmert transformation (e.g., Stuart & Ord, 1987, p. 350), S_k can be written as a quadratic form in $J - 1$ independent normal variates. This allows us to apply the results of Jennison & Turnbull (1991b) who show that the sequence $S_1, S_2, \ldots$ is Markov and derive its joint distribution, in which S_k is a multiple of a non-central chi-squared variate conditional on S_{k-1}. This joint distribution is quite tractable and can be used to calculate critical values giving tests with specified Type I error probabilities.

For boundaries analogous to the Pocock test of Section 2.4 with constant nominal significance levels, we set $c_k = C_P(p, K, \alpha)$, say, for $k = 1, \ldots, K$, where $p = J - 1$. For boundaries analogous to those of the O'Brien and Fleming test of Section 2.5, we set $c_k = (K/k) C_B(p, K, \alpha)$, $k = 1, \ldots, K$. Values of the constants $C_P(p, K, \alpha)$ and $C_B(p, K, \alpha)$ are provided in Table 2 of Jennison & Turnbull (1991b) for $p = 1$ to 5, $K = 1$ to 10, 20 and 50, and $\alpha = 0.01$, 0.05 and 0.10. An abbreviated version of this table with $\alpha = 0.05$ only is shown in Table 16.1.

If the group sizes or the numbers of subjects allocated to each arm within groups are unequal, tests can be based on the statistics

$$S_k = \frac{1}{\sigma^2} \sum_{j=1}^{J} n_{jk} (\bar{X}_{jk} - \bar{X}_{\cdot k})^2, \quad k = 1, \ldots, K, \tag{16.2}$$

where n_{jk} is the cumulative sample size on arm j at stage k and

$$\bar{X}_{\cdot k} = \sum_{j=1}^{J} n_{jk} \bar{X}_{jk} \Big/ \sum_{j=1}^{J} n_{jk}$$

is the overall mean. The marginal distribution of S_k is still χ^2_{J-1} and, in keeping with the significance level approach of Section 3.3, critical values $c_1, \ldots, c_K$ obtained assuming equally sized groups can be applied to the data actually observed to give an approximate test. As long as the imbalances are not too severe, the Type I error probability should remain close to its nominal level.

Proschan, Follmann & Geller (1994) have shown how (16.1) can be generalized to accommodate unequal variances. Again, the exact tables are no longer applicable and the same significance level approach could be used to obtain an approximate test. Alternatively, Proschan et al. (1994) suggest using simulation to obtain critical values.

Table 16.1 *Constants $C_P(p, K, \alpha)$ and $C_B(p, K, \alpha)$ for, respectively, Pocock-type and O'Brien & Fleming-type repeated χ^2-tests of homogeneity of J normal means. Tests have K analyses, the χ^2 statistic at each analysis has $p = J - 1$ degrees of freedom and the Type I error probability is $\alpha = 0.05$.*

Number of arms, J	*Degrees of freedom, p*	*Number of analyses, K*	$C_P(p, K, \alpha)^*$	$C_B(p, K, \alpha)^\dagger$
2	1	1	3.84	3.84
		2	4.74	3.91
		3	5.24	4.02
		4	5.58	4.10
		5	5.82	4.16
		6	6.02	4.21
		10	6.53	4.35
3	2	1	5.99	5.99
		2	7.08	6.02
		3	7.67	6.12
		4	8.06	6.20
		5	8.35	6.27
		6	8.58	6.33
		10	9.17	6.48
4	3	1	7.81	7.81
		2	9.04	7.83
		3	9.69	7.92
		4	10.13	7.99
		5	10.44	8.06
		6	10.69	8.11
		10	11.34	8.26
5	4	1	9.49	9.49
		2	10.82	9.50
		3	11.53	9.57
		4	12.00	9.64
		5	12.35	9.71
		6	12.62	9.77
		10	13.32	9.93
6	5	1	11.07	11.07
		2	12.49	11.08
		3	13.25	11.14
		4	13.75	11.21
		5	14.12	11.27
		6	14.41	11.33
		10	15.16	11.50

* Critical value c_k for the χ^2-statistic at analysis k is $C_P(p, K, \alpha), k = 1, \ldots, K$
† Critical value c_k for the χ^2-statistic at analysis k is $(K/k)C_B(p, K, \alpha), k = 1, \ldots, K$

16.2.2 Group Sequential F-Tests

In practice, the variance σ^2 will usually be unknown. In that case we replace σ^2 by its current estimate s_k^2 in (16.1) and monitor the F-statistics

$$F_k = \frac{n_k}{(J-1)s_k^2} \sum_{j=1}^{J} (\bar{X}_{jk} - \bar{X}_{\cdot k})^2, \quad k = 1, \ldots, K. \qquad (16.3)$$

A group sequential F-test would then stop to reject H_0 the first time $F_k \geq c_k$, or accept H_0 on reaching the final stage with $F_K < c_K$. Exact critical values $c_1, \ldots, c_K$ for which such a test has a specified Type I error probability α are not available in tables, but recursive formulae that could be used to compute them are given in Jennison & Turnbull (1991b, Section 2.3). Alternatively, approximate critical values can be obtained using the significance level approach of Chapter 3. In this prescription, standard tables of the F-distribution are used to find the values c_k satisfying

$$Pr\{F_{J-1,\, J(n_k-1)} \geq c_k\} = \alpha'_k, \quad k = 1, \ldots, K, \qquad (16.4)$$

where $F_{\nu_1,\, \nu_2}$ denotes an F-distribution on ν_1 and ν_2 degrees of freedom and α'_k is the nominal significance level at stage k of a group sequential chi-squared test. The values α'_k, $k = 1, \ldots, K$, can be found using constants from, say, our Table 16.1 or Table 2 of Jennison & Turnbull (1991b). This approach could also be used for unequal group sizes with the obvious modifications to (16.3) and (16.4). Proschan et al. (1994) show how to generalize the statistic (16.3) to accommodate unequal variances using separate (i.e., non-pooled) variance estimators within each treatment arm. They suggest using simulation to obtain critical values.

16.2.3 A Test for Trend

Another type of global statistic may be called for if treatment arms represent different levels of a single quantitative factor. For example, the treatments may be increasing levels of a particular drug, in which case it will be more appropriate to monitor a trend statistic of the form

$$Z_k = \frac{\sum_{j=1}^{J} (d_j - \bar{d})\bar{X}_{jk}}{\sqrt{\{\sum_{j=1}^{J} (d_j - \bar{d})^2\sigma^2/n_k\}}} \qquad (16.5)$$

where $d_1 \leq \ldots \leq d_J$ are specified constants. These d_j could be the dose levels in the J treatment arms, or one could simply set $d_j = j$ for $j = 1, \ldots, J$. It is straightforward to construct group sequential tests based on (16.5) since $Z_1, \ldots, Z_K$ have the canonical joint distribution (3.1) with

$$\theta = \sum_{j=1}^{J} (d_j - \bar{d})\mu_j \quad \text{and} \quad \mathcal{I}_k^{-1} = \sum_{j=1}^{J} (d_j - \bar{d})^2\sigma^2/n_k.$$

Hence, the methodology described in Chapters 3 to 10 may be applied directly. In particular, when σ^2 is unknown, group sequential t-tests can be applied with σ^2 replaced by s_k^2, the pooled within-groups variance estimate at analysis k. Use of a test based on (16.5) will be more powerful against alternatives in which the means form a monotonic sequence than the "omnibus" global statistic (16.1).

The same methodology could be applied if it was desired to monitor some other single linear combination of treatment arm means. As an example, it might be desired to monitor the main effect of a particular factor when treatment arms have a factorial structure and all other factors are of secondary importance. A nonparametric form of group sequential trend test has been considered by Lin & Liu (1992).

16.3 Monitoring Pairwise Comparisons

When a study has multiple treatment arms, it is likely there will be interest in monitoring several statistics simultaneously, rather than following a single global statistic as in Section 16. Some examples are:

(i) *All pairwise comparisons* Here, all $p = J(J-1)/2$ pairwise differences between treatment means are monitored and the corresponding null hypotheses, H_{ij}: $\mu_i = \mu_j$, $i \neq j$, are tested simultaneously.

(ii) *Comparisons with a control* One treatment, J say, is considered to be a standard against which the other $J-1$ are to be compared. All $J-1$ differences in means between the control arm and the remaining $J-1$ treatments are monitored simultaneously to test the $p = J-1$ null hypotheses H_j: $\mu_j = \mu_J$, $j = 1, \ldots, J-1$.

(iii) *Factorial or fractional factorial designs* Interest is in the main effects and possibly some interactions between factors. Null hypotheses are defined stating that all factors' main effects are zero. If interactions are also to be monitored, additions can be made to the family of null hypotheses. We denote by p the total number of separate linear hypotheses to be tested.

The factorial designs mentioned in the third example are becoming more common in clinical trials, particularly in nutritional and lifestyle intervention disease prevention trials. One example is the Linxian study (Blot et al., 1993) in which a fractional 2^4 design was employed to study the cancer prevention properties of four vitamin and mineral groups in a six year prospective intervention trial. Further examples are given by Natarajan et al. (1996).

In each of the three cases, there are p hypotheses to be tested. As in Chapter 15, we defined the experiment-wise error rate to be the probability of rejecting *at least one* true hypothesis. The experiment-wise error rate is said to be controlled *strongly* if it is no more than a specified overall level α, whatever the configuration of means μ_j, $j = 1, \ldots, J$. This requirement can be satisfied by a Bonferroni approach in which a group sequential test with Type I error probability α/p is run separately for each hypothesis and a hypothesis is rejected if it is rejected at any stage of the group sequential test. In examples (i) and (ii), the individual tests are two-sample tests, whereas in (iii), the appropriate linear contrast of treatment means is monitored, similar to the test of trend described in Section 16.2.3. The Tables 15.1 and 15.2 are convenient sources of constants needed to construct

Pocock or O'Brien & Fleming tests at levels α/p for $\alpha = 0.05$. Additional constants for $\alpha = 0.01$ are provided in Tables 1 and 2 of Follmann et al. (1994)

Example

Suppose a trial with $J = 4$ treatment arms is monitored using a $K = 5$ stage O'Brien & Fleming boundary and the experiment-wise error rate is set at 5%. Suppose observations are normally distributed with known variance. If we are interested in all six pairwise comparisons, we should monitor $p = 6$ two-sample statistics and, from Table 15.2, the critical value for each of the six standardized statistics at stage k is $c_k = C_B(5, 0.05/6)\sqrt{(5/k)} = 2.681\sqrt{(5/k)}$ for $k = 1, \ldots, 5$. On the other hand, if one of the treatments is a control, as in the hypertension trial example cited earlier, it might be considered appropriate simply to monitor the three pairwise differences with that control. In that case we use $C_B(5, 0.05/3) = 2.448$ from Table 15.2 and the critical value for each of the three standardized two-sample statistics is $c_k = 2.448\sqrt{(5/k)}$, $k = 1, \ldots, 5$.

If variances are unknown, the significance level approach of Section 3.3 can be employed. Then, at each stage k, the critical value c_k is converted to the corresponding percentile of the appropriate t-distribution, i.e., with tail probability $1 - \Phi(c_k)$, where Φ is the cdf of a standard normal distribution.

The Bonferroni procedure is conservative. Assuming equal allocation of subjects across treatment arms, and equal known variances, Follmann et al. (1994, Tables 1, 2) have derived critical values for procedures that have exact experiment-wise error rates equal to a specified value α. Based on 100,000 simulations, they tabulate constants needed to construct Pocock and O'Brien & Fleming boundaries for monitoring p pairwise differences in both situations (i) and (ii) above for $\alpha = 0.05$ and 0.01, $p = 2, \ldots, 5$, and $K = 1, \ldots, 6$. Follmann et al. (1994, p. 331) point out that the discrepancies between exact and Bonferroni-based critical values are surprisingly modest, the constants C_P and C_B differing in the second decimal place at most for all the situations they considered. Given that the Bonferroni procedure is more flexible, allowing unbalanced treatment allocation and indeed different boundary shapes for different pairwise comparisons if desired, it seems that little is lost in using the Bonferroni constants rather than the exact ones.

Notice that if the test statistic for a null hypothesis corresponding to a particular pairwise difference exceeds its boundary at an interim analysis, leading to a declaration that one treatment arm is inferior, we may wish to drop that arm from the study for ethical or economic reasons. Whether or not this happens, the procedures of this section are unaffected and the overall Type I error rate is still protected. This is unlike the group sequential tests based on global statistics in the previous section, whose construction assumes sampling will continue on all arms until the trial is stopped.

For case (ii), comparisons with a control, it is possible to increase the power of a group sequential Pocock-type of O'Brien & Fleming-type test based on exact or Bonferroni critical values by generalizing the "closed step-down" procedure of Marcus, Peritz & Gabriel (1976); see also Hochberg & Tamhane (1987, Section 2.4). This modification works by changing the critical values for remaining comparisons at later stages whenever any pairwise difference hypothesis is rejected. Follmann et al. (1994) prove that if a treatment arm is dropped at one stage because it has been shown to be inferior to the control, the experiment-wise error is preserved if critical values at subsequent stages are based on the *remaining* number of arms and the original number of analyses, K. Since the critical values are smaller for decreasing p, this must result in a more powerful procedure. In the above example, suppose one treatment of the three had been found inferior to the control at stage k_1. This treatment arm would be dropped from the study: it would receive no further subjects and comparisons involving this treatment would be excluded from future analyses. Then at stages $k > k_1$, the two remaining comparisons would use critical values $c_k = 2.303\sqrt{(5/k)}$ instead of $c_k = 2.448\sqrt{(5/k)}$. If another treatment arm is dropped at the next analysis, based on this new critical value, the one remaining comparison would subsequently use $c_k = 2.040\sqrt{(5/k)}$. Follmann et al. (1994) show the same step-down procedure preserves the experiment-wise error of α in case (i), all pairwise comparisons, but only when there are $J = 3$ arms. Their argument breaks down for $J \geq 4$ and the validity of the result is an open question.

Two well known multiple comparison procedures for all pairwise differences in the fixed sample case are Fisher's Least Significant Difference (LSD) method and the Newman-Keuls procedure; see Hochberg & Tamhane (1987). These methods have been generalized to the group sequential setting by Proschan et al. (1994).

In the analogue of the LSD procedure, initially the global statistic (16.1) or (16.3) is used to monitor the study at the specified error rate α. When, and only when, this statistic exceeds its boundary, the pairwise are differences examined using boundary values for unadjusted group sequential tests with two-sided Type I error probability α, as described in Chapters 2 and 3. Any treatment arm found inferior in a pairwise comparison at this stage is dropped from the study. At subsequent stages, only pairwise differences among the remaining treatment arms continue to be monitored using unadjusted two-sample group sequential tests, and any treatment found to be inferior is dropped. As an example, with $J = 4$ treatment arms, $K = 5$ analyses, $\alpha = 0.05$ and O'Brien & Fleming-type boundaries, we would start by using the global statistic (16.1) with boundary values $8.06(5/k)$ for $k = 1, \ldots, 5$. (The constant $C_B(3, 5, 0.05) = 8.06$ is obtained from Table 16.1.) If the boundary is exceeded, then at that and any subsequent stage, all pairwise differences are examined using a two-sample statistic such as (2.4) and critical values $2.04\sqrt{(5/k)}$ for $k = 1, \ldots, 5$. Here the constant $C_B(5, 0.05) = 2.04$ can be read from Table 2.3, or from the column in Table 15.2 for $p = 1$.

The generalization of the Newman-Keuls procedure is similar and is based on the range statistic instead of the chi-squared statistic. All pairwise absolute differences in means fall below a threshold c if and only if the range of the means falls below this threshold, so a range test can also be defined in terms of the difference between the largest and smallest sample means. At any stage, suppose there are J' arms that have not been dropped from the study. Then, the standardized two-sample statistic for comparing the largest and smallest sample means is compared with the level α critical value for $p = J'(J' - 1)/2$

comparisons. Exact values of this critical value can be obtained from Tables 1 and 2 of Follmann et al. (1994) or Table I of Proschan et al. (1994). Alternatively, one could use the slightly conservative Bonferroni-based values from Tables 15.1 and 15.2. If the difference between largest and smallest sample means is found to be significant, the exercise is repeated comparing the largest mean to the second smallest and the second largest to the smallest using critical values for the case of $J' - 1$ arms. This process is repeated until no further ranges are significant; for details, see Hochberg & Tamhane (1987, p. 66), who treat the fixed sample case. All arms found inferior by this process are dropped from the study and the procedure continues to the next stage, with only the ranges of contending arms continuing to be monitored.

As in the fixed sample case, the group sequential versions of the LSD and Newman-Keuls procedures only *weakly* protect the experiment-wise Type I error rate α. That is, the probability of *any* true hypothesis being rejected is no more than the specified α only under the global null hypothesis that all treatment means are equal. For other configurations of means μ_j, $j = 1, \ldots, J$, this probability may exceed α. For example, this can happen under either procedure if there are four treatment arms with means $\mu_1 = \mu_2 << \mu_3 = \mu_4$; then for either procedure, the global test will reject early and there is a probability of approximately 2α that at least one of the two true hypotheses $\mu_1 = \mu_2$ or $\mu_3 = \mu_4$ will be rejected. In the fixed sample case, Hochberg & Tamhane (1987, p. 69) show how the experiment-wise error can be strongly controlled at level α by reducing the nominal levels at which each component comparison is made; in principle, the same modification could be made to the group sequential versions.

16.4 Bibliography and Notes

Proschan et al. (1994) adapt the ideas presented here in the context of monitoring mean responses for multi-armed trials to survival time responses. The more technical details are given in Follmann et al. (1994, Appendix A.2).

Siegmund (1993) and Betensky (1996) propose a fully sequential design for comparing three treatments using a hybrid method, similar in spirit to the LSD procedure described above. Their procedure consists of two phases. In the first, a global statistic is monitored sequentially to test for homogeneity of the three means. If this hypothesis is accepted, the experiment terminates; otherwise, the least promising treatment arm is dropped and, in the second phase, a sequential test is performed with the remaining two treatments. Betensky (1997c) adapts the same procedure to accommodate survival time endpoints.

Hughes (1993) proposes a group sequential procedure based on two-sample statistics for pairwise comparisons with the aim of dividing the treatment arms into two subsets, one labeled inferior, the other superior. At interim analyses, treatments determined to be in the inferior group are dropped. If, at termination, only one arm is contained in the superior set, it is identified as the best one; otherwise all treatments in that set are declared superior. The procedure is in the same spirit as subset selection procedures, often used as screening methods to pick the most promising treatments for future study from a larger group of candidate treatments; see, for example, Bechhofer, Santner & Goldsman (1995, Chapter 3). In fact, in the ranking and selection literature, there is a considerable body of work on sequential and multi-stage procedures for identifying the best of several competing treatments. An indifference zone formulation is often adopted whereby, typically, designs must satisfy the requirement that the best treatment is selected with a pre-specified probability P^* whenever its mean exceeds that of the next best by a specified amount. Bechhofer et al. (1995, Chapter 2) survey the various procedures that have been proposed.

When there are multiple treatment arms, it becomes interesting to ask if gains can be made by unequal allocation of subjects. Of course, group sequential procedures in which arms can be dropped at interim analyses are, essentially, attempting to reduce sample sizes on the inferior arms. This is often highly desirable from an ethical viewpoint, and possibly also from an economic one. The more general class of designs in which the fractions of subjects randomly allocated to each treatment are allowed to depend on the accumulating results are called "adaptive allocation" designs or in some cases "multi-armed bandit" procedures. We discuss such designs in the next chapter.

CHAPTER 17

Adaptive Treatment Assignment

17.1 A Multi-Stage Adaptive Design

In this chapter we concentrate on the two-treatment parallel designs of Chapters 2 and 3, in particular, the unpaired two-treatment comparison of Section 3.1.1. It is not unusual for unequal randomization or drop-out of some subjects to produce unbalanced numbers of observations on the two treatments. We now consider intentional imbalance between treatments achieved by allowing treatment allocation in each stage to depend on previously observed outcomes. Such designs are said to use stage-wise data-dependent or stage-wise adaptive sampling rules.

Suppose we have responses $X_{Ai} \sim N(\mu_A, \sigma_A^2)$, $i = 1, 2, \ldots$, for subjects allocated to treatment A and $X_{Bi} \sim N(\mu_B, \sigma_B^2)$, $i = 1, 2, \ldots$, for those on treatment B, where the variances σ_A^2 and σ_B^2 are known but not necessarily equal. At each stage $k = 1, \ldots, K$ we collect m_{Ak} observations on treatment arm A and m_{Bk} on treatment arm B. The cumulative numbers of observations collected up to stage k on arms A and B are

$$n_{Ak} = \sum_{j=1}^{k} m_{Aj} \quad \text{and} \quad n_{Bk} = \sum_{j=1}^{k} m_{Bj}$$

and we denote the cumulative sample means by $\bar{X}_A^{(k)}$ and $\bar{X}_B^{(k)}$, respectively.

Let $\theta = \mu_A - \mu_B$ and suppose we wish to test H_0: $\theta = 0$. The standardized statistic at analysis k for testing H_0 is

$$Z_k = (\bar{X}_A^{(k)} - \bar{X}_B^{(k)})\sqrt{\mathcal{I}_k},$$

where

$$\mathcal{I}_k = (\sigma_A^2/n_{Ak} + \sigma_B^2/n_{Bk})^{-1}. \tag{17.1}$$

We can test H_0 using a group sequential two-sided test, with or without an inner wedge, or a group sequential one-sided test. In Chapters 2 to 6, we saw how to specify a boundary for $Z_1, \ldots, Z_K$ together with a particular information sequence, $\mathcal{I}_1, \ldots, \mathcal{I}_K$, to satisfy error probability requirements. If we opt for equal increments of information, we need $\mathcal{I}_k = (k/K)\mathcal{I}_K$, $k = 1, \ldots, K$, where the final information level $\mathcal{I}_K$ is determined using constants tabulated in Chapters 2 and 5 for two-sided tests and in Chapter 4 for one-sided tests.

In defining adaptive sampling rules, we shall assume $\mathcal{I}_1, \ldots, \mathcal{I}_K$ are pre-specified and design the sampling rules to produce these information levels. Thus, when planning the kth set of observations, group sizes m_{Ak} and m_{Bk} must be chosen to satisfy (17.1) with the pre-specified value of $\mathcal{I}_k$. There is still flexibility in the choice of m_{Ak} and m_{Bk} and we shall allow these to depend on the accumulated data through the current estimate of the treatment effect,

$$\hat{\theta}^{(k-1)} = \bar{X}_A^{(k-1)} - \bar{X}_B^{(k-1)}.$$

We show in Section 17.3 that, under such a sampling scheme, $\{Z_1, \ldots, Z_K\}$ have the canonical joint distribution (3.1), conditional on $\{\mathcal{I}_1, \ldots, \mathcal{I}_K\}$, and hence the required error probabilities are attained. However, the distribution (3.1) can fail to hold and error rates vary from their intended values if m_{Ak} and m_{Bk} depend on $\bar{X}_A^{(k-1)}$ and $\bar{X}_B^{(k-1)}$ in other ways.

The aim in using an adaptive allocation rule is to reduce the number of subjects assigned to the inferior treatment arm. Whether this is arm A or B is unknown initially but at any stage during the trial the current estimate of θ provides an indication of the relative merits of the two treatments, albeit subject to error, which can be used to determine adaptive treatment assignments. Reducing the expected number of subjects allocated to the inferior treatment, known as the "inferior treatment number" (ITN), usually leads to an increase in the total expected sample size or "average sample number" (ASN). A large ASN is also undesirable since it implies a long elapsed time before the trial can be concluded. As a device to balance the competing goals of reducing the ITN and ASN, one can aim to minimize the expected value of a loss function of the form

$$L(\theta) = u(\theta)\, n_{A\tau} + v(\theta)\, n_{B\tau}, \tag{17.2}$$

where τ denotes the stage at which the experiment terminates and $n_{A\tau}$ and $n_{B\tau}$ are the cumulative sample sizes on arms A and B at this point. Supposing a high response is desirable, the inferior treatment is A if $\theta < 0$ and B if $\theta > 0$. Thus, the weights $u(\theta)$ and $v(\theta)$ in (17.2) should be strictly positive with $v(\theta)$ increasing in θ for $\theta > 0$ and $u(\theta)$ increasing as θ decreases for $\theta < 0$. We shall consider the particular case

$$L(\theta) = \begin{cases} n_{A\tau} + a^{\theta/\delta}\, n_{B\tau} & \text{for } \theta \geq 0, \\ a^{-\theta/\delta}\, n_{A\tau} + n_{B\tau} & \text{for } \theta \leq 0, \end{cases} \tag{17.3}$$

where a is a chosen constant and δ the value of θ appearing in the test's power condition.

Since successive information levels are subject to the constraint (17.1), the allocation ratio minimizing (17.2) is

$$\frac{n_{A\tau}}{n_{B\tau}} = \frac{\sigma_A}{\sigma_B}\, w(\theta), \tag{17.4}$$

where

$$w(\theta) = \sqrt{\frac{v(\theta)}{u(\theta)}}.$$

Although this optimal ratio depends on the unknown θ, we can attempt to achieve it approximately using successive estimates of θ in the following adaptive rule.

Adaptive Sampling Rule

At the first stage, set

$$m_{A1} = \sigma_A\{\sigma_A + \sigma_B w(\tilde{\theta})\}\mathcal{I}_1 \quad \text{and}$$
$$m_{B1} = \sigma_B\{\sigma_A + \sigma_B w(\tilde{\theta})\}\mathcal{I}_1 / w(\tilde{\theta}), \tag{17.5}$$

where $\tilde{\theta}$ is a preliminary estimate of θ. If no such estimate of θ is available, one can use $w(\tilde{\theta}) = 1$ in (17.5). Of course, these allocations must be rounded to integer values.

In planning stage k $(2 \leq k \leq K)$, supposing the test has not yet terminated, we substitute the current estimate of θ in (17.4). The aim is, thus, to choose m_{Ak} and m_{Bk} so that the cumulative sample sizes at analysis k will be in the ratio

$$\frac{n_{Ak}}{n_{Bk}} = \frac{\sigma_A}{\sigma_B} w(\hat{\theta}^{(k-1)})$$

and achieve the specified information level by satisfying (17.1). This leads to group sizes

$$m_{Ak} = \sigma_A\{\sigma_A + \sigma_B w(\hat{\theta}^{(k-1)})\}\mathcal{I}_k - n_{A\,k-1} \quad \text{and}$$
$$m_{Bk} = \sigma_B\{\sigma_A + \sigma_B w(\hat{\theta}^{(k-1)})\}\mathcal{I}_k / w(\hat{\theta}^{(k-1)}) - n_{B\,k-1}, \tag{17.6}$$

which are again rounded to integers. If either of these values for m_{Ak} and m_{Bk} is negative, that allocation is set to zero and sufficient observations are taken on the other arm to satisfy (17.1).

One may prefer to set a minimum sample size, m^* say, for both arms at each stage. In this case, if either m_{Ak} or m_{Bk} as determined by (17.6) falls below m^*, that allocation is set to m^* and sufficient observations are taken on the other arm to satisfy (17.1). One reason for imposing a minimum group size on each treatment arm is to preserve at least some randomization in the treatment allocation and thereby maintain an element of "blinding". Another reason is concern about possible bias due to time trends in the patient population or treatment administration, although in this case a better strategy would be to include such time trends in a statistical model and use a suitable sequential procedure of the form we shall discuss in Section 17.2.

As illustrative examples, we consider one-sided group sequential tests from the power family of Section 4.2 with parameter $\Delta = 0$ and K equally spaced analyses. We assume equal variances, $\sigma_A^2 = \sigma_B^2$, and require Type I error $\alpha = 0.05$ and power $1 - \beta = 0.9$ at $\theta = \delta$. The boundary for $Z_1, \ldots, Z_K$ is given by (4.3) and the necessary information levels are $\mathcal{I}_k = (k/K)\mathcal{I}_K$, $k = 1, \ldots, K$, where $\mathcal{I}_K$ is given by (4.4). The constants $\tilde{C}_1(K, 0.05, 0.1, 0)$ and $\tilde{C}_2(K, 0.05, 0.1, 0)$ are obtained from Table 4.2. Equal sample sizes, $n_{A1} = n_{B1}$, are used in the initial stage and the adaptive allocation rule (17.6) is employed subsequently using the loss function (17.3), for which

$$w(\theta) = a^{\theta/(2\delta)}.$$

Table 17.1 *Properties of power family one-sided tests with* $\Delta = 0$ *using adaptive sampling in comparing two normal distributions with equal variances. The adaptive allocation rule* (17.6) *is employed with* $w(\theta) = a^{\theta/(2\delta)}$. *Tests have* K *groups of observations, Type I error probability* $\alpha = 0.05$ *at* $\theta = 0$, *and power* $1 - \beta = 0.9$ *at* $\theta = \delta$.
Expected sample sizes on treatments A and B, under selected values of θ, *are expressed as percentages of the sample size per treatment arm in a fixed sample test with equal treatment allocation and the same error probabilities. Estimates are based on* 250,000 *simulations and have standard errors of less than* 0.1.

		Expected sample size as percentage of fixed sample size							
		$a = 1$		$a = 1.5$		$a = 2$		$a = 4$	
	θ	A	B	A	B	A	B	A	B
$K = 2$									
	$-\delta$	52.7	52.7	52.7	52.6	52.7	52.6	52.8	52.6
	$-\delta/2$	57.3	57.3	57.7	57.0	58.0	56.8	58.7	56.3
	0	73.0	73.0	75.0	71.3	76.3	70.1	80.7	67.9
	$\delta/2$	88.5	88.5	93.0	84.5	96.7	82.1	107.2	76.9
	δ	81.4	81.4	86.2	77.5	89.9	75.0	101.5	70.1
	$3\delta/2$	62.7	62.7	64.6	61.0	66.3	60.0	71.3	58.1
	2δ	53.7	53.7	54.0	53.4	54.4	53.3	55.1	53.0
$K = 5$									
	$-\delta$	37.3	37.3	35.8	39.1	35.0	40.6	33.3	45.2
	$-\delta/2$	47.0	47.0	46.2	48.3	45.6	49.3	45.0	52.7
	0	63.8	63.8	65.0	62.9	66.0	62.5	69.3	62.1
	$\delta/2$	80.1	80.1	84.8	76.2	88.5	73.7	100.2	68.9
	δ	71.8	71.8	79.0	65.9	85.5	62.6	106.6	56.1
	$3\delta/2$	54.3	54.3	62.9	48.1	71.0	44.8	101.0	38.9
	2δ	43.7	43.7	52.5	37.7	61.3	34.7	96.9	29.9
$K = 10$									
	$-\delta$	33.4	33.4	30.9	36.6	29.6	39.7	27.2	51.5
	$-\delta/2$	43.0	43.0	41.7	44.7	41.0	46.2	39.9	52.1
	0	60.1	60.1	61.0	59.5	61.8	59.2	64.5	59.5
	$\delta/2$	77.0	77.0	81.3	73.1	84.9	70.9	95.9	66.3
	δ	68.2	68.2	75.3	62.7	81.3	59.3	102.0	53.0
	$3\delta/2$	50.2	50.2	58.5	44.4	66.1	41.0	97.3	35.5
	2δ	38.9	38.9	48.0	32.9	57.5	29.9	101.9	25.2

Table 17.1 displays expected sample sizes $E(n_{A\tau})$ and $E(n_{B\tau})$ for arms A and B under a range of values of θ. These are expressed as percentages of the sample size per treatment arm in a corresponding fixed sample test with equal treatment allocation. Results are for procedures with $K = 2, 5$ and 10 stages and with $a = 1$, 1.5, 2 and 4 in the loss function. The ITN is $E(n_{A\tau})$ when $\theta < 0$ and $E(n_{B\tau})$ when $\theta > 0$; the ASN is $\{E(n_{A\tau}) + E(n_{B\tau})\}/2$. When $a = 1$, the rule is non-adaptive and expected sample sizes coincide with those given in Table 4.2. It is evident from

the table that the rules with higher values of a can achieve substantial savings in ITN over the non-adaptive procedure with $a = 1$, although this does come at the expense of a higher ASN.

Further calculations show that, in many instances, expected sample sizes on each treatment arm are close to the values they would have if the optimal sampling ratio (17.4), with the *true* value of θ, were used throughout the study. In this idealized situation $E(n_{A\tau})$ and $E(n_{B\tau})$ would equal their values under a non-adaptive rule multiplied by factors $\{1+w(\theta)\}/2$ and $\{1+w(\theta)^{-1}\}/2$, respectively. As an example, for $K = 5$, $\theta = \delta$ and $a = 2$, we have $w(\theta) = \sqrt{2}$ and applying (17.4) with $\theta = \delta$ would give

$$E(n_{A\tau}) = \frac{(1+\sqrt{2})}{2} \times 71.8 = 86.7$$

and

$$E(n_{B\tau}) = \frac{(1+1/\sqrt{2})}{2} \times 71.8 = 61.3,$$

very close to the values 85.5 and 62.6 obtained under the adaptive rule in which θ is estimated as the study progresses. Departures from this pattern occur when a test is likely to terminate at an interim analysis before the sampling rule is able to adapt to estimates of θ. This is most evident for $K = 2$, where there is only one intermediate analysis, and under extreme values of θ for which the probability of early stopping is high.

If the variances σ_A^2 and σ_B^2 are unknown, an analogous procedure can be based on an approximate, unpooled two-sample t-statistic with group sequential boundaries defined through significance levels of the t-distribution as in Sections 3.8, 4.4, and 5.2.4. Allocations of observations at stages $k = 2, \ldots, K$ can be based on (17.6) with σ_A and σ_B replaced by estimates from data obtained in the previous $k-1$ stages. At the initial stage, preliminary estimates of σ_A and σ_B, as well as θ, must be used in (17.5). Note that if σ_A^2 and σ_B^2 are unequal, the optimal ratio (17.4) differs from unity even when $u(\theta) \equiv v(\theta)$. Consequently, adaptive allocation of observations to treatments can reduce both ASN and ITN, so adaptive sampling procedures can still be of considerable benefit when only a low ASN is deemed important.

17.2 A Multi-Stage Adaptive Design with Time Trends

The adaptive designs of Section 17.1 can lead to considerable imbalance in the sample sizes m_{Ak} and m_{Bk} within a group and this can cause problems if there is a possibility of time trends in the responses; see, for example, Peto (1985, p. 32). The ECMO study (Ware, 1989, p. 302) was criticized because a lack of concurrent control subjects in the second stage "raised the possibility of non-comparability of treatment groups". In fact, the methods of Section 17.1 can be extended to general normal linear regression models (see Jennison & Turnbull, 2000b) and linear or quadratic time trends can be incorporated as covariates, along with other concomitant variables. This approach could be followed to incorporate adaptive allocation in the two-treatment comparison adjusted for covariates described as the second example of Section 3.4.2. However, as an alternative approach, we now describe a modification of the procedure proposed in Section 17.1 which allows for arbitrary time trends in responses.

Suppose responses are independent and normally distributed as before, except now the observations at stage k have means $\mu_A + \gamma_k$ for treatment A and $\mu_B + \gamma_k$ for treatment B. It is desired to test the null hypothesis H_0: $\theta = 0$, where $\theta = \mu_A - \mu_B$, the $\gamma_1, \ldots, \gamma_K$ being treated as unknown nuisance parameters.

For $k = 1, \ldots, K$, let $\bar{X}_A^{(k)}$ denote the mean of the m_{Ak} responses on treatment arm A in the kth group, and similarly define $\bar{X}_B^{(k)}$ for treatment arm B. In each group $k = 1, \ldots, K$, the difference in mean responses from arms A and B, $\bar{X}_A^{(k)} - \bar{X}_B^{(k)}$, provides an unbiased estimate of θ. The maximum likelihood estimate of θ based on data accumulated up to stage k is the weighted average

$$\hat{\theta}^{(k)} = \frac{1}{w_1 + \ldots + w_k} \sum_{i=1}^{k} w_i (\bar{X}_A^{(i)} - \bar{X}_B^{(i)}) \qquad (17.7)$$

where the weights

$$w_k = \left(\frac{\sigma_A^2}{m_{Ak}} + \frac{\sigma_B^2}{m_{Bk}} \right)^{-1}, \quad k = 1, \ldots, K, \qquad (17.8)$$

are the reciprocals of the variances of the estimates $\bar{X}_A^{(k)} - \bar{X}_B^{(k)}$. Note that

$$Var(\hat{\theta}^{(k)}) = (w_1 + \ldots + w_k)^{-1}, \quad k = 1, \ldots, K.$$

Defining

$$\mathcal{I}_k = \sum_{i=1}^{k} w_i,$$

the standardized statistic for testing H_0 at stage k is $Z_k = \hat{\theta}^{(k)} \surd \mathcal{I}_k$, $k = 1, \ldots, K$. Assuming the sampling rule is designed to achieve pre-specified information levels $\{\mathcal{I}_1, \ldots, \mathcal{I}_K\}$, the joint distribution of $\{Z_1, \ldots, Z_K\}$ does not depend on the parameters $\gamma_1, \ldots, \gamma_K$ and follows the canonical joint distribution (3.1). Hence, as in Section 17.1, an information sequence $\{\mathcal{I}_1, \ldots, \mathcal{I}_K\}$ and group sequential boundary for $\{Z_1, \ldots, Z_K\}$ can be chosen to give a test meeting stated Type I error and power requirements.

As before, we obtain a sampling rule by attempting to minimize a loss function of the form (17.2) subject to attaining a fixed sequence of information levels $\mathcal{I}_1, \ldots, \mathcal{I}_K$. This constraint implies that m_{Ak} and m_{Bk} must satisfy (17.8) with $w_k = \mathcal{I}_k - \mathcal{I}_{k-1}$, or simply $w_k = \mathcal{I}_K / K$ in the case of equal information increments. If θ were known, the group sizes m_{Ak} and m_{Bk} should be in the optimal ratio

$$\frac{m_{Ak}}{m_{Bk}} = \frac{\sigma_A}{\sigma_B} w(\theta)$$

where, as before, $w(\theta) = \surd\{v(\theta)/u(\theta)\}$. This leads to allocations for the kth group, $k = 1, \ldots, K$, of

$$\begin{aligned} m_{Ak} &= \sigma_A \{\sigma_A + \sigma_B w(\theta)\} (\mathcal{I}_k - \mathcal{I}_{k-1}) \quad \text{and} \\ m_{Bk} &= \sigma_B \{\sigma_A + \sigma_B w(\theta)\} (\mathcal{I}_k - \mathcal{I}_{k-1}) / w(\theta), \end{aligned} \qquad (17.9)$$

where $\mathcal{I}_0$ is taken to be zero. Since θ is unknown, this sampling rule must be applied using successive estimates of θ. In the first stage, allocations are as in (17.5) and in subsequent stages, $k = 2, \ldots, K$, we use (17.9) with θ replaced by the current estimate $\hat{\theta}^{(k-1)}$, as given by (17.7).

One should expect this method to produce smaller reductions in ITN than the previous procedure which made no allowance for time trends, since there is no longer a mechanism for redressing sub-optimal allocation of observations in earlier groups when improved estimates of θ become available. This method can also be adapted to the case of unknown variances following the approach described in Section 17.1 for the procedure without time trends.

17.3 Validity of Adaptive Multi-stage Procedures

We now outline the theoretical results which justify the multi-stage adaptive procedures of Section 17.1. Similar theory provides the basis for procedures described in Section 17.2. We shall present results in terms of the score statistics $S_k = Z_k\sqrt{\mathcal{I}_k}$, $k = 1, \ldots, K$, which were introduced in Section 3.5.3. The joint distribution of the Z_ks follows directly from that of the S_ks.

The procedures of Section 17.1 and 17.2 are valid if the conditional joint distribution of $\{Z_1, \ldots, Z_K\}$ given $\{\mathcal{I}_1, \ldots, \mathcal{I}_K\}$ satisfies (3.1). We shall first produce an intermediate result concerning the joint distribution of $S_1, \ldots, S_K$ when $\mathcal{I}_k$ may depend on $S_1, \ldots, S_{k-1}$. We then obtain (3.1) by the simple device of restricting sampling rules so that they produce a pre-specified sequence of information levels, $\mathcal{I}_1, \ldots, \mathcal{I}_K$.

The Joint Distribution of $S_1, \ldots, S_K$

Suppose responses $X_{Ai} \sim N(\mu_A, \sigma^2)$ and $X_{Bi} \sim N(\mu_B, \sigma^2)$, $i = 1, 2, \ldots$, are observed on treatments A and B, respectively. For simplicity, we have assumed a common variance for the two response types but the results we present here extend to the case of unequal variances, σ_A^2 and σ_B^2, with only minor modifications. For $k = 1, \ldots, K$, we have

$$\begin{aligned}
\hat{\theta}^{(k)} &= \bar{X}_A^{(k)} - \bar{X}_B^{(k)}, \\
\mathcal{I}_k &= (\sigma^2/n_{Ak} + \sigma^2/n_{Bk})^{-1}, \\
Z_k &= (\bar{X}_A^{(k)} - \bar{X}_B^{(k)})\sqrt{\mathcal{I}_k}
\end{aligned}$$

and $S_k = Z_k\sqrt{\mathcal{I}_k}$.

Under a typical adaptive sampling rule, the choice of n_{Ak} and n_{Bk} will be based on the estimated treatment effect, $\hat{\theta}^{(k-1)} = S_{k-1}/\mathcal{I}_{k-1}$, and the current cumulative sample sizes, $n_{A\,k-1}$ and $n_{B\,k-1}$. In general, we can allow more than this: n_{Ak} and n_{Bk} may depend on $n_{A1}, \ldots, n_{A\,k-1}, n_{B1}, \ldots, n_{B\,k-1}$ and $S_1, \ldots, S_{k-1}$ but *not* on the scaled sample sum

$$W_{k-1} = \frac{1}{\sigma^2}\left(\sum_{i=1}^{n_{A\,k-1}} X_{Ai} + \sum_{i=1}^{n_{B\,k-1}} X_{Bi}\right).$$

Under these conditions, the joint distribution of $S_1, S_2, \ldots$ is given by

$$S_1 \,|\, \mathcal{I}_1 \sim N(\mathcal{I}_1 \theta,\, \mathcal{I}_1) \tag{17.10}$$

and

$$S_k - S_{k-1} \,|\, \mathcal{I}_1, \ldots, \mathcal{I}_k, S_1, \ldots, S_{k-1}$$

$$\sim N(\{\mathcal{I}_k - \mathcal{I}_{k-1}\}\theta,\, \mathcal{I}_k - \mathcal{I}_{k-1}) \quad \text{for } k \geq 2. \tag{17.11}$$

The key step in proving this result is to decompose $S_k - S_{k-1}$ as

$$\begin{aligned} S_k - S_{k-1} \;=\; & \frac{n_{Bk}}{n_{Ak} + n_{Bk}} \frac{1}{\sigma^2} \sum_{n_{Ak-1}+1}^{n_{Ak}} X_{Ai} \\ & - \frac{n_{Ak}}{n_{Ak} + n_{Bk}} \frac{1}{\sigma^2} \sum_{n_{Bk-1}+1}^{n_{Bk}} X_{Bi} \\ & + \frac{n_{Ak-1} n_{Bk} - n_{Bk-1} n_{Ak}}{(n_{Ak-1} + n_{Bk-1})(n_{Ak} + n_{Bk})} W_{k-1}. \end{aligned} \tag{17.12}$$

The first two terms in this decomposition involve only new data in the kth group of observations while the third term is a function of previously observed data. Note that if the ratio n_{Ak}/n_{Bk} remains constant across analyses, the third term is identically zero. Since the first two terms and the third term are based on separate sets of data, they are conditionally independent of each other given n_{Ak-1}, n_{Ak}, n_{Bk-1} and n_{Bk}. It can also be shown that W_{k-1} is conditionally independent of $S_1, \ldots, S_{k-1}$ given $n_{A1}, \ldots, n_{Ak-1}$ and $n_{B1}, \ldots, n_{Bk-1}$ with a

$$N(\{n_{Ak-1}\mu_A + n_{Bk-1}\mu_B\}/\sigma^2,\; \{n_{Ak-1} + n_{Bk-1}\}/\sigma^2)$$

conditional distribution. The result (17.11) follows from this expression for $S_k - S_{k-1}$ as the sum of three independent normal variables and some straightforward algebra. For full details we refer the reader to the complete proof provided by Jennison & Turnbull (2000b); this paper also extends the above theory to general normal linear models, showing that the sequence of score statistics for a linear combination of parameters, $\boldsymbol{c}^T \boldsymbol{\beta}$, satisfies (17.10) and (17.11) with $\mathcal{I}_k$ the information for $\boldsymbol{c}^T \boldsymbol{\beta}$ at analysis k, as long as the adaptive sampling rule depends on each $\widehat{\boldsymbol{\beta}}^{(k)}$ only through $\boldsymbol{c}^T \widehat{\boldsymbol{\beta}}^{(k)}$.

Inspection of the decomposition (17.12) shows why the choice of n_{Ak} and n_{Bk} should not be allowed to depend on W_{k-1}. Suppose, for example, $n_{Ak-1} = n_{Bk-1}$ and let a and b be a pair of integers with $b > a > n_{Ak-1}$. Then $n_{Ak} = a,\; n_{Bk} = b$ and $n_{Ak} = b,\; n_{Bk} = a$ both lead to the same $\mathcal{I}_k$ but the factor multiplying W_{k-1} in (17.12) is positive in the first case and negative in the second. If $n_{Ak} = a,\; n_{Bk} = b$ is chosen whenever W_{k-1} is greater than a specified value and $n_{Ak} = b,\; n_{Bk} = a$ otherwise, the distribution of the increment $S_k - S_{k-1}$ will be stochastically greater than its distribution when a choice between these two cases is made independently of W_{k-1}.

Achieving the Canonical Joint Distribution (3.1)

In order to ensure that the tests of Chapters 2 to 6 maintain their error probabilities when used in conjunction with adaptive sampling rules, we need the conditional distribution of $Z_k = S_k/\sqrt{\mathcal{I}_k}$, $k = 1, \ldots, K$, given $\mathcal{I}_1, \ldots, \mathcal{I}_K$ to have the canonical form (3.1). It is important to realize that the joint distribution of $S_1, \ldots, S_K$ given by (17.10) and (17.11) is not sufficient to ensure this conditional distribution. Suppose, for example, a sampling rule produces one value of $\mathcal{I}_2$ if S_1 is positive and another if S_1 is negative, then it is clear that the conditional distribution of S_1 given either value of $\mathcal{I}_2$ is not normal.

However, (17.10) and (17.11) do imply (3.1) if $\mathcal{I}_1, \ldots, \mathcal{I}_K$ are fixed independently of the values of $S_1, \ldots, S_K$. Thus, if a sampling rule is designed to ensure a pre-specified sequence of information levels, (3.1) is obtained automatically. The procedures described in Sections 17.1 and 17.2 are defined in this way, hence (3.1) holds and the tests have the same error probabilities as non-adaptive tests with the same information levels and boundaries for $Z_1, \ldots, Z_K$.

The restriction to a fixed sequence $\mathcal{I}_1, \ldots, \mathcal{I}_K$ can be relaxed a little to allow for perturbations in observed information due to randomness in actual group sizes. The key requirement that must be met is that $\mathcal{I}_k$ should be statistically independent of $S_1, \ldots, S_{k-1}$, for $k = 2, \ldots, K$. If information levels are variable, tests should be adapted accordingly using either the approximate methods of Chapters 2 to 6 or the error spending approach of Chapter 7.

17.4 Bibliography and Notes

There is considerable literature on statistical methodology for response-adaptive designs in sequential clinical trials. Early work has been reviewed by Hoel, Sobel & Weiss (1975), Simon (1977) and Iglewicz (1983) and more recent reviews are by Hardwick (1989) and Rosenberger & Lachin (1993). A variety of research topics are presented in twenty papers contained in the Proceedings of a 1992 conference on adaptive designs (Flournoy & Rosenberger, 1995).

The earliest ideas are due to Robbins (1952), who introduced the "two-armed bandit" problem in which it is desired to maximize return when presented with two alternative Bernoulli payoffs with unknown and unequal success probabilities. Specifically in the context of clinical trials, Anscombe (1963) and Colton (1963) proposed a two-stage design which allocates all patients in the second stage to the treatment appearing superior in the first stage. Cornfield, Halperin & Greenhouse (1969) generalized these ideas to multi-stage designs. Zelen (1969) introduced the "play-the-winner" (PW) design for comparing two dichotomous response distributions and this was extended to "randomized play-the-winner" (RPW) rules by Wei & Durham (1978). Rosenberger (1993, 1996) summarizes further developments and the use of biased coin randomization schemes for normal and survival outcomes. Yao & Wei (1996) discuss RPW rules in a group sequential setting; using simulation, they retrospectively examine what would have happened had these rules been applied to the binomial data of the ACTG076 maternal HIV transmission trial and the survival end-point of a VACURG prostatic cancer trial.

Robbins & Siegmund (1974) discuss adaptive allocation rules similar to those of Section 17.1 for the two-sample normal problem. They use an invariant sequential probability ratio test (SPRT) with continuous monitoring and are able to establish error rates by standard likelihood ratio arguments rather than the more detailed theory described in Section 17.3 for an arbitrary group sequential test. They then apply martingale arguments to obtain results on expected sample sizes. The SPRT with adaptive allocation was developed further by Louis (1975), who explicitly considered a loss function expressed as a weighted linear combination of ASN and ITN, and by Hayre (1979) who first used the loss function (17.2) with weights depending on the unknown difference θ. Louis (1977) and Hayre & Turnbull (1981a) apply similar adaptive SPRT-based designs to exponential survival data subject to censoring; in this case, the variance depends on the mean and the goals of reducing ASN and ITN are not necessarily in conflict, so adaptive sequential designs can be of particular benefit. Hayre & Turnbull (1981a) also consider other distributions, especially the binomial. It should be remarked that this class of designs is not only valuable in the hypothesis testing framework, but also for point and interval estimation; see Hayre & Turnbull (1981b,c).

If there are three or more treatment arms and the experimenter's goal is to select the best treatment, precise analysis of adaptive procedures becomes much more difficult. References in this area include Turnbull, Kaspi & Smith (1978), Jennison, Johnstone & Turnbull (1982) and, more recently, Coad (1995). The problem can be alternately modeled as a multi-armed bandit; see Gittins (1989).

Although many papers have been published on the methodology of adaptive sampling, there are few examples of its implementation in practice. Both logistical and ethical issues have been cited for this lack of usage; the arguments can be found in Bailar (1976), Simon (1977), Armitage (1985), Peto (1985), Royall (1991), Rosenberger & Lachin (1993) and particularly in Ware (1989) and the accompanying discussion. However, there have been a few trials where a response-adaptive design has been used, notably the ECMO trials reported by Cornell, Landenberger & Bartlett (1986) and Ware (1989) and two trials of anti-depression drugs sponsored by Eli Lilly and Co. (Tamura et al., 1994; Andersen, 1996), the latter being an interesting example of a four-armed adaptive trial.

CHAPTER 18

Bayesian Approaches

18.1 The Bayesian Paradigm

A very different framework for the design and analysis of group sequential trials arises if inference is made using the Bayesian paradigm. In this paradigm, uncertainty about θ, the parameter or parameters of interest, is expressed by considering it as a random variable with a probability distribution. At the start of the trial, this is called the *prior* distribution, with density $p_0(\theta)$, say. As data accumulate, this prior is updated to form the *posterior* distribution which summaries the current uncertainty about the value of θ. The updating is determined by Bayes Law, which states that the posterior density, $p(\theta \mid data)$ is given by the normalized product of the prior density and the likelihood $L(data \mid \theta)$, say, i.e.,

$$p(\theta \mid data) \propto L(data \mid \theta)\, p_0(\theta). \tag{18.1}$$

The constant of proportionality is such that the posterior density integrates to unity, or sums to unity if θ has a discrete distribution. At any stage, this posterior distribution can be used to draw inferences concerning θ. For instance, we may construct a *credible* set for θ with posterior probability equal to some pre-specified level $1 - 2\epsilon$. If θ is one-dimensional and $\epsilon = 0.025$, a 95% credible set, or Bayesian interval estimate, (θ_L, θ_U) satisfies (Lindley, 1965, p. 15)

$$Pr\{\theta_L < \theta < \theta_U \mid data\} = 0.95. \tag{18.2}$$

A one-sided or two-sided test for efficacy might be based on whether the interval excludes zero, or a test for equivalence could examine whether the interval lies completely within a specified range of equivalence.

To illustrate the calculations, consider the case of accumulating normal data giving rise to standardized statistics $Z_1, Z_2, \ldots$, with the canonical joint distribution (3.1). At any stage $k = 1, 2, \ldots$, the likelihood for the parameter θ is the normal density with mean θ and variance $\mathcal{I}_k^{-1}$ evaluated at $\hat{\theta}^{(k)} = Z_k/\sqrt{\mathcal{I}_k}$ (see Section 3.5.3). We shall discuss the choice of prior in detail later. For now, consider the convenient choice of a conjugate normal prior distribution $N(\mu_0, \sigma_0^2)$, where μ_0 and σ_0^2 are the specified prior mean and variance of θ. Using (18.1), the posterior distribution for θ at stage k is

$$N\left(\frac{\hat{\theta}^{(k)}\mathcal{I}_k + \mu_0\sigma_0^{-2}}{\mathcal{I}_k + \sigma_0^{-2}},\ \frac{1}{\mathcal{I}_k + \sigma_0^{-2}}\right) \tag{18.3}$$

and the 95% credible interval for θ is given by

$$\left(\frac{\hat{\theta}^{(k)}\mathcal{I}_k + \mu_0\sigma_0^{-2}}{\mathcal{I}_k + \sigma_0^{-2}} \pm 1.96 \frac{1}{\sqrt{\{\mathcal{I}_k + \sigma_0^{-2}\}}} \right). \tag{18.4}$$

Note that this interval is "shrunk" toward the prior mean μ_0 whereas the usual fixed sample frequentist confidence interval would be centered on the estimate $\hat{\theta}^{(k)}$. Often the prior mean μ_0 is taken to be zero, the value at the null hypothesis. In this case, the credible interval for θ is shrunk toward zero, a property regarded as desirable by some authors (Hughes & Pocock, 1988; Pocock & Hughes, 1989).

The limiting case as $\sigma_0 \to \infty$ gives a *reference* or *non-informative* improper uniform prior and the posterior distribution for θ reduces to $N(\hat{\theta}^{(k)}, \mathcal{I}_k^{-1})$. In this case, the credible interval (18.4) is numerically the same as a confidence interval unadjusted for multiple looks, although its interpretation is, of course, different.

Unlike the frequentist confidence intervals of Chapters 8 and 9, which condition on parameter values rather than on the observed data, the construction of a Bayes credible interval at termination or at any interim analysis does not depend on the sampling scheme used to obtain the data and the likelihood principle (e.g., Berger, 1985) is satisfied. The same comments apply to Bayesian P-values (Lindley, 1965, p. 58) of the type $Pr\{\theta < 0 \mid data\}$ evaluated under the posterior distribution. Hence, the techniques for inference both at interim analyses and upon termination are much more straightforward under the Bayesian paradigm.

18.2 Stopping Rules

Although Bayes inferences on termination are easily derived, the problems of design and, in particular, the decision of when to stop are not so straightforward. We shall consider the full Bayesian decision theoretic approach in subsequent sections. However, this methodology requires costs and utilities which are difficult to assess and an approach is often taken based only on the posterior distribution (18.1). One might, for example, stop a trial early if, at some intermediate stage k

$$(i)\ Pr\{\theta < 0 \mid data\} < \epsilon \quad \text{or} \quad (ii)\ Pr\{\theta > 0 \mid data\} < \epsilon, \tag{18.5}$$

where a typical value specified for ϵ might be 0.025. This is equivalent to stopping when a $1 - \epsilon$ credible region excludes zero. Rules similar to this have been proposed by Mehta & Cain (1984), Berry (1985) and Freedman & Spiegelhalter (1989).

The sequential design does not affect the Bayesian inference, so the credible interval (18.4) is still a correct summary in the Bayesian paradigm at the time of the kth analysis, whether or not the trial stops at this point. If, for example, condition (i) in (18.5) is satisfied, then the current posterior probability that $\theta < 0$ is less than ϵ, regardless of any stopping rule, formal or informal. This property leads to the statement by Berry (1987, p. 119) that there is "no price to pay for looking at data using a Bayesian approach". Nevertheless, the frequentist properties of Bayesian monitoring schemes can be quite surprising and, in particular, the Type I error rate is not controlled and can be grossly inflated.

Table 18.1 *False positive rates for the stopping rules* (18.5) *and* (18.6) *based on Bayesian posterior probabilities. Analyses are equally spaced.*

Number of analyses	*Type I error probability*	
K	*Non-informative prior* *	*Prior with 25% 'handicap'* †
1	0.05	0.03
2	0.08	0.04
3	0.11	0.05
4	0.13	0.05
5	0.14	0.05
10	0.19	0.06
20	0.25	0.07
50	0.32	0.09
∞	1.00	1.00

* Boundary: $|Z_k| > 1.96$ $k = 1, \ldots, K$
† Boundary given by (18.6) with $h = 0.25$ and $\alpha = 0.05$

For instance, in the normal example above, if we use the non-informative prior, letting $\sigma_0 \to \infty$ in (18.3), we see that the procedure (18.5) with $\epsilon = 0.025$ is equivalent to the repeated significance test rule which stops the first time that $|Z_k| > 1.96$. Table 18.1 shows the Type I error rate of this procedure as a function of K, the maximum number of analyses. This is also the probability, under $\theta = 0$, that the 95% credible interval on termination, $(\hat{\theta}^{(k)} \pm 1.96\,\mathcal{I}_k^{-1})$, which coincides with the unadjusted 95% frequentist confidence interval, will fail to include the true value $\theta = 0$.

Similar behavior of false positive rates for this form of procedure also occurs for other choices of prior. As an example, if a normal prior with zero mean and variance $\sigma_0^{-2} = \mathcal{I}_K/4$ is chosen, the Type I error rates are those given in the right hand column of Table 18.1. Here the analyses are assumed to be equally spaced with $\mathcal{I}_k = (k/K)\mathcal{I}_K$, $k = 1, \ldots, K$. This prior, which has been recommended by Grossman et al. (1994) and by Spiegelhalter et al. (1994, Section 8.1), corresponds to the situation in which a sample equal in size to 25% of the planned study has already been observed, prior to the study, and the mean of this sample is zero. We discuss this form of prior in Section 18.3 where it is referred to as a "handicap" prior. From Table 18.1, we see that for K around four or five, the error rate is approximately 0.05, for smaller K it is less, and for larger K it can be rather more.

A feature of Table 18.1 is that the false positive rate approaches unity as K tends to ∞. This phenomenon was termed "sampling to a foregone conclusion" by Cornfield (1966a,b), who reflected that "if one is concerned about the high probability of rejecting H_0, it must be because some probability of its truth is being entertained." Hence, for our normal example, he proposed using a mixed prior with a discrete probability mass p assigned to $\theta = 0$ and the remaining probability $1 - p$ distributed normally with mean zero and variance σ_0^2. With this prior, the posterior odds in favor of the hypothesis H_0: $\theta = 0$ are defined to be

$$\lambda = \frac{Pr\{\theta = 0 \mid data\}}{Pr\{\theta \neq 0 \mid data\}} = \frac{p}{1-p} RBO,$$

where

$$RBO = \sqrt{\{1 + \mathcal{I}_k \sigma_0^2\}} \exp\left(\frac{-Z_k^2}{2\{1 + (\mathcal{I}_k \sigma_0^2)^{-1}\}}\right)$$

is the ratio of the posterior to the prior odds for H_0, called the "relative betting odds" or RBO (Cornfield, 1969). This ratio is also known as the Bayes factor (Dickey, 1973). Suppose we use the previous rule that stops if $|Z_k| > 1.96$. Then, upon stopping with $\mathcal{I}_k$ large, the posterior odds λ are approximately equal to

$$\{p/(1-p)\} \sigma_0 \sqrt{\mathcal{I}_k} \exp(-1.96^2/2),$$

which now favor H_0 and not H_1 if $\mathcal{I}_k$ is sufficiently large. Hence, if decisions are based on the value of the RBO, large numbers of analyses do not result in almost certain rejection of H_0 and such a procedure is not subject to the threat of "sampling to a foregone conclusion". Cornfield (1966b) went on to propose a stopping rule based on parallel stopping boundaries for the RBO or, equivalently, the posterior odds λ. For such a procedure, stopping boundaries on the standardized Z_k scale diverge with sample size unlike the Pocock boundaries (Section 2.4), which are constant, or the O'Brien and Fleming boundaries (Section 2.5), which become narrower with sample size. Lachin (1981) has extended the Cornfield model to a composite null hypothesis by replacing the discrete prior mass at $\theta = 0$ under H_0 by a continuous prior supported on a small interval around zero.

Most Bayesians would be unhappy with the mixed prior approach of Cornfield, seeing the assignment of discrete mass to a single point as unrealistic; see remarks by Spiegelhalter & Freedman (1988, p. 461). It is fair to say that Cornfield's designs based on RBOs have not been adopted in recent practice and current Bayesian recommendations for monitoring (e.g., Freedman, Spiegelhalter & Parmar, 1994; Fayers, Ashby & Parmar, 1997) have been more along the lines of the rule (18.5). The principal concerns in the application of the Bayesian procedures we have described (which do not consider costs or utilities) are their frequentist properties and the choice of the prior. We shall take up the question of the prior in the next section. With regard to the Type I error rate and other frequentist properties, some proponents of the Bayesian approach cite the likelihood principle and argue that these are largely irrelevant; see, for example, Berry (1987) and Berger & Berry (1988). Other "pragmatic" Bayesians (e.g., Spiegelhalter, Freedman & Parmar, 1994) do admit a concern for controlling the false positive rate and propose use of priors that mollify the effect of Type I error inflation which Bayesian procedures might otherwise produce. Yet others, such as Pocock & Hughes (1989) "feel that control of the Type I error is a vital aid to restricting the flood of false positives in the medical literature." Regulatory agencies, such as the U.S. FDA, that oversee submissions based on pharmaceutical trials will likewise have a similar concern.

It has been noted that Bayesian inferences, being based on posterior probabilities, do not depend on monitoring or stopping rules. Hence, in the Bayesian paradigm, there is no necessity to set a maximum sample size. However, it is useful to have a target sample size and this can be based on "pre-posterior" analyses using predictive distributions (Spiegelhalter & Freedman, 1986). Suppose upon termination, we shall base a decision on the credible interval (18.2) and denote this (θ_L, θ_U). If $\theta > 0$ corresponds to a situation where we would wish to decide that a new treatment is preferable, our decision rule is to recommend the new treatment if $\theta_L > 0$, recommend against the new treatment if $\theta_U < 0$, and be "non-committal" if $\theta_L \leq 0 \leq \theta_U$. For a given sample size, the conditional probability of concluding with a recommendation for the new treatment given that it is preferable, i.e., $\theta > 0$, can be computed as

$$\frac{\int_0^\infty Pr\{\theta_L > 0 \mid \theta\}\, p_0(\theta)\, d\theta}{\int_0^\infty p_0(\theta)\, d\theta}.$$

A similar expression can be computed for the conditional probability of finding $\theta_U < 0$ and rejecting the new treatment given that it is inferior, i.e., $\theta < 0$. A target sample size can then be determined by ensuring that both of these probabilities exceed some prescribed level, such as 90%. Alternatively, the target sample size can be based on the predictive probability of a conclusive trial, i.e.,

$$1 - Pr\{\theta_L \leq 0 \leq \theta_U\} = 1 - \int_{-\infty}^{\infty} Pr\{\theta_L < 0 < \theta_U \mid \theta\}\, p_0(\theta)\, d\theta.$$

For further references in this area, see Spiegelhalter & Freedman (1986), Brown, Herson, Atkinson & Rozell (1987), and Moussa (1989).

18.3 Choice of Prior Distribution

A key to the Bayesian approach is that prior beliefs and external evidence can be summarized mathematically and are expressed in the form of a prior distribution for the unknown parameters. The issues concerning the choice of prior distribution are well reviewed in Spiegelhalter et al. (1994) and in the accompanying published discussion. This choice is especially important in the context of group sequential monitoring because data dependent stopping can greatly increase the sensitivity of Bayesian credible intervals to misspecification of the prior; see Rosenbaum & Rubin (1984). Ideally there would be a "single defendable prior" (Herson, 1994) but, almost by definition, a prior is subjective and there will be no single objective choice upon which all can agree. One avenue is simply to report the likelihood function, which each consumer combines with his or her individual personal prior in order to make inferences and decisions. However, this is usually impractical. Instead, a recommended strategy is to base decisions on a collection of analyses that result from a collection or "community" of priors. Kass & Greenhouse (1989, p. 312) point out that a purpose of a clinical trial is "to bring differing opinions to consensus" and simultaneous consideration of a variety of priors can assist in this aim. Fayers, Ashby & Parmar (1997) state that the prior distributions "should reflect the level of scepticism that is expressed by those clinicians one seeks to influence." We now list the types of prior that may be considered:

Clinical priors are supposed to reflect expert opinion. Priors are elicited via questionnaire (e.g., Freedman & Spiegelhalter, 1983; Chaloner et al., 1993) from clinicians knowledgeable in the field and averaged. An example of this process appears in the description of the CHART trial by Parmar et al. (1994). A problem with the approach is the representativeness of the chosen experts — who, by their involvement in the trial, may be too optimistic about a new proposed therapy (see, for example, Gilbert, McPeek & Mosteller 1977). Alternatively, clinical priors can be based on meta-analyses or overviews of historical information but, due to publication bias, these too may be overly optimistic.

Sceptical priors should represent one extreme in the range of opinion. As a working method of construction, Spiegelhalter et al. (1994) suggest a symmetric prior centered at zero with only a small probability, 5% for example, that the benefit, θ, exceeds a specified alternative hypothesis value $\theta_1 > 0$.

Enthusiastic priors act as a counterbalance to the sceptical prior. Operationally, an enthusiastic prior might be constructed by centering the distribution at the alternative θ_1, with only a small probability that $\theta < 0$. The presence of sceptical and enthusiastic priors in a collection has the effect of lessening the pressure to stop a trial prematurely in the face of early positive or negative results, respectively.

Reference or *Non-informative priors* attempt to be objective in that they endeavor to represent a lack of any prior opinion. In the normal data example we have been using, this would correspond to an improper uniform prior, the limit as $\sigma_0 \to 0$. This choice implies that the prior probability of θ lying in an interval around zero is the same as that for an equally wide interval centered at, say, 10^{10}, which might be regarded as very informative! Also the choice of the non-informative prior can depend on the parameterization, so what is supposed to be non-informative for θ can be quite informative for a function $g(\theta)$. For further discussion, see Jennison & Turnbull (1990, Section 3).

"Handicap" or "pragmatic Bayes" priors were proposed by Grossman et al. (1994) and Spiegelhalter et al. (1994) as a way to control frequentist properties of a Bayesian monitoring procedure. The prior is chosen so that the false positive rate is controlled at a given level α, e.g., 0.05, if there is to be a fixed maximum number, K, of planned analyses. Grossman et al. (1994) term this a "unified" method. In our normal data example, the unified method calls for a normal prior centered at zero with variance $\sigma_0^2 = (h\mathcal{I}_f)^{-1}$, where $\mathcal{I}_f$ is the information needed for a fixed sample, frequentist test with Type I error probability α and power $1-\beta$. The constant h is termed the *handicap*. Consider the Bayesian procedure that stops when the $1-\alpha$ credible region (given by (18.4) when $\alpha = 0.05$) first excludes zero, but with a maximum of K analyses. The handicap h is computed so that this procedure, if rigidly followed, has Type I error rate equal to α. Suppose the analyses are equally spaced with $\mathcal{I}_k = (k/K)\mathcal{I}_f$, $k = 1, \ldots, K$. Then, in terms of the standardized statistics, we have a two-sided test which stops to reject $H_0\colon \theta = 0$ at analysis k if

$$|Z_k| > \Phi^{-1}(1-\alpha/2)\sqrt{\{(k+hK)/k\}}, \quad k = 1, \ldots, K. \tag{18.6}$$

For $K = 1$, no handicap is needed, $h = 0$ and the prior is the improper, non-informative, uniform distribution arising as $\sigma_0 \to \infty$. Grossman et al. (1994) tabulate the values of h needed to achieve Type I error probability $\alpha = 0.05$ and 0.01 with $K = 2, \ldots, 10$ analyses. In the case of $\alpha = 0.05$, the handicap is $h = 0.16, 0.22, 0.25. 0.27$, and 0.33 for $K = 2, 3, 4, 5$, and 10, respectively. In the frequentist setting, the procedure can be viewed as simply an alternative to other two-sided tests such as those described in Chapter 2. However in the Bayesian paradigm, choosing a prior based on frequentist properties is somewhat paradoxical, and the procedure no longer possesses the property that inferences are independent of the sampling scheme; the dependence of the prior on the stopping rule and on K means that the likelihood principle is no longer obeyed.

Other similar ideas for priors have been described in the literature, such as the "cautious reasonable sceptical" prior of Kass & Greenhouse (1989) and the "open-minded" prior of George et al. (1994).

18.4 Discussion

The reporting of inferences arising from a collection of different priors can be cumbersome. However, at interim and terminal analyses, Fayers, Ashby & Parmar (1997, Table I) recommend presenting the posterior probability that θ exceeds a target value, θ_T say, in a two way table cross-classified by choice of prior, e.g., non-informative, sceptical, enthusiastic, and by target value, e.g., $\theta_T = 0$, $\theta_1/2$, or θ_1. These probabilities can then be used to guide the decisions of a data monitoring committee and communicated in scientific publications. However, the message can be problematic if the posterior probabilities disagree widely depending on the choice of prior.

A robust Bayesian methodology has been developed by Greenhouse & Wasserman (1995). Instead of proposing a single prior or several different priors, they propose using a class of priors indexed by a parameter γ, where $0 \leq \gamma \leq 1$. One such class is the family $\Gamma_\gamma = \{(1-\gamma)p_0(\theta) + \gamma Q;\ Q \in \mathcal{Q}\}$ where $\mathcal{Q}$ is the set of all priors and $p_0(\theta)$ is, say, the clinical prior. Bounds on posterior quantities of interest such as $Pr\{\theta > \theta_T \mid data\}$ for $\theta_T = 0$, $\theta_1/2$ or θ_1 over the family Γ_γ can then be plotted against γ as it varies from 0 to 1. Narrow bounds will indicate a robustness to the choice of prior.

A "backward" Bayes approach has been proposed by Carlin & Sargent (1996). They attempt to characterize the class of priors that lead to a given decision, such as stopping the trial and rejecting the null hypothesis, conditional on the observed data. This information can be helpful in the deliberations of a data monitoring committee, especially if the data and prior are in apparent conflict.

We referred earlier to the "unified" approach of Grossman et al. (1994) who considered frequentist properties, such as Type I error rates, of Bayesian procedures. Another way to reconcile Bayesian and frequentist procedures is to derive both as solutions to formal Bayes sequential decision problems with a prior distribution for the unknown parameter and costs for sampling and for an incorrect terminal decision. Anscombe (1963), Chernoff & Petkau (1981) and

Berry & Ho (1988) have used dynamic programming to solve Bayes sequential decision problems, although the difficulties of eliciting the required costs have been a deterrent to applying these methods in practice. Solving a Bayes decision problem is also a very useful route for finding frequentist group sequential test with certain optimality properties: by analyzing the risk function, it is evident that a Bayes optimal procedure minimizes the expected sampling cost subject to its attained error probabilities and this is precisely the type of property sought in an optimal frequentist test. Eales & Jennison (1992, 1995) construct optimal one-sided and two-sided tests, respectively, that minimize expected sample size under certain parameter values, subject to a fixed number of groups, a fixed maximum sample size and given error probabilities α and β. They use Bayes decision theory and dynamic programming to compute the optimal procedure without constraints on the error rates and search for a set of costs for which the optimal procedure also solves the constrained problem; we have already presented some of these results in Section 4.2.2. This method of optimization can be used in a reverse fashion to discover what priors and costs are implicit in a particular group sequential boundary. As stated in Eales & Jennison (1992, p. 16), "The fact that optimal frequentist tests are also optimal for a Bayes decision problem is a consequence of the complete class theorems of Brown, Cohen & Strawderman (1980); it also demonstrates an important underlying link between good Bayes and good frequentist methods."

The published discussion following the paper of Spiegelhalter et al. (1994) contains a good summary on the debate over the merits and faults of the Bayesian approach in the specific context of the design and analysis of clinical trials. An earlier commentary appears in Jennison & Turnbull (1990, Section 3). Although the subject is still under debate, it would seem that frequentist properties such as false positive rates *are* of great importance and that determination of sample sizes will continue to be based on frequentist ideas of requirements of Type I error probability and power at realistic alternatives. Bayesian posterior probabilities based on a family of priors may be cumbersome and perhaps confusing to a consumer reading reports of them in scientific publications. However, they can be very useful to diverse members of a data monitoring committee as an aid to making a stopping decision. A good example of this is described by Carlin et al. (1993) in the setting of a clinical trial for toxoplasmic encephalitis prophylaxis in AIDS patients. Robert (1994, Chapter 10) discusses the rationale of Bayesian methods in general and makes a strong case for their use, citing advantages in the representation of uncertainty, coherence of inference, and the ability of Bayesian methods "to borrow strength from previous studies through a prior distribution".

CHAPTER 19

Numerical Computations for Group Sequential Tests

19.1 Introduction

Numerical calculations for sequential tests with a discrete response date back to the two-stage acceptance sampling plans of Dodge and Romig (1929) and the multi-stage plans introduced by the Columbia University Research Group (Freeman et al., 1948) which developed into the United States military standard, MIL-STD-105E (1989). Computations for binary data were discussed in detail in Chapter 12. The computational task is greater in the analogous calculations for a continuous response where multiple integrals replace multiple sums. Armitage & Schneiderman (1958), Schneiderman (1961), Dunnett (1961) and Roseberry & Gehan (1964) computed properties of two-stage and three-stage procedures for normal observations with known variance and Armitage, McPherson & Rowe (1969) tackled sequential tests in earnest, obtaining accurate results for repeated significance tests with up to 200 analyses. Group sequential designs were proposed in the context of drug-screening trials with a dichotomous outcome by Schultz et al. (1973) and for clinical trials with continuous response variables by McPherson (1974) and Pocock (1977). Although the practical difference between sequential and group sequential analysis is substantial, computations for McPherson and Pocock's tests are essentially the same as for Armitage's (1975) repeated significance test with continuous monitoring and a small maximum sample size.

Research in the last two decades has produced a variety of group sequential testing boundaries, including error spending procedures to handle unpredictable group sizes, and methods for making frequentist inferences in the form of P-values and confidence intervals on termination of a group sequential test. In some instances, analytic approximations to the error probabilities and expected sample sizes of group sequential tests are available but, in general, direct numerical computation is needed to obtain accurate answers across the range of current methods.

Some details of numerical methods which can be used to compute properties of group sequential tests are available in the early papers of Armitage et al. (1969) and McPherson & Armitage (1971). In this chapter, we elaborate on these methods in the case of normally distributed observations with known variance. We shall work with the standardized statistics $Z_1, \dots, Z_K$, assuming these have the canonical joint distribution (3.1) given an information sequence $\mathcal{I}_1, \dots, \mathcal{I}_K$. Jennison (1994) has presented a description of group sequential computations in terms of the sample sums, or the score statistics $Z_k\sqrt{\mathcal{I}_k}$ in our terminology; we use similar notation in this chapter but for densities and conditional densities of different variables so care is required if these two treatments are to be studied together.

In Section 19.2 we describe how to compute the probability that a group sequential test crosses a given boundary at a certain analysis k. We apply this basic calculation in Section 19.3 to find properties of a specified test, and explain how to construct testing boundaries and choose sample sizes to attain particular Type I and II error probabilities. The implementation of error spending tests is dealt with in Section 19.4, where we also discuss how to find the target maximum information level needed to attain specified Type I error and power. In Section 19.5 we describe computations of the frequentist data summaries on termination of a group sequential tests presented in Chapter 8. We conclude with a brief discussion of extensions to the case of normal data with unknown variance and other response distributions, the design of group sequential tests with various optimality properties, and computer software currently available for designing and implementing group sequential trials.

19.2 The Basic Calculation

Suppose a group sequential test with a maximum of K analyses is defined in terms of standardized statistics $Z_1, \ldots, Z_K$ following the canonical joint distribution (3.1) for a given sequence of information levels $\mathcal{I}_1, \ldots, \mathcal{I}_K$. Let $\Delta_k = \mathcal{I}_k - \mathcal{I}_{k-1}$ for $k = 2, \ldots, K$. Then, $Z_1 \sim N(\theta\sqrt{\mathcal{I}_1}, 1)$ and for each $k = 2, \ldots, K$,

$$Z_k\sqrt{\mathcal{I}_k} - Z_{k-1}\sqrt{\mathcal{I}_{k-1}} \sim N(\theta\Delta_k, \Delta_k) \tag{19.1}$$

independently of $Z_1, \ldots, Z_{k-1}$.

We shall consider tests with continuation regions of the form (a_k, b_k), $k = 1, \ldots, K$. Most commonly used one-sided and two-sided hypothesis tests are of this form. The two-sided tests which permit early stopping to accept the null hypothesis discussed in Chapter 5 have continuation regions composed of two disjoint intervals and modified versions of the methods we shall describe can be applied to those tests.

A fundamental quantity to compute for a group sequential test is the probability of exiting by a specific boundary at a particular analysis. For each $k = 1, \ldots, K$, define

$$\psi_k(a_1, b_1, \ldots, a_k, b_k; \theta) = Pr_\theta\{a_1 < Z_1 < b_1, \ldots, a_{k-1} < Z_{k-1} < b_{k-1}, Z_k > b_k\} \tag{19.2}$$

and

$$\xi_k(a_1, b_1, \ldots, a_k, b_k; \theta) = Pr_\theta\{a_1 < Z_1 < b_1, \ldots, a_{k-1} < Z_{k-1} < b_{k-1}, Z_k < a_k\}. \tag{19.3}$$

These quantities will appear later in formulae for a test's error probabilities and expected sample size (more precisely, the expected information level on termination). They will also be used in constructing error spending boundaries and in computing P-values and confidence intervals on termination.

To evaluate (19.2) and (19.3), note that Z_1 has density

$$f_1(z_1; \theta) = \phi(z_1 - \theta\sqrt{\mathcal{I}_1}),$$

where $\phi(x) = \exp(-x^2/2)/\sqrt{(2\pi)}$ is the density at x of a standard normal variate. It follows from (19.1) that, for $k = 2, \ldots, K$, the conditional density of Z_k given $Z_1 = z_1, \ldots, Z_{k-1} = z_{k-1}$ depends only on z_{k-1} and is equal to

$$f_k(z_{k-1}, z_k; \theta) = \frac{\sqrt{\mathcal{I}_k}}{\sqrt{\Delta_k}}\,\phi\left(\frac{z_k\sqrt{\mathcal{I}_k} - z_{k-1}\sqrt{\mathcal{I}_{k-1}} - \theta\Delta_k}{\sqrt{\Delta_k}}\right). \tag{19.4}$$

Hence, for each $k = 2, \ldots, K$,

$$\begin{aligned} &\psi_k(a_1, b_1, \ldots, a_k, b_k; \theta) \\ &\quad = \int_{a_1}^{b_1} \cdots \int_{a_{k-1}}^{b_{k-1}} \int_{b_k}^{\infty} f_1(z_1; \theta) f_2(z_1, z_2; \theta) \ldots f_k(z_{k-1}, z_k; \theta)\, dz_k \ldots dz_1 \\ &\quad = \int_{a_1}^{b_1} \cdots \int_{a_{k-1}}^{b_{k-1}} f_1(z_1; \theta) f_2(z_1, z_2; \theta) \ldots f_{k-1}(z_{k-2}, z_{k-1}; \theta) \\ &\qquad\qquad \times e_{k-1}(z_{k-1}, b_k; \theta)\, dz_{k-1} \ldots dz_1 \end{aligned} \tag{19.5}$$

where

$$e_{k-1}(z_{k-1}, b_k; \theta) = \Phi\left(\frac{z_{k-1}\sqrt{\mathcal{I}_{k-1}} + \theta\Delta_k - b_k\sqrt{\mathcal{I}_k}}{\sqrt{\Delta_k}}\right). \tag{19.6}$$

Similarly, $\xi_k(a_1, b_1, \ldots, a_k, b_k; \theta)$ can be written as a $(k-1)$-fold multiple integral.

In Chapter 8 we defined functions $g_k(z_k; \theta)$, $k = 1, \ldots, K$, representing the sub-densities of $Z_1, \ldots, Z_K$, their integrals being less than unity for $k > 1$ due to early stopping at stages $1, \ldots, k-1$. Formally,

$$g_1(z_1; \theta) = f_1(z_1; \theta)$$

and, for a test with interval continuation regions,

$$g_k(z_k; \theta) = \int_{a_{k-1}}^{b_{k-1}} g_{k-1}(z_{k-1}; \theta)\, f_k(z_{k-1}, z_k; \theta)\, dz_{k-1}, \quad k = 2, \ldots, K.$$

Then, for example, we can write

$$\begin{aligned} \psi_k(a_1, b_1, \ldots, a_k, b_k; \theta) &= \int_{b_k}^{\infty} g_k(z_k; \theta)\, dz_k \\ &= \int_{a_{k-1}}^{b_{k-1}} \int_{b_k}^{\infty} g_{k-1}(z_{k-1}; \theta)\, f_k(z_{k-1}, z_k; \theta)\, dz_k\, dz_{k-1} \\ &= \int_{a_{k-1}}^{b_{k-1}} g_{k-1}(z_{k-1}; \theta)\, e_{k-1}(z_{k-1}, b_k; \theta)\, dz_{k-1}. \end{aligned}$$

In evaluating integrals numerically, we use a quadrature rule to replace each integral by a weighted sum. Thus, we approximate the integral of a function $q(z)$ from u to l as

$$\int_u^l q(z)dz \approx \sum_{i=1}^{m} w(i)\, q(z(i)),$$

where the the number of points at which q is evaluated and their locations $z(i)$ and weights $w(i)$, $i = 1, \ldots, m$, are chosen to ensure a sufficiently accurate approximation. We shall discuss the choice of grid points and weights later. First, we explain how the multiple summations in formulae such as (19.5) can be carried out efficiently. The integral on the right hand side of (19.5) is approximated by a $(k-1)$-fold sum to give

$$\psi_k(a_1, b_1, \ldots, a_k, b_k; \theta) \approx$$

$$\sum_{i_1=1}^{m_1} \cdots \sum_{i_{k-1}=1}^{m_{k-1}} w_1(i_1)\, f_1(z_1(i_1); \theta)\, w_2(i_2)\, f_2(z_1(i_1), z_2(i_2); \theta)$$

$$\ldots w_{k-1}(i_{k-1})\, f_{k-1}(z_{k-2}(i_{k-2}), z_{k-1}(i_{k-1}); \theta)$$

$$\times\, e_{k-1}(z_{k-1}(i_{k-1}), b_k; \theta). \tag{19.7}$$

For given $\{z_1(1), \ldots, z_1(m_1)\}, \ldots, \{z_K(1), \ldots, z_K(m_K)\}$, we define functions $h_1, \ldots, h_K$ by

$$h_1(i_1; \theta) = w_1(i_1)\, f_1(z_1(i_1); \theta), \quad i_1 = 1, \ldots, m_1,$$

and

$$h_k(i_k; \theta) = \sum_{i_{k-1}=1}^{m_{k-1}} h_{k-1}(i_{k-1}; \theta)\, w_k(i_k)\, f_k(z_{k-1}(i_{k-1}), z_k(i_k); \theta),$$

for each $i_k = 1, \ldots, m_k$ and $k = 2, \ldots, K$. Summing over i_1 for each i_2, the right hand side of (19.7) reduces to

$$\sum_{i_2=1}^{m_2} \cdots \sum_{i_{k-1}=1}^{m_{k-1}} h_2(i_2; \theta)\, w_3(i_3) f_3(z_2(i_2), z_3(i_3); \theta) \ldots$$

$$w_{k-1}(i_{k-1})\, f_{k-1}(z_{k-2}(i_{k-2}), z_{k-1}(i_{k-1}); \theta)\, e_{k-1}(z_{k-1}(i_{k-1}), b_k; \theta)$$

and further summations over $i_2, \ldots, i_{k-2}$ in turn yield

$$\psi_k(a_1, b_1, \ldots, a_k, b_k; \theta) \approx$$

$$\sum_{i_{k-1}=1}^{m_{k-1}} h_{k-1}(i_{k-1}; \theta)\, e_{k-1}(z_{k-1}(i_{k-1}), b_k; \theta). \tag{19.8}$$

The functions $h_1, \ldots, h_{K-1}$ can be evaluated in sequence and then used in formulae such as (19.8) to compute quantities of interest.

The progression from (19.7) to (19.8) parallels the iterative definition of the sub-densities $g_k(z_k; \theta)$ and it follows that the values $h_k(i_k; \theta)$, $i_k = 1, \ldots, m_k$, can be used to integrate the product of $g_k(z_k; \theta)$ and a function of z_k. For $1 \le k \le K$ and a general function $q(z_k)$,

$$\int_{a_1}^{b_1} \dots \int_{a_k}^{b_k} f_1(z_1;\theta)\, f_2(z_1, z_2;\theta) \dots f_k(z_{k-1}, z_k;\theta)\, q(z_k)\, dz_k \dots dz_1$$

$$= \int_{a_k}^{b_k} g_k(z_k;\theta)\, q(z_k)\, dz_k \approx \sum_{i_k=1}^{m_k} h_k(i_k;\theta)\, q(z_k(i_k)). \qquad (19.9)$$

The number of operations needed to compute functions $h_2, \dots, h_K$ is of order $m_1 m_2 + \dots + m_{K-1} m_K$; a lower order of operations is required to evaluate h_1 and any one-dimensional sum such as (19.8). By exploiting the special structure of the integrands in formulae such as (19.5), we have kept the total computational effort *linear* in K, whereas it would rise exponentially with K for general K-fold integrands.

We now consider the choice of grid points and their associated weights for each of the nested numerical integrations. In an expression such as (19.5), for each $j = 1, \dots, k-1$ the integral with respect to z_j has a positive integrand bounded above by the marginal density of Z_j in the absence of early stopping, which is normal with mean $\theta\sqrt{\mathcal{I}_j}$ and unit variance. This can be seen by noting that the integrand is increased if all other ranges of integration are extended to the whole real line and, in this case, since variables other than z_j are integrated over their full range, the result is the marginal density of Z_j. It is therefore reasonable to apply a numerical integration rule over z_j which is efficient for integrating the $N(\theta\sqrt{\mathcal{I}_j}, 1)$ density. The implementation of Simpson's rule described below provides $O(m^{-4})$ convergence as m, the number of grid points used in integrating this density over the whole real line or a subset of it, increases (see Chandler & Graham, 1988). This convergence rate also holds if the normal density is multiplied by a smooth bounded function, as is the case in expressions such as (19.5), and we have observed this rate of convergence empirically in calculations using increasing numbers of grid points.

We start by defining grid points and weights to integrate a function of z_j over the whole real line. Since the tails of the normal distribution decrease rapidly, it is appropriate to concentrate grid points in the center and allocate a smaller proportion, more widely spaced, to the tails. We have found it most effective to place two thirds of the grid points within three standard deviations of the normal mean and the remaining third in the tails. We create a set of $6r-1$ values, $x_1, \dots, x_{6r-1}$, defining elements on which to apply Simpson's rule, as follows:

$$x_i = \begin{cases} \theta\sqrt{\mathcal{I}_j} + \{-3 - 4\log(r/i)\}, & i = 1, \dots, r-1, \\ \theta\sqrt{\mathcal{I}_j} + \{-3 + 3(i-r)/2r\}, & i = r, \dots, 5r, \\ \theta\sqrt{\mathcal{I}_j} + \{3 + 4\log(r/(6r-i))\}, & i = 5r+1, \dots, 6r-1. \end{cases}$$

Here, the logarithmic spacing between the outer values and the expansion of the interval (x_1, x_{6r-1}) with r is required for $O(m^{-4})$ accuracy as the total number of grid points, m, increases. Other values may be used for the width of the middle interval, the factor multiplying $\log(r/i)$ and $\log(r/(6r-i))$ and the distribution of points between the middle interval and the tails, but we have found the above scheme to work as well as any.

In integrating the function $q(z_j)$ from $-\infty$ to ∞, we use $m_j = 12r - 3$ grid points. Odd numbered grid points are the x_i defined above, so $z_j(i_j) = x_{(i_j+1)/2}$ for $i_j = 1, 3, \ldots, m_j$, and we define the even numbered grid points as the midpoints of their neighbors,

$$z_j(i_j) = (z_j(i_j - 1) + z_j(i_j + 1))/2, \quad i_j = 2, 4, \ldots, m_j - 1.$$

We approximate the integral of $q(z_j)$ between the two odd numbered grid points $z_j(2i - 1)$ and $z_j(2i + 1)$ according to Simpson's rule as

$$\frac{d}{6}\, q(z_j(2i-1)) + \frac{4d}{6}\, q(z_j(2i)) + \frac{d}{6}\, (z_j(2i+1)),$$

where d is the interval length, $z_j(2i+1) - z_j(2i-1)$. Hence, the weights required for integrating over the whole real line are

$$w_j(i_j) = \begin{cases} \frac{1}{6}\,(z_j(3) - z_j(1)), & i_j = 1, \\ \frac{1}{6}\,(z_j(i_j+2) - z_j(i_j-2)), & i_j = 3, 5, \ldots, m_j - 2, \\ \frac{4}{6}\,(z_j(i_j+1) - z_j(i_j-1)), & i_j = 2, 4, \ldots, m_j - 1, \\ \frac{1}{6}\,(z_j(m_j) - z_j(m_j-2)), & i_j = m_j, \end{cases} \tag{19.10}$$

and using these gives the approximation

$$\int_{-\infty}^{\infty} q(z_j)\, dz_j \approx \sum_{i_j=1}^{m_j} w_j(i_j)\, q(z_j(i_j)).$$

The rapid decay of the tails of the normal density ensures that the absence of any contribution from values of z_j outside the range $(z_j(1), z_j(m_j))$ does not cause a significant lack of accuracy.

In order to integrate over a finite range (a_j, b_j) we take the same values $x_1, \ldots, x_{6r-1}$ defined above and trim off those outside (a_j, b_j), introducing new points at a_j and b_j if necessary. If $a_j < x_1$, we need make no adjustment at the left hand end; otherwise, we replace the largest x_i less than a_j by a_j and discard points x_i below this. Similarly, if $b_j > x_{6r-1}$, we do nothing at the right hand end, but otherwise we replace the smallest x_i greater than b_j by b_j and discard points x_i above this. The resulting values comprise our odd numbered grid points, $\{z_j(i_j);\, i_j = 1, 3, \ldots, m_j\}$, say, where $m_j \leq 12r-3$. We calculate even numbered grid points as the midpoints of their neighbors, as before, and weights for all points are again given by (19.10). The approximation to the integral is then

$$\int_{a_j}^{b_j} q(z_j)\, dz_j \approx \sum_{i_j=1}^{m_j} w_j(i_j)\, q(z_j(i_j)).$$

Using $r = 16$ in the above quadrature rule, giving a maximum of just less than 200 grid points per integral, we have found computed probabilities to be within 10^{-6} of their true values and about one decimal place of accuracy is lost in halving the value of r. Accuracy may be reduced if some increments in information are very small and we recommend using a higher value of r if $(\mathcal{I}_j - \mathcal{I}_{j-1})/\mathcal{I}_j$ is less than 0.01 for any j. Nevertheless, we have found the above method to provide accurate results over a wide range of group sequential tests with as many as 200 analyses.

19.3 Error Probabilities and Sample Size Distributions

19.3.1 Properties of a Given Test

The values of $\psi_k(a_1, b_1, \ldots, a_k, b_k; \theta)$ and $\xi_k(a_1, b_1, \ldots, a_k, b_k; \theta)$ for $k = 1, \ldots, K$ determine the distribution of the stopping time and associated decision for a group sequential test. Hence, we can obtain from them the test's error probabilities and expected information on termination for any θ.

Suppose, for example, a two-sided test of H_0: $\theta = 0$ has K analyses at information levels $\mathcal{I}_1, \ldots, \mathcal{I}_K$ with continuation regions $(a_1, b_1), \ldots, (a_K, b_K)$ for $Z_1, \ldots, Z_K$. Then, the test's Type I error probability is

$$Pr_{\theta=0}\{\text{Reject } H_0\} =$$

$$\sum_{k=1}^{K} \{\psi_k(a_1, b_1, \ldots, a_k, b_k; 0) + \xi_k(a_1, b_1, \ldots, a_k, b_k; 0)\}. \qquad (19.11)$$

If $\delta > 0$ is large enough that we can ignore the probability of crossing the lower boundary, the test's power when $\theta = \delta$ is

$$\sum_{k=1}^{K} \psi_k(a_1, b_1, \ldots, a_k, b_k; \delta) \qquad (19.12)$$

and power when $\theta = -\delta$ has the same form but with ξ_k rather than ψ_k and $-\delta$ in place of δ. The expected information on termination under a given value of θ, a quantity closely related to the test's expected sample size, is

$$\sum_{k=1}^{K-1} \{\psi_k(a_1, b_1, \ldots, a_k, b_k; \theta) + \xi_k(a_1, b_1, \ldots, a_k, b_k; \theta)\} \, \mathcal{I}_k +$$

$$[1 - \sum_{k=1}^{K-1} \{\psi_k(a_1, b_1, \ldots, a_k, b_k; \theta) + \xi_k(a_1, b_1, \ldots, a_k, b_k; \theta)\}] \, \mathcal{I}_K.$$

For a one-sided test of H_0: $\theta = 0$ against $\theta > 0$ with information levels $\mathcal{I}_1, \ldots, \mathcal{I}_K$ and continuation regions $(a_1, b_1), \ldots, (a_K, b_K)$, the Type I error probability and power at $\theta = \delta$ are

$$\sum_{k=1}^{K} \psi_k(a_1, b_1, \ldots, a_k, b_k; 0) \quad \text{and} \quad \sum_{k=1}^{K} \psi_k(a_1, b_1, \ldots, a_k, b_k; \delta)$$

respectively. The expected information on termination is given by the same expression as for the two-sided test.

If a test is to be evaluated under a number of values of θ, one may take advantage of the property

$$g_k(z_k; \theta_2) = g_k(z_k; \theta_1) \, l(z_k, \mathcal{I}_k; \theta_2, \theta_1) \qquad (19.13)$$

where

$$l(z_k, \mathcal{I}_k; \theta_2, \theta_1) = \exp\{(\theta_2 - \theta_1) z_k \sqrt{\mathcal{I}_k} - (\theta_2^2 - \theta_1^2)\mathcal{I}_k/2\}$$

is the likelihood ratio for the observation $Z_k = z_k$ under parameter values θ_2 and θ_1. This result is closely related to (8.3) and can be derived in a similar way from the recursive formulae for the functions $g_1, \ldots, g_K$. Using this with (19.9) we obtain

$$\int_{a_k}^{b_k} g_k(z_k;\theta_2) q(z_k)\, dz_k \approx \sum_{i_k=1}^{m_k} h_k(i_k;\theta_1)\, l(z_k(i_k), \mathcal{I}_k; \theta_2, \theta_1)\, q(z_k(i_k))$$

for a general function $q(z_k)$.

As an example, we can write probabilities of crossing the upper boundary under $\theta = \theta_2$ for each $k = 2, \ldots, K$ as

$$\psi_k(a_1, b_1, \ldots, a_k, b_k; \theta_2) \approx \sum_{i_{k-1}=1}^{m_{k-1}} h_{k-1}(i_{k-1};\theta_1) \times$$
$$l(z_{k-1}(i_{k-1}), \mathcal{I}_{k-1}; \theta_2, \theta_1)\, e_{k-1}(z_{k-1}(i_{k-1}), b_k; \theta_2)$$

as an alternative to (19.8). This allows us to calculate the functions $h_1, \ldots, h_{k-1}$ under one particular value $\theta = \theta_1$ and then use these to find probabilities $\psi_k(a_1, b_1, \ldots, a_k, b_k; \theta)$ under other values of θ at little additional cost. In doing this, for each $j = 1, \ldots, k-1$, a common set of grid points $z_j(i_j)$ is used for calculations under different values of θ. The results obtained are precisely those that would have been produced by direct application of Simpson's rule on these grid points to the integral representation of $\psi_k(a_1, b_1, \ldots, a_k, b_k; \theta)$ given in (19.5). Our remarks on numerical accuracy in Section 19.2 were based on the assumption that grid points are chosen for the particular value of θ being investigated. Since some loss of numerical accuracy is to be expected using similar numbers of grid points placed elsewhere over the ranges of $z_1, \ldots, z_{k-1}$, care should be taken to ensure there are adequate numbers of grid points in the appropriate regions for all θ values addressed in a common calculation.

19.3.2 Designing a Test with Specified Error Probabilities

The calculations described in Section 19.3.1 can be used to derive group sequential tests with specific properties. As an example, consider the Wang & Tsiatis family of two-sided tests of $H_0: \theta = 0$ introduced in Section 2.7.1, which contains Pocock and O'Brien & Fleming tests as special cases. The test with parameter Δ has boundaries for Z_k of the form

$$a_k = -c\,(k/K)^{\Delta - 1/2} \quad \text{and} \quad b_k = c\,(k/K)^{\Delta - 1/2}, \quad k = 1, \ldots, K,$$

and the constants $C_{WT}(K, \alpha, \Delta)$ tabulated in Section2.7.1 are the values of c for which the test with parameter Δ and K equally spaced analyses has two-sided Type I error probability α. Consideration of sample paths of $Z_1, \ldots, Z_K$ shows that the Type I error probability decreases as c increases. Hence a simple numerical search, using formula (19.11) to evaluate the Type I error rate for any given value of c, may be used to find $C_{WT}(K, \alpha, \Delta)$ for specified K, α and Δ.

In Chapter 2, we also tabulated constants R_P, R_B and R_{WT} for use in designing a test with the correct sample size to achieve power $1 - \beta$ at $\theta = \pm\delta$. Once again, these constants can be found by a numerical search, this time over the maximum information level. Suppose, in the Wang & Tsiatis family, K, α and Δ are specified and $C_{WT}(K, \alpha, \Delta)$ has been found. We need to find the value $\mathcal{I}_{max}$ such that (19.12) takes the value $1 - \beta$ when $\mathcal{I}_k = (k/K)\mathcal{I}_{max}$, $k = 1, \ldots, K$. The value of $\mathcal{I}_{max}$ affects the distribution of $\{Z_1, \ldots, Z_K\}$, and hence the power, through the means of the Z_ks and it can be shown that (19.12) increases with $\mathcal{I}_{max}$. Thus, it is straightforward to find the $\mathcal{I}_{max}$ required for given K, α, β and Δ. Taking the ratio of this $\mathcal{I}_{max}$ to the information level (3.6) required in a fixed sample test gives $R_{WT}(K, \alpha, \beta, \Delta)$.

The above derivation of two-sided tests is simplified by the separate treatment of Type I error and power. However, the task of finding constants $\tilde{C}_1(K, \alpha, \beta, \Delta)$, $\tilde{C}_2(K, \alpha, \beta, \Delta)$ and $\tilde{R}(K, \alpha, \beta, \Delta)$ for one-sided tests in the power family of Chapter 4 does not reduce to two separate problems. Instead, a pair of constants $\tilde{C}_1$ and $\tilde{C}_2$ must be found by a two-dimensional search. As explained in Section 19.3.1, there is no difficulty in computing the Type I error rate and power of the test defined by a particular pair of constants. The required values of $\tilde{C}_1$ and $\tilde{C}_2$ may therefore be obtained using a standard numerical routine to minimize the sum of squared differences between a test's Type I error and the target value α and between its power and the target β, the solution being found when this sum of squares is sufficiently close to zero. The constant $\tilde{R}$ is determined by $\tilde{C}_1$ and $\tilde{C}_2$ according to the formula stated in Section 4.2.1.

19.4 Tests Defined by Error Spending Functions

19.4.1 Implementation

The error spending tests of Chapter 7 require computation both in their design and their implementation. In applying the error spending approach, new boundary points must be calculated in response to the observed information level at each new analysis, as explained in Section 7.5. There, the expressions to be calculated were given in the form of integrals: the methods of Section 19.2 enable us to evaluate these integrals numerically.

For a two-sided test of H_0: $\theta = 0$, the boundary values for $Z_1, Z_2, \ldots$ are $\pm c_1, \pm c_2, \ldots$ and these are found in sequence as the study continues. At analysis k, the values $c_1, \ldots, c_{k-1}$ will have already been computed and we must find c_k as the solution to

$$\int_{c_k}^{\infty} g_k(z; 0)\, dz = \pi_k/2$$

or, equivalently,

$$\psi_k(-c_1, c_1, \ldots, -c_k, c_k; 0) = \pi_k/2,$$

where π_k is the two-sided Type I error probability assigned to analysis k. Applying (19.8), the problem becomes that of finding the value c_k for which

$$\sum_{i_{k-1}=1}^{m_{k-1}} h_{k-1}(i_{k-1}; 0)\, e_{k-1}(z_{k-1}(i_{k-1}), c_k; 0) = \pi_k/2. \qquad (19.14)$$

The $h_{k-1}(i_{k-1}; 0)$ can be computed in the usual way and, since the left hand side of (19.14) decreases as c_k increases, it is easy to find c_k by a numerical search. In fact, the derivative of the left hand side of (19.14) is readily computed since

$$\frac{d}{dc_k} e_{k-1}(z_{k-1}(i_{k-1}), c_k; 0) = -f_k(z_{k-1}(i_{k-1}), c_k; 0)$$

and using this derivative information in, say, a Newton-Raphson iteration can improve the speed of this search considerably.

The one-sided tests of Section 7.3 are defined by two error spending functions, one under the null hypothesis $\theta = 0$ and the other at the alternative $\theta = \delta$. Boundary values a_k and b_k are the solutions to

$$\int_{b_k}^{\infty} g_k(z; 0)\, dz = \pi_{1,k} \quad \text{and} \quad \int_{-\infty}^{a_k} g_k(z; \delta)\, dz = \pi_{2,k},$$

where $\pi_{1,k}$ and $\pi_{2,k}$ are the Type I and II error probabilities, respectively, assigned to analysis k. We can find a_k and b_k numerically by solving

$$\sum_{i_{k-1}=1}^{m_{k-1}} h_{k-1}(i_{k-1}; 0)\, e_{k-1}(z_{k-1}(i_{k-1}), b_k; 0) = \pi_{1,k}$$

and

$$\sum_{i_{k-1}=1}^{m_{k-1}} h_{k-1}(i_{k-1}; \delta)\, \{1 - e_{k-1}(z_{k-1}(i_{k-1}), a_k; \delta)\} = \pi_{2,k}$$

in essentially the same manner as the value c_k satisfying (19.14) was found for a two-sided test.

19.4.2 Design

We explained in Section 7.2.2 how a two-sided error spending test can be designed in the "maximum information" paradigm so as to achieve a specified power if information levels are equally spaced and reach the chosen target information level $\mathcal{I}_{max}$ at analysis K. As we vary $\mathcal{I}_{max}$, setting $\mathcal{I}_k = (k/K)\mathcal{I}_{max}$, $k = 1, \ldots, K$, the error probabilities allocated to each analysis and the sequence of critical values for $Z_1, \ldots, Z_K$ remain the same. The situation is therefore identical to that arising for parametric two-sided tests in Section 19.3.2 and the same type of search can be used to find the value of $\mathcal{I}_{max}$ for which power $1 - \beta$ is attained at $\theta = \pm\delta$.

A different approach is needed to design a one-sided error spending test. Again it is convenient to assume, for design purposes, that equally spaced information levels $\mathcal{I}_k = (k/K)\mathcal{I}_{max}$, $k = 1, \ldots, K$, will be observed. Initially, we must specify the Type I and Type II error spending functions $f(t)$ and $g(t)$, as defined in Section 7.3.1. Then, for a given target information level $\mathcal{I}_{max}$ and observed information sequence $\mathcal{I}_k = (k/K)\mathcal{I}_{max}$, we find values (a_k, b_k), $k = 1, \ldots, K$, to give cumulative Type I error probabilities $f(k/K)$ under H_0: $\theta = 0$ and Type II error probabilities $g(k/K)$ under $\theta = \delta$ at each analysis k. If the value of $\mathcal{I}_{max}$ is too low, this calculation will end with $a_K < b_K$, since the desired overall Type I and Type II error probabilities cannot be achieved simultaneously. If $\mathcal{I}_{max}$ is too high, the boundaries will cross, ending with $a_K > b_K$ or with $a_k > b_k$ at an earlier analysis. Learning which of these outcomes occurs for each proposed $\mathcal{I}_{max}$ is sufficient to implement a bisection search for the value of $\mathcal{I}_{max}$ under which the test terminates neatly at analysis K with $a_K = b_K$.

19.5 Analysis Following a Group Sequential Test

19.5.1 Point Estimation

The bias adjusted estimators discussed in Section 8.3 require evaluation under certain θ values of the bias of the MLE $\hat{\theta} = Z_T/\sqrt{\mathcal{I}_T}$, where T denotes the stage at which a test stops and Z_T the value of the standardized statistic at this point. This bias is $E_\theta(\hat{\theta}) - \theta$ where $E_\theta(\hat{\theta})$, given by (8.9), can be written as

$$E_\theta(\hat{\theta}) = \sum_{k=1}^{K} \left\{ \int_{-\infty}^{a_k} g_k(z_k;\theta)\,\frac{z_k}{\sqrt{\mathcal{I}_k}}\,dz_k + \int_{b_k}^{\infty} g_k(z_k;\theta)\,\frac{z_k}{\sqrt{\mathcal{I}_k}}\,dz_k \right\}.$$

A typical lower integral in this sum can be written as

$$\int_{a_{k-1}}^{b_{k-1}} \int_{-\infty}^{a_k} g_{k-1}(z_{k-1};\theta)\, f_k(z_{k-1}, z_k;\theta)\,\frac{z_k}{\sqrt{\mathcal{I}_k}}\,dz_k\,dz_{k-1}$$

and it follows from the definition of f_k in equation (19.4) and properties of the normal distribution (see Todd, Whitehead & Facey, 1996, p. 455) that this is equal to

$$\int_{a_{k-1}}^{b_{k-1}} g_{k-1}(z_{k-1};\theta)\, r_{k-1}(z_{k-1}, a_k;\theta)\,dz_{k-1}, \qquad (19.15)$$

where

$$r_{k-1}(z_{k-1}, a_k;\theta) = \frac{-\sqrt{\Delta_k}}{\mathcal{I}_k}\,\phi\left(\frac{a_k\sqrt{\mathcal{I}_k} - z_{k-1}\sqrt{\mathcal{I}_{k-1}} - \theta\Delta_k}{\sqrt{\Delta_k}}\right)$$

$$+ \frac{(z_{k-1}\sqrt{\mathcal{I}_{k-1}} + \theta\Delta_k)}{\mathcal{I}_k}\,\Phi\left(\frac{a_k\sqrt{\mathcal{I}_k} - z_{k-1}\sqrt{\mathcal{I}_{k-1}} - \theta\Delta_k}{\sqrt{\Delta_k}}\right).$$

Using (19.9), we can evaluate the integral (19.15) numerically as

$$\sum_{i_{k-1}=1}^{m_{k-1}} h_{k-1}(i_{k-1};\theta)\, r_{k-1}(z_{k-1}(i_{k-1}), a_k;\theta).$$

The upper integrals from b_k to ∞ can be computed in a similar manner and these results combined to give $E_\theta(\hat{\theta})$.

19.5.2 P-values

We defined frequentist P-values on termination of a group sequential test in Section 8.4. Suppose, for example, a test with continuation regions $(a_1, b_1), \ldots, (a_K, b_K)$ for $Z_1, \ldots, Z_K$ stops after crossing the upper boundary at analysis k^* with $Z_{k^*} = z^*$. The one-sided upper P-value for testing H_0: $\theta = 0$

based on the stage-wise ordering is then

$$\sum_{j=1}^{k^*-1} \psi_j(a_1, b_1, \ldots, a_j, b_j; 0) + \psi_{k^*}(a_1, b_1, \ldots, a_{k^*-1}, b_{k^*-1}, a_{k^*}, z^*; 0),$$

which can be calculated numerically by the methods of Section 19.2. One-sided lower P-values are found in the same manner and the two-sided P-value is twice the smaller of these two quantities.

Slightly different computations are required to find P-values for the other three orderings of the sample space discussed in Section 8.4. However, in each case the set of outcomes more extreme than that observed is a union of at most K semi-infinite intervals and upper and lower P-values are sums of terms ψ_j or ξ_j, as for the stage-wise ordering.

19.5.3 Confidence Intervals

In Section 8.5 we defined confidence intervals for a parameter θ on termination of a group sequential test, based on a specified ordering of the sample space. In computing such a confidence interval, the main task is to find values θ_L and θ_U satisfying (8.15) for the specified ordering. The calculations for each θ investigated as the roots θ_L and θ_U are sought are those needed to find one-sided upper and lower P-values, respectively, for testing a hypothesized value for θ.

Since the searches for θ_L and θ_U involve repeated calculations under a sequence of quite similar θ values, this is an ideal situation in which to use the likelihood ratio relation (19.13) to save computational effort.

An alternative way of reducing computation is to calculate derivatives of probabilities with respect to θ along with the probabilities themselves and exploit this derivative information in more efficient root-finding algorithms. Starting from the first integral expression for $\psi_k(a_1, b_1, \ldots, a_k, b_k; \theta)$ in (19.5), we have

$$\frac{d\psi_k}{d\theta} = \int_{a_1}^{b_1} \cdots \int_{a_{k-1}}^{b_{k-1}} \int_{b_k}^{\infty} \{f_1'(f_2 \ldots f_k) + f_1(f_2 \ldots f_k)'\}\, dz_k \ldots dz_1,$$

where, for conciseness, we have suppressed the arguments of ψ_k and $f_1, \ldots, f_K$. In this and subsequent formulae in this section, all primes denote derivatives with respect to θ.

Let $u_1(z_1; \theta) = f_1'(z_1; \theta)$ and $v_1(z_1; \theta) = f_1(z_1; \theta)$, and define functions u_k and v_k for $k = 2, \ldots, K$ by

$$u_k(z_k; \theta) = \int_{a_{k-1}}^{b_{k-1}} \{u_{k-1}(z_{k-1}; \theta)\, f_k(z_{k-1}, z_k; \theta) + v_{k-1}(z_{k-1}; \theta)\, f_k'(z_{k-1}, z_k; \theta)\}\, dz_{k-1}$$

and

$$v_k(z_k; \theta) = \int_{a_{k-1}}^{b_{k-1}} v_{k-1}(z_{k-1}; \theta)\, f_k(z_{k-1}, z_k; \theta)\, dz_{k-1}.$$

Then, again suppressing function arguments,

$$\frac{d\psi_k}{d\theta} = \int_{a_1}^{b_1} \dots \int_{a_{k-1}}^{b_{k-1}} \int_{b_k}^{\infty} \{u_1(f_2 \dots f_k) + v_1(f_2 \dots f_k)'\}\, dz_k \dots dz_1$$

$$\dots = \int_{a_j}^{b_j} \dots \int_{a_{k-1}}^{b_{k-1}} \int_{b_k}^{\infty} \{u_j(f_{j+1} \dots f_k) + v_j(f_{j+1} \dots f_k)'\}\, dz_k \dots dz_j$$

$$\dots = \int_{a_{k-1}}^{b_{k-1}} \int_{b_k}^{\infty} \{u_{k-1} f_k + v_{k-1} f_k'\}\, dz_k\, dz_{k-1}.$$

The numerical evaluation of $d\psi_k/d\theta$ parallels that of ψ_k itself, each integral over a continuation region (a_j, b_j) being replaced by a weighted sum over grid points $z_j(i_j)$, $i_j = 1, \dots, m_j$. Values of the functions $u_1, \dots, u_K$ and $v_1, \dots, v_K$ at the selected grid points are computed recursively. In fact, v_j is precisely the function g_j defined in Section 19.2 and the approximation to $v_j(i_j)$ multiplied by weight $w_j(i_j)$ is our previous $h_j(i_j)$. The approximation to $u_j(i_j)$ multiplied by $w_j(i_j)$ is a new function, readily obtained by additional calculations alongside those giving h_j. For further details of these computations see Jennison (1994).

19.6 Further Applications of Numerical Computation

19.6.1 Calculating Optimal Tests

The history of optimal sequential tests goes back to Wald & Wolfowitz's (1948) proof that the sequential probability ratio test (Wald, 1947) minimizes expected sample size at two parameter values subject to specified error probabilities being achieved at those points. This result concerns open-ended sequential tests with no upper limit on sample size. The search for optimality in group sequential tests requires a combination of analysis and numerical computation. A very effective computational method, proposed for binomial and normal responses by Weiss (1962), involves creating a Bayes decision problem and choosing the prior distributions and costs so that the Bayes procedure is also optimal with respect to desired frequentist criteria. Lai (1973) uses this approach to find an optimum sequential test with continuous monitoring of a normal response. Eales (1991), Eales & Jennison (1992, 1995) and Chang (1996) derive one-sided and two-sided group sequential tests of a normal mean θ which minimize expected sample size at a particular value of θ, averaged over several values of θ, or integrated with respect to a normal density for θ.

An experimenter may wish to see a number of different features in a good group sequential design rather than optimality in one specific sense. Nevertheless, the limits of optimal performance serve as useful benchmarks when judging the merit of a particular design: recall that we listed optimal expected sample sizes in Table 4.4 to show how well one-sided tests in the power family perform under two different θ values and we later compared expected sample sizes of one-sided error spending tests against the same results.

We illustrate the method used by Eales & Jennison (1992) in the derivation of a two-sided test between the hypotheses $H_0\colon \theta \le 0$ and $H_1\colon \theta > 0$ which minimizes the expected information on termination under $\theta = \delta/2$ subject to achieving error probabilities

$$Pr_{\theta=0}\{\text{Reject } H_0\} = Pr_{\theta=\delta}\{\text{Accept } H_0\} = \alpha$$

for some specified δ. Suppose K analyses at cumulative information levels $\mathcal{I}_1, \ldots, \mathcal{I}_K$ are allowed and standardized statistics $Z_1, \ldots, Z_K$ follow the canonical joint distribution (3.1). Our goal is to minimize $E_{\theta=\delta/2}(\mathcal{I}_T)$ where T is the analysis at which the test terminates. As a device for solving this problem, a Bayes sequential decision problem is created in which θ has the three point prior distribution, $\pi(0) = \pi(\delta/2) = \pi(\delta) = 1/3$, and a decision D_0: '$\theta \leq 0$' or D_1: '$\theta > 0$' is to be made with loss function $L(D_0, \delta) = L(D_1, 0) = d$, where $d > 0$, and $L(D, \theta) = 0$ otherwise. The sampling cost is $c(\theta)$ per unit of information, giving a total sampling cost $c(\theta)\mathcal{I}_T$, and we set $c(\delta/2) = 1$ and $c(\theta) = 0$ for $\theta \neq \delta/2$. The solution of this Bayes decision problem will minimize the expected total cost

$$\pi(\delta/2)E_{\theta=\delta/2}(\mathcal{I}_T) + d\pi(0)Pr_{\theta=0}\{D_1\} + d\pi(\delta)Pr_{\theta=\delta}\{D_0\}. \qquad (19.16)$$

For any given d, the Bayes problem can be solved by dynamic programming. In order to solve our original problem, we must find the value of d, d^* say, for which the Bayes optimal decision rule minimizing (19.16) also satisfies

$$Pr_{\theta=0}\{D_1\} = Pr_{\theta=\delta}\{D_0\} = \alpha. \qquad (19.17)$$

Clearly, the optimal rule for $d = d^*$ must minimize $E_{\theta=\delta/2}(\mathcal{I}_T)$ among all rules satisfying (19.17) and hence, equating decisions D_0 and D_1 with acceptance and rejection of H_0, respectively, we have the optimal group sequential test for our original problem.

In solving the Bayes decision problem of minimizing (19.16) for a given d, we need to determine the constants $c_1, \ldots, c_K$ such that stopping occurs at stage k with decision D_0 if $Z_k \leq (\delta/2)\sqrt{\mathcal{I}_k} - c_k$ and with decision D_1 if $Z_k \geq (\delta/2)\sqrt{\mathcal{I}_k} + c_k$. (Note that the problem is symmetric about $\theta = \delta/2$, where $E(Z_k)$ is equal to $(\delta/2)\sqrt{\mathcal{I}_k}$.) For $k = 1, \ldots, K$, let $\pi^{(k)}(\theta \mid z_k)$ denote the posterior distribution of θ, given $Z_k = z_k$. The minimum expected loss from stopping and making a decision at stage k when $Z_k = z_k$ is

$$\gamma^{(k)}(z_k) = d\min\{\pi^{(k)}(0 \mid z_k), \pi^{(k)}(\delta \mid z_k)\},$$

achieved by making decision D_1 when $z_k > (\delta/2)\sqrt{\mathcal{I}_k}$ and decision D_0 when $z_k < (\delta/2)\sqrt{\mathcal{I}_k}$. Let $\beta^{(k)}(z_k)$ denote the expected additional loss from continuing to sample at stage k when $Z_k = z_k$ and then proceeding optimally. Then, for $k = 1, \ldots, K-2$,

$$\beta^{(k)}(z_k) = (\mathcal{I}_{k+1} - \mathcal{I}_k)\pi^{(k)}(\delta/2 \mid z_k) + \int \min\{\beta^{(k+1)}(z_{k+1}), \gamma^{(k+1)}(z_{k+1})\}\, dF^{(k+1)}(z_{k+1} \mid z_k)$$

and

$$\beta^{(K-1)}(z_{K-1}) = (\mathcal{I}_K - \mathcal{I}_{K-1})\pi^{(K-1)}(\delta/2 \mid z_{K-1}) + \int \gamma^{(K)}(z_K)\, dF^{(K)}(z_K \mid z_{K-1}),$$

where $F^{(k+1)}(z_{k+1} \mid z_k)$, $k = 1, \ldots, K-1$, is the conditional cumulative distribution function of Z_{k+1} given $Z_k = z_k$.

By the usual backwards induction argument, c_k is the value such that $\beta^{(k)}((\delta/2)\sqrt{\mathcal{I}_k} + c_k) = \gamma^{(k)}((\delta/2)\sqrt{\mathcal{I}_k} + c_k)$. The functions $\beta^{(k)}(z_k)$ can be found recursively, starting at $k = K-1$. Values of $\beta^{(k)}(z_k)$ should be computed for a grid of values of z_k including $(\delta/2)\sqrt{\mathcal{I}_k} + c_k$ and $(\delta/2)\sqrt{\mathcal{I}_k} - c_k$; these are used in evaluating $\beta^{(k-1)}(z_{k-1})$ by numerical integration, first to find c_{k-1} by solving $\beta^{(k-1)}((\delta/2)\sqrt{\mathcal{I}_{k-1}} + c_{k-1}) = \gamma^{(k-1)}((\delta/2)\sqrt{\mathcal{I}_{k-1}} + c_{k-1})$, and then to calculate $\beta^{(k-1)}(z_{k-1})$ at a grid of values of z_{k-1}. The same grids of points and Simpson's rule weights can be used here as in Section 19.2.

The above strategy can be followed, with appropriately chosen prior $\pi(\theta)$ and cost of sampling function $c(\theta)$, to derive group sequential tests with a pre-specified sequence of information levels that minimize other criteria. For further details, see the references cited earlier in this section.

19.6.2 Other Response Distributions

The general approach we have described for normal data with known variance can be used to compute properties of group sequential tests for many other continuous response distributions. The key requirement is that the test should be defined in terms of a sequence of statistics, $T_1, \ldots, T_K$ say, which form a Markov process with tractable conditional distributions $T_{k+1} \mid T_k$. Denoting the density of T_1 by $f_1(t_1)$ and the conditional density of T_{k+1} given $T_k = t_k$ by $f_{k+1}(t_k, t_{k+1})$, $k = 1, \ldots, K-1$, the probability of exiting the upper boundary at analysis k is

$$\int_{a_1}^{b_1} \cdots \int_{a_{k-1}}^{b_{k-1}} \int_{b_k}^{\infty} f_1(t_1) f_2(t_1, t_2) \ldots f_k(t_{k-1}, t_k)\, dt_k \ldots dt_1,$$

an expression with the same form as that for $\psi_k(a_1, b_1, \ldots, a_k, b_k; \theta)$ in (19.5). This multiple integral can be evaluated numerically in a similar manner by a succession of summations. An example where this method is used to compute properties of group sequential χ^2 tests is described by Jennison & Turnbull (1991b).

In a group sequential t-test the appropriate statistic T_k is bivariate. Suppose, in the analysis of a normal linear model described in Section 11.4, that it is desired to test whether the scalar parameter $\theta = \boldsymbol{c}^T \boldsymbol{\beta}$ is equal to zero. The estimators at analysis k of θ and the variance scale factor σ^2 have marginal distributions

$$\hat{\theta}^{(k)} \sim N(\theta, \Gamma_k \sigma^2) \quad \text{and} \quad s_k^2 \sim \sigma^2 \chi^2_{\nu_k},$$

respectively, for appropriately specified Γ_k and ν_k. Let $T_{1k} = \hat{\theta}^{(k)}/\sigma$ and $T_{2k} = \nu_k s_k^2/\sigma^2$, then the results of Section 11.4 imply that the sequence $\{(T_{ik}, T_{2k}); k = 1, \ldots, K\}$, is Markov and, under H_0: $\theta = 0$,

$$T_{1,k+1} \mid T_{1k}, T_{2k} \sim N\left(\frac{\Gamma_{k+1}}{\Gamma_k} T_{1k},\ \Gamma_{k+1} - \frac{\Gamma_{k+1}^2}{\Gamma_k} \right)$$

and

$$T_{2,k+1} \mid T_{1,k+1}, T_{1k}, T_{2k} \sim T_{2k} + \frac{(T_{1,k+1} - T_{1k})^2}{\Gamma_k - \Gamma_{k+1}} + \chi^2_{\nu_{k+1}-\nu_k-1}.$$

Probabilities concerning the sequence of t-statistics, $T_{1k}/\surd(\Gamma_k T_{2k}/\nu_k)$, $k = 1, \ldots, K$, can be calculated numerically from these conditional distributions in much the same way as for normal data with known variance. Care must be taken in integrating over the conditional distribution for $T_{2,k+1}$ if the degrees of freedom $\nu_{k+1} - \nu_k - 1$ are low, especially if this number of degrees of freedom is odd since then the χ^2 density has an infinite $\{(\nu_{k+1} - \nu_k - 2)/2\}th$ derivative at zero. Calculations of this type reported by Jennison & Turnbull (1991b) produced the constants displayed in Table 11.1.

Bivariate statistics arise naturally in studies with two distinct endpoints. Jennison & Turnbull (1993c) describe group sequential procedures for monitoring efficacy and safety endpoints in a clinical trial. In their prototype problem, each pair of observations (Y_{1i}, Y_{2i}) has a bivariate normal distribution with $E(Y_{1i}) = \theta_1$, $E(Y_{2i}) = \theta_2$ and $Corr(Y_{1i}, Y_{2i}) = \rho$. A problem formulation with an element of equivalence testing (see Chapter 6) leads to a test between hypotheses H_0: '$\theta_1 \leq 0$ or $\theta_2 \leq 0$' and the alternative H_2: '$\theta_1 > 0$ and $\theta_2 > 0$'; with suitably defined response variables and parameters θ_1 and θ_2, H_2 represents situations in which a new treatment performs satisfactorily with regard to both efficacy and safety considerations. Again, a Markov sequence of statistic pairs can be constructed and probabilities of crossing boundaries calculated by iterated numerical integration.

The same computational approach may be used with more than two response variables but at a greatly increased computational cost. If each integral is replaced by a sum over m terms, the number of arithmetic operations required to assess a testing boundary for a d-variate response is of order m^{2d} but the numerical error, using Simpson's rule for each integral, remains of order m^{-4}. Thus, for high values of d, Monte Carlo simulation provides a better rate of convergence per numerical operation.

19.7 Computer Software

Two commercially available computer software packages for sequential design and analysis are EaSt (Cytel Software Corporation, 1992) and PEST 3 (Brunier & Whitehead, 1993). Briefly, EaSt provides Wang & Tsiatis (1987) boundaries for two-sided testing (see Section 2.7.1) and the power family tests of Pampallona & Tsiatis (1994) for one-sided testing and for two-sided testing with early stopping to accept H_0 (see Sections 4.2 and 5.2). EaSt also offers error spending methods (see Chapter 7) for one-sided and two-sided tests. The PEST 3 package implements the triangular test and double triangular test (Whitehead & Stratton, 1983; Whitehead, 1997) described in Sections 4.5 and 5.3, and the "restricted procedure" which can be used to produce O'Brien & Fleming (1979) boundaries (see Section 2.5). PEST 3 uses the "Christmas tree" adjustment to handle unequally spaced information levels. Both packages guide the user in designing and implementing a group sequential study and PEST 3 provides inference on termination, as described in our Chapter 8. Emerson (1996) provides a thorough review of the capabilities of these two packages and also discusses their general organization, documentation, user interface and ability to link with other statistical software. At the time of writing, new releases of both packages are imminent and both will have a variety of new features. In particular, the new version of EaSt, EaSt for Windows, (Cytel Software Corporation, 1999) will include methods for inference on termination.

As noted in Chapter 1, the module S+SeqTrial based on the Splus statistical software (MathSoft, 1998) is in development stage at the time of writing. The article by Halpern & Brown (1993) describes a computer program, available from those authors, for designing group sequential studies for survival endpoints.

FORTRAN routines implementing error-spending tests have been made available at the website `http://www.medsch.wisc.edu/landemets/` by the authors, David Reboussin, David DeMets, KyungMann Kim and K. K. Gordon Lan. Our own FORTRAN programs are available at the website `http://www.bath.ac.uk/~mascj/` at the University of Bath.

References

Sections in which the references are cited are shown in square brackets.

Alling, D.W. (1963). Early decision in the Wilcoxon two-sample test. *J. Amer. Statist. Assoc.*, **58**, 713–720. [10.1]

Alling, D.W. (1966). Closed sequential tests for binomial probabilities. *Biometrika*, **53**, 73–84. [10.1]

Altman, D.G. (1991). *Practical Statistics for Medical Research*, London: Chapman and Hall. [1.1]

Andersen, J.S. (1996). Clinical trial designs — made to order. *J. Biopharm. Statist.*, **6**, 515–522. [17.4]

Andersen, P.K. (1987). Conditional power calculations as an aid in the decision whether to continue a clinical trial. *Contr. Clin. Trials*, **8**, 67–74. [10.5, 10.6]

Anderson, S. and Hauck, W.W. (1990) Consideration of individual bioequivalence. *J. Pharmacokin. Biopharm.*, **18**, 259–273. [6.4]

Anderson, T.W. (1960). A modification of the sequential probability ratio test to reduce the sample size. *Ann. Math. Statist.*, **31**, 165–197. [1.3]

Anscombe, F.J. (1963). Sequential medical trials. *J. Amer. Statist. Assoc.*, **58**, 365–384. [17.4, 18.4]

Anthonisen, N.R. (1989). Lung Health Study. *Amer. Rev. Respiratory Diseases*, **140**, 871–872. [1.4]

Arghami, N.R. and Billard, L. (1991) A partial sequential t-test. *Sequential Analysis*, **10**, 181–197. [14.3]

Arghami, N.R. and Billard, L. (1992) Some sequential analogs of Stein's two-sample test. *J. Prob. Appl.*, **37**, 115–117. [14.3]

Armitage, P. (1954). Sequential tests in prophylactic and therapeutic trials, *Quarterly J. Med.*, **23**, 255–274. [1.4]

Armitage, P. (1957). Restricted sequential procedures. *Biometrika*, **44**, 9–56. [1.3, 8.4, 8.5]

Armitage, P. (1958a). Numerical studies in the sequential estimation of a binomial parameter. *Biometrika*, **45**, 1–15. [8.4, 8.5]

Armitage, P. (1958b). Sequential methods in clinical trials. *Amer. J. Public Health*, **48**, 1395–1402. [1.3]

Armitage, P. (1975). *Sequential Medical Trials*, Oxford: Blackwell. [1.3, 1.4, 1.6, 19.1]

Armitage, P. (1985). The search for optimality in clinical trials. *Intern. Statist. Rev.*, **53**, 15–24. [17.4]

Armitage, P. (1993). Interim analyses in clinical trials. In *Multiple Comparisons, Selection, and Applications in Biometry*, (Ed., F.M. Hoppe), New York: Marcel Dekker, 391–402. [1.3]

Armitage, P. and Berry, G. (1987). *Statistical Methods in Medical Research*, 2nd edn, Oxford: Blackwell. [1.1]

Armitage, P., McPherson, C.K. and Rowe, B.C. (1969). Repeated significance tests on accumulating data. *J. Roy. Statist. Soc. A.*, **132**, 235–244. [1.3, 2.4, 7.5, 8.2, 9.1, 19.1]

Armitage, P. and Schneiderman, M. (1958). Statistical problems in a mass screening program. *Ann. New York Academy Sci.*, **76**, 896–908. [1.3, 19.1]

Armitage, P., Stratton, I.M. and Worthington, H.V. (1985). Repeated significance tests for clinical trials with a fixed number of patients and variable follow-up. *Biometrics*, **41**, 353–359. [1.4, 9.3, 11.3, 11.7]

Aroian, L.A. (1968). Sequential analysis, direct method. *Technometrics* **10**, 125–132. [1.3]

Aroian, L.A. and Robison, D.E. (1969). Direct methods for exact truncated sequential tests of the mean for a normal distribution. *Technometrics*, **11**, 661–675. [1.3]

Ascher. H. and Feingold, H. (1984). *Repairable Systems Reliability*, New York: Marcel Dekker. [1.4]

Bailar, J.C. III. (1976). Patient assignment algorithms — an overview. In *Proceedings of the 9th International Biometric Conference, Vol. 1*, Raleigh: The Biometric Society, 189–206. [17.4]

Baillie, D.H. (1987a). Multivariate acceptance sampling — some applications to defence procurement. *The Statistician*, **36**, 465–478 (Correction **37**, 97 and **38**, 315) [15.7]

Baillie, D.H. (1987b). Multivariate acceptance sampling. In *Frontiers in Statistical Quality Control* **3** (Eds., H.J. Lenz, G.B. Wetherill and P.T. Wilrich), Wuerzberg-Vienna: Physica-Verlag.

Baker, A.G. (1950). Properties of some test in sequential analysis. *Biometrika*, **37**, 334–346. [14.3]

Barber, S. and Jennison, C. (1999). Symmetric tests and confidence intervals for survival probabilities and quantiles of censored survival data. *Biometrics*, **55**, 430–436. [13.7]

Barnard, G.A. (1946). Sequential tests in industrial statistics. *J. Roy. Statist. Soc. Suppl.*, **8**, 1–26. [1.3]

Bartky, W. (1943). Multiple sampling with constant probability. *Ann. Math. Statist.*, **14**, 363–377. [1.3]

Bather, J.A. (1985). On the allocation of treatments in sequential medical trials. *Intern. Statist. Rev.*, **53**, 1–13. [1.3]

Bather, J.A. (1988). Stopping rules and ordered families of distributions. *Sequential Analysis*, **7**, 111–126. [8.5]

Baum, C.W. and Veeravalli, V.V. (1994). A sequential procedure for multihypothesis testing. *IEEE Trans. Inform. Theory*, **40**, 1994–2007. [1.3]

Bechhofer, R.E., Kiefer, J. and Sobel, M. (1968). *Sequential Identification and Ranking Procedures*, Chicago: Univ. Chicago Press. [1.3]

Bechhofer, R.E., Santner, T.J. and Goldsman, D.M. (1995). *Design and Analysis of Experiments for Statistical Selection, Screening, and Multiple Comparisons*, New York: Wiley. [16.4]

Beck, G.J., Berg R.L., Coggins C.H., et al. (1991). Design and statistical issues of the modification of diet in renal-disease trial. *Contr. Clin. Trials*, **12**, 566–586. [1.1]

Berger, J.O. (1985). *Statistical Decision Theory and Bayesian Analysis*, 2nd end, New York: Springer. [18.1]

Berger, J.O. and Berry, D.A. (1988). Statistical analysis and the illusion of objectivity. *Amer. Scientist*, **76**, 159–165. [18.2]

Berry, D.A. (1985). Interim analysis in clinical trials: Classical vs. Bayesian approaches. *Statist. Med.*, **4**, 521–6. [18.2]

Berry, D.A. (1987). Interim analyses in clinical trials: The role of the likelihood principle. *The Amer. Statistician*, **41**, 117–122. [18.2]

Berry, D.A. and Fristedt, B. (1985). *Bandit Problems: Sequential Allocation of Experiments*, London: Chapman and Hall. [1.3]

Berry, D.A. and Ho, C.H. (1988). One-sided sequential stopping boundaries for clinical trials: A decision theoretic approach. *Biometrics*, **44**, 219–227. [1.3, 7.3, 18.4]

Betensky, R.A. (1996). An O'Brien-Fleming sequential trial for comparing three treatments. *Ann. Statist.*, **24**, 1765–1791. [16.4]

Betensky, R.A. (1997a). Conditional power calculations for early acceptance of H_0 embedded in sequential tests. *Statist. Med.*, **16**, 465–477. [10.6]

Betensky, R.A. (1997b). Early stopping to accept H0 based on conditional power: approximations and comparisons. *Biometrics*, **53**, 794–806. [10.6]

Betensky, R.A. (1997c). Sequential analysis of censored survival data with three treatment groups. *Biometrics*, **53**, 807–822. [16.4]

Betensky, R.A. (1998). Construction of a continuous stopping boundary from an alpha spending function. *Biometrics*, **54**, 1061–1071. [7.4]

Betensky, R.A. and Tierney, C. (1997). An examination of methods for sample size recalculation during an experiment. *Statist. Med.*, **16**, 2587–2598. [14.2]

Bilias, Y., Gu, M. and Ying, Z. (1997). Towards a general asymptotic theory for the Cox model with staggered entry. *Ann. Statist.*, **25**, 662–682. [13.8]

Birkett, M.A. and Day, S.J. (1994). Internal pilot studies for estimating sample size. *Statist. Med.*, **13**, 2455–2463. [14.2]

Blot, W.J. and Meeter, D.A. (1973). Sequential experimental design procedures. *J. Amer. Statist. Assoc.*, **68**, 586–593. [1.3]

Blot, W.J., Li, J., Taylor, P.R., Guo, W., Dawsey, S., Wang.G., Yang, C.S., Zheng, M., Gail, M., Li, G., Yu,Y., Liu, B., Tangrea, J., Sun, Y., Liu, F., Fraumeni, J.F., Zhang, Y. and Li, B. (1993). Nutrition intervention trials in Linxian, China: supplementations with specific vitamin/mineral combinations, cancer incidence, and disease specific mortality in the general population. *J. Nat. Cancer Inst.*, **85**, 1483–1492. [1.1, 16.3]

Blyth, C.R. and Still, H.A. (1983). Binomial confidence intervals. *J. Amer. Statist. Assoc.*, **78**, 108–116. [12.1, 12.2]

Bowker, A.H. and Lieberman, G.J. (1972). *Engineering Statistics*, 2nd ed., Englewood Cliffs: Prentice-Hall. [12.1]

Box, G.E.P., Hunter, W.G. and Hunter, J.S. (1978). *Statistics for Experimenters*, New York: Wiley. [1.1]

Braitman, L.E. (1993). Statistical estimates and clinical trials. *J. Biopharm. Statist.*, **3**, 249–256. [8.1]

Breslow, N.E. and Day, N.E. (1980). *Statistical Methods in Cancer Research, Vol. I: The Analysis of Case-Control Studies*, Lyon: Intern. Agency for Research on Cancer. [1.1, 12.3]

Breslow, N.E. and Day, N.E. (1987). *Statistical Methods in Cancer Research, Vol. II: The Design and Analysis of Cohort Studies*, Lyon: Intern. Agency for Research on Cancer. [1.1]

Brookmeyer, R. and Crowley, J. (1982). A confidence interval for the median survival time. *Biometrics*, **38**, 29–41. [9.1, 13.7]

Bross, I. (1952). Sequential medical plans. *Biometrics*, **8**, 188–205. [1.3]

Bross, I. (1958). Sequential clinical trials. *J. Chronic Diseases* **8**, 349–365. [1.3]

Brown, B.W., Herson, J., Atkinson, E.N. and Rozell, M.E. (1987). Projection from previous studies: A Bayesian and frequentist compromise. *Contr. Clin. Trials*, **8**, 29–44. [18.2]

Brown, L.D., Cohen, A. and Strawderman, W.E. (1980). Complete classes for sequential tests of hypotheses. *Ann. Statist.*, **8**, 377–398. (Correction **17**, 1414–1416). [18.4]

Browne, R.H. (1995). On the use of a pilot sample for sample size determination. *Statist. Med.*, **14**, 1933–1940. [14.2]

Brunier, H. and Whitehead, J. (1993). *PEST3.0 Operating Manual*, Univ. Reading, U.K. [1.6, 19.7]

Buckley, J. and James, I. (1979). Linear regression with censored data. *Biometrika*, **66**, 429–436. [11.6, 11.7]

Burdette, W.J. and Gehan, E.A. (1970). *Planning and Analysis of Clinical Studies*, Springfield, Illinois: Charles C. Thomas. [1.1]

Buyse, M.E., Staquet, M.J. and Sylvester, R.J. (1984). *Cancer Clin. Trials, Methods and Practice*, Oxford: Oxford Univ. Press. [1.1]

Byar, D.P. (1985). Prognostic variables for survival in a randomized comparison of treatments for prostatic cancer. In *Data* (Eds., D.F. Andrews and A.M. Hertzberg), New York: Springer-Verlag, 261–262. [13.8]

Canner, P.L. (1977). Monitoring treatment differences in long-term clinical trials. *Biometrics*, **33**, 603–615. [1.3, 2.3]

Cannon, C.P. (1997). Clinical perspectives on the use of multiple endpoints. *Contr. Clin. Trials*, **18**, 517–529. [15.1]

Carlin, B.P., Chaloner, K., Church, T., Louis, T.A. and Matts, J.P. (1993). Bayesian approaches for monitoring clinical trials with an application to toxoplasmic encephalitis prophylaxis. *The Statistician*, **42**, 355–367. [18.4]

Carlin, B.P. and Sargent, D.J. (1996). Robust Bayesian approaches for clinical trials monitoring. *Statist. Med.*, **15**, 1093–1106. [18.4]

Chaloner, K., Church, T., Louis, T.A. and Matts, J.P. (1993). Graphical elicitation of a prior distribution for a clinical trial. *The Statistician*, **42**, 341–353. [8.3]

Chandler, G.A. and Graham, I.G. (1988). The convergence of Nystrom methods for Weiner-Hopf equations. *Numerische Mathematik*, **52**, 345–364. [19.2]

Chang, M.N. (1989). Confidence intervals for a normal mean following a group sequential test. *Biometrics*, **45**, 247–254. [8.2, 8.4]

Chang, M.N. (1996). Optimal designs for group sequential clinical trials. *Commun. Statist. A.*, **25**, 361–379. [19.6]

Chang, M.N., Hwang, I.K. and Shih, W.J. (1998). Group sequential designs using both type I and type II error probability spending functions. *Commun. Statist. A.*, **27**, 1323–1339. [7.3]

Chatfield, C. and Collins, A.J. (1980). *Introduction to Multivariate Analysis*, London: Chapman and Hall. [15.3]

Chatterjee, S.K. and Sen, P.K. (1973). Nonparametric testing under progressive censoring. *Calcutta Statist. Assoc. Bull.*, **22**, 13–50. [10.2]

Checkoway, H., Pearce, N.E. and Crawford-Brown, D.J. (1989). *Research Methods in Occupational Epidemiology*, Oxford: Oxford Univ. Press. [1.1]

Chernoff, H. (1972). *Sequential Analysis and Optimal Design*, Philadelphia: SIAM. [1.3]

Chernoff, H. and Petkau, A.J. (1981). Sequential medical trials involving paired data. *Biometrika*, **68**, 119–132. [18.4]

Chinchilli, V.M. (1996). The assessment of individual and population bioequivalence. *J. Biopharm. Statist.*, **6**, 1–14. [6.1]

Choi, S.C., Smith, P.J. and Becker, D.P. (1985). Early decision in clinical trials when treatment differences are small. *Contr. Clin. Trials*, **6**, 280–288. [1.3, 10.3, 10.6]

Chow, S-C. and Liu, J-P. (1992). *Design and Analysis of Bioavailability and Bioequivalence Studies*, New York: Marcel Dekker. [1.1, 6.3]

Chow, S-C. and Liu, J-P. (1998). *Design and Analysis of Clinical Trials: Concepts and Methodologies*, New York: Wiley. [1.1]

Chuang, C-S. and Lai, T.L. (1998). Resampling methods for confidence intervals in group sequential trials. *Biometrika*, **85**, 317–332. [8.5]

Clark, L.C., Combs, G.F., Turnbull, B.W., Slate, E.H., Chalker, D.K., Chow, J., Davis, L.S., Glover, R.A., Graham, G.F., Gross, E.G., Krongrad, A., Lesher, J.L., Park, H.K., Sanders, B.B., Smith, C.L., Taylor, J.R. and the Nutritional Prevention of Cancer Study Group. (1996). Effects of selenium supplementation for cancer prevention in patients with carcinoma of the skin: A randomized clinical trial. *J. Amer. Med. Assoc.*, **276**, 1957–1963. [1.4, 10.5, 15.2]

Clopper, C.J. and Pearson, E.S. (1934). The use of confidence or fiducial limits illustrated in the case of the binomial. *Biometrika*, **26**, 404–413. [12.1]

Coad, D.S. (1995). Sequential allocation involving several treatments. In *Adaptive Designs* (Eds., N. Flournoy and W.F. Rosenberger), Hayward, California: Institute of Mathematical Statistics, 95–109. [17.4]

Cochran, W.G. and Cox, G.M. (1957). *Experimental Design*, 2nd ed., New York: Wiley. [1.1]

Coe, P.R. and Tamhane, A.C. (1993). Exact repeated confidence intervals for Bernoulli parameters in a group sequential clinical trial. *Contr. Clin. Trials*, **14**, 19–29. [9.5, 12.1, 12.2]

Colton, T. (1963). A model for selecting one of two medical treatments. *J. Amer. Statist. Assoc.*, **58**, 388–401. [17.4]

Conaway, M.R. and Petroni, G.R, (1995). Bivariate sequential designs for Phase II trials. *Biometrics*, **51**, 656–664. [15.7]

Cook, R.J. (1994). Interim monitoring of bivariate responses using repeated confidence intervals. *Contr. Clin. Trials*, **15**, 187–200. [15.6, 15.7]

Cook, R.J. (1996). Coupled error spending functions for parallel bivariate sequential tests. *Biometrics*, **52**, 442–450. [15.7]

Cook, R.J. and Farewell, V.T. (1994). Guidelines for monitoring efficacy and toxicity responses in clinical trials. *Biometrics*, **50**, 1146–1152. [15.6, 15.7]

Cook, R.J. and Farewell, V.T. (1996). Multiplicity considerations in the design and analysis of clinical trials. *J. Roy. Statist. Soc. A.*, **159**, 93–110. [15.7]

Cook, R.J. and Lawless, J.F. (1996). Interim monitoring of longitudinal comparative studies with recurrent event responses. *Biometrics*, **52**, 1311–1323. [11.7]

Cornell, R.G., Landenberger, B.D. and Bartlett, R.H. (1986). Randomized play-the-winner clinical trials. *Commun. Statist. A.*, **15**, 159–178. [17.4]

Cornfield, J. (1966a). Sequential trials, sequential analysis and the likelihood principle. *The Amer. Statistician*, **20**, 18–23. [18.2]

Cornfield, J. (1966b). A Bayesian test of some classical hypotheses — with applications to sequential clinical trials. *J. Amer. Statist. Assoc.*, **61**, 577–594. [18.2]

Cornfield, J. (1969). The Bayesian outlook and its application (with discussion). *Biometrics*, **25**, 617–657. [18.2]

Cornfield, J., Halperin, M. and Greenhouse, S.W. (1969). An adaptive procedure for sequential clinical trials. *J. Amer. Statist. Assoc.*, **64**, 759–770. [17.4]

Cox, D.R. (1972). Regression models and life tables (with discussion). *J. Roy. Statist. Soc. B.*, **34**, 187–220. [1.5, 3.5, 13.4, 13.6]

Cox, D.R.(1975). Partial likelihood. *Biometrika*, **62**, 269–276. [3.5]

Cox, D.R. (1989). Discussion of 'Interim analyses: The repeated confidence interval approach' (by C. Jennison and B.W. Turnbull). *J. Roy. Statist. Soc. B.*, **51**, 338. [15.2]

Cox, D.R. and Hinkley, D.V. (1974). *Theoretical Statistics*, London: Chapman and Hall. [11.6]

Cox, D.R. and Oakes, D. (1984). *Analysis of Survival Data*, London: Chapman and Hall. [1.3, 1.4]

Crow, E. (1956). Confidence intervals for a proportion. *Biometrika*, **43**, 423–435. [12.1]

Cutler, S.J. Greenhouse, S.W. Cornfield, J. and Schneiderman, M.A. (1966). The role of hypothesis testing in clinical trials. *J. Chron. Diseases*, **19**, 857–882. [1.3, 8.1]

Cytel Software Corporation. (1992). *EaSt: A software package for the design and analysis of group sequential clinical trials.* Cytel Software Corporation, Cambridge, Mass. [1.6, 19.7]

Cytel Software Corporation. (1999). *EaSt for Windows: A software package for the design and interim monitoring of group-sequential clinical trials*, Cytel Software Corporation, Cambridge, Mass. [1.6, 19.7]

Davis, B.R. and Hardy, R.J. (1992). Repeated confidence intervals and prediction intervals using stochastic curtailment. *Commun. in Statist. A.*, **21**, 351–368. [10.6]

Davis, C.E. (1978). A two sample Wilcoxon test for progressively censored data. *Commun. Statist. A.*, **7**, 389–398. [10.2]

Davis, C.E. (1997). Secondary endpoints can be validly analyzed, even if the primary endpoint does not provide clear statistical significance. *Contr. Clin. Trials*, **18**, 557–560. [15.2]

DeMets, D.L. (1984). Stopping guidelines vs stopping rules: A practitioner's point of view. *Commun. Statist. A.*, **13**, 2395–2418. [9.1]

DeMets, D.L. and Gail, M.H. (1985). Use of logrank tests and group sequential methods at fixed calendar times. *Biometrics*, **41**, 1039–1044. [3.7]

DeMets, D.L., Hardy, R., Friedman, L.M. and Lan, K.K.G. (1984). Statistical aspects of early termination in the Beta-Blocker Heart Attack Trial. *Contr. Clin. Trials*, **5**, 362–372. [7.2]

DeMets, D.L. and Ware, J.H. (1980). Group sequential methods for clinical trials with one-sided hypothesis. *Biometrika*, **67**, 651–660. [4.1]

DeMets, D.L. and Ware, J.H. (1982). Asymmetric group sequential boundaries for monitoring clinical trials. *Biometrika*, **69**, 661–663. [4.1]

Denne, J.S. (1996). Sequential procedures for sample size estimation. Ph.D. Thesis, Univ. of Bath, U.K. [14.3]

Denne, J.S. and Jennison, C. (1999a). Estimating the sample size for a t-test using an internal pilot. *Statist. Med.*, **18**, 1575–1585. [14.2]

Denne, J.S. and Jennison, C. (1999b). Improving the post-experimental properties of Stein's two-stage procedure. *Sequential Analysis*, **18**, 43–56. [14.2]

Denne, J.S. and Jennison, C. (1999c). A group sequential t-test with updating of sample size. *Biometrika*. To appear. [14.3]

Dickey, J. (1973). Scientific reporting and personal probabilities: Student's hypothesis. *J. Roy. Statist. Soc. B.*, **35**, 285–305. [18.2]

Dobbins, T.W. and Thiyagarajan, B. (1992). A retrospective assessment of the 75/75 rule in bioequivalence. *Statist. Med.*, **11**, 1333–1342. [6.4]

Dodge, H.F. and Romig, H.G. (1929). A method for sampling inspection. *Bell Syst. Tech. J.*, **8**, 613–631. [1.3, 19.1]

Duffy, D.E. and Santner, T.J. (1987). Confidence intervals for a binomial parameter based on multistage tests. *Biometrics*, **43**, 81–93. [1.3, 12.1]

Dunnett, C.W. (1961). The statistical theory of drug screening. In *Quantitative Methods in Pharmacology*, Amsterdam: North-Holland, 212–231. [1.3, 19.1]

Dunnett, C.W. and Gent, M. (1977). Significance testing to establish equivalence between treatments, with special reference to data in the form of 2×2 tables. *Biometrics*, **33**, 593–602. [1.1, 6.1, 6.3]

Durrleman, S and Simon, R. (1990). Planning and monitoring of equivalence studies. *Biometrics*, **46**, 329–336. [1.1, 6.5, 9.5]

Eales, J.D. (1991). Optimal Group Sequential Tests. Ph.D. dissertation, Univ. of Bath, U.K. [19.6]

Eales, J.D. and Jennison, C. (1992). An improved method for deriving optimal one-sided group sequential tests. *Biometrika*, **79**, 13–24. [1.3, 4.1, 4.2, 7.3, 18.4, 19.6]

Eales, J.D. and Jennison, C. (1995). Optimal two-sided group sequential tests. *Sequential Analysis*, **14**, 273–286. [1.3, 2.8, 18.4, 19.6]

Elashoff, R.M. and Beal, S. (1976). Two stage screening designs applied to chemical screening programs with binary data. *Annual Review of Biophysics and Bioengineering*, **5**, 561–587. [1.3]

Elfring, G.L. and Schultz, J.R. (1973). Group sequential designs for clinical trials. *Biometrics*, **29**, 471–477. [1.3, 2.3]

Emerson, S.S (1988). Parameter Estimation Following Group Sequential Hypothesis Testing. Ph.D. dissertation. Univ. of Washington, Seattle. [8.3, 8.5]

Emerson, S.S. (1993). Computation of the uniform minimum variance unbiased estimator of a normal mean following a group sequential trial. *Computers in Biomedical Research*, **26**, 68–73. [8.3]

Emerson, S.S. (1996). Statistical packages for group sequential methods. *The Amer. Statistician*, **50**, 183–192. [19.7]

Emerson, S.S. and Fleming, T.R. (1989). Symmetric group sequential designs. *Biometrics*, **45**, 905–923. [1.3, 4.1, 4.2, 4.3, 5.1]

Emerson, S.S. and Fleming, T.R. (1990). Parameter estimation following group sequential hypothesis testing. *Biometrika*, **77**, 875–892. [8.2, 8.3, 8.4, 8.5]

Emerson, S.S. and Kittelson, J.M. (1997). A computationally simpler algorithm for the UMVUE of a normal mean following a group sequential test. *Biometrics*, **53**, 365–369. [8.3]

Emlsee, S.K., Rogers, M.P., DeSimio, M.P. and Raines, R.A. (1997). Complete automatic target recognition system for tactical forward-looking infrared images. *Optical Engineering*, **36**, 2541–2548. [1.3]

Enas, G.G., Dornseif, B.E., Sampson, C.B., Rockhold, F.W. and Wuu, J. (1989). Monitoring versus interim analysis of clinical trials: A perspective from the pharmaceutical industry. *Contr. Clin. Trials*, **10**, 57–70. [1.2, 2.7, 14.1]

Etzioni, R. and Pepe, M. (1994). Monitoring of a pilot toxicity study with two adverse outcomes. *Statist. Med.*, **13**, 2311–2322. [15.7]

Facey, K.M. (1992). A sequential procedure for a Phase II efficacy trial in hypercholesterolemia. *Contr. Clin. Trials*, **13**, 122–133. [1.4, 14.3]

Fairbanks, K. and Madsen, R. (1982). P values for tests using a repeated significance test design. *Biometrika*, **69**, 69–74. [1.3, 8.4]

Fayers, P.M., Ashby, D. and Parmar, M.B. (1997). Bayesian data monitoring in clinical trials. *Statist. Med.*, **16**, 1413–1430. [18.2, 18.3, 18,4]

Federal Register (1985). Volume 50, No. 36, (22 February). [1.2]

Federal Register (1998). Volume 63, No. 179, 49583–49598, (16 September). [1.2]

Fisher, B., Costantino, J.P. Wickerham, D.I., et al. (1998). Tamoxifen for prevention of breast cancer: Report of the National Surgical Adjuvant Breast and Bowel Project P-1 Study. *J. Nat. Cancer Inst.*, **90**, 1371–1388. [9.1]

Fleiss, J.L. (1986). *The Design and Analysis of Clinical Experiments*, New York: Wiley. [1.1]

Fleming, T.R. (1982). One-sample multiple testing procedures for Phase II clinical trials. *Biometrics*, **38**, 143–151. [1.3, 12.1]

Fleming, T.R. (1992). Evaluating therapeutic interventions: Some issues and experiences (with discussion). *Statistical Science*, **7**, 428–456. [1.6, 9.5]

Fleming, T.R. and DeMets, D.L. (1993). Monitoring of clinical trials: Issues and recommendations. *Contr. Clin. Trials*, **14**, 183–197. [2.7, 7.4]

Fleming, T.R., Harrington, D.P. and O'Brien, P.C. (1984). Designs for group sequential tests. *Contr. Clin. Trials*, **5**, 348–361. [1.3, 2.8, 7.4]

Flournoy, N. and Rosenberger, W.F. (Eds.) (1995). *Adaptive Designs*, IMS Lecture Notes Monograph Series number 25, Hayward, California: Institute of Mathematical Statistics. [17.4]

Follmann, D.A., Proschan, M.A. and Geller, N.L. (1994). Monitoring pairwise comparisons in multi-armed clinical trials. *Biometrics* 50, 325–336. [16.1, 16.3, 16.4]

Food and Drug Administration (1985). *Guideline for Postmarketing Reporting of Adverse Drug Reactions.* Center for Drugs and Biologics, Food and Drug Administration, Rockville, Maryland. [1.2]

Food and Drug Administration (1988). *Guideline for the Format and Content of the Clinical and Statistical Sections of New Drug Applications.* Center for Drug Evaluation and Research, Food and Drug Administration, Rockville, Maryland. [1.2]

Food and Drug Administration (1998). E9: Statistical Principles for Clinical Trials. *Federal Register*, **63**(179), 49583–49598, (16 September, 1998). [1.2]

Freedman, L., Anderson, G., Kipnis, V., Prentice, R., Wang, C.Y., Rossouw, J., and Wittes, J. (1996). Approaches to monitoring the results of long-term disease prevention trials: Examples from the Women's Health Initiative. *Contr. Clin. Trials*, **17**, 509–525. [15.1]

Freedman, L.S. and Spiegelhalter, D.J. (1983). The assessment of subjective opinion and its use in relation to stopping rules for clinical trials. *The Statistician*, **32**, 153–160. [18.3]

Freedman, L.S. and Spiegelhalter, D.J. (1989). Comparison of Bayesian with group sequential for monitoring clinical trials. *Contr. Clin. Trials*, **10**, 357–367. [18.2]

Freedman, L.S., Spiegelhalter, D.J. and Parmar, M.K.B. (1994). The what, why and how of Bayesian clinical trial monitoring. *Statist. Med.*, **13**, 1371–1383. [18.2]

Freeman, H.A., Friedman, M., Mosteller, F. and Wallis, W.A. (1948). *Sampling Inspection.* McGraw-Hill, New York. [1.3, 19.1]

Freeman, P.R. (1989). Discussion of 'Interim analyses: The repeated confidence interval approach' (by C. Jennison and B.W. Turnbull). *J. Roy. Statist. Soc. B.*, **51**, 339. [9.1]

Freiman, J.A., Chalmers, T.C., Smith, H. and Kuebler, R.R. (1978). The importance of the Type II error, and sample size in the design of 71 "negative" trials. *New Engl. J. of Med.*, **299**, 690–694. [1.1]

Friedman, L.M., Furberg, C.D. and DeMets, D.L. (1998). *Fundamentals of Clinical Trials*, 3rd ed., New York: Springer. [1.1]

Fu, K.S. (1968). *Sequential Methods in Pattern Recognition and Learning*, New York: Academic Press. [1.3]

Gail, M.H., DeMets, D.L. and Slud, E.V. (1982) Simulation studies on increments of the two-sample logrank score test for survival time data, with application to group sequential boundaries. In *Survival Analysis* (Eds., J. Crowley and R.A. Johnson), Hayward, California: Institute of Mathematical Statistics, 287–301. [3.7]

Gange, S.J. and DeMets, D.L. (1996). Sequential monitoring of clinical trials with correlated responses. *Biometrika*, **83**, 157–167. [11.7]

Gart, J.J., Krewski, D., Lee, P.N., Tarone, R.E. and Wahrendorf, J. (1986). *Statistical Methods in Cancer Research, Vol. III: The Design and Analysis of Long-term Animal Experiments.* Intern. Agency for Research on Cancer, Lyon. [1.1]

Geary, D.N. (1988). Sequential testing in clinical trials with repeated measurements. *Biometrika*, **75**, 311–318. [11.3, 11.7]

Gehan, E.A. (1965). A generalized Wilcoxon test for comparing arbitrarily singly censored samples. *Biometrika*, **52**, 203–223. [13.8]

Gent, M. (1997). Discussion: Some issues in the construction and use of clusters of outcome events. *Contr. Clin. Trials*, **18**, 546–549 [15.1]

George, S.L. and Desu, M.M. (1974). Planning the size and duration of a clinical trial studying the time to some critical event. *J. Chron. Diseases*, **27**, 15–24. [10.5]

George, S.L., Li, C., Berry, D.A. and Green, M.R. (1994). Stopping a clinical trial early: Frequentist and Bayesian approaches applied to a CALGB trial in non-small-cell lung cancer. *Statist. Med.*, **13**, 1313–1327. [18.3]

Ghosh, B.K. (1991). A brief history of sequential analysis. In *Handbook of Sequential Analysis*, (Eds., B.K. Ghosh and P.K. Sen), New York: Marcel Dekker, 1–19. [1.3]

Ghosh, B.K. and Sen, P.K. (Eds.) (1991). *Handbook of Sequential Analysis*, New York: Marcel Dekker. [1.3]

Gilbert, J.P., McPeek, B. and Mosteller, F. (1977). Statistics and ethics in surgery and anaesthesia. *Science*, **198**, 684–689. [18.3]

Gittins, J.C. (1989). *Muli-Armed Bandit Allocation Indices*, Chichester: Wiley. [1.3, 17.4]

Goldhirsch, A., Coates, A.S., Castiglione-Gertsch, M. and Gelber, R.D. (1998). New treatments for breast cancer: Breakthroughs for patient care or just steps in the right direction? *Ann. Oncology*, **9**, 973–976. [9.1]

Gould, A.L. (1983). Abandoning lost causes (Early termination of unproductive clinical trials). *Proceedings of Biopharmaceutical Section*, American Statist. Assoc., Washington, D.C., 31–34. [1.2, 1.3, 5.1, 7.2]

Gould, A.L. (1992). Interim analyses for monitoring clinical trials that do not materially affect the Type I error rate. *Statist. Med.*, **11**, 55–66. [14.1, 14.2]

Gould, A.L. (1995a). Planning and revising the sample size for a trial. *Statist. Med.*, **14**, 1039–1051. [14.1]

Gould, A.L. (1995b). Group sequential extensions of a standard bioequivalence testing procedure. *J. Pharmacokinet. Biopharm.* **23**, 57–86. [6.5]

Gould, A.L. and Pecore, V.J. (1982). Group sequential methods for clinical trials allowing early acceptance of H_0 and incorporating costs. *Biometrika*, **69**, 75–80. [1.3, 5.1]

Gould, A.L. and Shih, W.J. (1992). Sample size re-estimation without unblinding for normally distributed outcomes with unknown variance. *Commun. Statist. A.*, **21**, 2833–2853. [14.1, 14.2, 14.3]

Gould, A.L. and Shih, W.J. (1998). Modifying the design of ongoing trials without unblinding. *Statist. Med.*, **17**, 89–100. [14.1, 14.3]

Greenhouse, J.B. and Wasserman, L. (1995). Robust Bayesian methods for monitoring clinical trials. *Statist. Med.*, **14**, 1379–1391. [18.4]

Grimmett, G.R. and Stirzaker, D.R. (1992). *Probability and Random Processes*, 2nd ed., Oxford: Clarendon Press. [10.2]

Grossman J., Parmar M.K.B., Spiegelhalter, D.J. and Freedman, L.S. (1994). A unified method for monitoring and analyzing controlled trials. *Statist. Med.*, **13**, 1815–1826. [18.2, 18.3, 18.4]

Gu, M. and Ying, Z. (1993). Sequential analysis for censored data. *J. Amer. Statist. Assoc.*, **88**, 890–898. [11.7]

Gu, M. and Ying, Z. (1995). Group sequential methods for survival data using partial likelihood score processes with covariate adjustment. *Statistica Sinica*, **5**, 793–804. [13.8]

Hall, P. (1981). Asymptotic theory of triple sampling for sequential estimation of a mean. *Ann. Statist.*, **9**, 1229–1238. [14.2]

Hall, W.J. (1962). Some sequential analogs of Stein's two-stage test. *Biometrika*, **49**, 367–378. [14.3]

Halperin, M., Lan, K.K.G., Ware, J.H., Johnson, N.J. and DeMets, D.L. (1982). An aid to data monitoring in long-term clinical trials. *Contr. Clin. Trials*, **3**, 311–23. [10.2, 10.6]

Halperin, M., Lan, K.K.G., Wright, E.C. and Foulkes, M.A. (1987). Stochastic curtailing for comparison of slopes in longitudinal studies. *Contr. Clin. Trials*, **8**, 315–326. [10.6, 11.3, 11.7]

Halperin, M. and Ware, J.H. (1974). Early decision in a censored Wilcoxon two-sample test for accumulating survival data. *J. Amer. Statist. Assoc.* **69**, 414–422. [10.1]

Halpern, J. and Brown, B.W. (1993). A computer program for designing clinical trials with arbitrary survival curves and group sequential testing. *Contr. Clin. Trials*, **14**, 109–122. [19.7]

Hamilton, D.C. and Lesperance, M.L. (1991). A consulting problem involving bivariate acceptance sampling by variables. *Canadian J. Statist.*, **19**, 109–117. [15.7]

Hardwick, J. (1989). Comment: recent progress in clinical trial designs that adapt for ethical purposes. *Statistical Science*, **4**, 327–336. [17.4]

Harrington, D. (1989). Discussion of 'Interim analyses: The repeated confidence interval approach' (by C. Jennison and B.W. Turnbull). *J. Roy. Statist. Soc. B.*, **51**, 346–347. [13.5]

Harrington, D.P., Fleming, T.R. and Green, S.J. (1982). Procedures for serial testing in censored survival data. In *Survival Analysis* (Eds., J. Crowley and R.A. Johnson), Hayward, California: Institute of Mathematical Statistics, 269–286. [3.7]

Hauck, W.W., Preston, P.E. and Bois, F.Y. (1997). A group sequential approach to crossover trials for average bioequivalence. *J. Biopharm. Statist.*, **7**, 87–96. [6.3, 6.5]

Haybittle, J.L. (1971). Repeated assessment of results in clinical trials of cancer treatment. *Brit. J. Radiology*, **44**, 793–797. [2.7]

Hayre, L.S. (1979). Two-population sequential tests with three hypotheses. *Biometrika*, **66**, 465–74. [17.4]

Hayre, L.S. and Turnbull, B.W. (1981a). A class of simple approximate sequential tests for adaptive comparison of two treatments. *Commun. Statist. A.*, **10**, 2339–2360. [17.4]

Hayre, L.S. and Turnbull, B.W. (1981b). Sequential estimation in two-armed exponential clinical trials. *Biometrika*, **68**, 411–416. [17.4]

Hayre, L.S. and Turnbull, B.W. (1981c). Estimation of the odds ratio in the two-armed bandit problem. *Biometrika*, **68**, 661–668. [17.4]

Herson, J. (1979). Predictive probability early termination for phase II clinical trials. *Biometrics*, **35**, 775–783. [1.3, 10.3, 10.6]

Herson, J. (1994). Discussion of 'Bayesian approaches to randomized trials' (by D.J. Spiegelhalter, L.S. Freedman and M.K.B. Parmar). *J. Roy. Statist. Soc. A.*, **157**, 396–397. [18.3]

Herson, J. and Wittes, J. (1993). The use of interim analysis in sample size adjustment. *Drug Information J.*, **27**, 753–760. [14.1, 14.2]

Hewett, J.E. and Spurrier, J.D. (1983). A survey of two stage tests of hypotheses: theory and applications. *Commun. Statist. A.*, **12**, 2307–2425. [1.3]

Hilsenbeck, S.G. (1988). Early termination of a Phase II clinical trial. *Contr. Clin. Trials*, **9**, 177–188. [10.6]

Hochberg, Y. and Marcus, R. (1983). Two-phase tests on a normal mean when variance is unknown. *J. Statist. Planning and Inference*, **7**, 233–242. [14.3]

Hochberg, Y. and Tamhane, A.C. (1987). *Multiple Comparison Procedures*, New York: Wiley. [16.3]

Hoel, D.G., Sobel, M. and Weiss, G.H. (1975). A survey of adaptive sampling for clinical trials. In *Perspectives in Biometry* (Ed., R. Elashoff), New York: Academic Press, 312–334. [17.4]

Hsu J.C., Hwang J.T.G., Liu H.K. and Ruberg, S.J. (1994). Confidence intervals associated with tests for bioequivalence *Biometrika*, **81**, 103–114. [9.5]

Hughes, M.D. (1993). Stopping guidelines for clinical trials with multiple treatments. *Statist. Med.*, **12**, 901–915. [16.4]

Hughes, M.D. and Pocock, S.J. (1988). Stopping rules and estimation problems in clinical trials. *Statist. Med.*, **7**, 1231–1242. [8.5, 18.1]

Hwang, I.K., Shih, W.J. and DeCani, J.S. (1990). Group sequential designs using a family of type I error probability spending functions. *Statist. Med.*, **9**, 1439–1445. [7.2]

Iglewicz, B. (1983). Alternative designs: sequential, multi-stage, decision theory and adaptive designs. In *Cancer Clinical Trials: Methods and Practice* (Eds., M.E. Buyse, J. Staquet and R.J. Sylvester), Oxford: Oxford Univ. Press, 312–334. [17.4]

Jackson, J.E. and Bradley, R.A. (1961). Sequential χ^2 and T^2 tests and their application to an acceptance sampling problem. *Technometrics*, **3**, 519–534. [15.7]

Jennison, C. (1987). Efficient group sequential tests with unpredictable group sizes. *Biometrika*, **74**, 155–165. [4.1, 7.3]

Jennison, C. (1992). Bootstrap tests and confidence intervals for a hazard ratio when the number of observed failures is small, with applications to group sequential survival studies. In *Computing Science and Statistics, Vol. 23* (Eds., C. Page and R. LePage), New York: Springer-Verlag, 89–97. [3.7, 10.4]

Jennison, C. (1994). Numerical computations for group sequential tests. In *Computing Science and Statistics, Vol. 25* (Eds., M. Tarter and M.D. Lock), Interface Foundation of America, 263–272. [19.1]

Jennison, C., Johnstone, I.M. and Turnbull, B.W. (1982). Asymptotically optimal procedures for sequential adaptive selection of the best of several normal means. In *Statistical Decision Theory and Related Topics III, Vol. 2* (Eds., S.S. Gupta and J.O. Berger), New York: Academic Press, 55–86. [17.4]

Jennison, C. and Turnbull, B.W. (1983). Confidence intervals for a binomial parameter following a multistage test with application to MIL-STD 105D and medical trials. *Technometrics*, **25**, 49–58. [1.3, 12.1]

Jennison, C. and Turnbull, B.W. (1984). Repeated confidence intervals for group sequential clinical trials. *Contr. Clin. Trials*, **5**, 33–45. [1.3, 3.7, 9.1, 13.5, 13.8]

Jennison, C. and Turnbull, B.W. (1985). Repeated confidence intervals for the median survival time. *Biometrika*, **72**, 619–625. [9.5, 13.7, 13.8]

Jennison, C. and Turnbull, B.W. (1989). Interim analyses: the repeated confidence interval approach (with discussion). *J. Roy. Statist. Soc. B.*, **51**, 305–361. [1.3, 7.2, 9.1, 9.2, 9.5, 12.1, 12.3, 12.5, 13.5]

Jennison, C. and Turnbull, B.W. (1990). Statistical approaches to interim monitoring of medical trials: A review and commentary. *Statistical Science*, **5**, 299–317. [7.2, 18.3, 18.4]

Jennison, C. and Turnbull, B.W. (1991a). Group sequential tests and repeated confidence intervals. In *Handbook of Sequential Analysis* (Eds., B.K. Ghosh and P.K. Sen), New York: Marcel Dekker, 283–311. [7.4]

Jennison, C. and Turnbull, B.W. (1991b). Exact calculations for sequential t, χ^2 and F tests. *Biometrika*, **78**, 133–141. [3.8, 11.5, 11.7, 15.3, 16.2, 19.6]

Jennison, C. and Turnbull, B.W. (1991c). A note on the asymptotic joint distribution of successive Mantel-Haenszel estimates of the odds ratio based on accumulating data. *Sequential Analysis*, **10**, 201–209. [9.5, 11.7, 12.3]

Jennison, C. and Turnbull, B.W. (1993a). One-sided sequential tests to establish equivalence between treatments with special reference to normal and binary responses. In *Multiple Comparisons, Selection, and Applications in Biometry* (Ed., F.M. Hoppe), New York: Marcel Dekker, 315–330. [6.5, 9.3, 9.5, 14.3]

Jennison, C. and Turnbull, B.W. (1993b). Sequential equivalence testing and repeated confidence intervals, with applications to normal and binary response. *Biometrics*, **49**, 31–43. [6.5, 9.3, 14.3]

Jennison, C. and Turnbull, B.W. (1993c). Group sequential tests for bivariate response: Interim analyses of clinical trials with both efficacy and safety endpoints. *Biometrics*, **49**, 741–752. [1.4, 15.1, 15.6, 15.7, 19.6]

Jennison, C. and Turnbull, B.W. (1997a). Group sequential analysis incorporating covariate information. *J. Amer. Statist. Assoc.*, **92**, 1330–1341. [3.5, 11.7, 13.4, 13.8]

Jennison, C. and Turnbull, B.W. (1997b). Distribution theory of group sequential t, χ^2 and F tests for general linear models. *Sequential Analysis*, **16**, 295–317. [11.4, 11.5, 11.7, 15.3]

Jennison, C. and Turnbull, B.W. (2000a) On group sequential tests for data in unequally sized groups and with unknown variance. *J. Statist. Planning and Inference*, **48**. To appear. [4.3, 5.1, 6.3]

Jennison, C. and Turnbull, B.W. (2000b). Group sequential tests with outcome-dependent treatment assignment. Unpublished manuscript. [17.2, 17.3]

Jiang, W. (1999). Group sequential procedures for repeated events data with frailty. *J. Biopharm. Statist.*, **9**, 379–399. [11.7]

Jiang, W., Turnbull, B.W. and Clark, L.C. (1999). Semiparametric regression models for repeated events with random effects and measurement error. *J. Amer. Statist. Assoc.*, **94**, 111–124. [1.4]

Johns, D. and Andersen, J.S. (1999). Use of predictive probabilities in Phase II and Phase III clinical trials. *J. Biopharm. Statist.*, **9**, 67–79. [10.6]

Jones, B. and Kenward, M.G. (1989). *Design and Analysis of Cross-Over Trials*, London: Chapman and Hall. [1.4, 6.3]

Ju, H.L. (1997). On TIER method for assessment of individual bioequivalence. *J. Biopharm. Statist.*, **7**, 63–85. [6.4]

Kalbfleisch, J.D. and Prentice, R.L. (1980). *The Statistical Analysis of Failure Time Data*, New York: Wiley. [1.3, 13.6]

Kaplan, E.L. and Meier, P. (1958). Nonparametric estimation from incomplete observations. *J. Amer. Statist. Assoc.*, **53**, 457–481. [1.5, 12.6, 13.1, 13.7]

Kass, R.E. and Greenhouse, J.B. (1989). Comments on 'Investigating therapies of potentially great benefit: ECMO' (by J.H. Ware). *Statistical Science* **4**, 310–317. [18.3]

Keaney, K.M. and Wei, L.J. (1994). Interim analyses based on median survival times. *Biometrika*, **81**, 279–286. [9.5, 13.7, 13.8]

Kiefer, J. and Weiss, L. (1957). Some properties of generalized sequential probability ratio tests. *Ann. Math. Statist.*, **28**, 57–74. [1.3]

Kim, K., Boucher, H. and Tsiatis, A.A. (1995). Design and analysis of group sequential logrank tests in maximum duration versus information trials. *Biometrics*, **51**, 988–1000. [7.2]

Kim, K. and DeMets, D.L. (1987a). Design and analysis of group sequential tests based on the type I error spending rate function. *Biometrika* **74**, 149–154. [1.3, 7.2]

Kim, K. and DeMets, D.L. (1987b). Confidence intervals following group sequential tests in clinical trials. *Biometrics*, **43**, 857–864. [1.3, 8.5]

Kim, K. and DeMets, D.L. (1992). Sample size determination for group sequential clinical trials with immediate response. *Statist. Med.*, **11**, 1391–1399. [1.4]

Kirkwood, T.B.L. (1981). Bioequivalence testing — a need to rethink (Reader Reaction). *Biometrics*, **37**, 589–591. [6.5]

Klein, J.P. and Moeschberger, M.L. (1997). *Survival Analysis*, New York: Springer. [13.3, 13.4]

Kleinbaum, D.G., Kupper, L.L. and Morgenstern, H. (1982). *Epidemiologic Research: Principles and Quantitative Methods*, Belmont, California: Lifetime Learning Publications. [1.1]

Koepcke, W. (1989). Analyses of group sequential clinical trials. *Contr. Clin. Trials*, **10**, 222S–230S. [9.5]

Kolata, G.B. (1979). Controversy over study of diabetes drugs continues for nearly a decade. *Science*, **203**, 986–990. [1.3]

Koziol, J.A. and Petkau, A.J. (1978). Sequential testing of the equality of two survival distributions using the modified Savage statistic. *Biometrika* **65**, 615–623. [10.2]

Lachin, J.M. (1981). Sequential clinical trials for normal variates using interval composite hypotheses. *Biometrics*, **37**, 87–101. [18.2]

Lai, T.L. (1973). Optimal stopping and sequential tests which minimize the maximum sample size. *Ann. Statist.*, **1**, 659–673. [1.3, 19.6]

Lai, T.L. (1984). Incorporating scientific, ethical and economic considerations into the design of clinical trials in the pharmaceutical industry: a sequential approach. *Commun. Statist. A.*, **13**, 2355–2368. [9.1]

Lai, T.L. (1991). Asymptotic optimality of generalized sequential likelihood ratio tests in some classical sequential testing problems. In *Handbook of Sequential Analysis* (Eds., B.K. Ghosh and P.K. Sen), New York: Marcel Dekker, 121–144. [1.3]

Lai,T.L. and Ying, Z. (1991). Large sample theory of a modified Buckley-James estimator for regression analysis with censored data. *Ann. Statist.*, **19**, 1370–1402. [11.6]

Lan, K.K.G. and DeMets, D.L. (1983). Discrete sequential boundaries for clinical trials. *Biometrika*, **70**, 659–663. [1.3, 7.2, 15.5]

Lan, K.K.G. and DeMets, D.L. (1989a). Changing frequency of interim analysis in sequential monitoring. *Biometrics*, **45**, 1017–1020. [7.4]

Lan, K.K.G. and DeMets, D.L. (1989b). Group sequential procedures: Calendar versus information time. *Statist. Med.*, **8**, 1191–1198. [7.2]

Lan, K.K.G. and Lachin, J.M. (1990). Implementation of group sequential logrank tests in a maximum duration trial. *Biometrics*, **46**, 759–770. [7.2]

Lan, K.K.G., Reboussin, D.M. and DeMets, D.L. (1994). Information and information fractions for design and sequential monitoring of clinical trials. *Commun. Statist. A.*, **23**, 403–420. [3.4, 7.2]

Lan, K.K.G., Rosenberger, W.F. and Lachin, J.M. (1993). Use of spending functions for occasional or continuous monitoring of data in clinical trials. *Statist. Med.*, **12**, 2219–2231. [7.2]

Lan, K.K.G., Simon, R. and Halperin, M. (1982). Stochastically curtailed tests in long-term clinical trials. *Commun. Statist.* **C, 1**, 207–219. [1.3, 10.2, 10.6]

Lan, K.K.G. and Wittes, J. (1988). The B-value: A tool for monitoring data. *Biometrics*, **44**, 579–585. [10.6]

Lan, K.K.G. and Zucker, D.M. (1993). Sequential monitoring of clinical trials. *Statist. Med.*, **12**, 753–766. [3.5]

Lee, J.W. and DeMets, D.L. (1991). Sequential comparison of changes with repeated measurements data. *J. Amer. Statist. Assoc.*, **86**, 757–762. [11.7]

Lee, J.W. and DeMets, D.L. (1992). Sequential rank tests with repeated measurements in clinical trials. *J. Amer. Statist. Assoc.*, **87**, 136–142. [11.7]

Lee, J.W. and Sather, H.N. (1995). Group sequential methods for comparison of cure rates in clinical trials. *Biometrics*, **51**, 756–763. [13.8]

Lee, Y.J., Staquet, M., Simon, R., Catane, R. and Muggia, F. (1979). Two stage plans for patient accrual in Phase II cancer clinical trials. *Cancer Treatment Reports*, **63**, 1721–1726. [1.3]

Li, Z. (1999). A group sequential test for survival trials: An alternative to rank-based procedures. *Biometrics*, **55**, 277–283. [13.8]

Lin, D.Y. (1991). Nonparametric sequential testing in clinical trials with incomplete multivariate observations. *Biometrika*, **78**, 120–131. [11.7, 15.5]

Lin, D.Y. (1992). Sequential log rank tests adjusting for covariates with the accelerated life model. *Biometrika*, **79**, 523–529. [13.8]

Lin, D.Y. and Liu, P.Y. (1992). Nonparametric sequential tests against ordered alternatives in multiple-armed clinical trials. *Biometrika*, **79**, 420–425. [16.2]

Lin, D.Y., Shen, L., Ying, Z. and Breslow, N.E. (1996). Group sequential designs for monitoring survival probabilities. *Biometrics*, **52**, 1033–1041. [13.7]

Lin, D.Y. and Wei, L.J. (1991). Repeated confidence intervals for a scale change in a sequential survival study, *Biometrics*, **47**, 289–294. [9.5]

Lin, D.Y., Wei, L.J. and DeMets, D.L. (1991). Exact statistical inference for group sequential trials. *Biometrics*, **47**, 1399–1408. [9.5, 12.2]

Lin, D.Y., Yao, Q. and Ying, Z. (1999). A general theory on stochastic curtailment for censored survival data. *J. Amer. Statist. Assoc.*, **94**, 510–521. [10.6, 13.8]

Lindley, D.V. (1965). *Introduction to Probability and Statistics from a Bayesian Viewpoint; Part 2, Inference.*, Cambridge: Cambridge Univ. Press. [18.1]

Liu, A. and Hall, W.J. (1999). Unbiased estimation following a group sequential test. *Biometrika*, **86**, 71–78. [8.3]

Lorden, G. (1976). 2-SPRT's and the modified Kiefer-Weiss problem of minimizing an expected sample size. *Ann. Statist.*, **4**, 281–291. [1.3, 4.1, 4.5]

Louis, T.A. (1975). Optimal allocation in sequential tests comparing the means of two Gaussian populations. *Biometrika*, **62**, 359–369. [17.4]

Louis, T.A. (1977). Sequential allocation in clinical trials comparing two exponential survival curves, *Biometrics*, **33**, 627–634. [17.4]

Madsen, R.W. and Fairbanks, K.B. (1983). P values for multistage and sequential tests. *Technometrics*, **25**, 285–293. [1.3]

Makuch, R. and Simon, R. (1982) Sample size requirements for comparing time-to-failure among *k* treatment groups. *J. Chronic Diseases*, **35**, 861–867. [10.5]

Mantel, N. (1966). Evaluation of survival data and two new rank order statistics arising in its consideration. *Cancer Chemotherapy Reports* **50**, 163–170. [3.7]

Mantel, N. and Haenszel, W. (1959). Statistical aspects of the analysis of data from retrospective studies of disease. *J. Nat. Cancer Inst.*, **22**, 719–748. [12.3]

Marcus, M.B. and Swerling, P. (1962). Sequential detection in radar with multiple resolution elements. *IRE Trans. Inform. Th.*, **IT-8**, 237–245. [1.3]

Marcus, R., Peritz, E. and Gabriel, K.R. (1976). On closed testing procedures with special reference to ordered analysis of variance. *Biometrika*, **63**, 655–660. [16.3]

Martinez, H., Habicht, J-P., Garza, C. and Mota, F. (1996). Clinical trial of a rice-powder oral rehydration beverage. *Food and Nutrition Bulletin*, **17**, 129-137. [1.4]

MathSoft, Inc. (1998). *S-PLUS*, version 4.5, Seattle, Washington: MathSoft Inc. [1.6, 13.6, 19.7]

McCullagh, P. and Nelder, J.A. (1989). *Generalized Linear Models*, 2nd ed., London: Chapman and Hall. [11.6]

McPherson, K. (1974). Statistics: the problem of examining accumulating data more than once. *New Engl. J. Med.*, **290**, 501–502. [1.3, 2.3, 19.1]

McPherson, K. and Armitage, P. (1971). Repeated significance tests on accumulating data when the null hypothesis is not true. *J. Roy. Statist. Soc. A.*, **134**, 15–25. [19.1]

Mehta, C.R. and Cain, K.C. (1984). Charts for early stopping of pilot studies. *J. Clinical Oncology*, **2**, 676–682. [18.2]

Meier, P. (1975). Statistics and medical experimentation. *Biometrics*, **31**, 511–529. [1.3, 9.1]

Metzler, C.M. (1974). Bioavailability — A problem in equivalence. *Biometrics*, **30**, 309–317. [6.5]

Miké, V. and Stanley, K.E. (Eds) (1982). *Statistics in Medical Research*, New York: Wiley. [1.1]

MIL-STD-105E (1989). *Military Standard Sampling Procedures and Tables for Inspection by Attributes.* U.S. Government Printing Office, Washington D.C. [1.2, 1.3, 12.1, 19.1]

MIL-STD-781C (1977). *Reliability Design Qualification and Production Acceptance Tests: Exponential Distribution.* U.S. Dept. of Defense, Washington D.C. [1.4]

Miller, R.G. (1981). *Survival Analysis*, New York: Wiley. [1.3]

Moussa, M.A.A. (1989). Exact, conditional and predictive power in planning clinical trials. *Contr. Clin. Trials*, **10**, 378–385. [18.2]

Natarajan, R., Turnbull, B.W., Slate, E.H. and Clark, L.C. (1996). A computer program for sample size and power calculations in the design of multi-arm and factorial clinical trials with survival time endpoints. *Computer Methods and Programs in Biomedicine*, **49**, 137–147. [13.4, 16.3]

O'Brien, P.C. (1984). Procedures for comparing samples with multiple endpoints. *Biometrics*, **40**, 1079–1087. [1.4, 15.1, 15.4, 15.5]

O'Brien, P.C. and Fleming, T.R. (1979). A multiple testing procedure for clinical trials. *Biometrics*, **35**, 549–556. [1.3, 2.3, 2.5, 4.1, 9.2, 12.2]

O'Neill, R.T. and Anello, C. (1978). Case-control studies: a sequential approach. *Amer. J. Epidemiology*, **108**, 415–424. [12.4,16.3]

Pampallona, S. and Tsiatis, A.A. (1994). Group sequential designs for one-sided and two-sided hypothesis testing with provision for early stopping in favor of the null hypothesis. *J. Statist. Planning and Inference*, **42**, 19–35. [4.1, 4.2, 5.1, 5.2]

Pampallona, S. Tsiatis A.A. and Kim, K. (1995). Spending functions for type I and Type II error probabilities of group sequential tests. Technical Report, Dept. of Biostatistics, Harvard School of Public Health, Boston. [7.3]

Parmar, M.K.B., Spiegelhalter, D.J., Freedman, L.S. and the CHART Steering Committee (1994). The CHART trials: Bayesian design and monitoring in practice. *Statist. Med.*, **13**, 1297–1312. [18.3]

Pasternack, B.S. (1984). A note on data monitoring, incomplete data and curtailed testing. *Contr. Clin. Trials*, **5**, 217–222. [10.6]

Pasternack, B.S. and Ogawa, J. (1961). The probability of reversal associated with a test procedure when data are incomplete. *J. Amer. Statist. Assoc.*, **56**, 125–134. [10.6]

Pasternack, B.S. and Shore, R.E. (1982). Sample sizes for individually matched case-control studies: A group sequential approach. *Amer. J. Epidemiology*, **115**, 778–784. [12.4]

Pawitan, Y. and Hallstrom, A. (1990). Statistical interim monitoring of the Cardiac Arrhythmia Suppression Trial. *Statist. Med.*, **9**, 1081–1090. [10.6]

Peace, K.E. (Ed.) (1992). *Biopharmaceutical Sequential Statistical Applications*, New York: Marcel Dekker. [1.6]

Pedersen, R. and Starbuck, R.R. (1992). Interim analysis in the development of an anti-inflammatory agent. In *Biopharmaceutical Sequential Statistical Applications* (Ed., K.E. Peace), New York: Marcel Dekker, 303–314. [14.1]

Pepe, M.S. and Anderson, G.L. (1992). Two-stage experimental designs: Early stopping with a negative result. *App. Statist.*, **41**, 181–190. [10.6]

Pepe, M.S. and Fleming, T.R. (1989). Weighted Kaplan-Meier statistics: A class of distance tests for censored data. *Biometrics*, **45**, 497–507. [13.8]

Peto, R. (1985). Discussion of papers by J.A. Bather and P. Armitage. *Intern. Statist. Rev.*, **53**, 31–34, [17.2, 17.4]

Peto, R. and Peto, J. (1972). Asymptotically efficient rank invariant procedures (with discussion). *J. Roy. Statist. Soc. A.*, **135**, 185–206. [3.7]

Peto, R., Pike, M.C., Armitage, P., Breslow, N.E., Cox, D.R., Howard, S.V., Mantel, N., McPherson, K., Peto, J. and Smith, P.G. (1976). Design and analysis of randomized clinical trials requiring prolonged observation of each patient. I. Introduction and Design. *Brit. J. of Cancer*, **34**, 585–612. [2.7]

Piantadosi, S. (1997). *Clinical Trials: A Methodologic Perspective*, New York: Wiley. [1.1]

Pinheiro, J.C. and DeMets, D.L. (1997). Estimating and reducing bias in group sequential designs with Gaussian independent increment structure. *Biometrika*, **84**, 831–845. [8.3]

PMA Biostatistics and Medical Ad Hoc Committee on Interim Analysis (1993). Interim analysis in the pharmaceutical industry. *Contr. Clinical Trials*, **14**, 160–173. [1.2]

Pocock, S.J. (1977). Group sequential methods in the design and analysis of clinical trials. *Biometrika*, **64**, 191–199. [1.3, 2.3, 2.4, 3.8, 4.1, 9.2, 11.5, 15.5, 19.1]

Pocock, S.J. (1982). Interim analyses for randomized clinical trials: The group sequential approach. *Biometrics*, **38**, 153–162. [2.8]

Pocock, S.J. (1983). *Clinical Trials: A Practical Approach*, New York: Wiley. [1.1, 3.4]

Pocock, S.J. (1996). The role of external evidence in data monitoring of a clinical trial (with discussion). *Statist. Med.*, **15**, 1285–1298. [9.1]

Pocock, S.J. (1997). Clinical trials with multiple outcomes: A statistical perspective on their design, analysis, and interpretation. *Contr. Clin. Trials*, **18**, 530–545. [15.7]

Pocock, S.J., Geller, N.L. and Tsiatis, A.A. (1987). The analysis of multiple endpoints in clinical trials. *Biometrics*, **43**, 487–498. [15.1, 15.3, 15.4]

Pocock, S.J. and Hughes, M.D. (1989). Practical problems in interim analyses, with particular regard to estimation. *Contr. Clin. Trials*, **10**, 209S–221S. [8.5, 18.1, 18.2]

Prentice, R.L. (1997). Discussion: On the role and analysis of secondary endpoints in clinical trials. *Contr. Clin. Trials*, **18**, 561–567. [15.2]

Prentice, R.L., Williams, B.J. and Peterson, A.V. (1981). On the regression analysis of multivariate failure time data. *Biometrika*, **68**, 373–379. [1.4]

Proschan, M.A. (1999). Properties of spending function boundaries. *Biometrika*, **86**, 466–473. [7.2, 9.1]

Proschan, M.A., Follmann, D.A and Geller, N.L. (1994). Monitoring multi-armed trials. *Statist. Med.*, **13**, 1441–1452. [16.2, 16.3, 16.4]

Proschan, M.A., Follmann, D.A. and Waclawiw, M.A. (1992). Effect of assumption violations on Type I error rate in group sequential monitoring. *Biometrics*, **48**, 1131–1143. [3.3, 7.4, 14.1]

Purich, E. (1980). *Bioavailability/Bioequivalency Regulation: An FDA Perspective in Drug Absorption and Disposition: Statistical Consideration* (Ed., K.S. Albert), American Statistical Association and Academy of Pharmaceutical Sciences, Washington, D.C., 115–137. [6.4]

Qu, R.P. and DeMets, D.L. (1997). Bias correction in group sequential analysis with correlated data. Tech. Rep. 123, Dept of Biostatistics, Univ. of Wisconsin.

Reboussin, D.M., Lan, K.K.G. and DeMets, D.L. (1992). Group sequential testing of longitudinal data. Technical Report No. 72, Dept of Biostatistics, Univ. of Wisconsin. [11.3, 11.7]

Reboussin, D.M., DeMets, D.L., Kim, K. and Lan, K.K.G. (1992). Programs for computing group sequential bounds using the Lan-DeMets method. Technical Report No. 60, Dept of Biostatistics, Univ. of Wisconsin. Biostatistics. [7.5, 19.7]

Robbins, H. (1952). Some aspects of the sequential design of experiments. *Bull. Amer. Math. Soc.*, **58**, 527–535. [17.4]

Robbins, H. (1970). Statistical methods related to the law of the iterated logarithm. *Ann. Math. Statist.*, **41**, 1397–1409. [9.1]

Robbins, H. and Siegmund, D.O. (1974). Sequential tests involving two populations. *J. Amer. Statist. Assoc.*, **69**, 132–139. [17.4]

Robert, C.P. (1994). *The Bayesian Choice.* Springer, New York. [18.4]

Robertson, T., Wright, F.T. and Dykstra, R.L. (1988). *Order Restricted Inference*, New York: Wiley. [15.5]

Robins, J., Breslow, N. and Greenland, S. (1986). Estimators of the Mantel-Haenszel variance consistent in both sparse-data and large-strata limiting models. *Biometrics*, **42**, 311–323. [12.3]

Rocke, D.M. (1984). On testing for bioequivalence. *Biometrics*, **40**, 225–230. [6.5]

Roseberry, T.D. and Gehan, E.A. (1964). Operating characteristic curves and accept-reject rules for two and three stage screening procedures. *Biometrics*, **20**, 73–84. [1.3, 19.1]

Rosenbaum, P.R. and Rubin, D.B. (1984). Sensitivity of Bayes inference with data dependent sampling rules. *The Amer. Statistician*, **38**, 106–109. [18.3]

Rosenberger, W.F. (1993). Asymptotic inference with response-adaptive treatment allocation designs. *Ann. Statist.*, **21**, 2098–2107. [17.4]

Rosenberger, W.F. (1996). New directions in adaptive designs. *Statistical Science*, **11**, 137–149. [17.4]

Rosenberger, W.F. and Lachin, J.M. (1993). The use of response-adaptive designs in clinical trials. *Contr. Clin. Trials*, **14**, 471–484. [17.4]

Rosner, G.L. and Tsiatis, A.A. (1988). Exact confidence intervals following a group sequential trial: A comparison of methods. *Biometrika*, **75**, 723–729. [8.4, 8.5]

Rothman, K.J. and Greenland, S. (1998). *Modern Epidemiology*, 2nd ed., Philadelphia: Lippincott-Raven. [1.1]

Royall, R.M. (1991). Ethics and statistics in randomized clinical trials (with discussion). *Statistical Science*, **6**, 52–88. [17.4]

Samuel-Cahn, E. (1980). Comparisons of sequential two-sided tests for normal hypothesis. *Commun. Statist. A.*, **9**, 277–290. [10.2]

Sandvik, L., Erikssen, J., Mowinckel, P. and Rødland, E.A. (1996). A method for determining the size of internal pilot studies. *Statist. Med.*, **15**, 1587–1590. [14.2]

SAS Institute Inc. (1996). *The SAS System*, version 6.12, Cary, North Carolina: SAS Insitite Inc. [13.6]

Schall, R. (1995). Assessment of individual and population bioequivalence using the probability that bioavailabilities are similar. *Biometrics* **51**, 615–626. [6.4]

Scharfstein, D.O. and Tsiatis, A.A. (1998). The use of simulation and bootstrap in information-based group sequential studies. *Statist. Med.*, **17**, 75–87. [7.2, 14.3]

Scharfstein, D.O., Tsiatis, A.A. and Robins, J.M. (1997). Semiparametric efficiency and its implication on the design and analysis of group sequential studies. *J. Amer. Statist. Assoc.*, **92**, 1342–1350. [7.2, 11.7, 13.8, 14.3]

Schervish, M.J. (1984). Algorithm AS 195: Multivariate normal probabilities with error bound. *App. Statist.*, **33**, 81–94. (Correction **34**(1985), 103–104.) [7.5, 11.1]

Schneiderman, M. (1961). Statistical problems in the screening search for anticancer drugs by the National Cancer Institute of the United States. In *Quantitative Methods in Pharmacology*, Amsterdam: North-Holland, 232–246. [1.3, 19.1]

Schoenfeld, D.A. and Richter, J.R. (1982). Nomograms for calculating the number of patients needed for a clinical trial with survival as an endpoint. *Biometrics*, **38**, 163–170. [10.5]

Schuirmann, D.J. (1987). A comparison of the two one-sided tests procedure and the power approach for assessing the equivalence of average bioavailability. *J. of Pharmacokinetics and Biopharmaceutics*, **15**, 657–680. [9.3]

Schultz, J.R., Nichol, F.R., Elfring, G.L. and Weed, S.D. (1973). Multiple-stage procedures for drug screening. *Biometrics*, **29**, 293–300. [1.3, 12.1, 19.1]

Sellke, T. and Siegmund, D. (1983). Sequential analysis of the proportional hazards model. *Biometrika*, **70**, 315–326. [13.8]

Selwyn, M.R., Dempster, A.P. and Hall, N.R. (1981). A Bayesian approach to bioequivalence for the 2 × 2 changeover design. *Biometrics*, **37**, 11–21. [6.5]

Shapiro, S.H. and Louis, T.A. (Eds.) (1983). *Clinical Trials: Issues and Approaches*, New York: Marcel Dekker. [1.1]

Shewhart, W.A. (1931). *Economic Control of Manufactured Product.* Van Nostrand, New York. [1.3]

Shih, W.J. (1992). Sample size re-estimation in clinical trials. In *Biopharmaceutical Sequential Statistical Applications* (Ed., K.E. Peace), New York: Marcel Dekker, 285–301. [14.1]

Siegmund, D. (1978). Estimation following sequential tests. *Biometrika* **65**, 341–349. [1.3, 8.4]

Siegmund, D. (1979). Corrected diffusion approximations in certain random walk problems. *Advances in Applied Probability*, **11**, 701–719. [4.5]

Siegmund, D. (1985). *Sequential Analysis.* Springer-Verlag, New York. [1.3, 8.2]

Siegmund, D. (1993). A sequential clinical trial for comparing three treatments. *Ann. Statist.*, **21**, 464–483. [16.4]

Simon, R. (1977). Adaptive treatment assignment methods and clinical trials. *Biometrics*, **33**, 743–749. [17.4]

Simon, R. (1986). Confidence intervals for reporting results of clinical trials. *Ann. Internal Medicine*, **105**, 429–435. [1.1]

Simon, R. (1993). Why confidence intervals are useful tools in clinical therapeutics. *J. Biopharm. Statist.*, **3**, 243–248. [8.1]

Slud, E.V. (1984). Sequential linear rank tests for two-sample censored survival data. *Ann. Statist.*, **12**, 551–571. [13.8]

Slud, E.V. and Wei, L-J (1982). Two-sample repeated significance tests based on the modified Wilcoxon statistic. *J. Amer. Statist. Assoc.*, **77**, 862–868. [1.3, 7.2, 7.4, 7.5, 11.7, 13.8]

Sobel, M. and Wald, A. (1949). A sequential decision procedure for choosing one of three hypotheses concerning the unknown mean of a normal distribution. *Ann. Math. Statist.*, **20**, 502–522. [5.3]

Spiegelhalter, D.J. and Freedman, L.S. (1986). A predictive approach to selecting the size of a clinical trial, based on subjective clinical opinion. *Statist. Med.*, **5**, 1–13. [18.2]

Spiegelhalter, D.J. and Freedman, L.S. (1988). Bayesian approaches to clinical trials (with discussion). In *Bayesian Statistics 3* (Eds., J.M. Bernardo, M.H. DeGroot, D.V. Lindley and A.F.M. Smith), Oxford: Oxford Univ. Press, 453–477. [18.2]

Spiegelhalter, D.J., Freedman, L.S. and Blackburn, P.R. (1986). Monitoring clinical trials: Conditional or predictive power? *Contr. Clin. Trials*, **7**, 8–17. [1.3, 10.3]

Spiegelhalter, D.J., Freedman, L.S. and Parmar, M.K.B. (1994). Bayesian approaches to clinical trials (with discussion). *J. Roy. Statist. Soc. A.*, **157**, 357–416. [1.3, 18.2, 18.3, 18.4]

Spitzer, W.O., Sackett, D.L., Sibley, J.C., Roberts, R.S., Gent, M., Kergin, D.J., Hackett, B.C. and Olynich, A. (1974). The Burlington randomized trial of the nurse practitioner. *New Engl. J. Med.*, **290**, 251–256. [1.1]

Stata Corporation. (1997). *Stata Statistical Software*, Release 5, College Station, Texas: Stata Corporation. [13.6]

Stein, C. (1945). A two-sample test for a linear hypothesis whose power is independent of the variance. *Ann. Math. Statist.*, **16**, 243–258. [14.2, 14.3]

Sterne, T.E. (1954). Some remarks on confidence or fiducial limits. *Biometrika*, **41**, 275–278. [12.1]

Stuart, A. and Ord, J.K. (1987). *Kendall's Advanced Theory of Statistics, Vol. 1*, 5th ed., London: Griffin. [16.2]

Su, J.Q. and Lachin, J.M. (1992). Group sequential distribution-free methods for the analysis of multivariate observations. *Biometrics*, **48**, 1033–1042. [9.5, 11.7, 15.5]

Tamura, R.N., Faries, D.E., Andersen, J.S. and Heiligenstein, J.H. (1994). A case study of an adaptive clinical trial in the treatment of out-patients with depressive disorder. *J. Amer. Statist. Assoc.*, **89**, 768–776. [17.4]

Tan, M. and Xiong, X. (1996). Continuous and group sequential conditional probability ratio tests for Phase II clinical trials. *Statist. Med.*, **15**, 2037–2052. [10.4, 10.6]

Tan, M., Xiong, X. and Kutner, M.H. (1998). Clinical trial designs based on sequential conditional probability ratio tests and reverse stochastic curtailing. *Biometrics*, **54**, 682–695. [10.4]

Tang, D., Geller, N.L. and Pocock, S.J. (1993). On the design and analysis of randomized clinical trials with multiple endpoints. *Biometrics*, **49**, 23–30. [15.4, 15.5]

Tang, D., Gnecco, C. and Geller, N.L. (1989a). Design of group sequential clinical trials with multiple endpoints. *J. Amer. Statist. Assoc.*, **84**, 776–779. [15.4]

Tang, D., Gnecco, C. and Geller, N.L. (1989b). An approximate likelihood ratio test for a normal mean vector with nonnegative components with application to clinical trials. *Biometrika*, **76**, 577–583. [15.5]

Thall, P.F., Simon, R.M. and Estey, E.H. (1995). Bayesian sequential monitoring for single-arm clinical trials with multiple outcomes. *Statist. Med.*, **14**, 357–379. [15.7]

The TIMI Study Group (1985). The thrombolysis in myocardial infarction (TIMI) trial: Phase I findings. *New Engl. J. Med.*, **312**, 932–936. [1.4]

Thomas, D.R. and Grunkemeier, G.L. (1975). Confidence interval estimation of survival probabilities for censored data. *J. Amer. Statist. Assoc.*, **70**, 865–871. [13.7]

Tilley, B.C., Marler, J., Geller, N.L., Lu, M., Legler, J., Brott, T., Lyden, P. and Grotta, J. (1996). Use of a global test for multiple outcomes in stroke trials with application to the National Institute of Neurological Disorders and Stroke t-PA stroke trial. *Stroke*, **27**, 2136–2142. [15.1]

Todd, S. and Whitehead, J. (1997). Confidence interval calculation for a sequential clinical trial of binary responses. *Biometrika*, **84**, 737–743. [19.5]

Todd, S., Whitehead, J. and Facey, K.M. (1996). Point and interval estimation following a sequential clinical trial. *Biometrika*, **83**, 453–461. [19.5]

Tsiatis, A.A. (1981). The asymptotic joint distribution of the efficient scores test for the proportional hazards model calculated over time. *Biometrika*, **68**, 311–315. [13.8]

Tsiatis, A.A. (1982). Group sequential methods for survival analysis with staggered entry. In *Survival Analysis* (Eds., J. Crowley and R.A. Johnson), Hayward, California: Institute of Mathematical Statistics, 257–268. [3.7]

Tsiatis, A.A., Boucher, H. and Kim, K. (1995). Sequential methods for parametric survival models. *Biometrika* **82**, 165–173. [11.7, 13.8]

Tsiatis, A.A., Rosner, G.L. and Mehta, C.R. (1984). Exact confidence intervals following a group sequential test. *Biometrics*, **40**, 797–803. [1.3, 8.1, 8.4, 8.5]

Tsiatis, A.A., Rosner, G.L. and Tritchler, D.L. (1985). Group sequential tests with censored survival data adjusting for covariates. *Biometrika* **72**, 365–373. [13.8]

Turnbull, B.W., Kaspi, H. and Smith R.L. (1978). Sequential adaptive sampling rules for selecting the best of several normal populations. *J. Statist. Comput. Simul.*, **7**, 133–150. [17.4]

Tygstrup, N., Lachin, J.M. and Juhl, E. (Eds) (1982). *The Randomized Clinical Trial and Therapeutic Decisions*, New York: Marcel Dekker. [1.1]

Veeravalli, V.V. and Baum, C.W. (1996). Hybrid acquisition of direct sequence CDMA signals. *Intern. J. Wireless Inform. Networks*, **3**, 55–65. [1.3]

Wald, A. (1947) *Sequential Analysis*, New York: Wiley. [1.3, 4.1, 4.3, 19.6]

Wald, A. and Wolfowitz, J. (1948). Optimum character of the sequential probability ratio test. *Ann. Math. Statist.*, **19**, 326–339. [1.3, 19.6]

Wang, S.K. and Tsiatis, A.A. (1987). Approximately optimal one-parameter boundaries for group sequential trials. *Biometrics*, **43**, 193–200. [1.3, 2.3, 2.7, 7.2]

Wang, Y. and Leung, D.H.Y. (1997). Bias reduction via resampling for estimation following sequential tests. *Sequential Analysis*, **16**, 249–267. [8.3]

Ware, J.H. (1989). Investigating therapies of potentially great benefit: ECMO (with discussion). *Statistical Science*, **4**, 298–340. [1.3, 17.2, 17.4]

Ware, J.H., Muller, J.E. and Braunwald, E. (1985). The futility index: An approach to the cost-effective termination of randomized clinical trials. *Amer. J. Med.*, **78**, 635–643. [10.2, 10.6]

Wei, L.J. and Durham, S. (1978). The randomized play-the-winner rule in medical trials. *J. Amer. Statist. Assoc.*, **73**, 840–843. [17.4]

Wei, L.J. and Johnson, W.E. (1985). Combining dependent tests with incomplete repeated measurements. *Biometrika*, **72**, 359–364. [15.5]

Wei, L.J., Su, J.Q.,and Lachin, M.J. (1990). Interim analyses with repeated measurements in a sequential clinical trial. *Biometrika*, **77**, 359–364. [11.7]

Weiss, L. (1962). On sequential tests which minimize the maximum expected sample size. *J. Amer. Statist. Assoc.*, **57**, 551–566. [19.6]

Westlake, W.J. (1972). Use of confidence intervals in analysis of comparative bioavailability trials. *J. Pharmaceut. Sciences*, **61**, 1340–1341. [6.3, 6.5]

Westlake, W.J. (1976). Symmetrical confidence intervals for bioequivalence trials. *Biometrics*, **32**, 741–744. [6.3, 6.5]

Westlake, W.J. (1979). Statistical aspects of comparative bioavailability trials. *Biometrics*, **35**, 272–280. [6.3]

Westlake, W.J. (1981). Bioequivalence testing — a need to rethink (Reader Reaction Response). *Biometrics*, **37**, 591–593. [6.5, 9.3]

Wetherill, G.B. and Glazebrook, K.D. (1986). *Sequential Methods in Statistics*, 3rd ed., London: Chapman and Hall. [1.3]

Whitehead, J. (1986a). On the bias of maximum likelihood estimation following a sequential test. *Biometrika* **73**, 573–581. [1.3, 8.3]

Whitehead, J. (1986b). Supplementary analysis at the conclusion of a sequential clinical trial. *Biometrics*, **42**, 461–471. [8.3, 15.7]

Whitehead, J. (1989). Sequential methods for monitoring declining quality, with applications to long-term storage of seeds. *Biometrics*, **45**, 13–22. [11.6, 12.5]

Whitehead, J. (1997). *The Design and Analysis of Sequential Clinical Trials*, Revised 2nd ed., Chichester: Wiley. [1.6, 3.4, 3.5, 4.1, 4.5, 5.1, 5.3]

Whitehead, J. and Stratton, I. (1983). Group sequential clinical trials with triangular continuation regions. *Biometrics*, **39**, 227–236. [1.3, 4.1, 4.5, 5.1, 5.3]

Williams, P.L. (1996). Sequential monitoring of clinical trials with multiple survival endpoints. *Statist. Med.*, **15**, 2341–2357. [15.7]

Wilson, E.B. and Burgess, A.R. (1971). Multiple sampling plans viewed as finite Markov chains. *Technometrics*, **13**, 371–383. [12.1]

Wittes, J. and Brittain, E. (1990). The role of internal pilot studies in increasing efficiency of clinical trials. *Statist. Med.*, **9**, 65–72. [14.1, 14.2]

Wu, M.C. and Lan, K.K.G. (1992). Sequential monotoring for comparison of changes in a response variable in clinical studies. *Biometrics* **48**, 765–779. [1.4, 11.3, 11.7]

Xiong, X. (1995). A class of sequential conditional probability ratio tests. *J. Amer. Statist. Assoc.*, **90**, 1463–1473. [10.4]

Yao, Q. and Wei, L.J. (1996). Play the winner for phase II/III trials. *Statist. Med.*, **15**, 2413–2423. [17.4]

Zelen, M. (1969). Play the winner rule and the controlled clinical trial. *J. Amer. Statist. Assoc.* **64**, 131–146. [1.3, 17.4]

Index